Introduction to

ORTHOTICS

A CLINICAL REASONING & PROBLEM-SOLVING APPROACH

Fifth Edition

BRENDA M. COPPARD, PhD, OTR/L, FAOTA

Professor, Associate Dean for Assessment,
Department of Occupational Therapy, Creighton University, Omaha, Nebraska

HELENE L. LOHMAN, OTD, OTR/L, FAOTA

Professor, Department of Occupational Therapy, Creighton University,
Omaha, Nebraska

ELSEVIER

Notices

Practitioners and researchers must always rely on their own experience and knowledge in evaluating and using any information, methods, compounds or experiments described herein. Because of rapid advances in the medical sciences, in particular, independent verification of diagnoses and drug dosages should be made. To the fullest extent of the law, no responsibility is assumed by Elsevier, authors, editors or contributors for any injury and/or damage to persons or property as a matter of products liability, negligence or otherwise, or from any use or operation of any methods, products, instructions, or ideas contained in the material herein.

Previous edition copyrighted 2015, 2008, 2001, 1996.

Library of Congress Control Number: 2018965674

Content Strategist: Lauren Willis
Senior Content Development Manager: Luke Held
Content Development Specialist: Kathleen Nahm
Publishing Services Manager: Julie Eddy
Senior Production Editor: Tracey Schriefer
Designer: Bridget Hoette

Printed in China

Last digit is the print number: 9   8   7   6   5   4

ELSEVIER

3251 Riverport Lane
St. Louis, Missouri 63043

Working together
to grow libraries in
developing countries

www.elsevier.com • www.bookaid.org

This work is dedicated to the late Roman Renner, my beloved father,
my family, and the Creighton community.

Brenda M. Coppard

This book is dedicated to my late husband, Michael, who passed away during
the time of our work on this edition. He was an occupational therapist
and an orthotist who inspired me to enhance my skills with orthotics.

Helene Lohman

Debbie Amini, EdD, OTR/L, FAOTA
Director of Professional Development
Business Operations
AOTA
Bethesda, Maryland

Salvador Bondoc, OTD, OTR/L, FAOTA
Professor and Chair
Department of Occupational Therapy
Quinnipiac University
Hamden, Connecticut

Paul Bonzani, BS/OT MHS, CHT
Assistant Clinical Professor
Occupational Therapy
University of New Hampshire
Durham, New Hampshire

Brenda M. Coppard, PhD, OTR/L, FAOTA
Professor of Occupational Therapy;
Associate Dean for Assessment
School of Pharmacy & Health Professions
Creighton University
Omaha, Nebraska

Yvette Elias, BS, OT/L, CNDT, ATRI-C, CHT
Clinical Specialist, Certified Hand Therapist
Department of Occupational Therapy
Nicklaus Children's Hospital
Miami, Florida

William Finley, BS Health Science, MS Occupational Therapy
Senior Clinical Instructor
Orthopedic Center
New York University Langone Medical
  Center
New York, New York;
Lead Instructor
Continuing Education
Gold Standard Seminars, LLC
Montclair, New Jersey;
Faculty
Physical Medicine and Rehabilitation
New York University Langone Medical
  Center
New York, New York

John P. Jackson, EdD
Chair and Program Director of MOT
  Program
Master of Occupational Therapy
Emory and Henry College
School of Health Sciences
Marion, Virginia

Elizabeth Kloczko, OTD, OTR/L
Clinical Assistant Professor
Department of Occupational Therapy
Quinnipiac University
Hamden, Connecticut

Debra Latour, OTD, MEd, BS
Assistant Professor of Practice
Division of Occupational Therapy
Western New England University
Springfield, Massachusetts;
Owner
Single-Handed Solutions, LLC
Springfield, Massachusetts

Helene L. Lohman, OTD, OTR/L, FAOTA
Professor
Occupational Therapy
Creighton University
Omaha, Nebraska

Marlene A. Riley, BA, MMS
Clinical Associate Professor
Department of Occupational Therapy &
  Occupational Science
Towson University
Towson, Maryland

Tara Ruppert, OTD
Assistant Professor
Occupational Therapy
College of Saint Mary
Omaha, Nebraska

Linda Scheirton, PhD
Professor
Occupational Therapy
Creighton University
Omaha, Nebraska;
Faculty Associate
Center for Health Policy and Ethics
Creighton University
Omaha, Nebraska

Kris Vacek, OTD, OTR/L
Dean
College of Health and Human Services
Rockhurst University
Kansas City, Missouri

Kristin Valdes, OTD, OT, CHT
Assistant Professor
Occupational Therapy
Gannon University
Ruskin, Florida

Audrey Yasukawa, BSE, MOT
Chief of Occupational Therapy
Developmental and Rehab Services
La Rabida Children's Hospital
Chicago, Illinois

EVIDENCE-BASED PRACTICE CHART CONTRIBUTORS

Andrea Coppola, OTD, OTR/L
Assistant Professor
Occupational Therapy
Springfield College
Springfield, Massachusetts

Whitney Henderson, OTD, MOT, OTR/L
Assistant Clinical Professor
Department of Occupational Therapy
University of Missouri-Columbia
Columbia, Missouri

PREFACE

Over two decades ago, as instructors in a professional occupational therapy program, we were unable to find an introductory orthotic textbook that addressed the development of orthotic theory and skills. This quest resulted in writing the first and subsequent editions of *Introduction to Orthotics: A Clinical Reasoning and Problem-Solving Approach.* Entry-level occupational therapy practitioners are expected to have fundamental skills in orthotic theory, design, and fabrication. It is unrealistic to assume that students gain these skills through observation and limited experience in didactic course work or fieldwork. With the growing emphasis in the health care environment on accountability, productivity, and efficacy, educators must determine the skills students need to apply theory to practice. The book emphasizes clinical reasoning to help students develop skills to critically and effectively provide orthotics in any area of practice. Additionally, laboratory activities intentionally guide the students to fabricate and evaluate a variety of orthoses. We know you have a choice in textbook selection and are hopeful you will consider this important textbook as required reading material for orthotic theory and practical skills.

Several features are improved in this fifth edition. Updated evidence-based orthotic provision is emphasized throughout the chapters, both in narrative and table formats. A focus on occupation-based orthotic intervention is present, and the Occupational Therapy Practice Framework terminology is incorporated throughout the book. In alignment with practice trends, new chapters address casting, orthoses for the shoulder, and professional issues related to upper extremity rehabilitation. The latest information from experts in the field, new patterns, and additional photographs enhance the book tremendously.

The fifth edition of *Introduction to Orthotics: A Clinical Reasoning and Problem-Solving Approach* is again designed with a pedagogy to facilitate the process of applying theory to practice in relationship to orthotic provision. The pedagogy employed within the book facilitates learning to meet the unique needs of students' preferred learning styles. Resources for students and educators on the Evolve website are expanded. Students have access to video clips, supplemental material for Chapter 13, and additional client resources, manufacturer resources, and tests and measures for Chapter 20. Educators have access to the image collection and a new test bank. The website provides visual and auditory instructions on orthotic provision.

Additional case studies stimulate clinical reasoning and problem-solving skills. Self-quizzes and review questions with answers provide the reader with excellent tools to test immediate recall of basic information. Readers are guided through orthotic fabrication in the laboratory with more illustrations and photographs than in the previous editions. The forms provided in the book present opportunities to promote reflection and to assist students' development of their self-assessment skills. Case studies, orthotic analyses, and documentation exercises are examples of learning activities designed to stimulate authentic problem solving. The learning exercises and laboratory experiences provide opportunities to test clinical reasoning and the technical skills of orthotic pattern design and fabrication.

This text is primarily designed for entry-level occupational therapy students, occupational therapy practitioners, and interdisciplinary practitioners who need development in orthotic provision, therapists re-entering the field, and students on fieldwork. Students continue to report they find the book beneficial because it facilitates the mastery of basic theory and furthermore the principles and techniques of orthotics skills that entry-level clinicians need for clinical competence. Instructors enthusiastically welcome the text because the text is targeted for entry-level occupational therapy students. Novice practitioners also report that the book enhances the development of knowledge and skills related to orthotics.

A cadre of expert contributors revised and expanded chapters that reflect current practice. This edition of *Introduction to Orthotics* contains 21 chapters. The first 5 chapters consist of foundations of orthotics; occupation-based orthotic provision; orthotic tools, processes, and techniques; anatomical and biomechanical principles; and assessment related to orthotic provision. These chapters provide fundamental information, which is built upon in subsequent chapters.

Chapter 6 addresses thorough clinical reasoning processes used in making decisions about practice involving orthotic design and construction. The material presented in this chapter relates to answering questions of case studies presented in subsequent chapters.

Chapters 7 through 12 present the theory, design, and fabrication process of common orthoses used in general clinical practice. Orthoses for the wrist, hand, thumb, elbow, and fingers are addressed. A new chapter in this edition is dedicated to the shoulder and orthotic provision.

The remaining chapters in the book are geared toward more specialized topics and to intermediate-to-advanced orthotic provision. Topics include mobilization orthoses, orthotic provision for nerve injuries, spasticity management orthoses, orthotics for elders and children, orthoses for the lower extremity, and prosthetics. We are pleased to offer two new chapters in this section. The chapter on casting offers knowledge and skills related to upper extremity casting. The last chapter of the book addresses professional issues related to hand therapy and orthotic provision. Written by a certified hand therapist, the chapter offers suggestions for professional development and career planning for the certification examination to those who are interested in this professional specialty area of practice.

A glossary of terms used throughout the book follows Chapter 21. This book contains two appendixes. Appendix A provides answers to quizzes, laboratory exercises, and case studies. Appendix B contains listings of web resources.

Although many therapists reviewed this book, each experienced therapist and physician may have a personal view on orthotic provision and therapeutic approaches and techniques. This book represents the authors' perspectives and is not intended to present the only correct approach. Thus therapists are encouraged to employ their clinical reasoning skills in practice.

We hope this fifth edition of the book complements your professional development and continued competence!

Brenda M. Coppard, PhD, OTR/L, FAOTA, and
Helene L. Lohman, OTD, OTR/L, FAOTA

ACKNOWLEDGMENTS

The completion of this fifth edition was made possible through the efforts of many individuals. We are grateful to Mojca Herman, MA, OTR/L, CHT, for the peer reviewing of drafts and revisions of chapters. We are grateful to Phil Beagle for his photography work. Additionally, we appreciate the talent and expertise of the following contributor authors to the current and previous editions: Debbie Amini, EdD, OTR/L, CHT; Omar Aragon, OTD, OTR/L; Janet Bailey, OTR/L, CHT; Serena M. Berger, MA, OTR; Shirley Blanchard, PhD, OTR/L, ABDA, FAOTA; Salvador Bondoc, OTD, OTR/L, FAOTA; Paul J. Bonzani, MHS, OTR/L, CHT; Maureen T. Cavanaugh, MS, OTR; Cynthia Cooper, MFA, MA, OTR/L, CHT; Andrea Coppola, OTD, MS, OTR/L; Lisa Deshaies, OTR/L, CHT; Beverly Duvall-Riley, MS, BSOT; Yvette Elias, OTR/L, CHT; Stefania Fatone, PhD; William Finley, MS, OTR/L, CSCS, CHT; Deanna J. Fish, MS, CPO; Sharon Flynn, PhD, OTR/L, CHUT; Linda Gabriel, PhD, OTR/L; Whitney Henderson, OTD, OTR/L; John Jackson, EdD, OTR, CHT; Karyn Kessler, OTR/L; Elizabeth Kloczko, OTS; Debra Latour, MEd, OTR/L; Dulcey G. Lima, OTR/L, CO; Michael Lohman, MEd, OTR/L, CO; Peggy Lynn, OTR, CHT; Ann McKie, OTR/L; Debra A. Monnin, OTR/L; Sally E. Poole, MA, OT, CHT; Debbie Rider, OTR/L, CHT; Marlene A. Riley, MMS, OTR, CHT; Christopher Robinson, MBA; Tara Ruppert, OTD, OTR/L, CHT; Susan Salzberg, MOT, OTR/L; Linda Scheirton, PhD; Deborah A. Schwartz, OTD, OTR/L, CHT; Lauren Sivula, OTS; Brittany Bennett Stryker, OTD, OTR/L, CO; Joan L. Sullivan, MA, OTR, CHT; Kris Vacek, OTD, OTR; Kristin Valdes, OTD, OT, CHT; Jean Wilwerding-Peck, OTR/L, CHT; Aviva Wolff, OTR/L, CHT; and Audrey Yasukawa, MOT, OTR/L.

We thank our families, colleagues, and friends for their continual support, encouragement, and patience. We also thank our students for enabling us to learn from them.

CONTENTS

Orthotic Foundations

Foundations of Orthotics

Brenda M. Coppard

CHAPTER OBJECTIVES

1. Define the terms *splint* and *orthosis*.
2. Identify the health professionals who may provide orthotic services.
3. Appreciate the historical development of orthotics as a therapeutic intervention.
4. Apply the Occupational Therapy Practice Framework (OTPF) to optimize evaluation and intervention for a client.
5. Describe how frame-of-reference approaches are applied to provision of orthoses.
6. Familiarize yourself with orthotic nomenclature of the past and present.
7. List the purposes of immobilization (static) orthoses.
8. List the purposes of mobilization (dynamic) orthoses.
9. Describe the six orthotic designs.
10. Define *evidence-based practice*.
11. Describe the steps involved in evidence-based practice.
12. Cite the hierarchy of evidence for critical appraisals of research.

KEY TERMS

dorsal	mobilization	torque transmission
evidence-based practice	orthosis	volar
immobilization	splint	

Maria is a student who is enrolled in an orthotics course. She is a bit anxious but is looking forward to gaining the knowledge and skills to be competent in orthotic provision. The instructor told Maria and her classmates that it takes time to build skills, and much practice is necessary.

The human upper extremity helps people carry out the activities that make their lives productive and meaningful. Dressing, bathing, typing, cooking, scrapbooking, and driving are a few of the activities that rely on the incredible complexity of the upper extremity. Therefore it is obvious that impairments of and disabilities affecting the upper extremity are often the domain of therapy intervention—including orthotic provision.

Determining orthotic design and fabricating hand orthoses are important aspects to providing optimal care for persons with upper extremity injuries and functional deficits. Fabrication of orthoses is both a science and an art. Therapists apply knowledge of occupation, pathology, physiology, kinesiology, anatomy, psychology, payment systems, and biomechanics to best design orthoses for persons. In addition, therapists consider and appreciate the aesthetic value of orthoses. People who are novices at making orthoses must be aware that each person is different, requiring a customized approach to orthoses. The use of occupation-based and evidence-based approaches to orthotic provision guides a therapist's consideration of a person's valued occupations. As a result, those occupations are used as both a means (e.g., as a medium for therapy) and an end to outcomes (e.g., intervention goals).[13]

Therapists develop and use clinical reasoning skills to effectively evaluate and treat clients with upper extremity conditions who may need orthotic interventions. This book emphasizes and fosters such knowledge and skills for those who are learning how to make orthoses in general practice areas. After therapists are knowledgeable in the science of orthotic design and fabrication, practical experience is essential for them to become comfortable and competent.

DEFINITION OF SPLINT AND ORTHOSIS

According to the American Society of Hand Therapists (ASHT)[4], a **splint** "refers to casts and strapping applied for reductions of fractures and dislocations. *Splinting* is a term that should not be utilized by therapists [who] are fabricating and issuing...orthoses. [Splinting] is used by physician offices for applying a cast. There are Current Procedural Terminology (CPT) codes for splinting that are used when

---

Note: This chapter includes content from previous contributions from Peggy Lynn, OTR, CHT.

billing for this purpose."[3] An **orthosis** is defined by ASHT[4] as a single device that is rigid or semirigid. Orthoses are applied to support a weak or deformed body part or to restrict or eliminate motion of a body part. Orthoses can be custom made or prefabricated. The terms *splint* and *orthosis* are often used synonymously. However, for payment purposes, therapists must use the proper term.

HISTORICAL SYNOPSIS OF ORTHOTIC INTERVENTION

Reports of primitive orthoses date back to ancient Egypt.[10] Decades ago, blacksmiths and carpenters constructed the first orthoses. Materials used to make the orthoses were limited to cloth, wood, leather, and metal.[25] Hand orthoses became an important intervention in physical rehabilitation during World War II. Survival rates of injured troops dramatically increased due to medical, pharmacological (e.g., the use of penicillin), and technological advances. During this period, occupational and physical therapists collaborated with orthotic technicians and physicians to provide orthoses to clients: Sterling Bunnell, MD, organized hand services at nine army hospitals in the United States.[10] In the mid-1940s under the guidance of Dr. Bunnell many orthoses were made and sold commercially. During the 1950s many children and adults needed orthoses to assist them in carrying out activities of daily living (ADLs) secondary to poliomyelitis.[21] During this time, orthoses were made of high-temperature plastics. With the advent of low-temperature thermoplastic materials in the 1960s, hand orthoses became a common intervention for clients.

Today some therapists and clinics specialize in hand therapy. Hand therapy evolved from a group of therapists in the 1970s who were interested in researching and rehabilitating clients with hand injuries.[6] In 1977 this group of therapy specialists established the ASHT. In 1991 the first certification examination in hand therapy was administered. Those therapists who pass the certification examination are credentialed as certified hand therapists (CHTs). The term *CHT* is not 100% accurate in that CHTs specialize in therapy for the upper extremity versus solely the hand.

Specialized organizations (e.g., American Society for Surgery of the Hand and ASHT) influence practice, research, and education in upper extremity orthoses.[8] For example, the ASHT Splint Classification System offered a uniform nomenclature in orthotics.[9]

PROFESSIONALS WHO MAKE ORTHOSES

A variety of health care professionals design and fabricate orthoses. Occupational therapists (OTs) and physical therapists (PTs) constitute a large group of health care providers whose services include orthotic design and fabrication. Certified occupational therapy assistants (COTAs) and physical therapy assistants (PTAs) also assist in the provision of orthotic services under the supervision or guidance of the OT and PT, respectively. PTs are frequently involved in providing

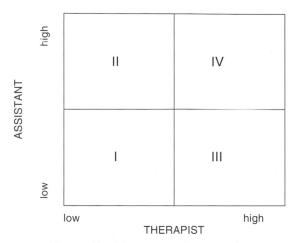

Fig. 1.1 Hand therapy experience matrix.

orthoses for the lower extremities. Certified orthotists (COs) are trained and skilled in the design, construction, and fitting of braces and orthoses prescribed by physicians. Dentists provide orthoses to address selective dental problems. Some nurses who have had special training fabricate orthoses, typically for patients in hospital burn units.

Cooper, Zarbock, and Zondlo[7] devised a hand therapy experience matrix to represent the collaborative roles for therapists and assistants (Fig. 1.1). Their model represents the therapist (axis x) and assistant (axis y) and the level of experience (low, high). In any therapist-assistant pairing, asking questions, seeking input, and sharing knowledge should be routine for a healthy collaborative relationship. The context and implications according to the quadrants include the following:

Quadrant I: Inexperienced therapist and assistant
- Will require obtaining information about diagnoses
- May require input and networking with an experienced therapist and/or physician

Quadrant II: Inexperienced therapist and experienced assistant
- Work collaboratively to develop an assessment and intervention plan similar to Quadrant I
- Therapist continues to supervise the assistant

Quadrant III: Experienced therapist and inexperienced assistant
- Therapist helps develop the assistant's knowledge and skills
- Therapist provides close supervision of assistant

Quadrant IV: Experienced therapist and experienced assistant
- Ideal pairing to continue specialization

Diagnoses that may require expertise include the following[7]:
- Complex crush injuries
- Complex regional pain syndrome (CRPS)
- Dupuytren release
- Flexor and extensor tendon injuries
- Joint replacements
- Nerve injury
- Replantations and revascularizations

- Severe burn injuries
- Severe wound infections

Orthotic design is based on scientific principles. A given diagnosis does not necessarily specify the orthosis required. Orthotic fabrication often requires creative problem solving. Such factors as a client's occupational needs and interests influence orthotic design, even among clients who have common diagnoses. Health care professionals who make orthoses must allow themselves to be creative and take calculated risks. Practice is needed to become proficient with the design and fabrication process. Students or therapists beginning to design and fabricate orthoses should be aware of personal expectations and realize that their skills will likely evolve with practice. Therapists experienced in orthotic provision tend to be more efficient with time and materials than novice students and therapists.

OCCUPATIONAL THERAPY THEORIES, MODELS, AND FRAME-OF-REFERENCE APPROACHES FOR ORTHOTIC INTERVENTION

The Occupational Therapy Practice Framework (OTPF) outlines the occupational therapy process of evaluation and intervention and highlights the emphasis on the use of occupation.[12] Performance areas of occupation as specified in the framework include the following: ADLs, instrumental activities of daily living (IADLs), education, work, play, leisure, and social participation. Performance areas of occupation place demands on a person's performance skills (i.e., motor skills, process skills, and communication/interaction skills). Therapists must consider the influence of performance patterns on occupation. Such patterns include habits, routines, and roles. Contexts affect occupational participation. Contexts include cultural, physical, social, personal, spiritual, temporal, and virtual dimensions. The engagement in an occupation involves activity demands placed on the individual. Activity demands include objects used and their properties, space demands, social demands, sequencing and timing, and required actions, body functions, and body structures. Client factors relate to a person's body functions and body structures. Table 1.1 provides examples of how the framework assists one in thinking about orthotic provision to a client.

Occupational therapy practice is guided by conceptual systems.[11,19] One such conceptual system is the Occupational Performance Model, which consists of performance areas, components, and contexts. A therapist using the Occupational Performance Model views a client's performance area or component while considering the context in which the person lives, works, and plays. The therapist is guided by several approaches in providing assessment and intervention. The therapist may apply the biomechanical, sensorimotor, and rehabilitative approaches. The biomechanical approach

---

TABLE 1.1	Examples[a] of the Occupational Therapy Practice Framework and Orthotic Provision	
Category	**Questions**
Performance in Areas of Occupation	
Activities of daily living (ADLs)	What ADLs will a person need to perform while wearing an orthosis? Will ADLs need to be modified because of orthotic provision?
Instrumental activities of daily living (IADLs)	What types of IADLs will the person wearing an orthosis have to carry out (e.g., child care, shopping, pet care)? Will IADLs need to be modified because of orthotic provision?
Education	Can the person who just received an orthosis read the brochure that explains the home program? What type of client education must be provided for optimum care?
Work	What paid or volunteer work does the client want or need to perform while wearing the orthosis? Will work activities need to be modified because of orthotic provision?
Play	Can a child who wears an orthosis interact with toys?
Leisure	Can the person who wears an orthosis engage in leisure activities? Do modifications in leisure equipment or activities need to be made for full participation?
Social participation	Will the orthosis provided cause an adolescent to withdraw from particular social situations because the orthosis draws unwanted attention?
Performance Skills	
Motor skills	Does the person have the coordination and strength to don and doff his new resting hand orthosis?
Process skills	Can the person who has developmental delays correctly complete the steps and sequence to don and doff an orthosis?
Communication/ interaction skills	Will the person who communicates via sign language be hindered in wearing an orthosis? Will the person feel like she can engage in sexual activity while wearing her orthosis?
Performance Patterns	
Habits	How will the therapist enable a habit for the person to take care of his orthosis?
Routines	How might ADL routines be interrupted because the orthosis interferes with established sequences?
Roles	What roles does the person fulfill, and will any related behaviors be affected by wearing an orthosis?
Contexts	
Cultural	What if the person does not believe the orthosis will help his condition?
Physical	Does the client have accessibility to transportation to the clinic for follow-up visits?

TABLE 1.1 Examples[a] of the Occupational Therapy Practice Framework and Orthotic Provision—cont'd

Category	Questions
Social	How might a caregiver be affected if the person receiving care is provided an orthosis?
Personal	What happens when a client needs an orthosis but has no means of paying for it?
Spiritual	How can the therapist tap into a client's motivation system to improve her outlook on the outcome of wearing an orthosis and receiving treatment?
Temporal	Should the client who has a 6-month life prognosis be issued an orthosis?
Virtual	Will the person who wears an orthosis be able to access his email?
Activity Demands	
Objects used and their properties	Will the teenager who is on the high school chess team be able to manipulate the chess pieces while wearing bilateral orthoses?
Space demands	Will wearing the orthosis impede a client's work tasks due to space restrictions?
Social demands	Will the teacher help the child don and doff an orthosis for participation in particular activities?
Sequencing and timing	Will the intensive care unit nursing staff be able to don and doff a client's orthosis according to the specified schedule?
Required actions	Can the client with arthritis thread the orthotic strap through the D-ring?
Required body functions	Does the client have the strength to lift her arm to dress while wearing an elbow orthosis?
Required body structures	How will the client with one arm amputated don and doff his orthosis?
Client Factors	
Body functions	Does the client have sensation to determine if a dynamic orthosis is exerting too much force on joints?

[a]Examples are inclusive, not exclusive.

uses biomechanical principles of kinetics and forces acting on the body. Sensorimotor approaches are used to inhibit or facilitate normal motor responses in persons whose central nervous systems have been damaged. The rehabilitation approach focuses on abilities rather than disabilities and facilitates returning persons to maximal function using their capabilities.[11] (See Self-Quiz 1.1.)

SELF-QUIZ 1.1[a]

Match the approach used in each of the following scenarios.
a. Biomechanical approach
b. Sensorimotor approach
c. Rehabilitation approach
1. _____ This approach is used on a child who has cerebral palsy. The goal of the orthosis is to decrease the amount of tone present.
2. _____ This approach allows a person who had a stroke to grasp the walker by using orthoses that are adapted to assist with grasp.
3. _____ This approach helps a person who had a tendon repair that resulted in flexor contractures of the metacarpophalangeal (MCP) joint regain full range of motion.

[a]See Appendix A for the answer key.

Each approach can incorporate orthoses as an intervention, depending on the rationale for orthotic provision. If the therapist is using the biomechanical approach, a dynamic (mobilization) hand orthosis may be chosen to apply kinetic forces to the person's body to increase range of motion (ROM). When the therapist chooses a sensorimotor approach, an orthosis may be used to manage spasticity. If a person wears a tenodesis orthosis to recreate grasp and release to maximize function in ADLs, the therapist is using the rehabilitation approach.[10]

BOX 1.1 Contextual and Subjective Dimensions of Occupation

Contextual Dimensions	Subjective Dimensions
• Temporal	• Restoration
• Circadian rhythms	• Eating
• Social schedules	• Sleeping
• Time (clocks)	• Self-care
• Patterns of occupations	• Hobbies
• Spatial	• Spirituality
• Physical body	• Pleasure
• Environmental conditions	• Play
• Object use	• Leisure
• Symbolic meanings of space	• Humor
• Sociocultural	• Ritual
• Identity	• Productivity
• Cultural diversity	• Challenge to avoid
• Genders	boredom
• Health care cultures	• Worth ethic
• Relationships	• Work identity
	• Stress

Pierce's notions[20] of contextual and subjective dimensions of occupation are powerful concepts for therapists to use for appropriate inclusion of orthotics into a client's care plan. Understanding how an orthosis affects a client's occupational engagement and participation is salient in meeting the client's needs and goals, which may result in increased adherence to the wearing schedule. Contextual dimensions include spatial, temporal, and sociocultural contexts.[13] Subjective dimensions include restoration, pleasure, and productivity. Box 1.1 explicates both contextual and subjective dimensions of occupation. Pierce's framework is used to structure questions for a client interview.

CATEGORIZATION OF ORTHOTICS

The Splint Classification System (SCS) of the ASHT was published in 1992.[14] The SCS uses the terms *splint* and *orthosis* interchangeably. The classification system defines splints or orthoses in relationship to the function the orthosis is performing on the body part, rather than the diagnosis or purpose of the orthosis. In 2004 the system was augmented with the inclusion of two device groups: splint-prostheses and prostheses.[12] Thus there are generally two types of terminology lexicons in practice: (1) terminology that preceded the SCS and (2) the SCS, which began in the 1990s. Not all clinics use the SCS orthotic terminology. Therapists must be familiar with the SCS and older, commonly used nomenclature.

According to the ASHT,[3] there are six orthotic classification divisions (Fig. 1.2):
- Identification of articular or nonarticular
- Location
- Direction
- Purpose
- Type
- Total number of joints

Identification of Articular or Nonarticular

The first element of the ASHT classification indicates whether or not an orthosis affects articular structures. Articular orthoses use three-point pressure systems "to affect a joint or joints

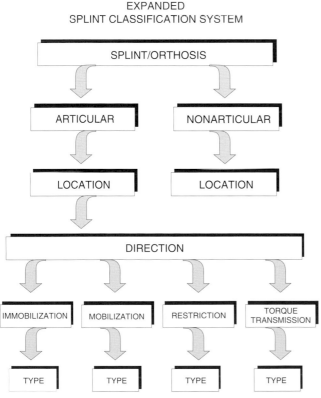

EXPANDED SPLINT CLASSIFICATION SYSTEM

SPLINT/ORTHOSIS

ARTICULAR → LOCATION → DIRECTION

NONARTICULAR → LOCATION

DIRECTION → IMMOBILIZATION → TYPE

MOBILIZATION → TYPE

RESTRICTION → TYPE

TORQUE TRANSMISSION → TYPE

Fig. 1.2 Expanded orthotic classification system division. (From Fess, E. F., Gettle, K. S., Philips, C. A., et al. [2005]. *Hand and upper extremity splinting: Principles and methods* [3rd ed.]. St. Louis, MO: Elsevier Mosby.)

by immobilizing, mobilizing, restricting, or transmitting torque."[3] Most orthoses are articular, and the term *articular* is often not specified in the technical name of the orthosis.

Nonarticular orthoses use a two-point pressure force to stabilize or immobilize a body segment.[3] Thus the term *nonarticular* should always be included in the name of the orthosis. Examples of nonarticular orthoses include those that affect the long bones of the body (e.g., humerus).

Location

Orthoses, whether articular or nonarticular, are further classified according to the location of primary anatomical parts included in the orthosis. For example, articular orthoses will include a joint name in the orthosis (e.g., elbow, thumb metacarpal [MP], index finger proximal interphalangeal [PIP]). Nonarticular orthoses are associated with one of the long bones (e.g., ulna, humerus, radius).

Direction

Direction classifications are applicable to articular orthoses only. Because all nonarticular orthoses work in the same manner, the direction is not specified. Direction is the primary kinematic function of orthoses. Such terms as *flexion, extension,* and *opposition* are used to classify orthoses according to direction. For example, an orthosis designed to flex the PIP joints of index, middle, ring, and small fingers would be named an *index–small-finger PIP flexion orthosis.*

Purpose

The fourth element in the ASHT classification system is purpose. The four purposes of orthoses are (1) mobilization, (2) immobilization, (3) restriction, and (4) torque transmission. The purpose of the orthosis indicates how the orthosis works. Examples include the following:
- Mobilization: Wrist/finger-MP extension mobilization orthosis
- Immobilization: Elbow immobilization orthosis
- Restriction: Elbow extension restriction orthosis
- Torque transmission: Finger PIP extension torque transmission orthosis, type 1 (2). (The number in parentheses indicates the total number of joints incorporated into the orthosis.)

Mobilization orthoses are designed to move or mobilize primary and secondary joints. **Immobilization** orthoses are designed to immobilize primary and secondary joints. Restrictive orthoses "limit a specific aspect of joint range of motion for the primary joints."[3] The purpose of **torque transmission** orthoses is to "(1) create motion of primary joints situated beyond the boundaries of the orthosis itself or (2) harness secondary 'driver' joint(s) to create motion of primary joints that may be situated longitudinally or transversely to the 'driver' joint(s)."[8] Torque transmission orthoses, illustrated in Fig. 1.3, are also referred to as *exercise orthoses.*

Type

The type classification specifies the secondary joints included in the orthosis. Secondary joints are often incorporated into the orthotic design to affect joints that are proximal, distal, or adjacent to the primary joint. There are 10 joint levels that constitute the upper extremity: shoulder, elbow, forearm, wrist, finger MP, finger PIP, finger distal interphalangeal (DIP), thumb carpometacarpal (CMC), thumb metacarpophalangeal (MCP), and thumb interphalangeal (IP) levels. Only joint levels are counted, not the number of individual joints. For example, if the wrist joint and multiple finger PIP joints are included as secondary joints in an orthosis, the type is defined as 2. (PIP joints account for one level, and the wrist joint accounts for another level, thus totaling two secondary joint levels.) The technical name for an orthosis that flexes the MCP joints of the index, middle, ring, and small fingers and incorporates the wrist and PIP joints is an *index–small-finger MCP flexion mobilization orthosis, type 2*. If no secondary joints are included in the orthotic design, the joint level is type 0.

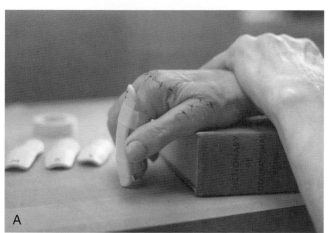

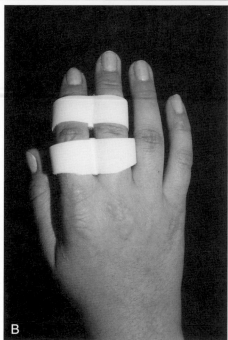

Fig. 1.3 Torque transmission orthoses may create motion of primary joints situated longitudinally (A) or transversely (B) according to secondary joints. (From Fess, E. E., Gettle, K. S., Philips, C. A., et al. [2005]. *Hand and upper extremity splinting: principles and methods* [3rd ed.]. St. Louis, MO: Elsevier Mosby.)

Total Number of Joints

The final ASHT classification level is the total number of individual joints incorporated into the orthotic design. The number of total joints incorporated in the orthosis follows the type indication. For example, if an elbow orthosis includes the wrist and MCPs as secondary joints, the orthosis would be called an *elbow flexion immobilization orthosis, type 2 (3)*. (The number in parentheses indicates the total number of individual joints incorporated into the orthosis.)

TERMINOLOGY OF ORTHOTIC DESIGNS

The purpose for an orthosis as a therapeutic intervention assists the therapist in determining its design. Several orthotic designs exist. Orthotic design classifications include the following[3,5]:
- Static
- Serial static
- Dropout
- Dynamic
- Static-progressive

Static orthoses have no movable parts.[3,5] In addition, static orthoses place tissues in a stress-free position to enhance healing and to minimize friction.[3,5] A static or immobilization orthosis (Fig. 1.4) can maintain a position to hold anatomical structures at the end of available ROM, thus exerting a mobilizing effect on a joint.[3,5] For example, a therapist fabricates an orthosis to position the wrist in maximum tolerated extension to increase extension of a stiff wrist. Because the orthosis positions the shortened wrist flexors at maximum length and holds them there, the tissue remodels in a lengthened form.[15]

Serial static orthoses (Fig. 1.5) require the remolding of a static orthosis. The serial static orthosis holds the joint or series of joints at the limit of tolerable range, thus promoting tissue remodeling. As the tissue remodels, the joint gains range, and the practitioner remolds the orthosis to once again place the joint at end range comfortably.

A dropout orthosis (Fig. 1.6) allows motion in one direction while blocking motion in another.[3] This type of orthosis may help a person regain lost ROM while preventing poor posture. For example, an orthosis may be designed to enhance wrist extension while blocking wrist flexion.[3,5]

Dynamic (mobilization) orthoses have one or more movable parts.[16,23] Elastic tension dynamic (mobilization) orthoses (Fig. 1.7) have self-adjusting or elastic components, which may include wire, rubber bands, or springs.[16] An orthosis that applies an elastic tension force to straighten an index finger PIP flexion contracture exemplifies an elastic tension/traction dynamic (mobilization) orthosis.

Static-progressive orthoses (Fig. 1.8) are types of dynamic (mobilization) orthoses. They incorporate the use of inelastic components, such as hook-and-loop tapes, outrigger line, progressive hinges, turnbuckles, and screws. The orthotic design incorporates the use of inelastic components to allow the client to adjust the amount of tension to prevent overstressing of tissue.[16] Chapter 13 more thoroughly addresses mobilization and torque transmission (dynamic) orthoses.

Many possibilities exist for orthotic design and fabrication. A therapist's creativity and skills are necessary for determining the best orthotic design. Therapists must stay updated on orthotic techniques and materials, which change rapidly. Reading professional literature and manufacturers' technical information helps therapists maintain knowledge about materials and techniques. A personal collection of reference books is also beneficial, and continuing-education courses and professional conferences provide ongoing updates on the latest theories and techniques.

EVIDENCE-BASED PRACTICE AND ORTHOTIC PROVISION

Calls for **evidence-based practice** have stemmed from medicine but have affected all health care delivery, including orthoses.[2,15,17,18,22] Sackett and colleagues[22] and Law[17] defined evidence-based practice as "the conscientious,

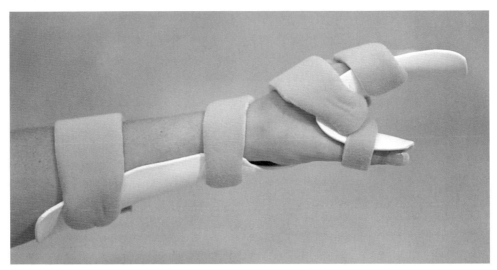

Fig. 1.4 Static immobilization orthosis. This static orthosis immobilizes the thumb, fingers, and wrist.

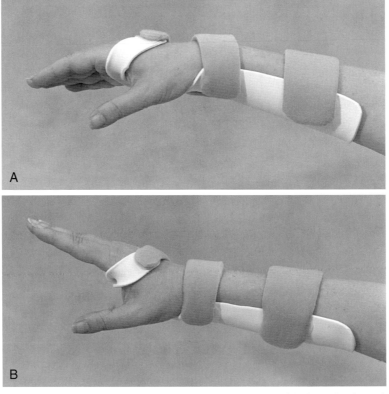

Fig. 1.5 Serial static orthoses (A and B). The therapist intermittently remolds the orthosis as the client gains wrist extension motion.

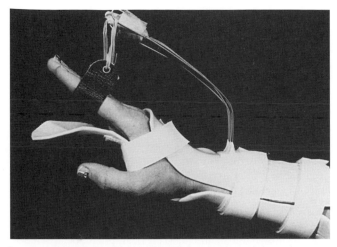

Fig. 1.6 Dropout orthosis. A **dorsal**–forearm-based dynamic extension orthosis immobilizes the wrist and rests all fingers in a neutral position. A **volar** block permits only the predetermined metacarpophalangeal joint flexion. (From Evans, R. B., & Burkhalter, W. E. [1986]. A study of the dynamic anatomy of extensor tendons and implications for treatment. *Journal of Hand Surgery, 11A,* 774.)

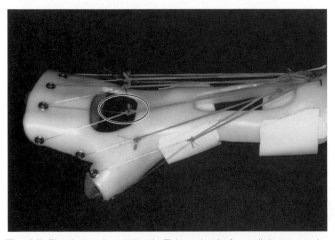

Fig. 1.7 Elastic tension orthosis This orthosis for radial nerve palsy has elastic rubber bands and inelastic filament traction. (Courtesy Dominique Thomas, RPT, MCMK, Saint Martin Duriage, France; from Fess, E. E., Gettle, K. S., Philips, C. A., et al. [2005]. *Hand and upper extremity splinting: principles and methods* [3rd ed.]. St. Louis, MO: Elsevier Mosby.)

explicit, and judicious use of current best evidence in making decisions about the care of individual clients. The practice of evidence-based medicine means integrating individual clinical expertise with the best available external clinical evidence from systematic research."

The aim of applying evidence-based practice is to "ensure that the interventions used are the most effective and the safest options."[22] Additionally, the American health care system increasingly emphasizes effectiveness and cost-efficiency and less credibility of provider preferences.[22] Essentially therapists apply the research process for practice. This process includes (1) formulating a clear question based on a client's problem, (2) searching the literature for pertinent research articles, (3) critically appraising the evidence for its validity and usefulness, and (4) implementing useful findings to the client case. Evidence-based practice is not about finding articles to support what a therapist does. Rather, it is reviewing a body of literature to guide the therapist in selecting the most appropriate assessment or intervention for an individual client.

Sackett and colleagues[22] and Law[17] outlined several myths of evidence-based practice and described the reality of each myth (Table 1.2). A misconception exists that evidence-based practice is impossible to implement or that it already exists. Although keeping current on all health care literature is impossible, practitioners should consistently review research findings related to their specific practice and even consider collecting their own data for evidence. Unfortunately, some practitioners rely primarily on their training or clinical experience to guide decision making. Novel clinical situations present a need for evidence-based practice.

Some argue that evidence-based practice leads to a "cookie-cutter" approach to clinical care. Evidence-based practice involves a critical appraisal of relevant research findings. It is not a top-down approach. Rather, it adopts a bottom-up approach that integrates external evidence with one's clinical experience and client choice. After reviewing the findings, practitioners must use clinical judgment to determine if, why, and how they will apply findings to an individual client case. Thus evidence-based practice is not a one-size-fits-all approach because all client cases are different.

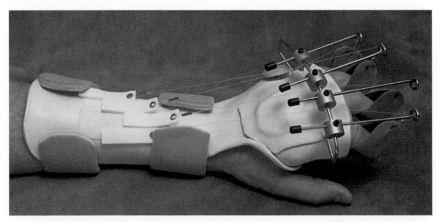

Fig. 1.8 Static progressive orthosis. An orthosis to increase proximal interphalangeal extension uses hook-and-loop mechanisms for adjustable tension.

Evidence-based practice is not intended to be a mechanism whereby all clinical decisions must be backed by a randomized controlled trial (RCT). Rather, the intent is to address efficacy and safety using the best current evidence to guide intervention for a client in the safest way possible. It is important to realize that efficacy and safety do not always result in a cost decrease.

Important to evidence-based practice is the ability of practitioners to appraise the quality of the evidence available. A hierarchy of evidence is based on the certainty of causation and the need to control bias (Fig. 1.9).[22,24] The highest quality (gold standard) of evidence is the meta-analysis of randomized controlled studies. Next in the hierarchy are randomized controlled trials (RCT). A well-designed cohort study is next in the hierarchy, followed by case-controlled studies and case reports. Last in the hierarchy is expert opinion or editorials. Box 1.2 presents a list of appraisal questions used to evaluate quantitative and qualitative research results.

Throughout this book the authors made an explicit effort to present the research relevant to each chapter topic. Note that the evidence is limited to the timing of this publication. Students and practitioners should review literature to determine applicability of contemporary publications. The Cochrane Library, Cumulative Index to Nursing and Allied Health Literature (CINAHL), EBSCOhost, EMB Reviews, MEDLINE, Embase (comprehensive pharmacological and biomedical database), OT SEARCH, OT CATs, OTseeker, Google Scholar, Health and Psychosocial Instruments (HaPI), Applied Social Sciences Index & Abstracts (ASSIA), and HealthSTAR are useful databases to access during searches for research.

TABLE 1.2 Evidence-Based Practice Myths and Realities

Myth	Reality
Evidence-based practice exists.	Practitioners spend too little time examining current research findings.
Evidence-based practice is difficult to integrate into practice.	Evidence-based practice can be implemented by busy practitioners.
Evidence-based practice is a "cookie-cutter" approach.	Evidence-based practice requires extensive clinical experience.
Evidence-based practice is focused on decreasing costs.	Evidence-based practice emphasizes the best clinical evidence for individual clients.

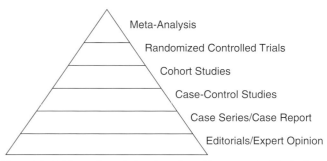

Fig. 1.9 Evidence-based levels of evidence. (Modified from http://ebp.lib.uic.edu/nursing/node/2?q=node/12 and Feree, N., & Kreider, C. M. [April 2011]. *Defining and applying strategies to find and critically assess the evidence.* Presentation at AOTA conference.)

BOX 1.2 Appraisal Questions Used to Evaluate Quantitative and Qualitative Research

Evaluating Quantitative Research

- Was the assignment of clients to treatments randomized?
- Were all subjects properly accounted for and attributed at the study's conclusion?
- Were subjects, health workers, and research personnel blinded to treatment?
- Were the groups similar to each other at the beginning of the trial?
- Aside from experimental intervention, were the groups treated equally?
- How large was the treatment effect?
- How precise was the treatment effect?
- Can the results be applied to my client care?
- Were all clinically important outcomes considered?
- Are the likely benefits worth the potential harms/costs?

Evaluating Qualitative Research

- Are the results trustworthy?
- Was the research question clearly articulated?
- Was the setting in which the research took place described?
- Were the sampling measures clearly described?
- Were methods to ensure the credibility of research used?
- Did the researchers address issues of confirmability and dependability?
- Was the collection of data prolonged and varied?
- Is there evidence of reflexivity?
- Was the research process subjected to internal or external audits?
- Were any steps taken to triangulate the outcomes?
- What were the primary findings?
- Were the results of the research kept separate from the conclusions drawn?
- If quantitative methods were appropriate as a supplement, were they used?
- Will the results help me care for my clients?

Data from Gray, J. A. M. (1997). *Evidence-based healthcare.* Edinburgh, Scotland: Churchill Livingstone; Krefting, L. (1990). Rigour in qualitative research: the assessment of trustworthiness. *American Journal of Occupational Therapy, 45,* 214–222; Rosenberg, W., & Donald, A. (1995). Evidence-based medicine: an approach to clinical problem-solving. *BMJ, 310,* 1122–1126.

REVIEW QUESTIONS

1. What health care professionals provide orthotic services to persons?
2. What are the three therapeutic approaches used in physical dysfunction? Give an example of how orthoses could be used as an intervention for each of the three approaches.
3. How might the OTPF[1] assist a therapist in orthotic provision?
4. What are the six divisions of the ASHT orthosis classification system?
5. For what purposes might an orthosis be used as part of an intervention plan?
6. What is evidence-based practice? How can it be applied to orthotic intervention?
7. In evidence-based practice, what is the hierarchy of evidence?

REFERENCES

1. American Occupational Therapy Association: Occupational therapy practice framework: doman and process, ed 3, *Am J Occup Ther* 68(Suppl):S1–S48, 2014.
2. American Occupational Therapy Association: *AOTA's evidence-based practice resources, using evidence to inform occupational therapy practice.* http://www.aota.org/Educate/Research/2011-EBP-Resources.aspx?FT=.pdf, April 2010.
3. American Society of Hand Therapists: *splint classification system*, Garner, NC, 1992, American Society of Hand Therapists.
4. American Society of Hand Therapists. http://www.-asht.org/practicemgmt/codingreimb.cfm
5. Bailey J, Cannon N, Colditz J, et al.: *Splint classification system*, Chicago, 1992, American Society of Hand Therapists.
6. Cailliet R: *Hand pain and impairment*, ed 4, Philadelphia, 1994, FA Davis.
7. Cooper C, Zarbock P, Zondlo JW: OTR and OTA collaboration in hand therapy, *AOTA Phy Dis Spec Int Sec Quart* 23:2–4, 2000.
8. Daus C: Helping hands: a look at the progression of hand therapy over the past 20 years, *Rehab Manag* 64–68, 1998.
9. Fess EE, Philips CA: *Hand splinting principles and methods*, ed 2, St. Louis, 1987, Mosby.
10. Fess EE: A history of splinting: to understand the present, view the past, *J Hand Ther* 15(2):97–132, 2002.
11. Fess EE, Gettle K, Philips C, et al.: *Hand and upper extremity splinting: principles and methods*, ed 3, St. Louis, 2004, Elsevier.
12. Fess EE, Gettle KS, Philips CA, et al.: A history of splinting. In Fess EE, Gettle KS, Philips CA, et al.: *Hand and upper extremity splinting: principles and methods*, St. Louis, 2005, Elsevier Mosby, pp 3–43.
13. Gray JM: Putting occupation into practice: occupation as ends, occupation as means, *Am J Occup Ther* 52(5):354–364, 1998.
14. Hill J, Presperin J: Deformity control. In Intagliata S, editor: *Spinal cord injury: a guide to functional outcomes in occupational therapy*, Rockville, MD, 1986, Aspen Publishers, pp 49–81.
15. Jansen CW: Outcomes, treatment effectiveness, efficacy, and evidence-based practice: examples from the world of splinting, *J Hand Ther* 15(2):136–143, 2002.
16. Malick MH: *Manual on dynamic hand splinting with thermoplastic material*, ed 2, Pittsburgh, 1982, Harmarville Rehabilitation Center.
17. Law M: Introduction to evidence based practice. In Law M, editor: *Evidence-based rehabilitation*, Thorofare, NJ, 2002, Slack, pp 3–12.
18. Lloyd-Smith W: Evidence-based practice and occupational therapy, *Br J Occup Ther* 60:474–478, 1997.
19. Pedretti LW: Occupational performance: a model for practice in physical dysfunction. In Pedretti LW, editor: *Occupational therapy: practice skills for physical dysfunction*, ed 4, St. Louis, 1996, Mosby, pp 3–12.
20. Pierce DE: *Occupation by design: building therapeutic power*, Philadelphia, 2003, FA Davis.
21. Rossi J: Concepts and current trends in hand splinting, *Occup Ther Health Care* 4(3–4):53–68, 1988.
22. Sackett DL, Rosenberg WM, Gray JA, et al.: Evidence-based medicine: what it is and what it isn't, *BMJ* 312(7023):71–72, 1996.
23. Schultz-Johnson K: Splinting the wrist: mobilization and protection, *J Hand Ther* 9(2):165–177, 1996.
24. Taylor MC: What is evidenced-based practice? *Br J Occup Ther* 60:470–474, 1997.
25. War Department: *Bandaging and splinting*, Washington, DC, 1944, United States Government Printing Office.

APPENDIX 1.1 CASE STUDY

Case Study 1.1[a]

Read the following scenario, and answer the questions based on information in this chapter.

Fred is a new therapist working in an outpatient care setting. He has an order to make a wrist immobilization orthosis for a person with a diagnosis of carpal tunnel syndrome who needs an orthosis to provide rest and protection.

1. According to the American Society of Hand Therapists (ASHT) orthotic terminology, which name appropriately indicates the orthosis indicated in the following figure?
   a. Forearm neutral mobilization, type 1 (2)
   b. Wrist neutral immobilization, type 1 (1)
   c. Wrist neutral immobilization, type 0 (1)

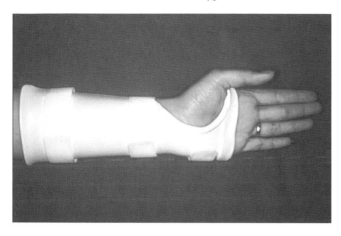

2. If Simon focuses on the person's ability to perform activities of daily living with the orthosis, what is the guiding approach?
   a. Rehabilitation
   b. Biomechanical
   c. Sensorimotor

3. Listed below are several types of evidence. Rank the studies in descending order (1 = highest level, 3 = lowest level).
   ___ a. Talking to a certified hand therapist about the protocol she believes is best for a particular client
   ___ b. A randomized control trial with one group of clients serving as the control group and another group of clients receiving a new type of treatment
   ___ c. A case study describing the treatment of an individual client

[a] See Appendix A for the answer key.

Occupation-Centered Orthotic Intervention

Debbie Amini

CHAPTER OBJECTIVES

1. Define *occupation-centered treatment* as it relates to orthotic design and fabrication.
2. Describe the influence of a client's occupational needs on orthotic design and selection.
3. Review evidence to support preservation of occupational engagement through orthotic intervention.
4. Describe how to use an occupation-centered approach to orthotic intervention.
5. Identify specific hand pathologies that can disrupt occupational performance and participation.
6. Describe orthotic design options to promote occupational engagement while ensuring safety of body structures and functions.
7. Apply knowledge of application of occupation-based practice to a case study.

KEY TERMS

client-centered intervention
context
occupation-based approach

occupation-centered orthotic
intervention
occupation-focused approach
occupational deprivation

occupational disruption
occupational profile
treatment protocol

Samuel is a 37-year-old self-employed builder who fell through an aging second-story floor approximately 5 months ago. His injuries included a fractured femur of his right leg, fractured metatarsals of his left foot, a compression fracture of his distal right dominant radius, and a volarly angulated fracture of his left nondominant radius. Because of these injuries, Samuel was immobilized in bilateral lower extremity casts, a cast on his left wrist, and an external fixator on his right wrist and unable to engage in his work activities.

One month following injury, Samuel began outpatient occupational therapy. He expressed a desire to return to his job as soon as possible due to the financial difficulty that he was experiencing from being unemployed and having no disability insurance. Using an occupation-centered lens, his occupational therapist helped him implement strategies to revive his company while addressing his client factor difficulties surrounding bilateral hand function. Samuel returned to work when his fractures were fully consolidated.

Unfortunately, through constant use of his left upper extremity, Samuel began to experience chronic wrist pain and painful snapping of his forearm with rotational movements. He was diagnosed with ulnocarpal impingement syndrome due to positive ulnar variance

in addition to a triangular fibrocartilage complex tear. Surgery was suggested, but it was expected to take him out of work for an additional 2 to 3 months. This was not acceptable to Samuel, who consulted with his occupational therapist in hopes of finding an alternate strategy that would allow him to work without pain until surgery became a feasible option. The occupational therapist and Samuel targeted his occupational goals and designed a custom forearm-based wrist orthosis that immobilized his wrist and allowed him to work without pain. Samuel plans to undergo a corrective surgery in approximately 1 year.

As stated eloquently by Mary Reilly, "Man, through the use of his hands as they are energized by mind and will, can influence the state of his own health."[26] This phrase reminds us that the hand, as directed by the mind and spirit, is integral to function. **Occupation-centered orthotic intervention** is an overarching paradigm for conducting occupational therapy assessment and intervention that promotes the ability of the individual with hand dysfunction to engage in desired life tasks and occupations.[14] An **occupation-focused approach** to orthotic intervention is attention to the occupational desires and needs of the individual, paired with the knowledge of the effects (or potential effect) of pathological

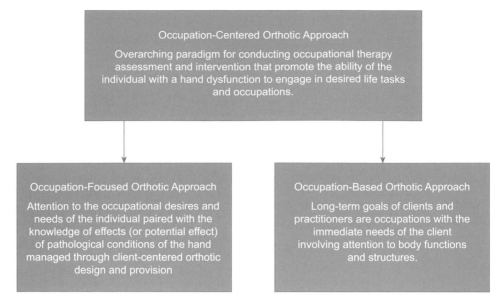

Fig. 2.1 Occupation-Centered Orthotic Approach (Occupation-Focused Orthotic Approach and Occupation-Based Orthotic Approach)

conditions of the hand, and managed through client-centered orthotic design and provision.[2] In addition to an occupation-focused perspective, an occupational therapist or occupational therapy assistant (practitioner) may also approach the provision of issuing orthotic devices from an occupation-based lens or approach. According to Fisher,[14] an **occupation-based approach** is one where the long-term goals of the client and practitioners are occupations, but the immediate needs of the client may involve attention to body functions and structures. In this case, interventions that may not be occupations per se must be appropriately integrated into the intervention plan.

In order to be occupation centered or occupation focused, a practitioner must first adopt a personal philosophy that supports occupation-centered practice. Please refer to Fig. 2.1 that explains these terms. **Occupation-centered practice,** which is also closely aligned with client-centered practice, is the acceptance of occupation as the central guiding paradigm of the profession, where practitioners assess, intervene, reason, and problem solve understanding the importance and power of occupation as the means and the end to what we do.[1,14] Multiple models of practice exist within this paradigm, including the Canadian Model of Occupational Performance and Engagement (CMOP-E)[30]; Person, Environment, Occupation Model; and the Model of Human Occupation and Occupational Adaptation. In addition, the practitioner should understand the tenets of the Occupational Therapy Practice Framework (OTPF), which provides a foundation for occupational therapy practice, and its relationship to the International Classification of Functioning, Disability and Health (ICF) within the United States.

The use of orthoses, an ancient technique of immobilization and mobilization, became associated with occupational therapy in the mid part of the twentieth century.[12] According to Fess, the most frequently recorded reasons for orthotic intervention include increasing function, preventing deformity, correcting deformity, protecting healing structures, restricting movement, and allowing tissue growth or remodeling.[13] From this description, it can be surmised that historically, orthotic intervention has been most closely aligned with the neuromusculoskeletal and movement-related body functions and body structures, described in the client factors category of the OTPF-3. Understanding orthotics exclusively from this perspective relegates their use to a preparatory method that is protocol and practitioner centric. But because body functions and body structures constitute only a part of the ability of the client to be an occupational being, the occupation-centered practitioner understands the importance of assisting the healing or mobility of the hand, with immediate and concurrent focus on the occupational needs of the client—those that transcend movement and strength of the body.

THREE LENS' OF OCCUPATION

This chapter provides definitions of client-centered/occupation-centered and occupation-based and occupation-focused practice and illustrates the process of combining these ways of thinking for orthotic intervention. In addition, outcome measures, assessment tools, intervention models, and orthotic options that promote occupational participation are described.

Client- and Occupation-Centered Practice With Orthotic Intervention

Client- and occupation centered practice are compatible, but a distinction is made between them.[24] **Client-centered** practice is defined as "an approach to service that embraces

---

BOX 2.1 Concepts and Actions of Client-Centered Practice

- Respect for clients and their families and choices they make
- Clients' and families' right to make decisions about daily occupations and therapy services
- A communication style that is focused on the person and includes provision of information, physical comfort, and emotional support
- Encourage client participation in all aspects of therapy service
- Individualized occupational therapy service delivery
- Enabling clients to solve occupational performance issues
- Attention to the person-environment-occupation relationship

---

a philosophy of respect for, and partnership with, people receiving services."[20] Law[18] outlined concepts and actions of client-centered practice that articulate the assumptions for shaping assessment and intervention with the client (Box 2.1). A client-centered perspective should inform occupation-centered practice.

Occupation-Based Approach

Many definitions of occupation-based practice exist within the literature. One definition states that it is "the degree to which occupation is used with reflective insight into how it is experienced by the individual, how it is used in natural contexts for that individual, and how much the resulting changes in occupational patterns are valued by the client."[15] Methods of employing empathy, reflection, interview, observation, and rigorous qualitative inquiry assist in understanding the occupations of others.[24] Christiansen and Townsend[7] described occupation-based occupational therapy as an approach to treatment that serves to facilitate engagement or participation in recognizable life endeavors. Pierce[24] described occupation-based treatment as including two conditions: (1) the occupation as viewed from the client's perspective and (2) the occupation occurring within a relevant context. This perspective supports the thinking of practitioners who are occupation based but address occupations from a bottom-up approach, where orthotics address the immediate needs of the pathology with focus on the eventuality of occupational participation.

Occupation-Focused Orthotic Approach

Occupation-focused orthotic intervention has a focus that supports the goals of the intervention plan and enables clients to engage in meaningful and relevant life endeavors as soon as possible. Unlike a more traditional medical and biomechanical model of orthotic intervention that may initially focus on body structures and functions or an occupation-based focus that seeks to address participation by affecting factors and skills, occupation-focused orthotic fabrication incorporates the client's occupational needs and desires, cognitive abilities, psychosocial status, and motivation as the priority

of intervention. When approaching the client from this perspective, the therapist incorporates client-centered thinking, appreciating that the client is an active participant in the treatment and decision-making process. Orthoses as occupation-focused and **client-centered intervention** focus on meeting client goals as opposed to therapist-designed or protocol-driven goals. Body structure healing is not the main priority; it is a priority equal to that of preservation of occupational engagement.

Occupation-focused orthotic intervention is part of a top-down versus bottom-up approach to occupational therapy intervention. According to Weinstock-Zlotnick and Hinojosa,[32] the therapist who engages in a top-down approach always begins treatment by examining a client's occupational performance and grounds treatment in a client-centered frame of reference. A therapist who uses a bottom-up approach first evaluates the pathology and then attempts to connect the body deficiencies to performance difficulties. The top-down approach is also consistent with both the OTPF and the Current Procedural Terminology (CPT) evaluation coding processes, which describe the creation of the occupational profile, a documented account of the client's occupational history and current occupational goals. The occupational profile is the first part in the occupational therapy evaluation process[3] (Box 2.2).

To achieve a needed balance between immediate attention to occupational participation and the needs of healing body structures, the occupation-centered practitioner can use multiple models or frames of reference to guide interventions. According to Ikiugu,[17] a practitioner may choose one primary model to guide selection of outcome measures, assessments, and interventions and then choose one or more additional secondary models that further inform assessment and intervention choices. It is recommended that the primary model chosen is an occupation-centered model with secondary models such as biomechanical or rehabilitation being used to inform the occupation-centered model and vice versa. This multifaceted yet occupation-centered perspective will ensure that chosen interventions are safe and effective in addressing desired occupational needs, which is the first and foremost priority.

Contexts and Environments

According to the OTPF, **context** and environment relate "to a variety of interrelated conditions within and surrounding the client that influence performance."[1] Occupational therapy is an approach that facilitates the individual's ability to participate in meaningful engagements within specific areas of occupation and varied contexts of living.[1] Context and environments, in addition to occupations, client factors, performance skills, and performance patterns, are a part of the domain of occupational therapy. **Contexts** include cultural, personal, temporal, and virtual aspects; environments include physical and social.[1] Thus therapists should consider both input from the client (views and perspective) and external conditions. Box 2.3 describes the contexts and environments as set forth in the OTPF-3.

BOX 2.2 Occupational Profile[1]

Occupational Profile	Marta
Reason the client is seeking service and concerns related to engagement in occupations	Marta is a 58-year-old single woman with a diagnosis of right medial epicondylitis who lives alone in an apartment. She was referred to occupational therapy by her orthopedic surgeon to address pain, weakness, and activities of daily living difficulties. At this time she reports that she is unable to engage in desired work, leisure, and housework tasks and is not comfortable caring for her new infant grandson.
Occupations in which the client is successful	Marta reports that she is fully independent in all self-care and hygiene activities and very light household chores such as microwaving meals and driving to the grocery store or her daughter's home. She states that she has pain during these activities but will complete them regardless.
Personal interests and values	Marta enjoys craft activities and playing games on her iPad when not working. Before the onset of medial epicondylitis, she had taken up adult coloring using gel pens and reports completing several books in less than a month.
Occupational history	Marta works full time at a small local pet store where she waits on customers, stocks shelves, and cleans animal cages. She enjoys her job and is seeking a promotion to a managerial position. She has worked at this shop for nearly 5 years but now reports difficulty with efficiency and managing heavy items.
Performance patterns (routines, roles, habits, and rituals)	Marta reports that her daily routine involves rising at 7 a.m., showering and dressing, and then making herself lunch for work. At 8 a.m. after eating a light breakfast she drives herself the 5 miles to her job. She works until 12 noon, takes a break for lunch, and completes her day at 5 p.m. She does not drink or smoke and reports no difficulties with participation in her religion.
What aspects of the client's environments or contexts does he or she see as supports to occupational engagement, barriers to occupational engagement	Marta has a daughter and son who are supportive even though they do not live with her. Both will immediately go to her home to help her manage her apartment whenever she calls them. Marta has concerns for her job due to her increasing difficulty and slowed pace. She worries that she will be passed over for a promotion when the current store manager retires next month. This has caused her a moderate level of emotional stress.
Client's priorities and desired targeted outcomes	Marta states that she would like to be pain-free so that she can participate fully in both work and household activities and get back to her crafts and caring for her grandson. She also does not want to miss her opportunity for promotion at work.

BOX 2.3 Description of Contexts

Context
- Cultural: The ethnicity, family values, attitudes, and beliefs of the individual
- Personal: Features of the person specific to them (age, gender, socioeconomic status, and so on)
- Temporal: Stages of life, time of day, time of year
- Virtual: Realistic simulation of an environment and the ability to communicate in cyberspace

Environments
- Physical: The physical environment in all respects
- Social: Relationships the individual has with other individuals, groups, organizations, or systems

From American Occupational Therapy Association. (2008). Occupational therapy practice framework: Domain and process. *American Journal of Occupational Therapy, 62,* 625–683.

Cultural Context

An often overlooked issue surrounding orthotic intervention is attention to the client's cultural needs. Unfortunately, to ignore culture is to potentially limit the involvement of clients in their orthotic programs. For example, there are cultures in which the need to rely on an orthosis is viewed as an admission of vulnerability or as a weakness in character. Such feelings can exist due to large group beliefs or within smaller family dynamic units. Orthotic intervention within this context must involve a great deal of client education and possibly education of family members. Issuing small, unobtrusive orthoses that allow as much function as possible may diminish embarrassment and a sense of personal weakness.

Personal Context

Personal context involves attention to issues such as age, gender, and educational and socioeconomic status. When clinicians who employ occupation-based orthotic intervention fabricate orthoses for older adults or children, they consider specific guidelines (see Chapters 16 and 17).

The choices in material selection and color may be different based on age and gender. For example, a child may prefer a bright-colored orthosis, whereas an adult executive may prefer a neutral-colored orthosis. Concerns may arise about the role educational level plays in orthotic design and provision. For clients who have difficulty understanding new and unfamiliar concepts, it is important to have an orthosis that is simple in design and can be donned and doffed easily. Precautions and instructions should be given in a clear manner.

Temporal Context

Temporal concerns are addressed through attention to issues such as comfort of the orthosis during hot summer months or the use of devices during holidays or special events such as proms or weddings. An example is the case of a bride-to-be who was 2 weeks postoperative for a flexor tendon repair of the index finger. The young woman asked repeatedly if she could take off her orthosis for 1 hour during her wedding. A compromise reached between the therapist and the client ensured that her hand would be safe during the ceremony. A shiny new orthosis was made specifically for her wedding day to immobilize the injured finger and wrist (modified Duran protocol). The therapist discarded the rubber-band/finger-hook component (modified Kleinert protocol). This change made the orthosis smaller and less obvious. The client was a happy bride, and her finger was well protected. Virtual context addresses the ability to access and use electronic devices. The ability to access devices (e.g., computers, iPads, radios, PDAs, MP3 players, cell phones) plays an important role in the lives of many people in the 21st century. Fine motor control is paramount when using these devices and should be preserved as much as possible to maximize electronic contact with the outside world for social participation, education, and work-related occupations. Attention to orthosis size and immobilizing only those joints required can facilitate the ability to manipulate small buttons and dials required to use such devices. For an orthosis to be accepted as a legitimate holistic device, it must work for clients within their context(s) and environments. Since contextual concerns are not always apparent to the practitioner, all clients should be asked if their orthoses are in any way inhibiting their ability to engage in any life experience. Most orthoses affect a person's ability to perform activities.

Social Environment

The social environment pertains to the ability of clients to meet the demands of their specific group or family. Social environments are an integral consideration for orthotic provision. For example, a new mother was given a wrist/thumb orthosis after being diagnosed with de Quervain tenosynovitis. The mother began to feel inadequate in her new role because she could not cuddle and feed the infant without contacting him with a rigid orthosis. In this case, it was suggested that a softer prefabricated orthosis or alternative wearing schedule be provided to maximize compliance with the orthotic program (Fig. 2.2).

Physical Environment

Knowledge of physical environments may contribute to an understanding of the need for orthotic provision, but the physical environment may also hamper consistent use if clients are unable to engage in required or desired activities. For example, if a client needs to drive to work and is unable to drive while wearing an orthosis, he might remove it despite the potential for reinjury. Fig. 2.3A depicts a young woman wearing an orthosis because she sustained a flexor digitorum profundus injury. She found that typing at her workplace while wearing the orthosis was creating shoulder discomfort. She asked the

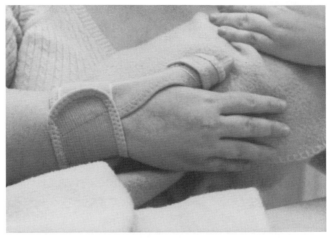

Fig. 2.2 Prefabricated thumb immobilization orthosis. It improves comfort while holding the infant.

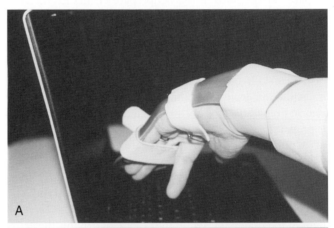

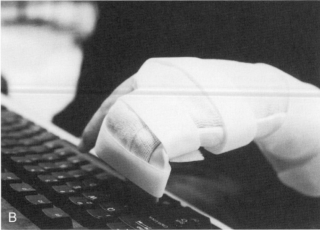

Fig. 2.3 A, Excessive pronation required to accurately press keys while using standard dorsal blocking orthosis. B, Improved ability to work on computer using modified volar-based protective orthosis.

therapist if she could remove her orthosis for work, and with physician approval the therapist created a modified protective orthosis (see Fig. 2.3B). The newly modified orthosis allowed improved function and protected the healing tendon.

Depending on its intended purpose, an orthosis might perpetuate dysfunction and may prolong the return to meaningful life engagement. Thus it is important to pay attention to the specifics of the client's personal environment and multiple contexts.

The impact is a matter of degree, and consideration needs to be given to the trade-off between how an orthosis enables clients (if only in the future) and how the orthosis presently disables them. Practitioners must be aware of the balance between enablement and disablement and must do their best to appropriately modify the orthosis or the wearing schedule to facilitate clients' occupational engagement. To ignore the interconnection of function is to practice a reductionist form of intervention, because it emphasizes only isolated skills and body structures without regard to engagement in selected activities.

Occupation-Centered Orthotics and Types of Intervention

The OTPF-3[1] describes several types of activities and occupations used as occupational therapy interventions: preparatory methods and tasks, activities, occupations, education and training, group intervention, and advocacy/self-advocacy. Preparatory methods and tasks prepare clients for the ability to engage in activities and occupations. They do not meet the definition of activities or occupations themselves and are either therapist-administered interventions or contrived engagements that address underlying client factors and performance skills only. Examples include exercise, inhibition or facilitation techniques, and positioning devices that are used in preparation for occupational participation. Examples of preparatory tasks include simulated activities (e.g., driving simulators) that begin to prepare the client for participation in actually driving a vehicle or cone stacking, which is often used to simulate reaching skills needed for placing items on kitchen shelves. Activities are goal directed and have an inherent purpose to the client; others readily understand them in the pragmatic sense. In the case of driving, the activity is under way when a client gets into a vehicle and drives. Occupation is the ultimate type of intervention. Clients participate in occupations within their natural environment and affix personal meaning to the experience. The ability to complete one's morning routine that includes driving to his or her place of employment is an occupation.

According to the OTPF-3, orthotics fabrication/provision is fundamentally a preparatory method. It is not an activity; it is initiated before occupational engagement and discontinued when hand function resumes. However, from an occupation-focused orthotic perspective, an orthotic intervention is not only a technique used in preparation for occupation. For appropriate clients, orthoses are an integral part of ongoing intervention to support occupational engagement through all types of intervention. For example, some clients may receive an orthosis to use as desired in a prophylactic manner to prevent the onset of pain while engaging in work and leisure pursuits that could otherwise lead to occupational dysfunction.

Orthotic Intervention as a Therapeutic Approach

In the OTPF-3[1] intervention approaches are defined as "specific strategies selected to direct the process of evaluation and intervention planning, selection and implementation on the basis of the client's desired outcome, evaluation data,

and evidence; approaches inform the selection of models and frames of reference."[1] These intervention approaches include:

- Create or promote health
- Establish or restore a skill or ability
- Maintain performance capabilities
- Modify context or activity demands through compensation and adaptation
- Prevent disability

From an occupation-based perspective, when orthoses enable occupation, they become an integral part of that occupation versus being a preparatory method only. Custom-fitted orthoses within the context of clients' occupational experience can promote health, remediate dysfunction, substitute for lost function, and prevent disability. When teamed with a full occupational profile, analysis of occupation, and knowledge of the appropriate use of orthoses for specific pathologies (supported by evidence of effectiveness), devices are selected to produce the outcomes that reach the goals collaboratively set by the client and the practitioner.

Orthotic Intervention as a Facilitator of Therapeutic Outcomes

As part of occupation-centered practice, orthotic intervention is a therapeutic approach interwoven through all levels of intervention. The OTPF[1] describes specific therapeutic outcomes expected from intervention. Outcomes are occupational performance (improvement and enhancement), participation, role competence, adaptation, health and wellness, prevention, quality of life, well-being, and occupational justice.[1]

Positive outcomes in occupational performance are the effect of successful intervention. Such outcomes are demonstrated either by improved performance within the presence of continued deficits resulting from injury or disease, or the enhancement of function when disease is not currently present. Orthotic intervention addresses both types of occupational performance outcomes (improvement and enhancement). Orthoses that improve function in a person with pathology result in an "increased independence and function in an ADL, IADL, education, work, play, leisure, or social participation."[1] For example, a wrist immobilization orthosis is prescribed for a person who has carpal tunnel syndrome. The orthosis positions the wrist to rest the inflamed anatomical structures and maximize the carpal tunnel space, thus decreasing pain and paresthesias and improving work performance. Orthoses that enhance function without specific pathology result in improved occupational performance from one's current status or prevention of potential problems. For example, some orthoses position the hands to prevent overuse syndromes resulting from hand-intensive repetitive or resistive tasks.

Role competence is the ability to satisfactorily complete desired roles (e.g., worker, parent, spouse, friend, and team member). Roles are maintained through orthotic intervention by minimizing the effects of pathology and facilitating upper extremity performance for role specific activities. For example, a mother who wears an orthosis for carpal tunnel syndrome should be able to hold her child's hand without extreme pain. Holding the child's hand makes her feel as though she is fulfilling her role as a mother.

Orthoses created to enhance adaptation to overcome occupational dysfunction address the dynamics of the challenges and the client's expected ability to overcome it. An example of orthotic intervention to improve adaptation might involve a client who experiences carpal ligament sprain but must continue working or risk losing employment. In this case a wrist immobilization orthosis that allows for digital movements may enable continued hand functions while resting the involved ligament.

Health and wellness are collectively described as the absence of infirmity and a "state of physical, mental, and social well-being."[1] Orthoses promote health and wellness of clients by minimizing the effects of physical disruption through protection and substitution. Enabling a healthy lifestyle that allows clients to experience a sense of wellness facilitates motivation and engagement in all desired occupations.

Prevention in the context of the OTPF involves the promotion of a healthy lifestyle at a policy creation, population, group, or person level.[1] When an external circumstance (e.g., environment, job requirement, and so on) exists with the potential for interference in occupational engagement, an orthotic program may be a solution to prevent the ill effects of the situation. If it is not feasible to modify the job demands, clients may benefit from the use of orthoses in a preventative role. For example, a wrist immobilization orthosis and an elbow strap are fitted to prevent lateral epicondylitis of the elbow for a client who works in a job that involves repetitive and resistive lifting of the wrist with a clenched fist. In addition, the worker is educated on modifying motions and posture that contribute to the condition.

One of the most difficult concepts to define is the concept of quality of life. Despite this, most individuals from Western cultures have a tacit understanding of its meaning and typically know it to be a condition that includes general health, physical, emotional, cognitive, role, and social function with an absence of signs and symptoms of pathology. Quality of life entails one's appraisal of abilities to engage in specific tasks that beneficially affect life and allows self-expressions that are socially valued.[11] One's state of being is determined by the ability of the client to be satisfied, engage in occupations, adapt to novel situations, and maintain health and wellness. Ultimately, orthotic intervention focused on therapeutic outcomes improves the quality of life through facilitating engagement in meaningful life occupations.

Well-being is a subjective state experienced by individuals when they are content with their own health, self-esteem, sense of belonging, security, and opportunities for self-determination.[1] An orthosis that reduces pain and allows engagement in needed and desired occupations will afford the individual control over his or her own health and make way for job and personal security, as well as ensuring opportunities for maintaining or creating self-determination. An example is the case of a hand-based thumb orthosis that allows the client to continue working as a data entry specialist at a place of employment that offers steady income and health benefits.

Occupational justice refers to the rights of people to be included in desired life pursuits, including education and movement within the community. When provided with orthoses that enable function, individuals who are at a disadvantage and cannot participate fully within society without a device may become empowered and able to take full advantage of all that society has to offer. For example, an individual who is not able to access a computer in the public library due to significant hand contractures may be able to search the Internet in this publically funded facility if an orthosis is provided that isolates the index finger of the dominant hand for one-finger typing.

THE INFLUENCE OF OCCUPATIONAL DESIRES ON ORTHOTIC DESIGN AND SELECTION

The **occupational profile** phase of the evaluation process described in the OTPF-3 involves learning about clients from a contextual and performance viewpoint.[1] For example, what are the interests and motivations of clients? Where do they work, live, and recreate? Tools (i.e., Canadian Occupational Performance Measure (COPM); Disabilities of the Arm, Shoulder, and Hand [DASH]; Patient-Rated Wrist Hand Evaluation [PRWHE]; and the Manual Ability Measure-20 [MAM-20]) that offer clients the opportunity to discuss their injuries in the context of their daily lives lend insight into the needs that must be addressed. Table 2.1 lists such tools. When used in conjunction with traditional methods of hand and upper extremity assessment (e.g., goniometers, dynamometers, and volumeters), they help therapists learn about the specific clients they treat and assist in orthotic selection and design.

The outcome measures listed in Table 2.1 emphasize client occupations and functions as the focus of intervention. Information obtained from such assessments supports the goal of occupation-based orthotic intervention, which is to improve the client's quality of life through the client's continued engagement in desired occupations.

An orthosis that focuses on client factors alone does not always treat the functional deficit. For example, a static orthosis to support the weak elbow of a client who has lost innervation of the biceps muscle protects the muscle yet allows only one angle of function of that joint. A dynamic flexion orthosis protects the muscle from end-range stretch yet allows the client the ability to change the arm angle through active extension and passive flexion. Assessment tools that measure physical client factors exclusively (e.g., goniometry, grip strength, volumeter, and so on) must remain as adjuncts to determine orthotic design, because physical functioning is an adjunct to occupational engagement.

Canadian Occupational Performance Measure

The COPM is an interview-based assessment tool for use in a client-centered approach.[19] The COPM assists the therapist in identifying problems in performance areas, such as those

TABLE 2.1   Client-Centered Outcome Measures

Tool	General Description	Contact Information
Manual Ability Measure-20 (MAM-20)[29]	A 20-item self-report questionnaire. Tool consists of two parts: (1) a client demographic sheet and (2) a self-report task list consisting of items that clients rate on a 4-point scale based on their perceived ability to complete tasks. It also includes a visual analog pain scale and column for indicating if skill can be completed with the noninvolved hand.	Chen, C.C., & Bode, R. K. (2010). Psychometric validation of the Manual Ability Measure-36 (MAM-36) in patients with neurologic and musculoskeletal disorders. *Archives of Physical Medicine and Rehabilitation, 91*(3), 414–420.
Canadian Occupational Performance Measure (COPM)[19]	The COPM is a client-centered approach to assessment of perceived functional abilities, interest, and satisfaction with occupations. This interview-based valid and reliable tool is scored and can be used to measure outcomes of treatment.	The COPM can be purchased through the Canadian Association of Occupational Therapists (CAOT) at http://www.caot.ca.
Disabilities of the Arm, Shoulder, and Hand (DASH) assessment[16]	DASH is a condition-specific tool. The DASH consists of 30 predetermined questions addressing function within performance areas. Clients are asked to rate their recent ability to complete skills on a scale of 1 (no difficulty) to 5 (unable). The DASH assists with the development of the occupational profile through its valid and reliable measure of clients' functional abilities.	Visit the DASH/QuickDASH website at http://www.dash.iwh.on.ca.
Patient-Rated Wrist Hand Evaluation (PRWHE)[21]	The PRWHE is a condition-specific tool through which the client rates pain and function in 15 preselected items.	MacDermid, J.C., & Tottenham, V. (2004). Responsiveness of the disability of the arm, shoulder, and hand (DASH) and patient-rated wrist/hand evaluation (PRWHE) in evaluating change after hand therapy. *Journal of Hand Therapy, 17,* 18–23.

described by the OTPF-3. In addition, clients' perceptions of their ability to perform the identified problem area and their satisfaction with their abilities are determined when using the COPM.[19] Therapists can use the COPM with clients from all age groups and with any type of disability. Parents or family members can serve as proxies if the client is unable to take part in the interview process (e.g., if the client has dementia). When the COPM is readministered, objective documentation of the functional effects of orthotic intervention through comparison of preintervention and postintervention scores is made.

When the COPM is used, contextual issues arise during the client interview about satisfaction with function. Clients may indicate why certain activities create personal dissatisfaction despite their ability to perform them. An example is the case of a woman who resides in an assisted living setting. During administration of the COPM, she identifies that she is able to don her orthosis by using her teeth to tighten and loosen the straps. She needs to remove the orthosis to use utensils during meals. However, she is embarrassed to do this in front of other residents while at the dining table. The use of the COPM uncovers issues that are pertinent to individual clients and must be considered by the therapist.

Disabilities of the Arm, Shoulder, and Hand

The DASH is a condition-specific tool that measures a client's perception of how current upper extremity disability has affected function.[10] The DASH consists of 30 predetermined questions that explore function within performance areas.

The client is asked to rate on a scale of 1 (no difficulty) to 5 (unable) his or her current ability to complete particular skills, such as opening a jar or turning a key. The DASH assists the therapist in gathering data for an occupational profile of functional abilities. The focus of the assessment is not on body structures or on the signs and symptoms of a particular diagnostic condition. Rather, the merit of the DASH is the information obtained is about the client's functional abilities.

An interview, although not mandated by the DASH, should become part of the process to enhance the therapist's understanding of the identified problems. The therapist must also determine why a functional problem exists and how it may be affecting quality of life. The DASH is an objective means of measuring client outcomes when readministered following orthosis provision or other treatment interventions.

When selecting the DASH as a measure of occupational performance, the therapist may consider several additional facts. For example, the performance areas measured are predetermined in the questionnaire and may limit the client's responses. In addition, the DASH does not specifically address contextual issues or client satisfaction or provide insight into the emotional state of the client. Additional information can be obtained through interview to gain insight needed for proper orthotic design and selection.

Patient-Rated Wrist Hand Evaluation

The PRWHE is a condition-specific tool through which clients rate their pain and functional abilities in 15 preselected areas.[21] PRWHE assists with the development of the occupational profile through obtaining information about clients' functional abilities. The functional areas identified in the PRWHE are generally much broader than those in the DASH. Similar to the DASH, the PRWHE's questions to elicit such information are not open-ended questions as in the COPM. Information about pain levels during activity and client satisfaction of the aesthetics of the upper limb are gathered during the PRWHE assessment.

The PRWHE does not specifically require an inquiry into the details of function, but such information would certainly assist the therapist and make the assessment process more occupation based. The PRWHE does not include questions related to context. Therefore the therapist should include such questions in treatment planning discussions.

The Manual Ability Measure-20

The MAM-20 was developed by occupational therapists[3] and can be used with both musculoskeletally and neurologically based hand function deficits. The tool was originally described in 2005 in the *Journal of Hand Surgery* (British and European volume) as the Manual Ability Measure-16. The tool consists of two parts: (1) a client demographic sheet and (2) a self-report task list consisting of items that clients rate on a 4-point scale based on their perceived ability to complete the task. The rating scale ranges from 1, "cannot do," to 4, "easy." The 0 (zero) option indicates "almost never do (even prior to condition)." The tool also includes a visual analog pain scale and a column to indicate if a task is being completed with the opposite hand. The MAM-20 takes a positive wellness stance and addresses function versus dysfunction. The client scores higher when higher levels of function are present. Research has supported the validity and reliability of the MAM-20.[4]

Analysis Phase

Following the data collection part of the evaluation process, the analysis of occupational performance occurs. If a therapist uses one of the aforementioned tools, analysis of the performance process has been initiated. Further questions will be asked based on the answers of previous questions. The therapist continues to gain specific insight into how orthotic intervention can be used to remediate the reported dysfunction.

During the analysis phase the therapist may actually want to see the client perform several functions to gain additional insight into how activity affects, or is impacted by, the diagnosis or pathology. For example, a client states that he cannot write because of thumb carpometacarpal (CMC) joint pain. Therefore the therapist asks the client to show how he is able to hold the pen while describing the type of discomfort experienced with writing. The therapist begins orthotic design analysis by holding the client's thumb in a supported position to simulate the effect of a hand-based orthosis. The client actively participates in the process by giving feedback to the therapist during orthotic design and fabrication.

After a client-centered occupation-based profile and analysis is completed, an occupation-based orthotic intervention plan is developed. Measuring only physical factors to create a client profile results in a therapist seeing only the upper extremity and not the client. The upper extremity does not dictate the quality of life. Rather, the mind, spirit, and body do so collectively! (See Self-Quiz 2.1.)

EVIDENCE TO SUPPORT PRESERVATION OF OCCUPATIONAL ENGAGEMENT AND PARTICIPATION

Fundamental to occupational therapy treatment is the belief that individuals must retain their ability to engage in meaningful occupations or risk further detriment to their subjective experience of quality of life. If humans behaved as automatons (completing activities without drive, interest, or attention), correcting deficits would become reductionist and mechanical. A reductionistic approach could guarantee that an adaptive device or exercise could correct any problem and immediately lead to the continuation of the required task (much like replacing a spark plug to allow a car to start). Fortunately, humans are not automatons, and occupational therapy exists to support the ability of the individual to engage in and maintain participation in desired occupations.

The literature supports the premise that any temporary or permanent disruption in the ability to engage in meaningful occupations can be detrimental. For example, with a flexor tendon repair therapists must follow protocols to facilitate appropriate tissue healing. Such protocols typically restrict the hand from performing functional pursuits for a minimum of 6 to 8 weeks. However, occupational dysfunction must be effectively minimized as soon as possible to maintain quality of life.[22]

 SELF-QUIZ 2.1[a]

Answer the following questions.

1. Consider an orthotic intervention plan with a client of a different culture than yours. What factors of orthotic design and provision may need special attention to ensure acceptance, compliance, and understanding?

2. When designing orthoses to match the occupational needs of a young child, what performance areas and personal contextual factors will you be interested in addressing?

[a]See Appendix A for answers.

Evidence to Support Occupational Engagement

Supported by research, in addition to anecdotal experiences and reports of therapists, is the importance of multidimensional engagement in meaningful occupations. Described by Wilcock and Hocking,[34] the term **occupational deprivation** is a state wherein clients are unable to engage in chosen meaningful life occupations due to factors outside their control. Disability, incarceration, and geographical isolation are but a few circumstances that create occupational deprivation. Depression, isolation, difficulty with social interaction, inactivity, and boredom leading to a diminished sense of self can result from occupational deprivation.[7] **Occupational disruption** is a temporary and less severe condition that is also caused by an unexpected change in the ability to engage in meaningful activities.[7] Additional studies conducted by behavioral scientists interested in how individual differences, personality, and lifestyle factors influence well-being have shown that engagement in occupations can influence happiness and life satisfaction.[6]

Ecological models of adaptation suggest that people thrive when their personalities and needs are matched with environments or situations that enable them to remain engaged, interested, and challenged.[5] Walters and Moore[31] found that among the unemployed, involvement in meaningful leisure activities (not simply busywork activities) decreased the sense of occupational deprivation.

Palmadottir[23] completed a qualitative study that explored clients' perspectives on their occupational therapy experience. Positive outcomes of therapy were experienced by clients when treatment was client centered and held purpose and meaning for them. Thus, when a client who has an upper extremity functional deficit receives an orthosis, the orthosis should meet the immediate needs of the injury while meeting the client's desire for occupational engagement.

According to Clark and colleagues,[8] older adults from federally subsidized housing complexes realized positive outcomes in life satisfaction, role functioning, and physical and emotional health after receiving lifestyle interventions. These interventions include education for safety, time use, and cultural awareness, goal setting, and activities for social participation. The ability to engage in this program and the occupations targeted can be facilitated through orthoses that prevent or correct occupational dysfunction resulting from upper extremity changes associated with aging (e.g., joint changes, pain, weakness) or pathological conditions (e.g., arthritis, fractures, carpal tunnel syndrome).

Research offers evidence that orthoses of all types and for all purposes are indeed effective in reaching the goals of improved function.[9,25,27,28,33] Refer to the chapters throughout this book for current evidence related to specific orthoses. Three examples are presented to demonstrate such evidence of client-centered and occupation-based orthotic intervention. One study was conducted on the effects of orthotic intervention of the CMC joint of individuals with basal joint osteoarthritis. Two orthoses were provided to determine client preference and effects of custom versus prefabricated orthoses. Both orthoses demonstrated modest improvements in hand function. The prefabricated orthosis was the preferred orthosis, although the custom-made orthosis decreased

pain slightly more. According to the authors, this reinforces the client-centered approach to orthotic intervention in that clients can be given a choice in orthotic design knowing that both types are effective in enhancing occupational engagement.[27]

Thiele and colleagues[28] found that individuals using wrist immobilization orthoses for pain control during functional activities did have positive results in pain reduction, occupational performance, and strength. In addition, it was found that customized leather orthoses were preferred to commercially available fabric orthoses.

A nocturnal wrist extension orthosis was found to be effective in reducing the symptoms of carpal tunnel syndrome experienced by midwestern auto assembly plant workers.[33] This evidence leads us to conclude that orthotic intervention with attention to occupational needs can and should be used to preserve quality of life.

UTILIZING AN OCCUPATION-CENTERED APPROACH TO ORTHOTIC INTERVENTION

With guiding philosophies in place, the therapist using an occupation-based approach to orthotic intervention begins the following problem-solving process of orthotic design and fabrication.

Step 1: Referral

The clinical decision-making process begins with the referral. Some orthotic referrals come from physicians who specialize in hand conditions. A referral may contain details about the diagnosis or requested orthosis. However, some orders may be from physicians who do not specialize in the treatment of the hand. If this is the case, the physician may depend on the expertise of the therapist and may simply order an orthosis without detailing specifics. An orthotic intervention order for a client with a condition may also rely on the knowledge and creativity of the therapist. At this step the therapist must begin to consider the diagnosis, the contextual issues of the client, and the type of orthosis that must be fabricated.

Step 2: Client-Centered and Occupation-Based Evaluation

Therapists use outcome measures (such as, the COPM, DASH, MAM-20, or PRWHE) to learn which occupations clients desire to complete during orthotic wear, which occupations orthoses can support, and which occupations the orthoses will eventually help accomplish. The therapist and the client use this information for goal prioritization and orthotic design in Step 4.

Step 3: Understand/Assess the Condition and Consider Intervention Options

Review biology, cause, course, and traditional interventions of the person's condition, including protocols and healing time frames. Assess the client's physical status.

Research orthotic options, and determine possible modifications to result in increased occupational engagement without sacrificing orthotic effectiveness. When an orthosis is ordered to prevent an injury, the therapist must analyze any activities that may be impacted by wearing the orthosis and determining how it may affect occupational performance.

Step 4: Analyze Assessment Findings for Orthotic Design

Analyze information about pathology and **treatment protocols** to reconcile needs of tissue healing and function (occupational engagement). Consider whether the condition is acute or chronic. Acute injuries are those that have occurred recently and are expected to heal within a relatively brief time period. Acute conditions may require orthoses to preserve and protect healing structures. Examples include tendon or nerve repair, fractures, carpal tunnel release, de Quervain release, Dupuytren release, or other immediate postsurgical conditions requiring mobilization or immobilization through orthotic intervention.

If the condition is acute, orthotic intervention adheres to protocols and knowledge of client occupational status and desires. Determine if the client is able to engage in desired occupations within the orthosis. If the client can engage in occupations while wearing the orthosis, continue with a custom occupation-based treatment plan in addition to orthotic intervention.

Step 5: Determining Orthotic Design

If the client is unable to complete desired activities and functions within the orthosis, the therapist must determine modifications or alternative orthotic designs to facilitate function. Environmental modifications or adaptations may be needed to accommodate lack of function if no further changes can be made to the orthosis.

Fig. 2.4A is an example of a finger-based trigger finger orthosis that allows unrestricted ability of the client to engage in a craft activity. Compare the orthosis shown in Fig. 2.4B with the orthosis shown in Fig. 2.4C. The orthosis in Fig. 2.4B was previously issued and limited mobility of the ulnar side of the hand and diminished comfort and activity satisfaction.

To ensure that an occupation-based approach to orthotic intervention has been undertaken, the occupation-based orthotic intervention checklist can be used (Form 2.1). This checklist focuses the therapist's attention on client-centered occupation-based practice. Using the checklist helps ensure that the client does not experience occupational deprivation or disruption.

ORTHOTIC DESIGN OPTIONS TO PROMOTE OCCUPATIONAL ENGAGEMENT AND PARTICIPATION

The characteristics of an orthosis have an influence on a client's ability to function. The therapist faces the challenge

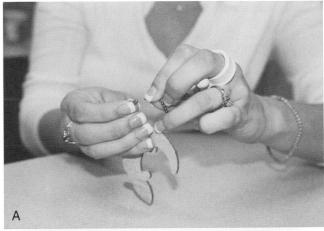

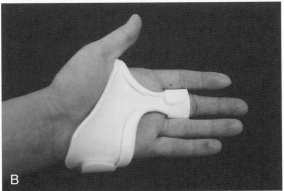

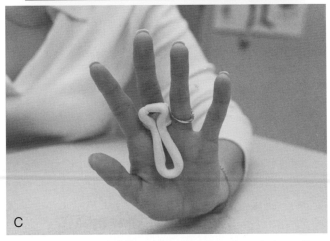

Fig. 2.4 A, Functional ability while using finger-based trigger finger orthosis. B, Confining hand-based trigger finger orthosis. C, Finger based metacarpophalangeal blocking trigger finger orthosis.

of trying to help restore or protect the client's involved anatomical structure while preserving the client's performance. To achieve optimal occupational outcomes, specific designs and materials must be used to fabricate orthoses that are user friendly. The therapist must employ clinical reasoning that considers the impact on the injured tissue and the desires of the client. Such consideration results in an orthosis that best protects the anatomical structure at the same time it preserves the contextual and functional needs of the client.

SUMMARY

Engagement in relevant life activities to enhance and maintain quality of life is a concept to be considered with orthotic provision. The premise that orthotic intervention of the hand and upper extremity can improve the overall function of the hand is supported in the literature. Hence orthotic intervention that includes attention to the functional desires of the client is a valid occupation-centered treatment approach that enhances life satisfaction and facilitates therapeutic outcomes.

⚡ PATIENT SAFETY

Based on sound clinical reasoning (refer to Chapters 5 and 6), therapists may create orthoses to enhance occupational participation that may deviate from common orthotic designs that follow standard hand therapy protocols. The therapist should evaluate this creative design to judge whether the orthosis is appropriate for the client. When in doubt, therapists must seek and gain approval from the treating physician to ensure that the orthosis modification will not cause harm or create the potential for injury during activity. It is the therapist's responsibility to give the rationale for the design to the physician and any compelling literature to support the proposed intervention.

REVIEW QUESTIONS

1. According to this chapter, what is the definition of *occupation-centered orthotic intervention*?
2. What is occupational deprivation, and how is it impacted by occupation-centered orthotic intervention?
3. What are the reasons therapists provide orthoses to clients who have upper extremity pathology?
4. Why is it important for the client to be an active participant in the orthotic process?
5. Why is attention to the context of the client integral to occupation-centered orthotic intervention?
6. What could occur if concern for patient safety is not present when selecting orthoses used for individuals with acute conditions of the hand or upper extremity?
7. Why should a therapist be knowledgeable about tissue healing and treatment protocols despite the fact that such factors do not imply occupation-focused treatment?

REFERENCES

1. American Occupational Therapy Association: Occupational therapy practice framework: domain and process, *Am J Occup Ther* 68(Suppl):S1–S48, 2014.
2. Amini D: The occupational basis for splinting, *Adv Occup Ther Pract* 21:11, 2005.
3. Brennan C, McGuire MJ, Metzler C: New occupational therapy evaluation CPT codes: coding overview and guidelines on code selection, *OT Practice* 21(22):CE1–CE8, 2016.
4. Chen CC, Bode RK: Psychometric validation of the Manual Ability Measure-36 (MAM-36) in patients with neurologic and musculoskeletal disorders, *Arch Phys Med Rehabil* 91(3):414–420, 2010.
5. Christiansen C: Three perspectives on balance in occupation. In Zemke R, Clark F, editors: *Occupational science: the evolving discipline*, Philadelphia, 1996, FA Davis, pp 431–451.
6. Christiansen CH, Backman C, Little BR, et al.: Occupations and subjective well-being: a study of personal projects, *Am J Occup Ther* 53(1):91–100, 1999.
7. Christiansen C, Townsend E: *Introduction to occupation: the art and science of living*, Upper Saddle River, NJ, 2009, Pearson Education.
8. Clark F, Jackson J, Carlson M, et al.: Effectiveness of a lifestyle intervention in promoting the well-being of independently living older people: results of the Well Elderly 2 Randomized Controlled Trial, *J Epidemiol Community Health* 66(9):782–790, 2012.
9. Carruthers KH, et al.: Casting and splinting management for hand injuries in the in-season contact sport athlete, *Sports Health*, 2017:1941738117700133.
10. Institute for Work & Health: *The DASH outcome measure* (website). Retrieved from www.dash.iwh.on.ca.
11. Fayers P, Machin D: *Quality of life: the assessment, analysis and interpretation of patient reported outcomes*, ed 2, West Sussex, 2007, John Wiley & Sons Ltd.
12. Fess EE: A history of splinting: to understand the present, view the past, *J Hand Ther* 15(2):97–132, 2002.
13. Fess EE, Gettle KS, Philips CA, et al.: *Hand and upper extremity splinting: principles and methods*, ed 3, St. Louis, 2005, Elsevier Mosby.
14. Fisher AG: Occupation-centered, occupation-based, occupation-focused: Same, same or different, *Scand J Occup Ther* 21:96–107, 2014.
15. Goldstein-Lohman H, Kratz A, Pierce D: A study of occupation-based practice. In Pierce D, editor: *Occupation by design: building therapeutic power*, Philadelphia, 2003, FA Davis, pp 239–261.
16. Hudak PL, Amadio PC, Bombardier C: Development of an upper extremity outcome measure: the DASH (disabilities of the arm, shoulder and hand), *The Upper Extremity Collaborative Group (UECG)* 29:602–608, 1996.
17. Ikiugu MN, Smallfield S, Condit C: A framework for combining theoretical conceptual practice models in occupational therapy practice, *Can J Occup Ther* 76(3):162–170, 2009.
18. Law M, editor: *Client-centered occupational therapy*, Thorofare, NJ, 1998, Slack.
19. Law M, Baptiste S, Carswell A, et al.: *Canadian occupational performance measure*, Ottawa, ON, 2014, CAOT.
20. Law M, Baptiste S, Mills J: Client-centered practice: what does it mean and does it make a difference? *Can J Occup Ther* 62(5):250–257, 1995.

21. MacDermid JC, Tottenham V: Responsiveness of the disability of the arm, shoulder, and hand (DASH) and patient-rated wrist/hand evaluation (PRWHE) in evaluating change after hand therapy, *J Hand Ther* 17(1):18–23, 2004.

22. McKee P, Rivard A: Orthoses as enablers of occupation: client-centered splinting for better outcomes, *Can J Occup Ther* 71(5):306–314, 2004.

23. Palmadottir G: Client perspectives on occupational therapy in rehabilitation services, *Scand J Occup Ther* 10:157–166, 2003.

24. Pierce D: *Occupational science for occupational therapy*, Thorofare, New Jersey, 2013, Slack, Inc.

25. Ramsey L, Winder RJ, McVeigh JG: The effectiveness of working wrist splints in adults with rheumatoid arthritis: a mixed methods systematic review, *J Rehabil Med* 46(6):481–492, 2014.

26. Reilly M: Occupational therapy can be one of the great ideas of 20th century medicine, *Am J Occup Ther* 16:1–9, 1962.

27. Sillem H, Backman CL, Miller WC, et al.: Comparison of two carpometacarpal stabilizing splints for individuals with thumb osteoarthritis, *J Hand Ther* 24(3):216–226, 2011.

28. Thiele J, Nimmo R, Rowell W, et al.: A randomized single blind crossover trial comparing leather and commercial wrist splints for treating chronic wrist pain in adults, *BMC Musculoskelet Disord* 10:129, 2009.

29. Thomas JJ, Fowler D: Convergent validity: the relationship between perceived pain and the manual ability measure–20 (MAM–20), *Am J Occup Ther* 69(Suppl 1), 2015.

30. Townsend EA, Polatajko HJ: *Enabling occupation ii: advancing an occupational therapy vision for health, well-being & justice through occupation*, Ottawa, ON, 2007, CAOT ACE.

31. Walters L, Moore K: Reducing latent deprivation during unemployment: the role of meaningful leisure activity, *J Occup Organ Psychol* 75:15–18, 2002.

32. Weinstock-Zlotnick G, Hinojosa J: Bottom-up or top-down evaluation: is one better than the other? *Am J Occup Ther* 58(5):594–599, 2004.

33. Werner R, Franzblau A, Gell N: Randomized controlled trial of nocturnal splinting for active workers with symptoms of carpal tunnel syndrome, *Arch Phys Med Rehabil* 86(1):1–7, 2005.

34. Wilcock A, Hocking C: *An occupational perspective of health*, ed 3, Thorofare, NJ, 2015, Slack.

APPENDIX 2.1 CASE STUDIES

Case Study 2.1[a]

Read the following scenario, and use your clinical reasoning skills to answer the questions based on information in this chapter.

Natasha is a 68-year-old woman who is legally blind. Natasha underwent a metacarpophalangeal (MCP) joint silicone arthroplasty procedure for long, ring, and small fingers of her left hand due to severe rheumatoid arthritis 3 days ago. You received an order to fabricate "forearm-based dynamic extension orthosis to hold the fingers in neutral alignment but allow flexion and extension of the MCPs throughout the day." Natasha attends her first therapy appointment accompanied by her husband, who is now her primary caregiver.

1. During the initial session, you attempt to conduct an interview using the Canadian Occupational Performance Measure (COPM) with Natasha. Her answers seem unrealistic, and you suspect that she is not providing accurate information. What steps can you take to verify that the information you obtained is reflective of her current level of function?

   _____

   _____

2. How will you be certain that Natasha is able to read and comprehend the printed orthosis care sheet?

   _____

   _____

3. How will you be certain that Natasha is able to follow the home exercise program pamphlet?

   _____

   _____

4. You design a creative way to allow safe range of motion exercises while maintaining neutral alignment of the digits. How will you ensure that the orthosis modification is appropriate and will not cause harm?

   _____

   _____

Case Study 2.2[a]

Read the following scenario, and use your clinical reasoning skills to answer the questions based on information in this chapter.

Graysen is a 29-year-old man with a 2-year status post multiple trauma, which was secondary to an improvised explosive device blast in Kabul, Afghanistan. Graysen was referred to occupational therapy by his current orthopedic physician for treatment of residual hand and upper extremity dysfunction and difficulty participating in desired occupations. An occupational therapist evaluated him using goniometry, dynamometry, the Nine Hole Peg Test, and the Canadian Occupational Performance Measure (COPM). The results of the range-of-motion measurements indicate full passive motion in flexion and extension with 75% impairment of active flexion of all digits and full active extension of all digits of both hands. Thumbs are functional yet lack 10% of passive and active motion. Grip strength testing indicated 15 pounds of force bilaterally with 5 pounds of lateral pinch strength. The Nine Hole Peg Test indicated impaired fine motor coordination with a score of 60 seconds on the left nondominant hand and 72 seconds on the right hand using lateral pinch only.

Graysen indicated three areas of functional concern while completing the COPM. These include the inability to (1) complete independent bill paying, (2) use the computer to communicate with friends and family on social network sites, and (3) prepare his plate for independent eating. Graysen has scored his ability and satisfaction with these skills as follows (10 = high; 1 = low).

- Bill paying:
  1. Performance: 2
  2. Satisfaction: 3
- Computer use and social communication:
  1. Performance: 2
  2. Satisfaction: 1
- Eating/plate preparation:
  1. Performance: 3
  2. Satisfaction: 4
- Average scores:
  1. Performance: 8/3, 2.6 average
  2. Satisfaction: 7/3, 2.3 average

1. According to the information presented previously, what areas should be addressed first to assist Graysen with occupational satisfaction? Why?

   _____

2. What approach to treatment facilitates the most expedient return to function? Why?

   _____

3. What components of this assessment indicate a concern for the occupational participation and context of the client?

   _____

4. What occupational areas would you need to consider for Graysen's orthotic design?

   _____

Case Study 2.3[a]

Read the following scenario, and use your clinical reasoning skills to answer the questions based on information in this chapter.

Irene is a 63-year-old married female. She does not work outside of the home but is very involved in civic organizations such as volunteering for Boys and Girls Club. She and her husband, who recently retired as the vice president of a local bank, purchased a historic home in the downtown area of their city. They installed a swimming pool as swimming is another important leisure and health pursuit of Irene. Approximately 3 weeks ago, while walking her dog on an uneven sidewalk, Irene sustained a fracture to her dominant right elbow and

---

[a] See Appendix A for the answer key.

[a] See Appendix A for the answer key.

underwent an open reduction and internal fixation procedure with Kirschner wire to secure the bone fragments for healing.

At this time Irene is keeping occupied by having multiple friends visit throughout the day. They spend many hours at poolside discussing politics and national events. Her husband currently transports Irene to all of her doctor appointments and assists her with some activities such as grocery shopping.

Irene is being seen for the first time in occupational therapy today to begin active mobilization of the elbow joint and to address occupational concerns.

The half-cast orthosis provided by the physician was effective in immobilizing and protecting the joint, yet Irene reported to the therapist the following difficulties:

- General dependency for all self-care and transportation
  - Unable to attend volunteer and church activities
  - Unable to engage in desired swimming activities due to water-soluble orthosis/cast
- Dependency in application of orthosis (elastic wrap required)
- Limited wrist mobility due to length of orthosis/cast

- Bulkiness of orthosis/cast creating difficulty with dressing into long-sleeve shirts and jackets
- Heaviness of orthosis/cast, leading to shoulder soreness

1. What additional information should the therapist acquire to create an occupation-centered treatment plan for Irene?
2. Identify an appropriate outcome measure that could be used in the case of Irene.
3. Using an occupation-focused approach, what would be the first change that you would make to the orthosis that Irene is currently using? Why?
4. How would your answer to question 3 change if you decided to use an occupation-based approach to her care due to the severity of the elbow fracture?

APPENDIX 2.2 FORM

Form 2.1 Occupation-Based Orthotic Intervention Checklist

1. Orthosis meets requirements of protocol for specific pathology; ensuring attention to bodily functions and structures.	Yes ○	No ○	NA ○
2. If indicated, orthotic design is approved with referring physician.	Yes ○	No ○	NA ○
3. Orthosis allows client to engage in all desired occupation-based tasks through support of activity demands.	Yes ○	No ○	NA ○
4. Orthosis supports client habits, roles, and routines.	Yes ○	No ○	NA ○
5. Orthotic design fits client's cultural needs.	Yes ○	No ○	NA ○
6. Orthotic design fits with temporal needs, including season, age of client, and duration of use.	Yes ○	No ○	NA ○
7. Orthotic design takes into consideration the client's physical environment.	Yes ○	No ○	NA ○
8. Orthotic design supports the client's social pursuits.	Yes ○	No ○	NA ○
9. Client's personal needs are addressed through orthotic design.	Yes ○	No ○	NA ○
10. Client is able to engage in the virtual world (e.g., cellular phone, PDA, computer use).	Yes ○	No ○	NA ○
11. Orthosis is comfortable.	Yes ○	No ○	NA ○
12. Client verbalizes understanding of orthosis use, care, precautions, and rationale for use.	Yes ○	No ○	NA ○
13. Client demonstrates the ability to don and doff orthosis.	Yes ○	No ○	NA ○
14. Adaptations to the physical environment are made to ensure function in desired occupations.	Yes ○	No ○	NA ○
15. Client indicates satisfaction with orthotic design and functionality within orthosis.	Yes ○	No ○	NA ○

MATCHING ACTIVITY OF OCCUPATION-CENTERED ORTHOTIC INTERVENTION[a]

Matching: Match the terms from the chapter text in column A to the best description in column B.

Column A		Column B	
1	Biomechanical____	A	Occupation focused
2	Client factors addressed initially	B	Assessment that measures change in functional status over time
3	Rest and sleep		
4	Social	C	Occupation based
5	Cultural	D	Client-centered practice
6	Addressing occupations concurrent with factors	E	Secondary model
7	Paradigm guiding practice	F	Occupation centered
8	Creating an occupational profile	G	Context
9	Outcome measure	H	Tool used to measure client factors
10	Assessment	I	Environment
		J	An occupation that can be disrupted by pain

[a] See Appendix A for the answer key.

Orthotic Processes, Tools, and Techniques

Brenda M. Coppard

CHAPTER OBJECTIVES

1. Categorize orthotic materials according to their properties.
2. Recognize tools commonly used to make orthoses.
3. Identify various methods to optimally prepare a client for orthotic intervention.
4. Explain the process of cutting and molding an orthosis.
5. List common items that should be available to a therapist for making orthoses.
6. List the advantages and disadvantages of using prefabricated orthoses.
7. Explain the reasons for selecting a soft orthosis over a prefabricated orthosis.
8. Explain three ways to adjust a static progressive force on prefabricated orthoses.
9. Relate an example of how a person's occupational performance might influence prefabricated orthosis selection.

KEY TERMS

handling characteristics
hard end feel
heat gun

memory
performance characteristics
physical agent modality (PAM)

soft end feel
thermoplastic material

Lola is a new therapist beginning her first week of practice in an outpatient clinic. She receives her first referral for a client who needs evaluation and intervention, including the provision of an orthosis. Lola's heart beats quickly, and for a few seconds she panics! Then she calms down and remembers her education whereby she gained foundational knowledge and skills required for orthotic intervention. With a clear head, she rises to the challenge.

Britt became employed a week ago at an outpatient therapy clinic. He received an order to fabricate a wrist immobilization orthosis for a male construction worker recently diagnosed with carpal tunnel syndrome. Britt felt confident making the pattern and molding the orthosis on the client. However, when Britt initiated removal of the orthosis from the client, he realized the thermoplastic material stuck to the client's arm hair! Britt was embarrassed and began thinking about how to remove the orthosis without causing the client discomfort.

Therapists who offer orthotic intervention must have competency in a variety of processes, tools, and techniques to avoid situations like the one that Britt encountered. This chapter presents commonly used processes, tools, and techniques related to making orthoses. Orthotic intervention is used for variety of clients who require custom-made or prefabricated orthoses.

THERMOPLASTIC MATERIALS

Low-temperature thermoplastic (LTT) materials are most commonly used to fabricate orthoses. The materials are considered "low temperature" because they soften in water heated between 135°F and 180°F.[19] The therapist can usually safely place the softened material directly against a person's skin while the plastic is still moldable. LTT materials compare to high-temperature thermoplastics that become soft when warmed to greater than 250°F[27] and cannot touch a person's skin while moldable without causing a thermal injury. When LTT material is heated, it becomes pliable and then hardens to its original rigidity after cooling. The first commonly available LTT material was Orthoplast. Currently many types of thermoplastic materials are available from several companies. Clinics stock various types of materials based on patient population, common diagnoses, therapists' preferences, and availability.

In addition to orthotic fabrication, LTT material is commonly used to adapt devices for improving function. For example, thermoplastic material may be heated and wrapped around pens, handles, utensils, and other tools to build up the circumference and decrease the required motion needed to use such items.

Therapists select the best type of **thermoplastic material** for orthotic fabrication. Decisions are based on such factors as cost, properties of the thermoplastic material, familiarity with orthotic materials, and therapeutic goals. One type of thermoplastic material is not the best choice for every type or size of orthosis. If a therapist has not had experience with a particular thermoplastic material, it is beneficial to read the manufacturer's technical literature describing the material's content and properties. Practice using new materials before fabricating orthoses on clients can avoid disastrous effects.[11]

THERMOPLASTIC MATERIAL CONTENT AND PROPERTIES

Thermoplastic materials are elastic, plastic, a combination of plastic and rubberlike, and rubberlike.[16] Thermoplastic materials that are elastic based have some amount of memory. (Memory is addressed later in this section.) Typically, elastic thermoplastic material has a coating to prevent the material from adhering to itself. (Most thermoplastic materials have a nonstick coating, but there are a few that specify that they do not.) Elastic materials have a longer working time than other types of materials and tend to shrink during the cooling phase.

Thermoplastic materials with a high plastic content are drapable and have a low resistance to stretch. Plastic-based materials are often used because they result in a highly conforming orthosis. Applying LLT with a high plastic content requires great skill in handling the material (e.g., avoiding fingerprints and stretch) during heating, cutting, moving, positioning, draping, and molding. Thus for novice practitioners positioning the client in a gravity-assisted position is best to prevent overstretching of the material.

Thermoplastic materials that are described as rubbery or rubberlike tend to be more resistant to stretching and fingerprinting. These materials are less conforming than their more drapable plastic counterparts. Therapists should not confuse resistance to stretch during the molding process with the rigidity of the orthosis upon completion. Materials that are quite drapable become extremely rigid when cooled and set. In addition, the more contours that an orthosis has, the more rigid it will be.

Some LTT materials are engineered to include an antimicrobial protection. Orthoses can create a moist surface on the skin where mold and mildew can form. When skin cells and perspiration remain in a relatively oxygen-free environment for hours at a time, it is conducive to microbe growth and results in odor. Daily cleansing with isopropyl alcohol on the inside surface of the orthosis effectively combats this problem. Thermoplastic materials containing the antimicrobial protection offer a defense against microorganisms. The antimicrobial protection does not wash or peel off.

Each type of thermoplastic material has unique properties,[9] which are categorized by handling and performance characteristics. **Handling characteristics** refer to the thermoplastic material properties when heated and softened, and **performance characteristics** refer to the thermoplastic material properties after the material has cooled and hardened.

Handling Characteristics
Memory

Memory is a property that describes a material's ability to return to its preheated (original) shape, size, and thickness when reheated. The property ranges from 100% to little or no memory capabilities.[16] Materials with 100% memory return to their original size and thickness when reheated. Materials with little to no memory do not recover their original thickness and size when reheated or stretched.

Most materials with memory turn translucent (clear) during heating. Using the translucent quality as an indicator, the therapist easily determines that the material is adequately heated; thus it prevents overheating or underheating. The ability to see through the material also assists the therapist with properly positioning and contouring the material on the client.

Memory allows therapists to reheat and reshape orthoses several times without the material stretching excessively. Materials with memory must be constantly molded throughout the cooling process to sustain maximal conformability to the underlying body part. Novice or inexperienced therapists who wish to correct errors in a poorly molded orthosis frequently use materials with memory. Materials with memory accommodate the need to redo or revise an orthosis multiple times while using the same piece of material over and over. LTT material with memory is often used to make orthoses for clients who have high tone or stiff joints because the memory allows therapists to serially adjust a joint(s) into a different position. Clinicians use a serial adjustment approach when they intermittently remold to a person's limb to accommodate changes in range of motion.

Materials with memory may pose problems when a therapist is attempting to make fine adjustments. For example, spot heating a small portion may inadvertently change the entire orthosis because of shrinkage. Therapists must carefully control duration of heat exposure. It may be best in these situations to either reimmerse the entire orthosis in water and repeat the molding process, or prevent the problem and select a different type of LTT material.

Drape and Contour

Drape and contour is the degree of ease with which a material conforms to the underlying shape without manual assistance. The degree of drape or contour varies among different types of material. The duration of heating is important. The longer the material heats, the softer it becomes, and the more vulnerable it becomes to gravity and stretch. When a material with high drape is placed on a surface, gravity assists the material in draping and contouring to the underlying surface. Material exhibiting high drape must be handled with care after heating. Therapists avoid holding the plastic in a position whereby gravity affects the plastic and results in a stretched, thin piece of plastic. Thus, therapists carefully take the thermoplastic material out of the pan in a horizontal rather than vertical position. When cutting an orthotic pattern from the softened plastic, it is positioned on a clean countertop to cut the pattern from the material. This cutting placement also avoids stretching the material. Material with high drape is difficult to use for large orthoses and is most successful on a cooperative person who can place the body part in a gravity-assisted position.

Thermoplastic materials with high drape may be more difficult for beginning practitioners because the materials must be handled gently, and often the material is handled too aggressively. Successful molding requires therapists to refrain from pushing the material during shaping. Instead, the material should be lightly stroked into place. Light touch and constant movement of therapists' hands result in orthoses that are cosmetically appealing. Materials with low drape require firm pressure during the molding process. Therefore, persons with painful joints or soft-tissue damage have better tolerance for materials with high drape.

Elasticity

Elasticity is a material's resistance to stretch and its tendency to return to its original shape after stretch. Materials with elasticity have a slight tendency to rebound to their original shapes during molding. Materials with a high resistance to stretch can be worked more aggressively than materials that stretch easily. As a result, resistance to stretch is a helpful property when one is working with uncooperative persons, those with high tone, or when an orthosis includes multiple joints and placement covers larger surface areas (i.e., forearm, wrist, ulnar border of hand, and thumb in one orthosis). Low elastic (high plastic) materials stretch easily and become thin. Therefore, light touch must be used.

Bonding

Self-bonding or self-adherence is the degree to which material sticks to itself when properly heated. Some materials are coated; others are not. Coated materials always require surface preparation with a bonding agent or solvent to remove the coating. Self-bonding (uncoated) materials may not require surface preparation.

Coated materials tack at the edges, because the coating covers only the surface and not the edges. Often the tacked edges can be pried apart after the material is completely cool. If a coated material is stretched, it becomes tackier and is more likely to bond. When heating self-bonding material, the therapist is cautious that the material does not overlap on itself during the heating or draping process. If the material overlaps, it sticks to itself. Noncoated materials may adhere to paper towels, towels, bandages, and even the hair on a client's extremity! Thus, it may be necessary to apply an oil-based lotion to the client's extremity before the application of the material. To facilitate handling of the material, therapists often wet their hands and scissors with water or lotion to prevent sticking.

All thermoplastic material, whether coated or uncoated, forms stronger bonds when surfaces are prepared with a solvent or bonding agent (which removes the coating from the material). A bonding agent or solvent is a chemical that is brushed onto surfaces of both softened plastic areas that require a bond. In some cases, therapists roughen the two surfaces that will have contact with each other. This procedure, called *scoring*, is carefully done with the end of a scissors, an awl, or a utility knife. After surfaces are scored, they are softened and then brushed with a bonding agent and adhered together. The sequence is important to follow. If bonding agent is applied to the scored material and then placed in water, fumes develop and the bonding agent is diluted. Self-adherence is an important characteristic for mobilization orthoses to secure outriggers to bases of the orthoses (see Chapter 13) and when the plastic must attach to itself to provide support—for example, when wrapping around the thumb as in a thumb spica orthosis (see Chapter 8).

Self-Finishing Edges

A self-finishing edge is a handling characteristic that allows any cut edge to seal and leave a smooth rounded surface if the material is cut when warm. This handling characteristic saves time for therapists because they do not have to manually flare or smooth the edges.

Other Considerations

Other handling characteristics include heating time, working time, and shrinkage. The time required to heat thermoplastic materials to a working temperature must be monitored closely, because material left too long in hot water often becomes excessively soft and stretchy. To prevent burns and discomfort, therapists must be cognizant of the material's temperature before applying it to a person's skin. After material that is ⅛-inch thick is sufficiently heated, it is usually pliable for approximately 3 to 5 minutes. Some materials allow up to 4 to 6 minutes of working time. Materials thinner than ⅛ inch and those that are perforated heat and cool more quickly.[17] Properties are described in the manufacturer's product documents.

Shrinkage is an important consideration when therapists are properly fitting any orthosis, but particularly with a circumferential design. Plastics shrink slightly as they cool. During the molding and cooling time, precautions must be taken to avoid a shrinkage-induced problem, such as difficulty removing a thumb or finger from a circumferential component of an orthosis.

Performance Characteristics
Conformability

Conformability is a performance characteristic that refers to the ability of thermoplastic material to fit intimately onto contoured areas. Material that drapes easily and conforms to a high degree is impressionable and picks up the client's fingerprints and crease marks (as well as therapists' fingerprints). Orthoses that intimately conform to persons are more comfortable because they distribute pressure best and reduce the likelihood of the orthosis migrating on the extremity.

Flexibility

A thermoplastic material with a high degree of flexibility can take stresses repeatedly. Flexibility is an important characteristic for circumferential orthoses because these orthoses must be pulled open for each application and removal.

Durability

Durability is the length of time thermoplastic material will last—or its shelf life. Rubber-based materials are more likely to become brittle with age than are plastic-based materials.

Rigidity

Materials having a high degree of rigidity are strong and resistant to repeated stress. Rigidity is especially important for medium- to large-size orthoses (such as orthoses for elbows or forearms). Large orthoses require rigid material to support the weight of larger joints. In smaller orthoses, rigidity is important if the plastic must stabilize a joint. Rigidity can be enhanced by contouring an orthosis intimately to the underlying body shape.[35] Most LTT materials cannot tolerate the repeated forces involved in weight bearing on an orthosis, such as for foot orthoses. Most foot orthoses will have fatigue cracks within a few weeks.[10] Rather the person should be provided with an ankle-foot orthosis made from high-temperature material.

Perforations

Theoretically, perforations in material allow for air exchange to the underlying skin. Various perforation patterns are available (e.g., mini-, maxi-, and micro-perforated). Perforated materials are also designed to reduce the weight of orthoses. Several precautions must be taken if one is working with perforated materials.[35] Perforated material should not be stretched, because stretching enlarges the holes in the plastic and thereby decreases its strength and pressure distribution. When cutting a pattern out of perforated material, therapists cut between the perforations to prevent uneven or sharp edges that occur when cutting through a perforation. If this cannot be avoided, the edges of the orthosis should be smoothed, lined with a thin padding material such as moleskin, or with purchased edging material.

Finish, Color, and Thickness

Finish refers to the texture of the endproduct. Some thermoplastics have a smooth finish, whereas others have a grainy texture. Generally, coated materials are easier to keep clean because the coating resists soiling.[16]

The *color* of the thermoplastic material may affect a person's acceptance and satisfaction with the orthosis and compliance with the wearing schedule. Dark-colored orthoses tend to show less soiling and appear cleaner than white orthoses. Brightly colored orthoses tend to be popular with children and youth. Colored materials may be used to facilitate attention to one side of the body as with unilateral neglect.[8] In addition, colored orthoses are easily seen and therefore useful in preventing loss (e.g., laundry) in institutional settings. For example, it is easier to see a blue orthosis in white bed linen than to see a white orthosis in white bed linen.

A common thickness for thermoplastic material is $\frac{1}{8}$ inch. However, if the weight of the entire orthosis is a concern, a thinner plastic may be used—reducing the bulkiness of the orthosis and possibly increasing the person's comfort and improving adherence to the wearing schedule. Some thermoplastic materials are available in thicknesses of $\frac{1}{16}$, $\frac{3}{32}$, and $\frac{3}{16}$ inch. Thinner thermoplastic materials are commonly used for small orthoses, arthritic joints, and pediatric orthoses. The $\frac{3}{16}$-inch thickness is commonly used for lower extremity orthoses and fracture braces.[12] Keep in mind that plastics thinner than $\frac{1}{8}$ inch soften and harden more quickly than thicker materials. Therefore, therapists who are novices in orthotic intervention may find it easier to use $\frac{1}{8}$-inch-thick materials than thinner materials.[10] Table 3.1 lists property guidelines for thermoplastic materials. (See Laboratory Exercise 3.1.)

PROCESS: MAKING THE ORTHOSIS

Orthotic Patterns

Making an accurate pattern for an orthosis is necessary for success. It is important initially to spend the appropriate amount of time and attention when making a well-fitting pattern. In the long run, it saves the practitioner's time and the materials involved in adjustments or fabricating an entirely new orthosis. A pattern is made for each person who needs an orthosis. Generic patterns rarely fit persons correctly without adjustments. Having several sizes of generic patterns cut out of aluminum foil for trial fittings may speed up the pattern process. A standard adult pattern can be reduced on a copy machine for pediatric-size patterns.

To make a custom pattern, the therapist traces the outline of the person's hand (or corresponding body part) on a paper towel, foil, or parchment paper, making certain that the hand is flat and in a neutral position. If the person's hand is unable to flatten on the paper, or if it is too painful to make the pattern on the involved hand, the contralateral hand may be used to draw the pattern and fit the pattern and orthosis. If the contralateral hand cannot be used, the therapist may hold the paper in a manner to contour to the hand position. The therapist marks on the paper any anatomical landmarks needed for the pattern before the hand is removed. The therapist then draws the pattern over the outline of the hand, cuts out the pattern with scissors, and completes final sizing. The therapist must hold the pencil or drawing utensil at a 90 degree angle to the paper and maintain that angle when tracing the hand to ensure the best pattern result.

Fitting the Pattern to the Client

As shown in Fig. 3.1, moistening the paper pattern and applying it to the person's hand helps the therapist determine which adjustments are required. Patterns made from aluminum foil work well to contour the pattern to the extremity. If the pattern is too large in areas, the therapist can adjust by marking the pattern with a pencil and cutting or folding the paper. Sometimes it is necessary to make a new pattern or to retrace a pattern that is too small or requires major adjustments. Always ensure that the pattern fits the person before tracing it onto and cutting it out of the thermoplastic material. It is well worth the time to make an accurate pattern because any ill-fitting pattern directly affects the finished product.

TABLE 3.1 Thermoplastic Property Guidelines[a]

Thermoplastic Name	Degree of Heating Temperature (°F)	Thermoplastic Name	Degree of Heating Temperature (°F)
Memory		Roylan Polyform	150–170
Roylan Aquaplast ProDrape-T	160–170	Polyform	150–160
Roylan Aquaplast-T Resilient	150–170	Roylan Polyflex II	160-170
Roylan Aquaplast-T	160–170	Polyflex	150–160
Colours	150–160	Omega Max	140–160
Encore	140–160	Orfit	135
FiberForm Soft	150–160	Orfit NS (nonstick)	150
FiberForm Stiff	150–160	Orfit Natural NS (nonstick)	150
Encore	160	Orfit Soft-Fit NS (nonstick)	150
Prism	160	Orthoplast II	150–160
Spectrum	140–145	Roylan Aquaplast-T Watercolors	160–170
Omega Black	160		
Omega Max	140–160	**Moderate Drape and Contour**	
Omega Plus	140–160	Roylan Aquaplast-T	160–170
Orfibrace	150	Roylan Ezeform	150–170
Orfilight	150	Roylan Ezeform	150–160
Orfit NS (nonstick)	150	Clinic	160
Orfit Natural NS (nonstick)	150	Preferred	160
Orfit Soft-Fit NS (nonstick)	150	Prism	160
Orfit Classic Stiff	135	Spectrum	160
Prism	140–160	Vanilla	160
Rebound	150–160	Orfibrace	150
Roylan Aquaplast-T Watercolors	160–170	Orfilight	150
		Prism	140–160
Rigidity		Solaris	160
Colours	150–160	Roylan Aquaplast-T Watercolors	160–170
Excel	150–160		
Roylan Ezeform	150–170	**Resistance to Drape**	
FiberForm Soft	150–160	Roylan Aquaplast Original Resilient	150–170
FiberForm Stiff	150–160	Caraform	140–145
Infinity	150–160	Colours	150–160
Marque-Easy	150–160	FiberForm Soft	150–160
Clinic	160	FiberForm Stiff	150–160
Clinic	160	Omega Black	160
Preferred	160	Omega Plus	140–160
Spectrum	160	Rebound	150–160
Vanilla	160	Roylan Synergy	160–170
Omega Max	140–160		
Omega Plus	140–160	**Resistance to Stretch**	
Orfibrace	150	Aquaplast Original Resilient	150–170
Roylan Polyform	150–160	Roylan Aquaplast Resilient-T	150–170
Solaris	160	Colours	150–160
		Excel	150–160
High Drape and Contour		Roylan Ezeform	150–170
Roylan Aquaplast ProDrape-T	160–170	FiberForm Soft	150–160
Contour Form	140–145	FiberForm Stiff	150–160
Encore	140–160	Infinity	150–160
Excel	150–160	Prism	160
Roylan Ezeform	160–170	Spectrum	160
Infinity	150–160	Vanilla	160
Marque-Easy	150–160	Omega Black	160
Encore	160	Omega Max	140–160
Clinic	160	Omega Plus	140–160
Clinic D	160	Orfibrace	150
Flexx (with powder coating that provides a light tack that holds the material in place while warm)	150–160	Rebound	150–160
		Roylan San-Splint	150-170
		Solaris	160
NCM Spectrum	160	Roylan Synergy	160–170

Continued

TABLE 3.1	Thermoplastic Property Guidelines[a]—cont'd		
Thermoplastic Name	Degree of Heating Temperature (°F)	**Thermoplastic Name**	Degree of Heating Temperature (°F)
Self-Adherence		Prism	140–160
Roylan Aquaplast Original	160–170	Rebound	150–160
Contour Colors	140–145	Solaris	160
Contour Form	140–145	Spectrum	160
Encore	140–160	Roylan Synergy	160–170
Roylan Ezeform	150–170		
Marque-Easy	150–160	**Antimicrobial Defense**	
Clinic (with dry heat)	160	Aquaplast ProDrape-T with antimicrobial built in	160–170
Vanilla (with dry heat)	160	Aquaplast-T with antimicrobial built in	160–170
Spectrum	140–145	Polyflex II with antimicrobial built in	150–160
Omega Max	140–160	Polyform with antimicrobial built in	150–160
Orfilight (with dry heat)	150	TailorSplint with antimicrobial built in	150–160
Orfit Soft	135		
Orfit Stiff	135		

[a]Not all-inclusive.
Resources: https://www.ncmedical.com/; https://www.orfit.com/; https://www.performancehealth.com; https://www.medwest.ca; http://remingtonmedical.com

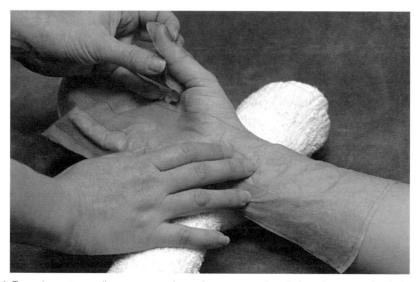

Fig. 3.1 To make pattern adjustments, moisten the paper, and apply it to the extremity during fitting.

Throughout this book, detailed instructions are provided for making a variety of orthotic patterns. Remember that therapists with experience and competency may find it unnecessary to identify all landmarks as indicated by the detailed instructions. Form 3.1 lists suggestions helpful to a beginning practitioner when drawing and fitting patterns.

Fabricating the Orthosis From the Pattern

After making and fitting the pattern to the client, the therapist places it on the sheet of thermoplastic material in a way to conserve material and then traces the pattern on the thermoplastic material with a pencil. (Conserving materials ultimately saves expenses for the clinic or hospital.) Pencil lines do not show up on all plastics. Using an awl to "scratch" the pattern outline on the plastic works well. Another option is to use a grease pencil or china pencil. However, if using a grease pencil, the therapist should cut just inside the drawn line as it is difficult to remove the grease pencil markings. Caution should also be taken when an ink pen is used because the ink may smear onto the plastic. With much effort and on some occasions, the ink might be removed with chlorine. Another option with thermoplastic materials that have memory and are difficult to draw on, such as Aquaplast, is to first cut the pattern out of paper towel or aluminum foil. Then after the thermoplastic material has softened in water and dried off, place the pattern piece on top of the material, and cut around it.

Once the pattern is outlined on a sheet of material, a rectangle slightly larger than the pattern is cut with a utility knife

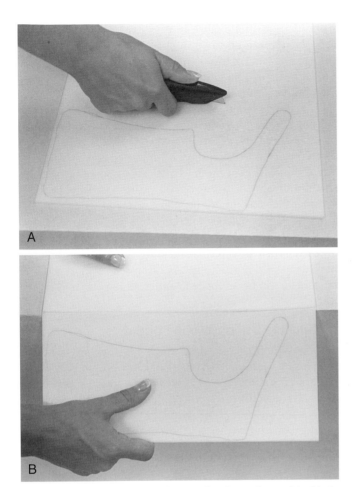

Fig. 3.2 A, A utility knife is used to cut the sheet of material with the pattern outline on it in such a way that the thermoplastic material fits in the hydrocollator or fry pan. B, The score from the utility knife is pressed against a countertop.

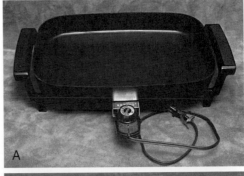

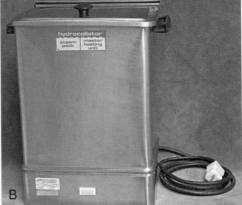

Fig. 3.3 Soften thermoplastic material in (A) an electric fry pan or (B) a hydrocollator.

(Fig. 3.2). After the cut is made, the material is folded over the edge of a countertop. If unbroken, the material is turned over to the other side and folded over the countertop's edge. Any unbroken line is then cut with a utility knife or scissors.

Heating the Thermoplastic Material

Thermoplastic material is softened in an electric fry pan, commercially available orthotic pan, or hydrocollator filled with water heated to approximately 135°F to 180°F (Fig. 3.3). (Some materials can be heated in a microwave oven or in a fry pan without water.) To ensure temperature consistency, the temperature dial should be marked to indicate the correct setting of 160°F by using a hook-and-loop (Velcro) dot or piece of tape. When softening materials vertically in a hydrocollator, the therapist must realize the potential for problems associated with material stretching due to gravity's effects. If a fry pan is used, the water height in the pan should be a minimum of three-fourths full (approximately 2 inches deep).

Adequate water height allows a therapist to submerge portions of the orthosis later when making adjustments. If the thermoplastic material is larger than the fry pan, a portion of the material should be heated. When soft, place the material on a wet paper towel or dry cloth towel. The remaining hard material is placed in the fry pan for softening. A nonstick mesh may be placed in the bottom of a fry pan to prevent the plastic from sticking to any materials or particles. However, it can create a mesh imprint on some plastics. When the thermoplastic piece is large (and especially when it is a high-stretch material), it is a great advantage to lift the thermoplastic material out of the pan on the mesh or a hefty paper towel, or with two spatulas. This keeps the plastic flat and minimizes stretch.

Cutting the Thermoplastic Material

After removing the thermoplastic material from the water with a spatula or on the mesh, the therapist places the material on a flat surface and cuts the material with either curved- or flat-edged orthotic scissors (Fig. 3.4). The therapist uses sharp scissors and cuts with long blade strokes (as opposed to using only the tips of the scissors). When cutting, the therapist must not completely close or collapse the blades of the scissors. Novice orthotic fabricators should practice their cutting skills before attempting to fabricate an orthosis for a client. When cutting the thermoplastic material, the therapist should be careful to push away excess thermoplastic material pieces to prevent them from adhering to the thermoplastic portion needed for the actual orthosis.

Scissors must be sharpened annually and possibly more often, depending on use. Dedicating scissors for specific materials prolongs the edge of the blade. For example, one pair of scissors is used to cut plastic, another for paper, another for adhesive-backed products, and so on. Nonstick scissors that cut through adhesive-backed hook and loop are

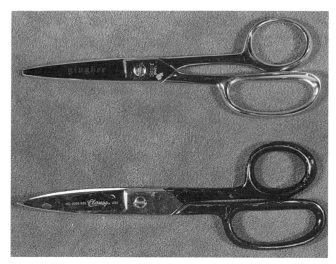

Fig. 3.4 Sharp round- or flat-edged scissors work well for cutting thermoplastic.

commercially available.[11,18] These scissors are designed to protect the blades and are easily cleaned with water. Adhesive remover or solvent will remove adhesive that builds up on traditional scissor blades. Sharp scissors in a variety of sizes (e.g., fingernail scissors) are helpful for intricate contoured cutting and trimming.

Reheating the Thermoplastic Material and Positioning the Client

After the pattern is cut from the material, it is reheated. During reheating the therapist positions the person to the desired joint position(s). To expedite the process, it is beneficial to practice positioning with the client. Visualize the desired joint position(s), and practice "eyeballing" or estimating the position so that it can be done quickly without using a goniometer. If the therapist anticipates positioning challenges and needs to spend time solving problems, positioning should occur before the material is reheated to prevent the material from overheating.[24] The therapist completes any prepadding of bony prominences and covers dressings and padding before the molding process. (The LTT sticks to the dressings and padding if not covered with stockinette.)

Several client positioning options exist. The client is placed in a position that is comfortable, especially for the shoulder and elbow. A therapist may use a gravity-assisted position for volar-based hand/wrist orthoses by having the person rest the dorsal wrist area on a towel roll while the forearm is in supination to maintain proper wrist positioning. Alternatively, a therapist may ask the person to rest the elbow on a table and work with the hand while it is in a vertical position. The vertical position allows for easier visual inspection or when taking joint measurements, but the material may stretch with the effects from gravity.

For persons with joint stiffness, a warm water soak or whirlpool, ultrasound, paraffin dip, or hot pack can be used before positioning for the orthotic-making process. For persons experiencing significant pain and who are taking pain

medications, orthotic fabrication is easiest when pain medications are taken 30 to 60 minutes before the session. This timing helps control the client's pain during orthotic fabrication. (Clients taking pain medications should avoid driving themselves to and from therapy.) For persons with hypertonicity, it may be effective to apply a hot pack on the joint that needs to be positioned in the orthosis. Then the joint is positioned, and the orthosis is applied in a submaximal range. When the orthotic fabrication is completed after warming or after a **physical agent modality (PAM)** session, the joints are usually more mobile. However, the orthosis may not be tolerated after the preconditioning effect wears off. Thus, the therapist must find a balance to complete a gentle warm-up and avoid aggressive preconditioning treatments.[24] Goniometers are used, when possible, to measure joint angles for optimal therapeutic positioning. As discussed, with experience joint angles can be "eyeballed," and a goniometer may not be needed.

Molding the Orthosis to the Client

Once positioning is accomplished, the therapist retrieves the softened thermoplastic material . Any hot water is wiped off on a paper towel, a fabric towel, or a pillow that has a dark-colored pillowcase on it. (The dark-colored pillowcase helps identify any small scraps or snips of material from previous orthotic intervention activities that may adhere to the thermoplastic material.) The therapist checks the temperature of the softened plastic and finally applies the thermoplastic material to the person's extremity. The thermoplastic material may be extremely warm, and thus the therapist uses caution to prevent skin burn or discomfort. For persons with fragile skin who are at risk of burns, the extremity may be covered with stockinette before the thermoplastic material is applied. Another option is to apply a double layer of wet paper towel pieces over the skin. The therapist always immediately asks the client if the material is too warm—regardless of what technique is used and even when precautions are taken. Some thermoplastic materials stick to hair on the person's skin, but this situation can be avoided by using a stockinette or applying an oil-based lotion on the skin before application of the thermoplastic material. Note that lotions must not be used on open wounds.

⚡ **PATIENT SAFETY**

Use caution when placing the warm thermoplastic material on the client. Use caution to prevent skin burn or discomfort. For persons with fragile skin who are at risk of burns, cover the extremity with a stockinette or a double layer of wet paper towels before applying the thermoplastic material. Regardless, any person can benefit from the double layer of wet paper towels for protection with orthotic fabrication. Some thermoplastic materials stick to hair on the person's skin, but this situation can be avoided by using a stockinette or applying lotion to the skin before the application of the splinting material.

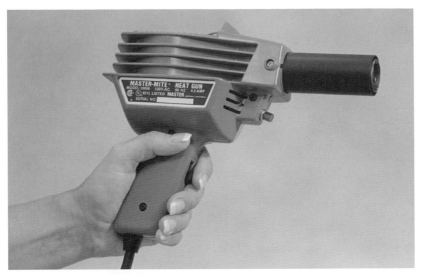

Fig. 3.5 A heat gun is used for spot heating.

Therapists may choose to hasten the cooling process to maintain joint position and the orthotic shape. Several options exist. First, a therapist can use an environmentally friendly cold spray. Cold spray is an agent that serves as a surface coolant. Cold spray should not be used near persons who have severe allergies or who have respiratory problems. Because the spray is flammable, it should be properly stored.

A second option is to dip the person's extremity with the orthosis into a tub of cold water. This must be done cautiously with persons who have hypertonicity because the cold temperature may cause a rapid increase in the amount of tone, thus altering joint position. Similar to using a tub of cold water, the therapist may carefully walk the person wearing the orthosis to a sink and run cold water over the orthosis.

Third, a therapist may use frozen Theraband and wrap it around the orthosis to hasten cooling. An Ace bandage immersed in ice water and then wrapped around the orthosis may also speed cooling.[35] However, the bandages often leave imprints on the thermoplastic material.

Making Adjustments

Adjustments are made to an orthosis by using a variety of techniques and equipment. While the thermoplastic material is still warm, a therapist adjusts the orthosis—such as marking a trim line with one's fingernail or a pencil. Before complete cooling, stretching small areas of the orthosis is possible. The amount of allowable stretch depends on the property of the material and the cooling time that has elapsed. If the plastic is too cool to cut with scissors, the therapist quickly dips the area in hot water to resoften. A professional-grade metal turkey baster or ladle assists in directly applying hot water to modify a small or difficult-to-immerse area of the orthosis.

A **heat gun** (Fig. 3.5) is also used to make adjustments. A heat gun has a switch for off, cool, and hot. After using a heat gun, before turning it to the off position, the therapist sets the switch to the cool setting. The cool setting allows the motor to cool down and protects the motor from overheating. When a heat gun is on the hot setting, caution must be used to avoid burning of materials surrounding it and to avoid skin burns from reaching over the flow of the hot air.

Heat guns must be used with care. Because heat guns warm unevenly, therapists should not use them for major heating and trimming. Use of heat guns to soften a large area on an orthosis may result in a buckle or a hot-cold line. A hot-cold line develops when a portion of plastic is heated and its adjacent line or area is cool. A buckle can form where the hot area stretched, and the cooled material did not. Heat guns are helpful for softening small focused areas for finishing touches. When using a heat gun, it is best to continually move the heat gun's air projection in a circular pattern on the area of the orthosis to be softened; otherwise it can burn the material. In addition, the area to be softened should be heated on both sides of the plastic. Attachments for the heat gun's nozzle are available to focus the direction of hot air flow. Small heat guns are available and may assist in spot heating thinner plastics and areas of the orthosis that have attachments that cannot be exposed to heat (i.e., orthotic outrigger line).[24,25]

Strapping

After achieving a correct fit, the therapist uses strapping materials to secure the orthosis onto the person's extremity. Many strapping materials are available commercially. Velcro hook and loop, with or without an adhesive backing, is commonly used for portions of the strapping mechanism. Velcro is available in a variety of colors and widths. Therapists trim Velcro to a desired width or shape. For cutting self-adhesive Velcro, employ sharp scissors other than those used to cut thermoplastic material. The adhesive backing from strapping materials often accumulates on the scissor blades and makes the scissors a poor cutting tool. The adhesive can be removed with solvent, or the therapist can use nonstick scissors. With self-adhesive Velcro hook the corners are rounded. Rounded corners decrease the chance of corners peeling off the orthosis. Precut self-adhesive Velcro hook dots are commercially

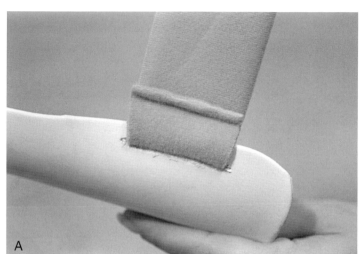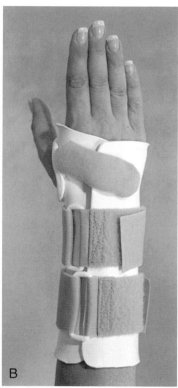

Fig. 3.6 A, Strap is threaded through a slit in forearm trough. The strap is overlapped upon itself and securely sewn. B, D-ring strapping mechanism.

available and save therapists' time in cutting and rounding corners, and they keep adhesive off scissors. Clinic aides or volunteers may cut self-adhesive Velcro hook pieces that have rounded corners to save therapists' time. Briefly heating the adhesive backing and the site of attachment on the orthosis with a heat gun increases the bond of the hook or loop to the thermoplastic material.

Alternative pressure-sensitive straps, which attach to the Velcro hook, are available. Soft padded strapping materials add comfort; however, they tend to be less durable than Velcro loop. Some padded strapping materials, when cut, are self-sealing for a more finished look. Soft straps without self-sealing edges tend to tear apart with use over time. The therapist may cut extra straps and give them to the client to take home if necessary. Commercially sold orthotic strapping kits provide all the straps needed for a forearm-based orthosis in one convenient package.

Another consideration is the patient's skin integrity with choosing the amount of softness with strapping material. Spiral or continuous strapping is used to evenly distribute pressure along the orthosis. A spiral or continuous strap is a piece of soft strapping that spirals around the forearm portion of an orthosis. Rather than several individual pieces of Velcro hook being cut to attach to selected places on the orthosis, a long strip of Velcro hook can be used on both sides of the forearm trough. The spiral or continuous strap attaches to the Velcro hook. Spiral or continuous straps can be used in conjunction with compression gloves for persons who have edema. The spiral strapping and glove prevent the trapping of distal edema.

To prevent the person wearing the orthosis from losing straps, the therapist may attach one end of the strap to the orthosis with a rivet or strong adhesive glue. Another helpful technique is to heat the end of a metal butter knife with a heat gun and push it through the thermoplastic material to make a slit the width of the strapping material. The area is cooled, and the knife is removed. The therapist threads the strap through the slit, folds the strap end over itself, and sews the strap together (Fig. 3.6A). D-ring straps are available commercially. D-ring straps afford the greatest control over strap tension and distal migration of the orthosis (see Fig. 3.6B).

Strap placement is critical to a proper fit. Many therapists fail to place the straps strategically for joint control and render the orthosis useless.[24] Schultz-Johnson particularly stresses strap placement at the wrist, rather than proximal to the wrist.

Padding and Avoiding Pressure Areas

Therapists modify portions of orthoses that may potentially cause pressure areas or irritations. The therapist can use a heat gun to push out areas of the thermoplastic material that may irritate bony prominences. If padding is used, any bony prominences must be padded before the orthosis is formed. Padding must not be added as an afterthought. Padding over an area(s) or lining of an entire orthosis may prevent irritation. Sufficient space must be made available for the thickness of the padding. Otherwise, the pressure may increase over the area.

Use of a self-adhesive gel disk (other paddings work as well) is helpful to cushion bony prominences, such as the ulnar head.

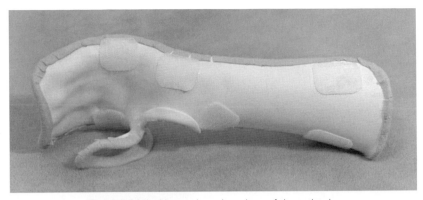

Fig. 3.7 Moleskin overlaps the edges of the orthosis.

TABLE 3.2   Padding Categorization Guidelines

Padding Name	Density	Durability	Surface Texture	Self-Adhesive
BioPad	Thin	Short	Soft	Yes
Contour foam	Semidense	Medium	Textured	Yes
Elasto-Gel splint pads	Dense	Medium	Semisoft	Yes
Firm foam padding	Dense	Long	Semisoft	Yes
Hapla padding	Semidense	Long	Textured	Yes
Luxafoam	Semidense	Medium	Soft	Yes
Microtape	Thin	Medium	Soft	Yes
Moleskin	Thin	Long	Soft	Yes
Orthopedic adhesive	Dense	Long	Semisoft	Yes
Orthopedic felt	Dense	Long	Semisoft	No
Plastazote padding	Semidense	Medium	Semisoft	No
Reston foam padding	Thin	Short	Semisoft	Yes
Silopad pressure	Dense	Long	Semisoft	Yes
Slo-Foam padding	Semidense	Medium	Textured	No
Splint cushion	Semidense	Medium	Semisoft	Yes
Splint pad	Semidense	Long	Textured	Yes
Soft splint padding	Thin	Medium	Soft	Yes
Sorbothane	Dense	Medium	Semisoft	No
Terry cushion	Thin	Long	Textured	Yes

From North Coast Medical (https://www.ncmedical.com/); Performance Health (https://performancehealth.com).

To use gel disks, the therapist adheres the disk to the person's skin and then forms the orthosis over the gel disk. Upon cooling of the orthosis, the gel disk is removed from the person and adhered to the corresponding area in the interior of the orthosis. To bubble out or dome areas over bony prominences, a therapist can place elastomer putty over the prominence before applying the warm thermoplastic material to the client.

If an entire orthosis is lined with padding, the therapist uses the orthotic pattern to cut out the padding needed. Tracing the pattern ¼ to ½ inch larger on the padding is completed if the intention is to overlap the self-adhesive padding over the edges of the orthosis, as shown in Fig. 3.7.

Gel lining is often used within the interior of the orthosis to assist in managing scars. Two types of gel lining are available: silicone gel and polymer gel. Silicone gel sheets, which are flexible and washable, can be cut with scissors into any shape. The silicone gel sheets are often positioned in conjunction with pressure garments or orthoses, or they are positioned with self-adherent wrap (e.g., Coban). Persons using silicone gel sheets are monitored for the development of rashes, skin irritations, and maceration. Polymer gel sheets are filled with mineral oil, which is released into the skin to soften "normal," hypertrophic, or keloid scars. Polymer gel sheets adhere to the skin and can be used with pressure garments or orthoses.

Various padding systems are commercially available in a variety of densities, durability, cell structures, and surface textures.[15] Padding with self-adhesive backing is available and saves the therapist's time and use of materials because glue does not have to be used to adhere the padding to an orthosis. While some cushioning and padding materials have an adhesive backing for easy application, other types of padding are applied to any flat sheet of thermoplastic material and put in a heavyweight sealable plastic bag before immersion in hot water. The padding is adhered to the thermoplastic material before molding the orthosis on the client. Putting the plastic with the padding adhered to it in a plastic bag prevents the padding from getting wet and can save the therapist time. Table 3.2 outlines padding products.

Padding has either closed or open cells. Closed-cell padding resists absorption of odors and perspiration, and it can easily be wiped clean. Open-cell padding allows for absorption. Because of low durability and soiling, padding used in an orthosis may require periodic replacement. Some types of padding are virtually impossible to remove from an orthosis. Thus when padding needs replacement, so does the orthosis.

Edge Finishing

Edges of an orthosis should be smooth and rolled or flared to prevent pressure areas on the person's extremity. The therapist may use a heat gun or heated water in a fry pan or hydrocollator to heat, soften, and smooth edges. Therapists can moisten their fingertips with water or lotion help avoid finger imprints on the plastic. Most of the newer thermoplastic materials have self-finishing edges. When the warm plastic is cut, it does not require detailed finishing other than that necessary to flare the edges slightly.

Reinforcement

Strength of an orthosis increases when the plastic is curved. Thus, a plastic that has curves is stronger than a flat piece of thermoplastic material. When the thermoplastic material is stretched too thin or is too flexible to adequately support an area such as the wrist, reinforcement is needed. If an area of an orthosis requires reinforcement, an additional piece of material bonded to the outside of the orthosis increases the strength. A ridge molded in the reinforcement piece provides additional strength (Fig. 3.8).

PREFABRICATED ORTHOSES

In addition to making custom-made orthoses, options exist for use of prefabricated orthoses. The manufacturing of commercially available prefabricated orthoses is market driven. Therefore, changes in style or materials may appear from year to year. Styles and materials are also affected by the manufacturing processes. Manufacturers are slow to change materials and design even when the market requests it. When a material, cut, or style of a prefabricated orthosis does not sell well, it may be discontinued or replaced with a different design. Vendors often attempt to manufacture prefabricated orthoses for broad populations. Based on research evidence, custom-made orthoses are preferred for some diagnostic conditions.

Manufacturing for a specific population is often costly and not financially rewarding unless that "specific population" has a large market. Improvements in the quality of prefabricated orthoses are affected by market economics, which stimulate companies to manufacture better products in terms of comfort, durability, and therapeutics. Current catalogs serve as the ultimate reference to what is available. Vendors offering prefabricated orthoses are listed at the end of this chapter.

In addition to market economics, the proliferation of various styles of prefabricated orthoses is attributed to two factors. First, the proliferation of prefabricated orthoses can be influenced by the third-party payers' willingness to

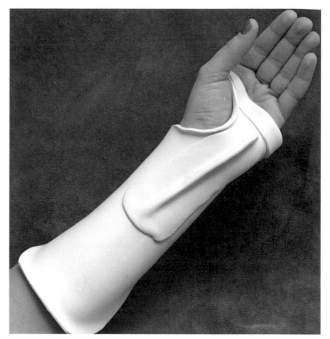

Fig. 3.8 Orthosis reinforcement. This ridge on the reinforcement piece adds strength.

reimburse for orthoses. Pediatric orthoses marketed for orthopedic needs tend to be smaller versions of adult-size orthoses.

Another reason for the proliferation of prefabricated orthoses involves the conceptual advances in design, technology, and the recognition that a need for these types of orthoses exists. For example, the refinement of wrist and thumb prefabricated orthoses has been influenced by the advancement of ergonomic knowledge and the public's awareness of the incidence and effects of cumulative trauma disorders. The development of 3-D printing is an example of a technological advancement that is beginning to influence orthotic and prosthetic provision, particularly in pediatrics.[5] The use of 3-D printing is intended to provide a lower-cost option for serial applications of pediatric prostheses and orthoses due to the child's growth.

Prefabricated orthoses are available from numerous vendors in a variety of styles, materials, and sizes. Prefabricated orthoses are available for the head, neck, joints of the upper and lower extremities, and trunk. Typically, prefabricated orthoses are ordered by size—and in some cases for right or left extremities. The therapist is responsible for using the manufacturer's measurement instructions to provide the correct size. Some orthoses have a universal size, meaning that one orthosis fits the right or left hand. Before deciding to provide a prefabricated orthosis for a client, the therapist must be aware of the advantages and disadvantages of prefabricated orthoses.

Advantages and Disadvantages of Prefabricated Orthoses

The advantages and disadvantages of using prefabricated orthoses are listed in Box 3.1.

BOX 3.1 Advantages and Disadvantages of Using Soft and Prefabricated Orthoses

Advantages	Disadvantages
• May save time and effort (if the orthosis fits the person well) • Immediate feedback from client in terms of satisfaction and therapeutic fit • Variety of material choices • Some clients prefer the sports-brace appearance	• Unique fit is often compromised • Little control over therapeutic positioning of joints • Expensive to stock a variety of sizes and designs • Prefabricated and soft splints usually made for a few target populations (cannot address all conditions requiring unique or creative splint designs)

Advantages

An obvious advantage of using a prefabricated orthosis is saving of the therapist's time and effort. The time required to design a pattern, trace and cut the pattern from plastic, and mold the orthosis to the person is saved when a prefabricated orthosis is used. However, keep in mind the time and expense involved in ordering and paying for the prefabricated orthoses. The costs and wage hours involved in processing an order through a large facility are considerable. Many clinics stock commonly used prefabricated orthoses in their inventory. Maintaining the inventory requires time, storage space, and overhead cost.

If a prefabricated orthosis is in a clinic's inventory, the ability to immediately assess the orthosis in terms of therapeutic timeliness and customer satisfaction is an advantage. After orthotic application, the client is readily able to see and feel the orthosis. When fabricating a custom orthosis, the therapist may find that it does not meet the client's expectations or needs. When this occurs, a considerable amount of time and effort is expended in modifying the current orthosis or in designing and fabricating an entirely new orthosis. With prefabricated orthoses, an educated trial-and-error process can be used to find the best orthosis to meet the client's goals and therapeutic needs.

A third advantage is the variety of materials used to make prefabricated orthoses. Many prefabricated orthotic materials offer sophisticated technology that cannot be duplicated in the clinic. For example, a prefabricated orthosis made from high-temperature thermoplastic material is often more durable than a counterpart made of LTT material. Softer materials (combinations of fabric and foam) may be more acceptable to persons, especially those with rheumatoid arthritis.

Research about custom-made versus prefabricated orthoses is mixed. Soft orthoses can be more comfortable or as comfortable as LTT custom-made orthoses. In a study comparing soft versus hard resting hand orthoses in 39 persons with rheumatoid arthritis, Callinan and Mathiowetz[3] found that compliance with wearing the orthosis was significantly better with the soft orthosis (82%) than with the hard orthosis

(67%). In a systematic review that specifically addressed interventions for trapeziometacarpal osteoarthritis, prefabricated polychloroprene (Neoprene) orthoses and custom-made thermoplastic orthoses were found to equally reduce pain.[1] Some research outcomes showed no differences among prefabricated and custom orthoses, and the lowest-cost orthosis was recommended.[6] Therapists must realize that a person who needs rigid immobilization for comfort will not prefer a soft orthosis, because soft orthoses allow for some mobility to occur. Some clients may think that the sports-brace appearance of a prefabricated orthosis is more aesthetically pleasing than the medical appearance of a custom-fabricated orthosis. For these clients, adherence to the wearing schedule may increase.

Disadvantages

Several disadvantages of prefabricated orthoses exist. A major disadvantage of using a prefabricated orthosis is that a custom, unique fit is often compromised. Soft prefabricated orthoses vary in how much they can be adjusted. If a high degree of conformity or a specialized design or position is needed, a prefabricated orthosis will usually not meet the person's needs. LTT prefabricated orthoses can be spot heated and adjusted somewhat (Fig. 3.9), but they will never conform like a custom-made orthosis of the same material. Some prefabricated orthoses require adjustments. For example, thumb orthoses may require adjustment of the palmar bar to prevent chafing in the thumb web space. Other preformed orthoses must be adjusted by trimming the forearm troughs for proper strap application.

The second disadvantage of prefabricated orthoses is related to the therapist's lack of control over customization. Because most prefabricated orthoses are made for the public, therapeutic positions for conditions may not be included in the designs. For example, some thumb prefabricated orthoses position the thumb in radial abduction, and the condition may warrant palmar abduction. Thus, when using prefabricated orthoses, therapists often have little or no control over joint angle positioning. Often a therapeutic protocol or specific client need prescribes a specific joint angle for positioning. In such instances the therapist must select a prefabricated orthosis that is designed with the appropriate joint angle(s) or choose one that can be adjusted to the correct angle. If unavailable, a custom orthosis is warranted. For example, therapists must use prefabricated orthoses cautiously with persons who have fluctuating edema. The orthosis and its strapping system must accommodate the extremity's changing size. In addition, when conditions require therapists to create unique orthotic designs, the desired prefabricated orthoses may not always be commercially available.

A third disadvantage of using a prefabricated orthosis is that the orthosis may not be in a clinic's stock, and it may have to be ordered. Many clinics cannot afford to stock an extensive array of prefabricated orthoses because of cost and storage restrictions. When an orthosis must be applied immediately and the prefabricated orthosis is not in the clinic's stock, a time delay for ordering it is unacceptable. A custom-made

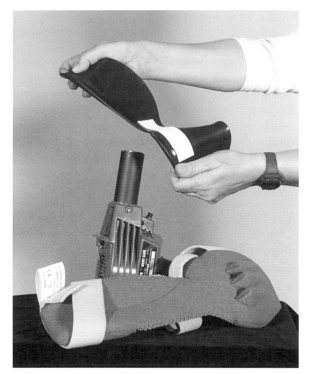

Fig. 3.9 Adjustments can be made to commercial low-temperature thermoplastic orthoses with the use of a heat gun. (Courtesy Medical Media Service, Veterans Administration Medical Center, Durham, North Carolina.)

orthosis should be fabricated instead of waiting for the prefabricated orthosis to arrive.

Once the advantages and disadvantages are weighed, a decision is made regarding whether to use a prefabricated or a custom-made orthosis. The therapist engages in a clinical reasoning process to select the most appropriate orthosis.

Selecting an Orthosis

Therapists rarely use custom or prefabricated orthoses for 100% of their clientele. The therapist uses clinical reasoning based on a frame of reference to select the most appropriate orthosis. Outcome research continues to address custom versus prefabricated orthosis usage. To determine whether to use a prefabricated or a custom-made orthosis, the therapist must know the specific orthotic needs of the person and determine how best to accomplish them. Some questions to ask are:

- Would a soft material or an LTT best meet the person's needs?
- How would the function and fit of a prefabricated orthosis compare with that of a custom-made orthosis?

To properly evaluate whether a prefabricated orthosis or a custom-made orthosis would best meet a person's needs, the factors and questions discussed in the following sections must be considered and answered.

Diagnosis

Therapists provide orthoses to people, not diagnoses. However, one must be well versed in clinical conditions that often require orthotic intervention. Questions about orthotic intervention and diagnoses include:

- Is a prefabricated orthosis available for the diagnosis?
- Which orthotic design meets the therapeutic goals?
- Is there a match between the therapeutic goals and the design of a prefabricated or soft orthosis?
- What evidence exists to indicate a particular orthotic design for a particular diagnostic category?

For example, if a therapist must provide an orthosis to immobilize a wrist joint in neutral position, a prefabricated orthosis must have the ability to position and immobilize the wrist in the required neutral position rather than extension.

Age of the Person

Think about age-related issues that impact orthotic intervention. Consider questions such as:

- Is the client at an age where he or she may have an opinion about the orthotic cosmesis?
- What special considerations are there for an older adult or a young child? (See Chapters 16 and 17.)
- What are the person's age-related activities and roles?
- How might orthotic provision affect the activities and roles?

For example, an adolescent who is self-conscious may be unwilling to wear a custom-made elastic tension radial nerve orthosis at school because of its appearance. However, the adolescent might agree to wear a prefabricated wrist orthosis because of its less conspicuous sportsbrace appearance.

Medical Complications

Medical complications often impact orthotic design. Considerations include:

- Does the person have compromised skin integrity, vascular supply, or sensation?
- Is the person experiencing pain, edema, contractures, or cognitive impairments?
- Are there incision sites to avoid?

Medical conditions are considered because they may influence orthotic design. For example, the therapist may choose an orthosis with wide elastic straps to accommodate the change in the extremity's circumference for a person who has fluctuating edema.

Goals

Clients have goals—things they wish to do and symptoms they want to eliminate. Therapists should consider the following questions:

- What are the client's goals?
- What are the therapeutic goals?
- What activities and roles are important to the client?

The therapist determines the client's priorities and goals from an interview with the client and/or caregivers and guardians. The therapist facilitates clients' adherence to an orthotic wear schedule by understanding each person's capabilities and expectations.

Orthotic Design

Choosing an orthotic design is individualized for each client. Questions to consider include:

- Which joints must be immobilized or mobilized?
- What are the therapeutic goals?
- How will the orthosis achieve the desired therapeutic goals?

It is important to avoid immobilizing unnecessary joints. Any orthosis that limits active range of motion may result in joint stiffness and muscle weakness. For example, if the hand is solely involved, use a hand-based orthosis to avoid limiting wrist motion.

Occupational Performance

Clients lead lives that are filled with participation in meaningful activities and occupations. Participation in such activities is important. The therapist should reflect on the following questions:

- Does the orthosis affect the client's occupational performance?
- Does the orthosis maintain, improve, or eliminate occupational performance?
- Does wearing the orthosis interfere with participation in valued activities?

Occupational performance is considered, regardless of the age of the client. Stern and colleagues[32] studied 42 persons with rheumatoid arthritis and reported that the "major use of wrist orthoses occurs during instrumental activities of daily living where greater stresses are placed on the wrist."[32] In another study of people with thumb carpometacarpal osteoarthritis, researchers concluded that client-centered treatment strategies are useful to control pain during meaningful activities.[26] Therapists ask the client about his or her occupational participation and provide opportunities for the client to engage in such activities while wearing the orthosis. Functional problems that occur while wearing the orthosis require clinical reasoning. Resolution of functional problems may lead to a modification of performance technique, an adjustment in the wearing schedule, or a change in the orthotic design.

Client's or Caregiver's Ability to Adhere to Orthotic Instructions

Clients and caregivers must be educated on issues related to orthotic intervention. One should consider the following questions:

- What is the client's health literacy level and insight into his or her condition? (See Chapter 5 for health literacy assessments.)
- Is the person or caregiver capable of following written and verbal instruction?
- Is the person motivated to adhere to the wearing schedule? Are there any factors that may influence adherence?

The five determinants of adherence include health system factors, socioeconomic factors, therapy-related factors, patient-related factors, and condition-related factors.[36] Forgetfulness, fear, cultural beliefs, desire to be normal, trust of therapist, values, therapeutic priorities, and confusion about the orthotic purpose and schedule may influence adherence to a therapeutic plan.[29] A therapist should consider a person's motivation, cognitive functioning, and physical ability when determining an orthotic design and schedule.

Maximizing adherence to therapy-related interventions includes ensuring orthoses are comfortable and esthetically pleasing; incorporating occupationally meaningful activities into therapy; and preparing clients that some aspects of therapy may cause discomfort or pain early on, but these feelings do not signify further damage or injury. Furthermore, maximizing adherence involves communicating with medical staff to ensure appropriate and effective pain medications are prescribed (especially in the early stages of rehabilitation) and sharing stories and examples of previous clients who successfully adapted activities during orthotic wear.[16] Adherence tends to increase with proper education.[2,16] For example, persons receiving education often have a better outcome if instructions are presented in verbal and written formats.[22] Therapists often explain to clients that long-term gains are usually worth short-term inconveniences. When adherence is a problem, the orthotic intervention may require modification.

Independence With Orthotic Regimen

A client's follow-through with a therapeutic intervention is important to achieving optimal outcomes. If there is no caregiver, can the client independently apply and remove the orthosis? Can the person monitor for precautions, such as the development of numbness, reddened areas, pressure sores, rash, and so on? For example, Fred (an 80-year-old man) needs a bilateral resting hand orthosis to reduce pain from an exacerbation of rheumatoid arthritis. His 79-year-old wife is forgetful. Fred's therapist designs a wearing schedule so that Fred can elicit assistance from his wife. The therapist recommends putting the orthosis on the bed so that Fred can remind his wife to assist him in donning the orthosis before bedtime.

Comfort

If an orthosis is uncomfortable to the client, chances are it will not be worn. Therapists should ask questions related to comfort, including:

- Does the person report that the orthosis is comfortable?
- Does the person have any condition, such as rheumatoid arthritis, that may warrant special attention to comfort?
- Are there insensate areas that may be at risk when wearing the orthosis, and what adjustments need to be made to address this?

Therapists monitor the comfort of an orthosis on each client. If the orthosis is not comfortable, a person is not likely to wear it. In studying three prefabricated wrist supports for persons with rheumatoid arthritis, Stern and colleagues[33] concluded that "satisfaction appears to be based not only on therapeutic effect, but also the comfort and ease of its use."

Environment

Where people live, work, and recreate has an impact on orthotic intervention. Therapists must consider the following:

- In what type of environment will the person be wearing the orthosis?
- How might the environment affect orthotic wear and care?

Industrial settings. Industrial settings may warrant orthoses made of more durable materials, such as leather, high-temperature thermoplastics, or metal. For example, orthoses may need extra cushioning to buffer vibration from machinery or tools that often aggravate cumulative trauma disorders.

Long-term care settings. Therapists providing prefabricated orthoses to residents in long-term care settings must consider the influence of multiple caretakers and the fragile skin of many older adults. The following suggestions may assist in dealing with multiple caretakers and older adults' fragile skin. Orthoses should be labeled with the person's name. To avoid strap loss, consider attaching them to the orthosis, or choose a prefabricated orthosis with attached straps. Select orthotic materials that are durable and easy to keep clean. Orthoses made from colored, thermoplastic material provide a contrast and may be more easily identified and distinguished from white or neutral-colored backgrounds.

School settings. Several factors relating to pediatric orthoses must be considered by the therapist. Pediatric prefabricated orthoses should be made of materials that are easy to clean. Orthoses for children should be durable. Consider attaching straps to the orthosis, or choose a prefabricated orthosis with attached straps. Because multiple caretakers (parents and school personnel) are typically involved in the application and wear schedule, instructions for wear and care should be clear and easy to follow. When the child is old enough, personal and parental preferences should be considered during orthotic selection. If the orthosis is for long-term use, the therapist must remember that the child will grow. If possible, the therapist should select an orthosis that can be adjusted to avoid the expense of purchasing a new orthosis. In addition, orthoses with components that may scratch or be swallowed by the child should be avoided.

Education Format

Educating the client and/or caregiver on the orthotic intervention plan is linked to outcomes.

Utilizing approaches that consider health literacy to ease understanding is helpful (refer to Chapter 6). The therapist must consider:

* What education does the client and caregiver need to adhere to the orthotic-wearing schedule?
* What is the learning style of the client and caregiver?
* How can the therapist adjust the educational format to match the client's and caregiver's learning styles?

Educating clients and caregivers in methods consistent with their preferred learning style may increase compliance. Learning styles include kinesthetic, visual, and auditory.[4]

Written instructions should include the purpose of the orthosis, wearing schedule, care, precautions, and emergency contact information. Because correct use of an orthosis affects intervention outcomes, the client should demonstrate an understanding of instructions in the presence of the therapist. A therapist may complete a follow-up phone call at a suitable interval to detect any problems encountered by the client or caregiver about the orthosis (see Chapter 6).[20]

Fitting and Adjusting

If a decision is made to use a prefabricated orthosis and a selection is made, the therapist evaluates the orthosis for size, fit, and function. Like custom orthoses, a particular prefabricated orthotic design does not work for every client. As professionals who provide orthoses to clients, therapists have an obligation and duty to fit the orthosis to the client rather than fitting the client to the orthosis. The implications of this duty suggest that clinics should stock a variety of commercial orthotic designs. Although a large clinic's overhead is expensive, limiting choices may result in poor client compliance.[34] When a variety of orthotic designs are available, a trial-and-error approach can be used with commercial orthoses because most clients are able to report their preference for an orthosis after a few minutes of wear. When fitting a client with a commercial orthosis, the therapist asks the following questions[34]:

* Does the orthosis feel secure on your extremity?
* Does the orthosis or its straps rub or irritate you anywhere?
* When wearing the orthosis, does your skin feel too hot?
* What activities will you be doing while wearing your orthosis?
* When you move your extremity while wearing the orthosis, do you experience any pain?
* Does the orthosis feel comfortable after wearing it for 20 to 30 minutes?

In addition to fit and size, therapists evaluate the effect of the prefabricated orthosis on function. Outcomes of comparison studies addressing custom-made versus prefabricated orthoses are mixed.[8,13,14,28,32,33] More research is warranted to make conclusions.

Technical Tips for Custom Adjustments to Prefabricated Orthoses

The following points describe common adjustments made to commercial LTT orthoses. High-temperature thermoplastic orthoses cannot be adjusted using equipment such as heat guns and hydrocollators. The provider must be competent to adjust high-temperature thermoplastic orthoses, as is a certified orthotist/prosthetist.

1. Therapists should ensure that orthoses do not irritate soft tissue, reduce circulation, or cause paresthesias.[33] Adjustments may include flaring ends, bubbling out pressure areas, or the addition of padding.
2. Although soft orthoses are intended to be used as is, minor modifications to customize the fit to a person can be accomplished. Some soft orthoses can be trimmed with scissors to customize fit. If a soft orthosis has stitching to hold layers together, it will need to be resewn. (Note that it is beneficial to have a sewing machine in the clinic.)
3. Modification methods for preformed orthoses include heating, cutting, or reshaping portions of the LTT orthosis. Minor modifications can be made with the use of a heat gun, fry pan, or hydrocollator to soften LTT preformed orthoses for trimming or slight stretching.

- Some elastic traction/tension prefabricated orthoses may be adjusted by bending and repositioning portions of wire, metal, or foam orthotic components. Occasionally, technical literature accompanying the orthosis describes how to adjust the amount of traction. Often traction is adjusted with the use of an Allen wrench on the rotating wheels of a hinge joint, as shown in Fig. 3.10. When there are no instructions describing how to adjust prefabricated orthoses, the therapist uses creative problem-solving skills to accomplish the desired changes.
- When a static prefabricated orthosis is used and serial adjustments are required to accommodate increases in passive range of motion (PROM), the orthosis must be reheated and remolded to the client. It is advantageous to select a prefabricated orthosis made of material that has memory properties to allow for the serial adjustments.
- The amount of force provided by some static-progressive orthoses is made through mechanical adjustment of the force-generating device. Force may be adjusted by manipulating the orthotic turnbuckle, bolt, or hinge.
- The force exerted by elastic traction components of a prefabricated orthosis is also made through adjustments of the force-generating device. Therapists adjust the forces by changing elastic component length by gradually moving the placement of the Neoprene or rubber band–like straps on an orthosis throughout the day, as shown in Fig. 3.11.
- Adding components to prefabricated orthoses can be helpful. For example, putty-elastomer inserts that serve as finger separators can be used in a resting hand orthosis. Finger separators add contour in the hand area to maintain the arches. A therapist may choose to add other components, such as wicking lining or padding.
- Prefabricated orthoses can be modified by replacing parts of them with more adjustable materials. For example, if a wrist orthosis has a metal stay, replacing it

with an LTT stay results in a custom fit with the correct therapeutic position.
- It is often necessary to customize strapping mechanisms of prefabricated orthoses. The number and placement of straps are adjusted to best secure the orthosis on the person. Straps must be secured properly, but not so tightly as to restrict circulation. Straps coursing through web spaces must not irritate soft tissue. The research by Stern and colleagues[33] on commercial wrist orthoses indicates that clients with stiff joints experienced difficulty threading straps through D-rings. Clients reported having to use their teeth to manipulate straps. Straps that are too long also appear to be troublesome because they catch on clothing.[33]
- Stern and colleagues[31] showed that although commercial orthoses are often critiqued for being too short, some persons prefer shorter forearm troughs. Shorter orthoses seem to be preferred by clients when wrist support, not immobilization, is needed.

After the necessary adjustments are completed and a proper fit is accomplished, a therapist determines the wearing schedule.

Wearing Schedule

Although there are no easy answers about wearing protocols, experienced therapists have several guidelines for decision making as they tailor wearing schedules to each client.[23] Evidence from the literature also provides information about wearing schedules.

- For orthoses designed to increase PROM, light tension exerted by an orthosis over a long period of time is preferable to high tension for short periods of time.
- For joints with **hard end feels** (i.e., an abrupt, hard stop to movement when bone contacts bone during PROM) and PROM limitations, more hours of orthotic wear are warranted than for joints with **soft end feels** (i.e., a soft compression of tissue is felt when two body surfaces approximate each other).

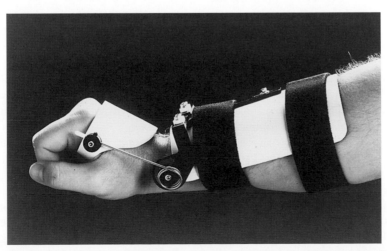

Fig. 3.10 Tension is adjusted with an Allen wrench on the rotating wheels on the hinge joint of this orthosis.

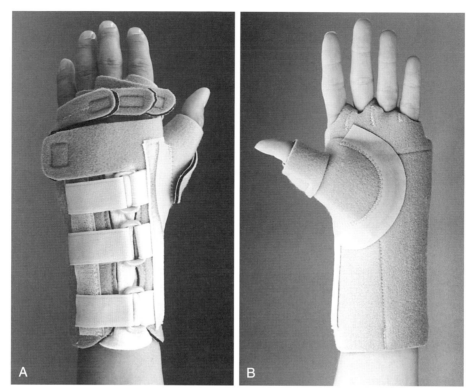

Fig. 3.11 A, The Rolyan In-Line orthosis with thumb support can be adjusted by loosening or tightening the Neoprene straps. B, Volar view of the Rolyan In-Line orthosis with thumb support. (Courtesy Patterson Medical, Warrenville, Illinois.)

- Persons tolerate static orthoses (including serial and static-progressive orthoses) better than dynamic orthoses during sleep.
- When treatment goals are considered, wearing schedules should allow for facilitation of active motion, functional use of joints, and hygiene when appropriate.

As with any orthotic provision, the orthotic-wearing schedule is given in verbal and written formats to the person and caregiver(s). The wearing schedule depends on the person's condition and impairments and the severity (chronic or acute) of the problem. The wearing schedule also depends on the therapeutic goal of the orthosis, the demands of the environment, and the ability of the person and caregiver(s).

Care of Prefabricated Orthoses

Always check the manufacturer's instructions for cleaning the orthosis. Give the client the manufacturer's instructions on orthotic care. If a client is visually impaired, make an enlarged copy of the instructions. For soft orthoses the manufacturer usually recommends hand washing and air drying, because the agitation and heat of some washers and dryers can ruin soft orthoses. Because air drying the soft orthoses takes time, occasionally two of the same orthosis are provided so that the person can alternate wear during cleaning and drying. The inside of LTT orthoses should be wiped out with rubbing alcohol. The outside of LTT orthoses can be cleaned with toothpaste or nonabrasive cleaning agents and rinsed with tepid water. Clients and caregivers should be reminded that

LTT orthoses soften in extreme heat, as in a car interior or on a windowsill or radiator.

Precautions for Patient Safety

In addition to selecting, fitting, and scheduling the wear of a prefabricated orthosis, the therapist educates the client or caregiver about any precautions and how to monitor for them. There are several precautions to be aware of with the use of commercial orthoses. These are discussed in the following section.

Dermatological Issues Related to Orthotic Wear

Latex sensitivity. Some prefabricated orthoses and thermoplastic materials contain latex. Latex-sensitive people, including clients and medical professionals, are being identified.[7,19] Therapists should request a list of both latex and latex-free products from the suppliers of commercial orthoses used. Typically, because manufacturers are more aware of latex sensitivity, most products do not contain latex but warrant checking.

Allergic contact dermatitis. Dermatological issues related to Neoprene orthoses exist. Allergic contact dermatitis (ACD) and miliaria rubra (prickly heat) are associated in some persons when wearing Neoprene orthoses.[30] ACD symptoms include itching, skin eruptions, swelling, and skin hemorrhages. Miliaria rubra presents with small, red, elevated, inflamed papules and a tingling and burning sensation. Before using commercial or custom Neoprene orthoses, therapists should question clients about dermatological reactions and allergies. If a person reacts to a Neoprene orthosis, wear should be discontinued, and the therapist should notify the manufacturer. An interface, such as polypropylene stockinette, may resolve the problem.

Clients need to be instructed not only in proper orthotic care but in hygiene of the body part included in the orthosis. Intermittent removal of the orthosis to wash the body part, the application of cornstarch, or the provision of wicking liners may help minimize dermatological problems. Time of year and ambient temperatures are considered by the therapist. For example, Neoprene may provide desired warmth to stiff joints and increase comfort while improving active and passive range of motion. However, during extreme summer temperatures, the Neoprene orthosis may cause more perspiration and increase the risk of skin maceration if inappropriately monitored.

Ordering Commercial Orthoses

A variety of vendors sell prefabricated orthoses. Companies often sell similar orthotic designs, but the item names can be quite different. To keep abreast of the newest commercial orthoses, therapists browse through vendor catalogs or websites, communicate with vendor sales representatives, and seek out vendor exhibits during professional meetings and conferences for the ideal "hands-on" experience. Vendors often distribute samples upon request to therapists and clinics.

It is most beneficial to the therapist and the client when a clinic has a variety of commercial orthotic designs and sizes for right and left extremities. Keeping a large stock in a clinic is expensive. To cover the overhead expense of stocking and storing prefabricated orthoses, a percentage markup of the prefabricated orthosis is often charged in addition to the therapist's time and materials used for adjustments. Clinics' data about the most common diagnoses and past products are used to determine what to order to maintain an appropriate inventory. Many products have a "shelf life," or a time period whereby the materials age and may become brittle, less elastic, or discolored. Thus, the clinic's inventory must be used before the shelf life limit to be cost efficient.

ORTHOTIC WORKROOM OR CART

Having a well-organized and stocked orthotic area benefits the therapist who makes decisions about the orthotic design and constructs the orthosis in a timely manner. Clients who need orthotic intervention also benefit from a well-stocked orthotic supply inventory. Readily available materials and tools expedite the orthotic-making process.

Clinics should consider the services commonly rendered and stock their materials accordingly. In addition to a stocked orthotic inventory, therapists may find it useful to have a mobile cart organized for orthotic provision in a client's room or in another portion of the health care setting. The cart is used to readily transport orthotic supplies to the client, rather than a client coming to the therapist. For therapists who travel from clinic to clinic, suitcases on rollers are ideal to store and transport orthotic supplies. Orthotic carts or cases should contain items such as:

- Paper towels
- Pencils/awl/grease pencils
- Masking tape
- Thermoplastic material
- Fry pan
- Scissors (various sizes)
- Strapping materials, including Ace bandages
- Padding materials
- Heat gun
- Spatulas, metal turkey baster
- Thermometer
- Pliers
- Revolving hole punch
- Glue
- Goniometer
- Solvent or bonding agent
- Other specialized supplies as needed (e.g., finger loops, outrigger wire, outrigger line, springs, turnbuckles, rubber bands, and so on)

DOCUMENTATION AND REASSESSMENT

Orthotic provision must be well documented. Documentation assists in third-party reimbursement, communication to other health care providers, and demonstration of efficacy of the intervention. Documentation includes several elements, such as the type, purpose, and anatomical location of the orthosis. Therapists document that they educated clients using oral and written instructions. The topics of client education are documented and include the wearing schedule, orthotic care, precautions, and any home program activities. Finally, the therapist's judgment of how receptive and to what extent the client understood the instructions is documented.

In follow-up visits, documentation includes any changes in the orthotic design and wearing schedule. In addition, the therapist notes whether problems with adherence are apparent. The therapist determines whether the range of motion is increasing with orthotic wearing time and draws conclusions about orthotic efficacy or adherence to the program. Function with and without the orthosis should be documented. For example, the therapist determines whether the person can independently perform some type of function because of wearing the orthosis. The therapist must listen to the client's reports of functional problems and solve problems to remediate or compensate for the functional deficit. If function or range of motion is not increased, the therapist must consider orthotic revision or redesign or counseling the client on the importance of wearing the orthosis.

The therapist performs reassessments regularly until the person is weaned from the orthosis or discharged from services. Facilities use different methods of documentation, and the therapist should be familiar with the routine method of the facility. (Refer to the documentation portion of Chapter 6 for more information.)

REVIEW QUESTIONS

1. What are six handling characteristics of thermoplastics?
2. What are six performance characteristics of thermoplastics?
3. At what temperature range are LTT materials softened?
4. What steps are involved in making a pattern for an orthosis?
5. What equipment can be used to soften thermoplastic materials?
6. How can a therapist prevent a tacky thermoplastic from sticking to the hair on a person's arms?
7. What are the purposes of using a heat gun?
8. Why should a therapist use a bonding agent?
9. Why should the edges of an orthosis be rolled or flared?

REFERENCES

1. Aebischer B, Elsig S, Taeymans J: Effectiveness of physical and occupational therapy on pain, function and quality of life in patients with trapeziometacarpal osteoarthritis – a systematic review and meta-analysis, *Hand Ther* 21(1):5, 2015.
2. Agnew PJ, Maas F: Compliance in wearing wrist working splints in rheumatoid arthritis, *Occup Ther J Res* 15(3):165–180, 1995.
3. Callinan N, Mathiowetz V: Soft versus hard resting hand splints in rheumatoid arthritis: pain relief, preference and compliance, *Am J Occup Ther* 50(5):347–353, 1996.
4. Fleming ND, Mills C: Helping students understand how they learn, *The Teaching Professor* vol. 3–4, 1993.
5. Ganesan B, Al-Jumaily A, Luximon A: 3D printing technology applications in occupational therapy, *Phys Med Rehabil Int* 3(3):1085–1088, 2016.
6. Grenier ML, Mendonca R, Dalley P: The effectiveness of orthoses in the conservative management of thumb CMC joint osteoarthritis: an analysis of function pinch strength, *J Hand Ther* 29:307–313, 2016.
7. Jack M: Latex allergies: a new infection control issue, *Can J Infect Control* 9(3):67–70, 1994.
8. Jansen CW, Olson SL, Hasson SM: The effect of use of a wrist orthosis during functional activities on surface electromyography of the wrist extensors in normal subjects, *J Hand Ther* 10(4):283–289, 1997.
9. Lee DB: Objective and subjective observations of low-temperature thermoplastic materials, *J Hand Ther* 8(2):138–143, 1995.
10. McKee P, Morgan L: Orthotic materials. In McKee P, Morgan L, editors: *Orthotics in rehabilitation*, Philadelphia, 1998, FA Davis.
11. MedWest: https://www.medwest.ca.
12. Melvin JL: *Rheumatic disease in the adult and child: occupational therapy and rehabilitation*, Philadelphia, 1989, FA Davis.
13. Mullen TM: Radiographic and functional analysis of movement allowed by four wrist immobilization devices. *Doctoral dissertation*, 2008, Western Michigan University, pp 77. https://doi.org/10.1002/art.24866.
14. Nordenskiöld U: Elastic wrist orthoses: reduction of pain and increase in grip force for women with rheumatoid arthritis, *Arthritis Care Res* 3(3):158–162, 1990.
15. North Coast Medical: https://www.ncmedical.com/.
16. O'Brien L: The evidence on ways to improve patient's adherence in hand therapy, *J Hand Ther* 25(3):247–250, 2012.
17. Orfit: https://www.orfit.com/.
18. Performance Health: http://www.performancehealth.com.
19. Personius CD: Patients, health care workers, and latex allergy, *Med Lab Obs* 27(3):30–32, 1995.
20. Racelis MC, Lombardo K, Verdin J: Impact of telephone reinforcement of risk reduction education on patient compliance, *J Vasc Nurs* 16(1):16–20, 1998.
21. Remington Medical: http://remintonmedical.com.
22. Schneiders AG, Zusman M, Singer KP: Exercise therapy compliance in acute low back pain patients, *Man Ther* 3(3):147–152, 1998.
23. Schultz-Johnson K: Splinting: a problem-solving approach. In Stanley BG, Tribuzi SM, editors: *Concepts in hand rehabilitation*, Philadelphia, 1992, FA Davis.
24. Schultz-Johnson K: *Personal communication*, 1999.
25. Schultz-Johnson K: *Personal communication*, 2006.
26. Shankland B, Beaton D, Ahmed S, Nedelec B: Effects of client-centered multimodal treatment on impairment, function, and satisfaction of people with thumb carpometacarpal osteoarthritis, *J Hand Ther* 30:307–313, 2017.
27. Shurr DG, Michael JW: *Prosthetics and orthotics*, Upper Saddle River, NJ, 2002, Prentice Hall.
28. Sillen H, Backman CL, Miller L, William C, Li L: Comparison of two carpometacarpal stabilizing splints for individuals with thumb osteoarthritis, *J Hand Ther* 24(3):216–226, 2011.
29. Smith-Forbes EV, Howell DM, Willoughby J, Armstrong H, Pitts DG, Uhl TL: Adherence of individuals in upper extremity rehabilitation: a qualitative study, *Arch Phys Med Rehabil* 97(8), 2016. 1262–1128.
30. Stern EB, Callinan N, Hank M, et al.: Neoprene splinting: dermatological issues, *Am J Occup Ther* 52(7):573–578, 1998.
31. Stern EB, Sines B, Teague TR: Commercial wrist extensor orthoses: hand function, comfort and interference across five styles, *J Hand Ther* 7:237–244, 1994.
32. Stern EB, Ytterberg S, Krug HE, et al.: Finger dexterity and hand function: effect of three commercial wrist extensor orthoses on patients with rheumatoid arthritis, *Arthritis Care Res* 9(3):197–205, 1996.
33. Stern EB, Ytterberg SR, Krug HE, et al.: Commercial wrist extensor orthoses: a descriptive study of use and preference in patients with rheumatoid arthritis, *Arthritis Care Res* 10(1):27 35, 1997.
34. Sussman C, Bates-Jensen BM: *Wound care: a collaborative practice manual for physical therapists and nurses*, Philadelphia, 1998, Lippincott Williams & Wilkins.
35. Wilton JC: *Hand splinting principles of design and fabrication*, Philadelphia, 1997, Saunders.
36. World Health Organization: *Adherence to long-term therapies: evidence for action*, Geneva, 2003, World Health Organization.

APPENDIX 3.1 LABORATORY EXERCISE

Laboratory Exercise 3.1 Low-Temperature Thermoplastics

Cut small squares of different thermoplastic materials. Soften them in water, and experiment with the plastics so that you can answer the following questions for each type of thermoplastic material.

Name of the thermoplastic material: _____

1. Does it contour and drape to the hand?   Yes ○   No ○
2. Does it appear to be strong when cool?   Yes ○   No ○
3. Can its edges be rolled easily?   Yes ○   No ○
4. Does it discolor when heated?   Yes ○   No ○
5. Does it take fingerprints easily?   Yes ○   No ○
6. Does it bond to itself?   Yes ○   No ○
7. Can it revert to original shape after being reheated several times?   Yes ○   No ○

APPENDIX 3.2 FORM

Form 3.1 Hints for Drawing and Fitting a Splint Pattern

- Explain the pattern-making process to the person.

- Ask or assist the person to remove any jewelry from the area that will be in the orthosis.

- Wash the area that will be fitted with an orthosis if it is dirty.

- If applying an orthosis over bandages or foam, cover the extremity with stockinette or a moist paper towel to prevent the plastic from sticking to the bandages.

- Position the affected extremity on a paper towel in a flat, natural resting position. The wrist should be in a neutral position with a slight ulnar deviation. The fingers should be extended and slightly abducted.

- To trace the outline of the person's extremity, keep the pencil at a 90-degree angle to the paper.

- Mark the landmarks needed to draw the pattern before the person removes the extremity from the paper.

- For a more accurate pattern, the paper towel can be wet and placed on the area for evaluation of the pattern, or aluminum foil can be used.

- Folding the paper towel to mark adjustments in the pattern can help with evaluation of the pattern.

- When evaluating the pattern fit of a forearm-based orthosis on the person, look for the following:

  - Half the circumference of body parts for the width of troughs

  - Two-thirds the length of the forearm

  - The length and width of metacarpal or palmar bars

  - The correct use of hand creases for landmarks

  - The amount of support to the wrist, fingers, and thenar and hypothenar eminences

- When tracing the pattern onto the thermoplastic material, do not use an ink pen because the ink may smear when the material is placed in the hot water to soften. Rather, use a pencil, grease pencil, or awl to mark the pattern outline on the material.

APPENDIX 3.3 SOURCES OF VENDORS

AliMed
1-800-225-2610
https://www.alimed.com/

Allegro Medical
1-800-861-3211
https://www.allegromedical.com

Benik Corporation
1-800-442-8910
https://benik.com/

Biodynamic Technologies
1-800-879-2276
https://www.biodynamictech.com

Chesapeake Medical Products
1-888-560-2674
http://www.chesapeakemedical.com

Core Products International, Inc.
1-877-249-1251
https://www.coreproducts.com/

DeRoyal
1-800-251-9864
http://www.deroyal.com/

3-Point Products
1-410-604-6393
https://www.3pointproducts.com/

Dynasplint
1-800-638-6771
http://www.dynasplint.ca/en/

Joint Active Systems
1-800-879-0117
http://www.jointactivesystems.com/For-Professionals/

Joint Jack Company
1-860-657-1200
http://jointjackcompany.com/

North Coast Medical, Inc.
1-800-821-9319
https://www.ncmedical.com/

Performance Health
1-800-323-5547
https://www.performancehealth.com

Restorative Care of America, Inc. (RCAI)
1-800-627-1595
http://www.rcai.com/

Tetra Medical Supply Corporation
1-800-621-4041
https://www.tetramed.com/

4

Anatomical and Biomechanical Principles Related to Orthotic Provision

Brenda M. Coppard

CHAPTER OBJECTIVES

1. Define the anatomical terminology used in orthotic prescriptions.
2. Relate anatomy of the upper extremity to orthotic design.
3. Identify arches of the hand.
4. Identify creases of the hand.
5. Articulate the importance of the hand's arches and creases to orthotic intervention.
6. Recall actions and nerve innervations of upper extremity musculature.
7. Differentiate among prehensile and grasp patterns of the hand.
8. Apply basic biomechanical principles to orthotic design.
9. Describe the correct width and length for a forearm orthosis.
10. Describe appropriate uses of padding in an orthosis.
11. Explain the reason that orthotic edges should be rolled or flared.
12. Relate the concept of contour to orthotic fabrication.
13. Describe the change in skin and soft tissue mechanics with scar tissue, material application, edema, contractures, wounds, and infection.

KEY TERMS

aponeurosis	prehension	ulnar
degrees of freedom	pressure	viscoelasticity
dorsal	radial	volar
grasp	stress	zones of the hand
mechanical advantage	three-point pressure	
plasticity	torque	

Brad is a new practitioner in a rural hospital. He commonly receives referrals to see clients who initially were clients in larger health facilities. These clients are typically post-surgery and opt for follow-up therapy at the local, smaller and rural hospital. Brad has a strong knowledge base of anatomical and biomechanical principles. He often reflects on the hours he spent studying diligently, and he is happy that he did so for this client population. He is able to refer to resources from his collection of books in his professional library that began when he was a student.

BASIC ANATOMICAL REVIEW FOR ORTHOTIC INTERVENTION

Orthotic intervention requires sound knowledge of anatomical terminology and structures, biomechanics, and the way in which pathological conditions impact function. Knowledge of anatomical structures is necessary in the choice and fabrication process of an orthosis. Anatomical knowledge influences the therapeutic intervention and home program. The

following is a brief overview of anatomical terminology, proximal-to-distal structures, and landmarks of the upper extremity pertinent to the orthotic process. The overview is neither comprehensive nor all-inclusive. For more depth and breadth in anatomical review, access an anatomy text, anatomical atlases, anatomy websites, or software programs that show and explain anatomical structures.

Terminology

Knowing anatomical location terminology is extremely important when a therapist receives a prescription for an orthosis or is reading professional literature about orthotic interventions. In rehabilitation settings the word *arm* usually refers to the segment of the upper extremity from the shoulder to the elbow (humerus). The term *antecubital fossa* refers to the depression at the bend of the elbow. *Forearm* is used to describe the portion of the upper extremity from the elbow to the wrist, which includes the radius and ulna. *Carpal* or *carpus* refers to the wrist or the carpal bones. A variety of terms are used to refer to the thumb and fingers (phalanges). Such terms include *thumb, index, middle* or *long, ring,* and

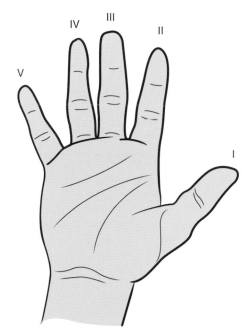

Fig. 4.1 Numbering system used for the digits of the hand.

little fingers. A numbering system is used to refer to the digits (Fig. 4.1). The thumb is digit I, the index finger is digit II, the middle (or long) finger is digit III, the ring finger is digit IV, and the little finger is digit V.

The terms *palmar* and **volar** are used interchangeably and refer to the front or anterior aspect of the hand and forearm in relationship to the anatomical position. The term **dorsal** refers to the back or posterior aspect of the hand and forearm in relationship to the anatomical position. The term **radial** indicates the thumb side, and the term **ulnar** refers to the side of the fifth digit (little finger). Therefore, when a therapist receives an order for a dorsal wrist orthosis, the physician has ordered an orthosis that is to be applied on the back of the hand and wrist. Another example of location terminology in an orthotic prescription is a radial gutter thumb immobilization (thumb spica) orthosis. This type of orthosis is applied to the thumb side of the hand and forearm.

Literature addressing hand injuries and rehabilitation protocols often refers to zones of the hand. Fig. 4.2 diagrams the **zones of the hand**.[18] Table 4.1 presents the zones' borders. Therapists should be familiar with these zones for understanding literature, conversing with other health providers, and documenting pertinent information.

SHOULDER JOINT

The shoulder complex consists of seven joints, including the glenohumeral, suprahumeral, acromioclavicular, scapulocostal, sternoclavicular, costosternal, and costovertebral joints.[10] The suprahumeral and scapulocostal joints are pseudojoints, but they contribute to the shoulder's function. Mobility of the shoulder is a compilation of all seven joints. Because the shoulder is extremely mobile, stability is sacrificed. This is evident when one considers that the head of the humerus articulates with approximately a third of the glenoid fossa.

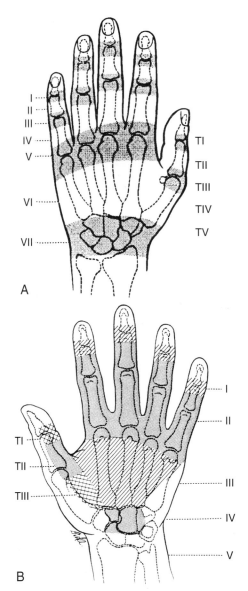

Fig. 4.2 Zones of the hand for (A) extensor and (B) flexor tendons. (From Kleinert, H.E., Schepel, S., & Gill, T. [1981]. Flexor tendon injuries. *Surgical Clinics of North America, 61*[2], 267.)

The shoulder complex allows motion in three planes, including flexion, extension, abduction, adduction, and internal and external rotation.

The scapula is intimately involved with movement at the shoulder. *Scapulohumeral rhythm* is a term used to describe the coordinated series of synchronous motions, such as shoulder abduction and elevation.

A complex of ligaments and tendons provides stability to the shoulder. Shoulder ligaments are named according to the bones they connect. The ligaments of the shoulder complex include the coracohumeral ligament and the superior, middle, and inferior glenohumeral ligaments.[17] The rotator cuff muscles contribute to the dynamic stability of the shoulder by compressing the humeral head into the glenoid fossa.[28] The rotator cuff muscles include the supraspinatus, infraspinatus, teres minor, and subscapularis. Table 4.2 lists the muscles involved with scapular and shoulder movements.

TABLE 4.1 Tendon Injury Zones of the Hand

	Flexor Tendon Zone Borders	Extensor Tendon Zone Borders
Zone I	Extends flexor digitorum profundus (FDP) distal to flexor digitorum superficialis (FDS) on middle phalanx	Over the distal interphalangeal (DIP) joints
Zone II (no man's land)	Extends from proximal end of the digital fibrous sheath to the distal end of the A1 pulley	Over the middle phalanx
Zone III	Extends from proximal end of the finger pulley system to the distal end of the transverse carpal ligament	Over the apex of the proximal interphalangeal (PIP) joint
Zone IV	Entails the carpal tunnel, extending from the distal to the proximal borders of the transverse carpal ligament	Over the proximal phalanx
Zone V	Extends from the proximal border of the transverse carpal ligament to the musculotendinous junctions of the flexor tendons	Over the apex of the metacarpophalangeal (MCP) joint
Zone VI	—	Over the dorsum of the hand
Zone VII	—	Under the extensor tendon retinaculum
Zone VIII	—	The distal forearm
Thumb zone TI	Distal to the interphalangeal (IP) joint	Over the IP joint
Thumb zone TII	Annular ligament to IP joint	Over the proximal phalanx
Thumb zone TIII	The thenar eminence	Over the MCP joint
Thumb zone TIV	—	Over the first metacarpal
Thumb zone TV	—	Under the extensor tendon retinaculum
Thumb zone TVI	—	The distal forearm

ELBOW JOINT

The elbow joint complex consists of the humeroradial, humeroulnar, and proximal radioulnar joints. The humeroradial joint is an articulation between the humerus and the radius. The humeroradial joint has two degrees of freedom that allow for elbow flexion and extension and forearm supination and pronation. The humerus articulates with the ulna at the humeroulnar joint. Flexion and extension movements take place at the humeroulnar joint. Elbow flexion and extension are limited by the articular surfaces of the trochlea of the ulna and the capitulum of the humerus.

The medial and lateral collateral ligaments strengthen the elbow capsule. The radial collateral, lateral ulnar, accessory lateral collateral, and annular ligaments constitute the ligamentous structure of the elbow.

Muscles acting on the elbow can be categorized as functional groups: flexors, extensors, flexor-pronators, and extensor-supinators. Table 4.3 lists the muscles in these groups and their innervation.

WRIST JOINT

The wrist joint is frequently incorporated into an orthotic design. Knowledge of the wrist joint structure is required to appropriately choose and fabricate an orthosis that meets therapeutic goals and objectives. The osseous structure of the wrist and hand consists of the ulna, radius, and eight carpal bones. Several joints are associated with the wrist complex, including the radiocarpal, midcarpal, and distal radioulnar joints.

The carpal bones are arranged in two rows (Fig. 4.3). The proximal row of carpal bones includes the scaphoid

(navicular), lunate, and triquetrum. The pisiform bone is considered a sesamoid bone.[28] The distal row of carpal bones consists of the trapezium, trapezoid, capitate, and hamate. The distal row of carpal bones articulates with the metacarpals.

The radius articulates with the lunate and scaphoid in the proximal row of carpal bones. This articulation is the radiocarpal joint, which is mobile. The radiocarpal joint (Fig. 4.4) is formed by the articulation of the distal head of the radius and the scaphoid and lunate bones. The ulnar styloid is attached to the triquetrum by a complex of ligaments and fibrocartilage. The ligaments bridge the ulna and radius and separate the distal radioulnar joint and the ulna from the radiocarpal joint. Motions of the radiocarpal joint include flexion, extension, and radial and ulnar deviation. The majority of wrist extension occurs at the midcarpal joint with less movement occurring at the radiocarpal joint.[17]

The midcarpal joint (see Fig. 4.4) is the articulation between the distal and proximal carpal rows. The joint exists, although there are no interosseous ligaments between the proximal and distal rows of carpals.[8] The joint capsules remain separate. However, the radiocarpal joint capsule attaches to the edge of the articular disk, which is distal to the ulna.[23] The wrist motions of flexion, extension, and radial and ulnar deviation also take place at this joint. The majority of wrist flexion occurs at the radiocarpal joint. The midcarpal joint contributes less movement for wrist flexion.[17]

The distal radioulnar joint is an articulation between the head of the ulna and the distal radius. Forearm supination and pronation occur at the distal radioulnar joint.

Wrist stability is provided by the close-packed positions of the carpal bones and the interosseous ligaments.[28] The intrinsic intercarpal ligaments connect carpal bone to carpal

TABLE 4.2 Muscles Contributing to Scapular and Shoulder Motions

Movement	Muscles	Innervation
Scapular elevation	Upper trapezius	Accessory, CN 1 third and fourth cervical; dorsal
	Levator scapulae	scapular
Scapular depression	Lower trapezius	Accessory CN 1
Scapular lateral rotation	Serratus anterior	Long thoracic
Scapular medial rotation	Rhomboids	Dorsal scapular
Scapular abduction	Serratus anterior	Long thoracic
Scapular adduction	Middle and lower trapezius	Accessory CN 1
	Rhomboids	Dorsal scapular
Shoulder flexion	Anterior deltoid	Axillary
	Coracobrachialis	Musculocutaneous
Shoulder extension	Teres major	Lower subscapular
	Latissimus dorsi	Thoracodorsal
Shoulder abduction	Middle deltoid	Axillary
	Supraspinatus	Suprascapular
Shoulder adduction	Pectoralis major	Medial and lateral
	Latissimus dorsi	Pectoral
	Teres major	Thoracodorsal
	Coracobrachialis	Lower subscapular
		Musculocutaneous
Shoulder external rotation	Infraspinatus	Suprascapular
	Teres minor	Axillary

TABLE 4.3 Elbow and Forearm Musculature Actions and Nerve Supply

Muscle Group	Innervation
Flexors	
Biceps	Musculocutaneous
Brachialis	Musculocutaneous, radial
Brachioradialis	Radial
Extensors	
Triceps	Radial
Anconeus	Radial
Supinators	
Supinator	Posterior
Interosseous branch of supinator	Radial
Pronators	
Pronator teres	Median
Pronator quadratus	Anterior
Interosseous branch of pronator quadratus	Median

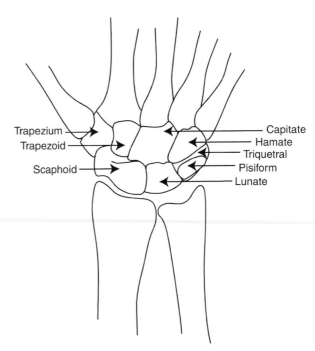

Fig. 4.3 Carpal bones. Proximal row: scaphoid, lunate, pisiform, and triquetrum. Distal row: trapezium, trapezoid, capitate, and hamate. (From Pedretti, L. W. [Ed.]. [1996]. *Occupational therapy: Practice skills for physical dysfunction* [4th ed., p. 320]. St. Louis, MO: Mosby.)

bone. The extrinsic ligaments of the carpal bones connect with the radius, ulna, and metacarpals. The ligaments on the volar aspect of the wrist are thick and strong, providing stability. The dorsal ligaments are thin and less developed.[28] In addition, the intercarpal ligaments of the distal row form a stable fixed transverse arch.[12] Ligaments of the wrist cover the volar, dorsal, radial, and ulnar areas. The ligaments in the wrist serve to stabilize joints, guide motion,

limit motion, and transmit forces to the hand and forearm. These ligaments also assist in prevention of dislocations. The wrist contributes to the hand's mobility and stability. Having two **degrees of freedom** (movements occur in two planes), the wrist is capable of flexing, extending, and deviating radially and ulnarly.

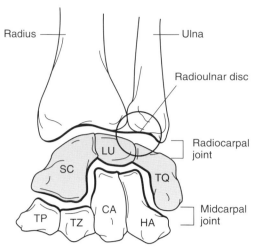

Fig. 4.4 Radiocarpal and midcarpal joints. *CA,* Capitate; *HA,* hamate; *LU,* lunate; *SC,* scaphoid; *TP,* trapezium; *TQ,* triquetrum; *TZ,* trapezoid. (From Norkin, C., & Levangie, P. [1983]. *Joint structure and function: A comprehensive analysis* [p. 217]. Philadelphia, PA: FA Davis.)

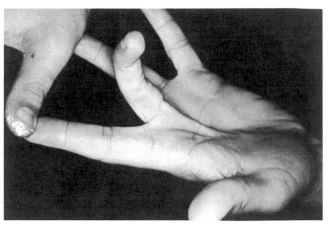

Fig. 4.5 Bowstringing of the flexor tendons. (From Stewart-Pettengill, K. M., & van Strien, G. [2002]. Postoperative management of flexor tendon injuries. In E. J. Mackin, A. D. Callahan, T. M. Skirven, et al. [Eds.], *Rehabilitation of the hand: Surgery and therapy* [5th ed., p. 434]. St. Louis, MO:, Mosby.)

FINGER AND THUMB JOINTS

Cutaneous and Connective Coverings of the Hand

The skin is the protective covering of the body. There are unique characteristics of volar and dorsal skin, which are functionally relevant. The skin on the palmar surface of the hand is thick, immobile, and hairless. It contains sensory receptors and sweat glands. The palmar skin attaches to the underlying palmar **aponeurosis,** which facilitates grasp.[7] Palmar skin differs from the skin on the dorsal surface of the hand. The dorsal skin is thin, supple, and quite mobile. Thus it is often the site for edema accumulation. The skin on the dorsum of the hand accommodates to the extremes of the fingers' flexion and extension movements. The hair follicles on the dorsum of the hand assist in protecting and activating touch receptors when the hair is moved slightly.[7]

Palmar Fascia

The superficial layer of palmar fascia in the hand is thin. Its composition is highly fibrous and is tightly bound to the deep fascia. The deep fascia thickens at the wrist and forms the palmar carpal ligament and the flexor retinaculum. The fascia thins over the thenar and hypothenar eminences but thickens over the midpalmar area and on the volar surfaces of the fingers. The fascia forms the palmar aponeurosis and the fibrous digital sheaths.[8]

The superficial palmar aponeurosis consists of longitudinal fibers that are continuous with the flexor retinaculum and palmaris longus tendon. The flexor tendons course under the flexor retinaculum. With absence of the flexor retinaculum, as in carpal tunnel release, bowstringing of the tendons may occur at the wrist level (Fig. 4.5). The distal borders of the superficial palmar aponeurosis fuse with the fibrous digital sheaths. The deep layer of the aponeurosis consists of transverse fibers, which are continuous with the thenar and hypothenar fascias. Distally, the deep layer forms the superficial transverse metacarpal ligament.[8] The extensor retinaculum is a fibrous band that bridges over the extensor tendons. The deep and superficial layers of the aponeurosis form this retinaculum.

Functionally, the fascial structure of the hand protects, cushions, restrains, conforms, and maintains the hand's arches.[7] For example, therapists often fabricate orthoses for persons post-surgery who have Dupuytren disease, a condition in which the palmar fascia thickens and shortens.

Joint Structure

Orthoses often immobilize or mobilize joints of the fingers and thumb. Therefore, therapists must have knowledge of these joints. The hand skeleton comprises five polyarticulated rays (digits/fingers) (Fig. 4.6). The radial ray or first ray (thumb) is the shortest and includes three bones: a metacarpal and two phalanges. Joints of the thumb include the carpometacarpal (CMC) joint, the metacarpophalangeal (MP) joint, and the interphalangeal (IP) joint (see Fig. 4.6 for hand and finger joints with exception of showing CMC joint). Functionally, the thumb is the most mobile of the digits. The thumb significantly enhances functional ability by its ability to oppose the pads of the fingers, which is needed for prehension and grasp. The thumb has three degrees of freedom, allowing for flexion, extension, abduction, adduction, and opposition. The second through fifth rays comprise four bones: a metacarpal and three phalanges. Joints of the fingers include the MCP joint, proximal interphalangeal (PIP) joint, and the distal interphalangeal (DIP) joint. The digits are unequal in length. Specific finger length varies among people. For example, some people's index finger is longer than the ring finger and vice versa. In any case, the respective finger lengths contribute to the hand's functional capabilities.

The thumb's metacarpotrapezial or CMC joint is saddle shaped and has two degrees of freedom, allowing for flexion, extension, abduction, and adduction movements. The CMC

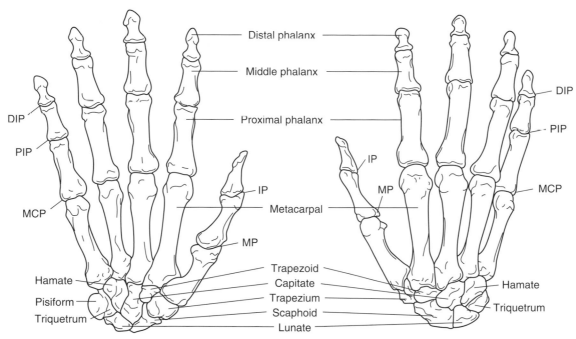

Fig. 4.6 Joints of the fingers and thumb.

joints of the fingers have one degree of freedom to allow for small amounts of flexion and extension.

The fingers' and thumb's MCP joints have two degrees of freedom: flexion, extension, abduction, and adduction. The convex metacarpal heads articulate with shallow concave bases of the proximal phalanges. Fibrocartilaginous volar plates extend the articular surfaces on the base of the phalanges. As the finger's MCP joint is flexed, the volar plate slides proximally under the metacarpal. This mechanism allows for significant range of motion. The volar plate movement is controlled by accessory collateral ligaments and the metacarpal pulley for the long flexor tendons to blend with these structures.

During extension the MCP joint moves medially and laterally. During MCP extension the collateral ligaments are slack. When digits II through V are extended at the MCP joints, finger abduction movement is free. Conversely, when the MCP joints of digits II through V are flexed, abduction is extremely limited. The medial and lateral collateral ligaments of the metacarpal heads become taut and limit the distance by which the heads can be separated for abduction to occur. Mechanically, this provides stability during grasp.

Digits II through V have two IP joints: a PIP joint and a DIP joint. The thumb has only one IP joint. The IP joints have one degree of freedom, contributing to flexion and extension motions. IP joints have a volar plate mechanism similar to the MCP joints, with the addition of check reign ligaments. The check reign ligaments limit hyperextension.

Table 4.4 provides a review of muscle actions and nerve supply of the wrist and hand.[13] Muscles originating in the forearm are referred to as extrinsic muscles. Intrinsic muscles originate within the hand. Each group contributes to upper extremity function.

EXTRINSIC MUSCLES OF THE HAND

Extrinsic muscles acting on the wrist and hand are further categorized as extensor and flexor groups. Extrinsic muscles of the wrist and hand are listed in Box 4.1. Extrinsic flexor muscles are most prominent on the medial side of the upper forearm. The function of extrinsic flexor muscles includes flexion of joints between the muscles' respective origin and insertion. Extrinsic muscles of the hand and forearm accomplish flexion and extension of the wrist and the phalanges (fingers). For example, the flexor digitorum superficialis (FDS) flexes the PIP joints of digits II through V, whereas the flexor digitorum profundus (FDP) primarily flexes the DIP joints of digits II through V.

Because these extrinsic muscle tendons pass on the palmar side of the MCP joints, they tend to produce flexion of these joints. During grasp, flexion of the MCPs is necessary to obtain the proper shape of the hand. However, flexion of the wrist is undesirable because it decreases the grip force—this is why many protocols require the wrist to be in 20 to 30 degrees of extension because this position facilitates a stronger grip than a flexed wrist position. The synergic contraction of the wrist extensors during finger flexion prevents wrist flexion during grasp. The force of the extensor contraction is proportionate to the strength of the grip. The stronger the grip, the stronger the wrist extensors contract.[25] Digit extension and flexion are a combined effort from extrinsic and intrinsic muscles.

At the level of the wrist, the extensor tendons organize into six compartments.[16] The first compartment consists of tendons from the abductor pollicis longus (APL) and extensor pollicis brevis (EPB). When the radial side of the wrist is palpated, it is possible to feel the taut tendons of the APL and EPB.

TABLE 4.4 Wrist and Hand Musculature Actions and Nerve Supply

Muscle	Actions	Nerve
Flexor carpi radialis	Wrist flexion, wrist radial deviation	Median
Palmaris longus	Wrist flexion, tenses palmar fascia	Median
Flexor carpi ulnaris	Wrist flexion, wrist ulnar deviation	Ulnar
Extensor carpi radialis longus (ECRL)	Wrist radial deviation, wrist extension	Radial
Extensor carpi radialis brevis (ECRB)	Wrist extension, wrist radial deviation	Radial
Extensor carpi ulnaris (ECU)	Wrist extension, wrist ulnar deviation	Radial
Flexor digitorum superficialis (FDS)	Finger proximal interphalangeal (PIP) flexion	Median
Flexor digitorum profundus (FDP)	Finger distal interphalangeal (DIP) flexion	Median, ulnar
Extensor digitorum communis (EDC)	Finger metacarpophalangeal (MCP) extension	Radial
Extensor indicis proprius (EIP)	Index finger MCP extension	Radial
Extensor digiti minimi (EDM)	Little finger MCP extension	Radial
Interosseous	Finger MCP abduction	Ulnar
Dorsal palmar	Finger MCP adduction	Ulnar
Lumbricals	Finger MCP flexion and interphalangeal (IP) extension	Median, ulnar
Abductor digiti minimi	Little finger MCP abduction	Ulnar
Opponens digiti minimi	Little finger opposition	Ulnar
Flexor digiti minimi	Little finger MCP flexion	Ulnar
Flexor pollicis longus	Thumb IP flexion	Median
Flexor pollicis brevis	Thumb MCP flexion	Median, ulnar
Extensor pollicis longus (EPL)	Thumb IP extension	Radial
Extensor pollicis brevis (EPB)	Thumb MCP extension	Radial
Abductor pollicis longus (APL)	Thumb radial abduction	Radial
Abductor pollicis brevis	Thumb palmar abduction	Median
Adductor pollicis	Thumb adduction	Ulnar
Opponens pollicis	Thumb opposition	Median

BOX 4.1 Extrinsic Muscles of the Wrist and Hand

- Extensor digitorum
- Extensor pollicis longus (EPL)
- Flexor digitorum profundus (FDP)
- Flexor pollicis longus
- Extensor digiti minimi (EDM)
- Extensor carpi radialis longus (ECRL)
- Extensor carpi ulnaris (ECU)
- Palmaris longus
- Flexor digitorum superficialis (FDS)
- Extensor pollicis brevis (EPB)
- Extensor indicis proprius (EIP)
- Abductor pollicis longus (APL)
- Extensor carpi radialis brevis (ECRB)
- Flexor carpi radialis
- Flexor carpi ulnaris

The second compartment contains tendons of the extensor carpi radialis longus (ECRL) and brevis (ECRB). A therapist can palpate the tendons on the dorsoradial aspect of the wrist by applying resistance to an extended wrist.

The third compartment houses the tendon of the extensor pollicis longus (EPL). This tendon passes around the Lister tubercle of the radius and inserts on the dorsal base of the distal phalanx of the thumb.

The fourth compartment includes the four extensor digitorum communis (EDC) tendons and the extensor indicis proprius (EIP) tendon, which are the MCP joint extensors of the fingers.

The fifth compartment includes the extensor digiti minimi (EDM), which extends the little finger's MCP joint. The EDM acts alone to extend the little finger.

The sixth compartment consists of the extensor carpi ulnaris (ECU), which inserts at the dorsal base of the fifth metacarpal. A taut tendon can be palpated over the ulnar side of the wrist just distal to the ulnar head.

Unlike the other fingers, the index and little fingers have dual extensor systems consisting of the EIP and the EDM in conjunction with the EDC. The EIP and EDM tendons lie on the ulnar side of the EDC tendons. Each finger has a FDS and FDP tendon. Five annular (or A) pulleys and four cruciate (or C) pulleys prevent the flexor tendons from bowstringing (Fig. 4.7).

In relationship to orthotic fabrication, when pathology affects extrinsic musculature, the orthotic design often incorporates the wrist and hand. This wrist-hand orthotic design is necessary because the extrinsic muscles cross the wrist and hand joints.

INTRINSIC MUSCLES OF THE HAND AND WRIST

The intrinsic muscles of the thumb and fingers are listed in Box 4.2. The intrinsic muscles are the muscles of the thenar

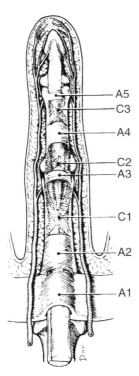

Fig. 4.7 Annular *(A)* and cruciate *(C)* pulley system of the hand. The digital flexor sheath is formed by five annular *(A)* pulleys and three cruciate *(C)* bands. The second and fourth annular pulleys are the most important for function. (From Tubiana, R., Thomine, J. M., & Mackin, E. [1996]. *Examination of the hand and wrist* [p. 81]. St. Louis, MO: Mosby.)

BOX 4.2   Intrinsic Muscles of the Hand

Central Compartment Muscles	Thenar Compartment Muscles	Hypothenar Compartment Muscles
Lumbricals	Opponens pollicis	Opponens digiti minimi
Palmar interossei	Abductor pollicis brevis	Abductor digiti minimi
Dorsal interossei	Adductor pollicis	Flexor digiti minimi brevis
	Flexor pollicis brevis	Palmaris brevis

and hypothenar eminences, the lumbricals, and the interossei. Intrinsic muscles are grouped according to those of the thenar eminence, the hypothenar eminence, and the central muscles between the thenar and hypothenar eminences. The function of these intrinsic hand muscles produces flexion of the proximal phalanx and extension of the middle and distal phalanges, which contribute to the precise finger movements required for coordination.

The thenar eminence consists of the opponens pollicis, flexor pollicis brevis, adductor pollicis, and abductor pollicis brevis. The thenar eminence contributes to thumb opposition, which functionally allows for grasp and prehensile patterns. The thumb seldom acts alone except when pressing objects and playing instruments.[25]

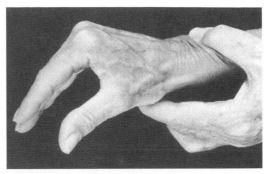

Fig. 4.8 Intrinsic plus position of the hand. Metacarpophalangeal flexion with proximal interphalangeal extension. (From Tubiana, R., Thomine, J. M., & Mackin, E. [1996]. *Examination of the hand and wrist* [p. 308]. St. Louis, MO: Mosby.)

However, without a thumb the hand is virtually nonfunctional.

The hypothenar eminence includes the abductor digiti minimi, the flexor digiti minimi, the palmaris brevis, and the opponens digiti minimi. Similar to the thenar muscles, the hypothenar muscles also assist in rotating the fifth digit during grasp.[3]

The muscles of the central compartment include lumbricals and palmar and dorsal interossei. The interossei muscles are complex with variations in their origins and insertions.[3] There are four dorsal interossei and three palmar interossei muscles. The four lumbricals are weaker than the interossei. The lumbricals originate on the radial aspect of the FDP tendons and insert on the extensor expansion of the finger. They are the only muscles in the human body with a moving origin and insertion. The primary function of the lumbricals is to flex the MCP joints.[28]

Normally the interossei extend the PIP and DIP joints when the MCP joint is in extension. The dorsal interossei produce finger abduction, and the palmar interossei produce finger adduction. Functionally, the first dorsal interossei is a strong abductor of the index finger, which assists in properly positioning the hand for pinching. Research shows the interossei are active during grasp and power grip in addition to pinch.[19] With function of the interossei and lumbricals, a person can place the hand in an intrinsic plus position. An intrinsic plus position is established when the MCP joints are flexed and the PIP joints are fully extended (Fig. 4.8). This position is sometimes referred to as a "table top" position. Some injuries may result in an intrinsic minus hand caused by paralysis or contractures (Fig. 4.9). With an intrinsic minus hand the person loses the cupping shape of the hand.[3] In addition, the intrinsic musculature may waste or atrophy. In relationship to orthotic provision, if intrinsic muscles are solely affected, the orthotic design often involves immobilizing or mobilizing only the finger joints as opposed to incorporating the wrist. To facilitate function and prevent deformity, joint positioning in orthoses frequently warrants an intrinsic plus posture rather than an intrinsic minus position. Throughout this textbook several orthoses include the hand positioned in an intrinsic plus position.

ARCHES OF THE HAND

The hand has three arches, which contribute to a strong functional grasp. The arches include (1) the longitudinal arch, (2) the distal transverse arch, and (3) the proximal transverse arch (Fig. 4.10). Because of their functional significance, these arches require attention during the orthotic fabrication process for their preservation. Therapists should never position the hand in a flat posture in an orthosis because doing so compromises function and creates deformity. Especially in cases of muscle atrophy (as with a tendon or nerve injury), the orthosis should maintain the integrity and mobility of the arches.

The proximal transverse arch is fixed and consists of the distal row of carpal bones. The proximal transverse arch is a rigid arch acting as a stable pivot point for the wrist and long-finger flexor muscles.[12] The transverse carpal ligament and the bones of the proximal transverse arch form the carpal tunnel. The finger flexor tendons pass beneath the transverse carpal ligament. The transverse carpal ligament provides mechanical advantage to the finger flexor tendons by serving as a pulley.[2]

The distal transverse arch, which deepens with flexion of the fingers, is mobile and passes through the metacarpal heads.[2] An orthosis must allow for the functional movement of the distal arch to maintain or increase normal hand function.[12]

The longitudinal arch allows the DIP, PIP, and MCP joints to flex.[16] This arch follows the longitudinal axes of each finger. Because of the mobility of their base, the first, fourth, and fifth metacarpals move in relationship to the shape and size of an object placed in the palm. **Grasp** is the result of holding an object against the rigid portion of the hand provided by the second and third digits. The flattening and cupping motions of the palm allow the hand to pick up and handle objects of various sizes.

ANATOMICAL LANDMARKS OF THE HAND

Creases of the Hand

The creases of the hand are critical landmarks for orthotic pattern making and molding. Therefore knowledge of the creases and their functional implications is important. Three flexion creases are located on the palmar surface of digits II through V, and additional creases are located on the palmar surface of the hand and wrist (Fig. 4.11).

The three primary palmar creases are the distal, proximal, and thenar creases. As shown in Fig. 4.11, the distal palmar crease extends transversely from the fifth MCP joint to a point midway between the third and second MCP joints.[9] This crease is the landmark for the distal edge of the palmar portion of an orthosis intended to immobilize the wrist while allowing motion of the MCPs.[20] By positioning the orthosis proximal to the distal palmar crease, the therapist makes full MCP joint flexion possible. Proximal to the distal palmar crease is the proximal palmar crease, which is used as a guide

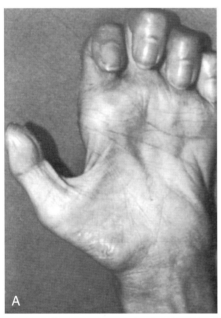

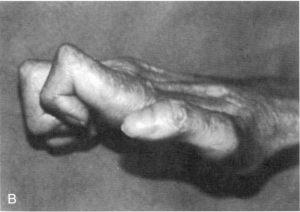

Fig. 4.9 A, Intrinsic minus position of the hand. B, Notice loss of normal arches of the hand and wasting of all intrinsic musculature resulting from a long-standing low median and ulnar nerve palsy. (From Aulicino, P. L. [2002]. Clinical examination of the hand. In E. J. Mackin, A. D. Callahan, T. M. Skirven, et al. [Eds.]. *Rehabilitation of the hand: Surgery and therapy* [5th ed., p. 130]. St. Louis, MO: Mosby)

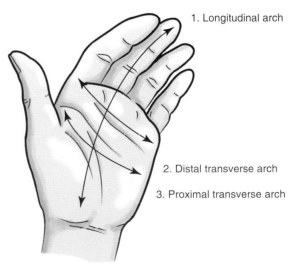

1. Longitudinal arch

2. Distal transverse arch

3. Proximal transverse arch

Fig. 4.10 Arches of the hand.

during orthotic fabrication. An orthosis must be proximal to the proximal palmar crease at the index finger, or the MCP joint will not be free to move into flexion.

The thenar crease begins at the proximal palmar crease near the radial side of the second digit and curves around the base of the thenar eminence (see Fig. 4.11).[9] To allow for thumb motion, this crease should define the limit of the orthosis' edge. If the orthosis extends beyond the thenar crease toward the thumb, thumb opposition and palmar abduction of the CMC joint are inhibited.

The two palmar (or volar) wrist creases are the distal and proximal wrist creases. The distal wrist crease extends from the pisiform bone to the tubercle of the trapezium (see Fig. 4.11) and forms a line that separates the proximal and distal rows of the carpal bones. The proximal wrist crease corresponds to the radiocarpal joint and delineates the proximal border of the carpal bones, which articulates with the distal radius.[9] The distal and proximal wrist creases assist in locating the axis of the wrist motion.[13] Wrist creases serve as a guide when fabricating hand-based orthoses that allow for wrist motion. Such wrist creases should not be covered by the orthosis to allow for full wrist flexion and extension.

The three digital palmar flexion creases are on the palmar aspect of digits II through V (Fig. 4.11). The distal digital crease (or DIP crease) marks the DIP joint axis, and the middle digital crease (or PIP crease) marks the PIP joint axis. The proximal digital crease (or MCP crease) is distal to the MCP joint axis at the base of the proximal phalanx. The creation of the proximal and distal palmar creases results from the thick palmar skin folding due to the force allowing full MCP flexion.[2] The flexion axis of the IP joint of the thumb corresponds to the IP crease of the thumb. Similarly, the MCP crease describes the axis of thumb MCP joint flexion.

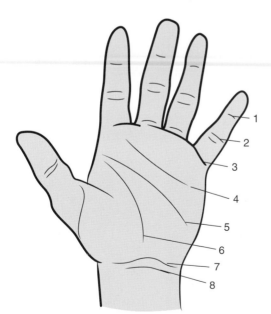

Fig. 4.11 Creases of the hand. *1,* Distal digital (distal interphalangeal) crease; *2,* middle digital (proximal interphalangeal) crease; *3,* proximal digital (metacarpophalangeal) crease; *4,* distal palmar crease; *5,* proximal palmar crease; *6,* thenar crease; *7,* distal wrist crease; *8,* proximal wrist crease.

The creases are close to but not always directly over bony joints.[12] When providing an orthosis to immobilize a particular joint, the therapist must be sure to include the corresponding joint flexion crease within the orthosis so as to provide adequate support for immobilization. Conversely, when attempting to mobilize a specific joint, the therapist must not incorporate the corresponding flexion crease in the orthosis to allow for full range of motion.[16] When one is working with persons who have moderate to severe edema, the creases may dissipate. Creases may also dissipate with disuse associated with paralysis or disuse resulting from pain, stiffness, or psychological problems.

GRASP AND PREHENSILE PATTERNS

The normal hand can perform many prehensile patterns in which the thumb is a crucial factor. Therapists must be knowledgeable about prehensile and grasp patterns, especially when providing orthoses to assist the performance of these patterns.

Even though hand movements are extremely complex, they are categorized into several basic prehensile and grasp patterns, including fingertip prehension, palmar prehension, lateral prehension, cylindrical grasp, spherical grasp, hook grasp,[25] and intrinsic plus grasp.[5] Fig. 4.12 depicts these types of prehensile and grip patterns. Remember that finer prehensile movements require less strength than grasp movements. Pedretti[22] remarked, "The grasp and prehension patterns that may be provided by hand orthoses are determined by the muscles that are functioning, potential and present deformities, and how the hand is to be used."

Fingertip **prehension** is the contact of the pad of the index or middle finger with the pad of the thumb.[25] This movement, which clients use to pick up small objects such as beads and pins, is the weakest of the pinch patterns and requires fine motor coordination. An orthosis to facilitate the fingertip prehension for a person with arthritis may include a static orthosis to block (stabilize) the thumb IP joint in slight flexion (Fig. 4.13).[5]

Palmar prehension, also known as the *tripod* or *three jaw chuck pinch*,[5,13] is the contact of the thumb pad with the pads of the middle and index fingers. People use palmar prehension for holding pencils and picking up small spherical objects. Orthoses to facilitate palmar prehension include thumb spica orthoses that position the thumb in palmar abduction, which may be hand or forearm based (Fig. 4.14).

Lateral prehension, the strongest of the pinch patterns, is the contact between the thumb pad and the lateral aspect of the index finger.[25] Clients typically use this pattern for holding keys. Orthoses that position the hand for lateral prehension include thumb spica orthoses that place the thumb in slight radial abduction (Fig. 4.15).

Cylindrical grasp is used for holding cylindrical-shaped objects, such as soda cans, pan handles, and cylindrical tools.[25] The object contacts in the palm of the hand, and the adducted fingers flex around the object to maintain a grasp. Orthotic provision to encourage such motions as thumb opposition or finger and thumb joint flexion may contribute to a person's ability to regain cylindrical grasp (Fig. 4.16).

The spherical grasp is used to hold round objects, such as balls and spherical-shaped fruit.[25] The object rests against the palm of the hand, and the abducted five digits flex around the object. Orthoses that enhance spherical grasp include orthoses addressing such motions as finger and thumb abduction (Fig. 4.17).

The hook grasp, which is accomplished by the fingers only, involves the carrying of such items as briefcases and suitcases by the handles.[25] The PIPs and DIPs flex around the object, and the thumb often remains passive in this type of grasp. With ulnar and median nerve damage, this position may be avoided rather than encouraged. However, for PIP and DIP joints lacking flexion a therapist may fabricate mobilization (dynamic) flexion orthoses to gain range of motion in these joints.

The intrinsic plus grip is characterized by MCP flexion and PIP and DIP extension. The thumb is positioned in palmar abduction for opposition with the third and fourth fingers.[5] This grasp is helpful when holding flat objects, such as books, trays, or sandwiches. The intrinsic plus grip is not present with ulnar and median nerve injuries. A therapist may facilitate the grasp by using a figure-eight orthosis, shown in Fig. 4.18.

BIOMECHANICAL PRINCIPLES FOR ORTHOTIC INTERVENTION

Orthotic fabrication involves application of external forces on the hand, and thus understanding basic biomechanical principles is important for the therapist when constructing and fitting orthoses. Correct biomechanics of orthotic design results in an optimal fit and reduces risks of skin irritation and pressure areas, which ultimately may lead to client

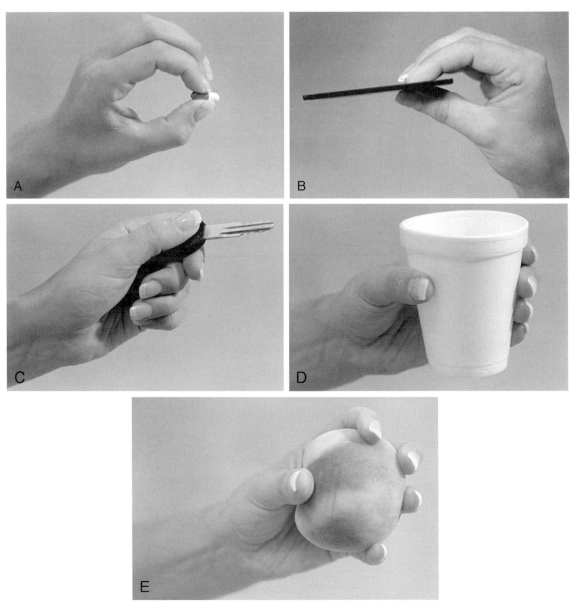

Fig. 4.12 Prehensile and grip patterns of the hand. A, Fingertip prehension. B, Palmar prehension. C, Lateral prehension. D, Cylindrical grasp. E, Spherical grasp. F, Hook grasp. G, Intrinsic plus grasp.

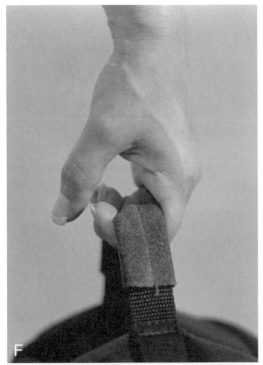

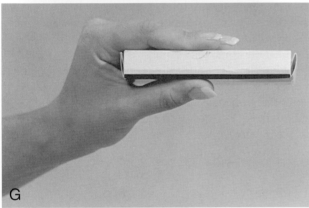

Fig. 4.12, cont'd

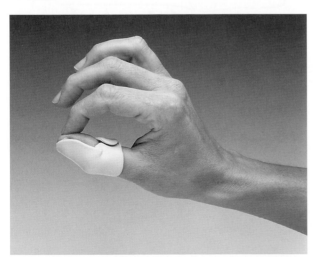

Fig. 4.13 Static orthosis to block the thumb interphalangeal joint in slight flexion to facilitate tip pinch. (From Pedretti, L. W. [Ed.]. [1996]. *Occupational therapy: Practice skills for physical dysfunction* [4th ed., p. 327]. St. Louis, MO: Mosby.)

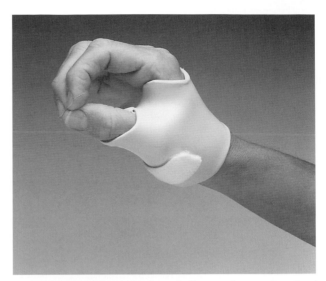

Fig. 4.14 Thumb spica orthosis to facilitate palmar prehension by positioning the thumb in opposition to the index and long fingers. (From Pedretti, L. W. [Ed.]. [1996]. *Occupational therapy: Practice skills for physical dysfunction* [4th ed., p. 327]. St. Louis, MO: Mosby.)

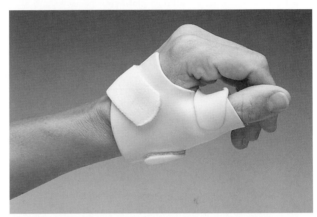

Fig. 4.15 Thumb spica orthosis to facilitate lateral prehension by positioning the thumb in lateral opposition to the index finger. (From Pedretti, L. W. [Ed.]. [1996]. *Occupational therapy: Practice skills for physical dysfunction* [4th ed., p. 327]. St. Louis, MO: Mosby.)

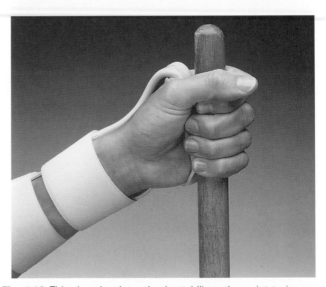

Fig. 4.16 This dorsal wrist orthosis stabilizes the wrist to increase grip force and minimizes coverage of the palm. (From Pedretti, L. W. [Ed.]. [1996]. *Occupational therapy: Practice skills for physical dysfunction* [4th ed., p. 328]. St. Louis, MO: Mosby.)

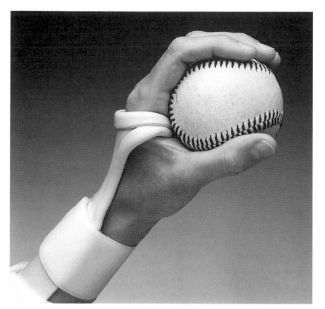

Fig. 4.17 This dorsal wrist orthosis stabilizes the wrist and allows metacarpophalangeal mobility required for a spherical grasp. (From Pedretti, L. W. [Ed.]. [1996]. *Occupational therapy: Practice skills for physical dysfunction* [4th ed., p. 328]. St. Louis, MO: Mosby.)

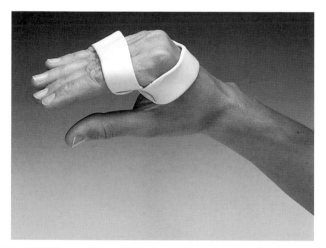

Fig. 4.18 Figure-eight orthosis to facilitate an intrinsic plus grasp. (From Pedretti, L. W. [Ed.]. [1996]. *Occupational therapy: Practice skills for physical dysfunction* [4th ed., p. 328]. St. Louis, MO: Mosby.)

comfort, compliance, and function. In addition, knowledgeable manipulation of biomechanics increases the orthoses' efficiency and improves orthoses' durability while decreasing cost and frustration.[15]

Three-Point Pressure

Most orthoses use a three-point pressure system to affect a joint motion. A **three-point pressure** system consists of three individual linear forces in which the middle force is directed in an opposite direction from the other two forces, as depicted in Fig. 4.19. Three-point pressure systems in orthoses are used for different purposes.[2,15] For example, an orthosis affecting extension or flexion of a joint exerts forces in one plane or unidirectionally, as shown in Fig. 4.20. Three-point systems can be applied to multiple directions. In other words, an orthosis may immobilize one joint while mobilizing an adjacent joint. An example of a multidirectional three-point pressure system is a circumferential wrist orthosis, shown in Fig. 4.21.

Mechanical Advantage

Orthoses incorporate lever systems, which incorporate forces, resistance, axes of motion, and moment arms. Orthoses that serve as levers use a proximal input force (F_i), two moment arms, and an axis or fulcrum to move a distal output force.[15] Similar to a teeter-totter, the force side of an orthosis' lever equals the resistance side of the lever. The sum of the proximal (F_i) and the distal (F_o) forces equals the magnitude (F_m) of the middle opposing force. The system's balance is defined as:

$$F_i \times d_i = F_o \times d_o$$

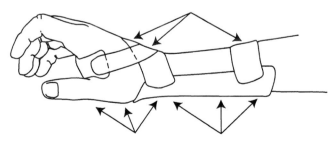

Fig. 4.19 Three-point pressure system is created by an orthosis' surface and properly placed straps to secure the orthosis and ensure proper force for immobilization. (From Pedretti, L. W. [Ed.]. [1996]. *Occupational therapy: Practice skills for physical dysfunction* [4th ed., p. 336]. St. Louis, MO: Mosby.)

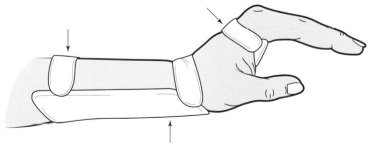

Fig. 4.20 Unidirectional three-point pressure system. (From Fess, E. E., & Philips, C.A. [1987]. *Hand splinting: Principles and methods* [2nd ed., p. 4]. St. Louis: Mosby.)

In this equation, F_i is the input force, and d_i is the input distance (or the proximal force moment arm). F_o is the resistance (or output) force, and d_o is the output distance (or the resistance moment arm). **Mechanical advantage** is defined as:

$$\frac{d_i}{d_o}$$

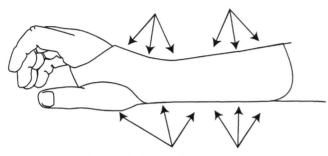

Fig. 4.21 Multidirectional three-point pressure systems. (From Pedretti, L. W. [Ed.]. [1996]. *Occupational therapy: Practice skills for physical dysfunction* [4th ed., p. 336]. St. Louis, MO: Mosby.)

Mechanical advantage principles can be applied and adjusted when the therapist is designing an orthosis. For example, when designing a volar-based wrist immobilization orthosis, increasing the length of the forearm trough decreases force on the proximal anterior forearm (Fig. 4.22). Mechanical advantage results in a more comfortable orthosis for the client. Application of this concept involves consideration of the anatomical segment length in designing the orthosis. For example, the length of an orthosis' forearm trough should be approximately two-thirds the length of the forearm. Persons wearing volar-based orthoses should be able to flex their elbows fully without interference.[4] The width of a thumb or forearm trough should be half the circumference of the thumb or forearm. The muscle bulk of an extremity gradually increases more proximal to the body, and the orthosis' trough should widen proportionately as it courses proximally. When making an orthotic pattern, the therapist must maintain at least one-half the circumference of the thumb or forearm for a correct fit.

Torque

Torque is a biomechanical principle defined as the "extent to which a force tends to cause rotation of an object (body part)

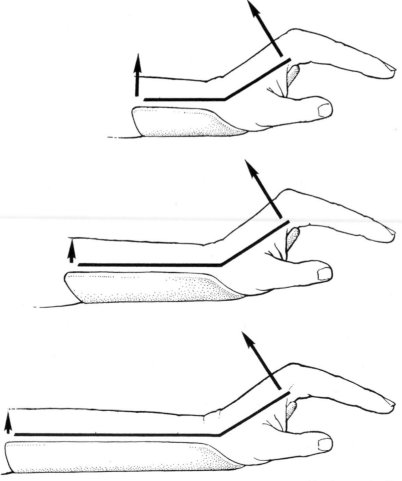

Fig. 4.22 A longer forearm trough decreases the resultant pressure caused by the proximally transferred weight of the hand to the anterior forearm. (From Fess, E. E., Gettle, K. S., Philips, C. A., et al. [2005]. Mechanical principles. In E. E. Fess, & C. A. Philips [Eds.], *Hand splinting: Principles and methods* [3rd ed., p. 167]. St. Louis, MO: Mosby.)

about an axis."[21] Other terms used synonymously include *moment arm* or *moment of force*. Torque is the product of the applied force (F) multiplied by the perpendicular distance from the axis of rotation to the line of application of force (d). The equation for torque is:

$$Torque = F \times d$$

It is important to consider torque for dynamic or mobilization orthoses (see Chapter 13).

Pressure and Stress

There are four ways in which skin and soft tissue can be damaged by force or **pressure**:
- Degree
- Duration
- Repetition
- Direction

Degree and Duration of Stress

Generally, low **stress** can be tolerated for longer periods of time, whereas high stress over long periods of time causes damage.[6] It must be noted that *low stress* and *high stress* are generic and imprecise terms. Generally, the tissue that least tolerates pressure is the skin. Skin becomes ischemic as load increases. Low stress can be damaging if it is continuous and can eventually cause capillary damage and lead to ischemia. The effects of continuous low force from constricting circumferential bandages and orthoses and their straps can be damaging at times. However, if a system can be devised to distribute pressure over a larger area of skin, a higher load can be exerted on a ligament, adhesion, tendon, or muscle. Such an orthotic design may include a longer trough or a circumferential component.

Repetitive Stress

If a stress is repetitively applied in moderate amounts, it can lead to inflammation and skin breakdown.[6] An example of a repetitive stress may be seen in a person wearing a dynamic flexion orthosis that has rubber band traction. If the person continually flexes the finger against the tension, the tissue may become inflamed after some time. If inflammation or redness occurs, the tension is adjusted by relaxing the traction. Persons with traumatic hand injuries or pathology may not be able to tolerate the repetitive amounts of stress a normal person could tolerate. Poor tolerance is usually a result of damaged vascular and lymph structures.

High stress may quickly result in tissue damage.[6] High stress can be applied to the skin from any object, such as an orthosis or bandage. The smaller or sharper the object is, the greater the amount of stress is produced. High stress should be avoided at all times. For example, if a dynamic orthosis is applying too much stress to a joint, circulation may be restricted (potentially leading to tissue damage).

Direction of Stress

During orthotic fabrication, consider the direction of stress or force on the skin and soft tissue. There are three directions of force to consider: (1) tension, (2) compression, and (3) shear.[15] Compression stress results from forces pressing inwardly on an object (Fig. 4.23A). Tension occurs when forces on an object are applied opposite each other (Fig. 4.23B). Shear force occurs "when parallel forces are applied in an equal and opposite direction across opposite faces of a structure"[15] (Fig. 4.23C). Researchers suggest that shear stress is the most damaging to skin.[6]

Therapists must recognize and know how to use the stress of orthoses in such a way as to not create soft-tissue damage. Generally, avoid excessive stress or pressure from orthoses by employing wide troughs placed far from the fulcrum of movement while using an appropriate amount of tension on structures.[2] To determine the appropriate amount of tension on structures, the orthosis' tension should be sufficient to take the joint to a comfortable joint end range. This means that the tension in the orthosis should bring the joint just to the maximum comfortable position (flexion, extension, deviation, or rotation) that is tolerable. This position should be one the client can tolerate for long periods of time. The client may need to work up to a longer wearing time, but the goal is usually at least 4 hours per day.

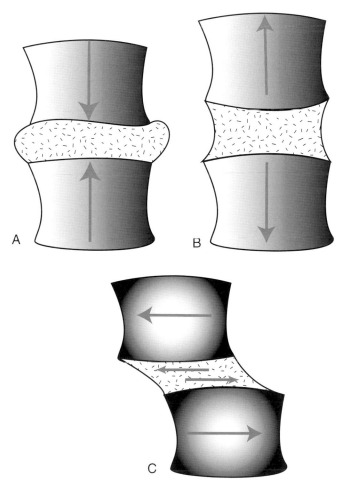

Fig. 4.23 A, Compression is a force pushing tissues together. B, Tension occurs when forces pull in opposite directions (tensile forces). C, Shear forces are parallel to the surfaces they affect. (From Greene, D. P., & Roberts, S. L. [2005]. *Kinesiology movement in the context of activity* [2nd ed., p. 21]. St. Louis, MO: Mosby.)

Ideally, the 4 hours will be continuous, but it can be broken up as necessary. Ask clients to try to wear their orthoses to improve passive range of motion (PROM) during sleep. However, this depends on their cognitive, sensory, and substance abuse status. The rationale for this wearing schedule is based on studies that show that low-load prolonged stress at the end range is very effective in increasing PROM. Technically, for dense scars or for tissue that has adaptively shortened over a long period of time, higher tension forces can be used as long as the pressure is well distributed along the skin. The skin is the structure that is the "weak link." The skin cannot tolerate the tension in the orthosis and becomes ischemic and therefore painful. If the pressure is well distributed, higher forces can be used and the tissue lengthens more quickly as a result.

Several examples depict the effects of force on soft tissues.[15] For example, after repair of a tendon rupture a therapist may employ early mobilization with a small amount of tension to facilitate the alignment of collagen fibers for improving tensile strength of the healing tendon. The tendon may be re-ruptured if the tension and repetition applied are not well controlled. An orthosis may be applied to assist in controlling fluctuating edema in the upper extremity. However, if the orthosis applies too much compression force on the underlying soft tissue over too much time, the orthosis may restrict vascularity, possibly leading to soft-tissue necrosis. Shear stress between a healing tendon and its sheath must be carefully monitored to minimize and control adhesion shape.

The concepts of stress are considered with orthotic intervention. Orthoses and straps apply external forces on tissues that in turn affect forces or stresses exerted internally.[15] The formula for pressure is:

$$Pressure = \frac{Total\ force}{Area\ of\ force\ application}$$

Ideally, orthoses should be contoured and cover a large surface area to decrease pressure and the risk of pressure sores.[11] Straps should be as wide as possible to distribute pressure appropriately and to prevent restriction of circulation or trapping of edema.

Thermoplastic orthoses can cause pressure points over areas with minimal soft tissue or over bony prominences. To avoid this risk, the therapist uses an orthotic design that is wider and longer.[16] A larger design is more comfortable, because it decreases the force concentrated on the hand and arm by increasing the surface area of the orthosis' force application.

Continuous well-distributed pressure is the goal of an orthosis, but pressure over any bony prominence should be nonexistent.[9] Therapists should be cautious of pressure over bony prominences, such as the radial and ulnar styloids and the dorsal-aspect MCPs and the PIPs (Fig. 4.24). Therapists can use heat guns to alleviate pressure exerted by the orthosis. This is done by heating the plastic in problem areas and pushing the plastic away from the bony prominence. Another technique for avoiding pressure on bony prominences is to place the orthosis over padding, gel pads, or elastomer positioned over bony prominences. A frequent mistake in orthotic fabrication occurs when a pad is placed over the localized pressure area after the orthosis is formed.[6] Remember that padding takes up space, reducing the circumference measurement of the orthosis and increasing the pressure over an area. Plan for the addition of padding before application of the thermoplastic material. The orthotic design must accommodate the thickness of the padding.

Moist substances, such as perspiration and wound drainage, can cause skin maceration, irritation, and breakdown. Bandages help absorb the moisture but require frequent changing for infection control.[1] Some types of stockinettes are more effective in wicking moisture away from skin. Polypropylene and thick terry liners are much more effective than cotton or common synthetic stockinettes. Therapists can fabricate an orthosis over extremities covered with a stockinette or bandages, but the orthosis should be altered if the bulk of dressings or bandages changes.

Rolled or round edges on the proximal and distal ends of the orthosis cause less pressure than straight edges.[9,21] Imperfect edges are potential causes of pressure areas and therefore should be smoothed.

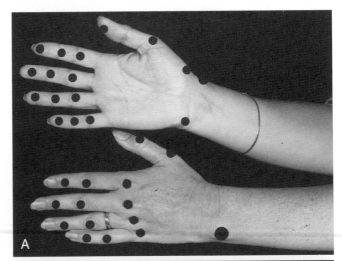

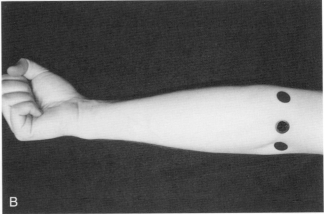

Fig. 4.24 A and B, Bony sites susceptible to pressure, which may cause soft-tissue damage. (From Fess, E. E., Gettle, K. S., Philips C. A., et al. [2005]. Principles of fit. In E. E. Fess & C. A. Philips [Eds.]. *Hand splinting: Principles and methods* [3rd ed., p. 261]. St. Louis, MO: Mosby.)

CONTOUR

When flat, thermoplastic materials are flexible and can be bent. Curving and contouring thermoplastic material to an underlying surface changes the mechanical characteristics of the material.[21,27] Contoured thermoplastic material is stronger and is better able to handle externally applied forces (Fig. 4.25). Thermoplastic materials have varying degrees of drapability and conformity properties, which may affect the degree of contour the therapist is able to obtain in an orthosis.

MECHANICS OF SKIN AND SOFT TISSUE

Therapists often use orthoses to effect a change in skin and soft tissue, which may address performance deficits. It is important to have a basic understanding of the mechanics of normal soft tissue and skin. In addition, one should know when and how the mechanics change in the presence of scar tissue, materials (bandages, orthoses, cuffs), edema, contractures, wounds, and infection.

Normal skin and soft tissue have properties of plasticity and viscoelasticity, which allow them to resist breakdown under stress in normal situations.[6] **Plasticity** refers to the extent the skin can mold and reshape to different surfaces. **Viscoelasticity** refers to the skin's degree of viscosity and elasticity, which enables the skin to resist stress. The skin and soft tissue tolerate some force or stress, but beyond a certain point the skin breaks down.[29]

When edema is present, the hand's normal soft tissue undergoes mechanical changes because of the volume of viscous fluid present.[6,26] Prolonged or excessive edema can lead to permanent deformity. Therefore, edema must be managed in conjunction with orthotic application (e.g., elevating the affected extremity, moving unaffected joints to actively contract the muscles to facilitate venous blood return from the extremity).[21] Orthoses often assist in controlling edema. Because of the increase in volume of fluid, swollen skin, joints, and tendons have an increase in friction in relation to the resistance to movement. "Swollen tissue, then, in addition to its increased viscosity, is limited in its ability to be elongated, compressed, or compliant. This is why a hand never has a normal range of motion as long as there is edema in the tissue in and under the skin."[6]

Properties of thermoplastic material are selected carefully as they can affect skin and soft tissue.[24] For example, when orthoses are secured on the extremity using elastic bandages, they have the potential to apply high amounts of stress and may lead to constriction in the vascular and lymphatic circulation. A therapist must consider the amount of pressure applied to skin and tissue, especially when a second wrap of an elastic bandage covers an initial wrap. The pressure applied by the second wrap is doubled. Pressure occurs even when bandages are applied in a figure-eight fashion. Another consideration is the effect that bandages have on motion. Movement while bandages are worn can further concentrate pressure, particularly over bony prominences. If appropriate, bandages should be removed while exercises are being performed.

Finger cuffs or loops used with mobilization orthoses increase pressure on the underlying skin and tissue. Bell-Krotoski and colleagues[6] caution that using very flexible finger cuffs could increase the shear stress on fingers. Leather finger loops may be an appropriate choice because they simulate normal skin by being flexible while providing some firmness to decrease the shear stress. Finger loops should be as wide as possible to avoid edge shear and to distribute pressure (Fig. 4.26). Chapter 13 addresses finger loops in more depth.

In joints with flexion contractures, skin on the dorsum of the joints grows with elongation tension on the skin.[6] Skin on the volar surface of the joints is reabsorbed by a reduction in the elongation tension. There is a natural balance of tension in the skin and muscles. Skin will adjust to the tension required of it. Not only will skin lose length (contracture), but it grows new cells to lengthen. The use of stretch gradually produces these changes. If skin is stretched to the point of microtrauma, a scar forms. When skin stretches, it releases proteins that result in scar formation. The scar tissue decreases the elasticity of the skin. To counteract excessive scarring, therapists use scar massage, mobilization techniques, and gentle stretch.

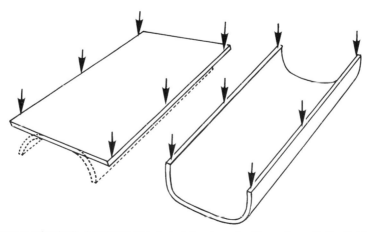

Fig. 4.25 Contour mechanically increases the material's strength. (From Fess, E. E., Gettle, K. S., Philips C. A., et al. [2005]. Mechanical principles. In E. E. Fess & C. A. Philips [Eds.], *Hand splinting: Principles and methods* [3rd ed., p. 178]. St. Louis, MO: Mosby.)

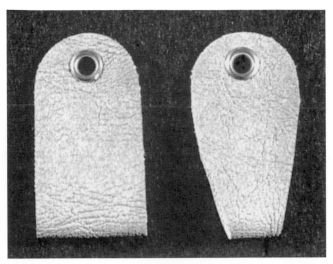

Fig. 4.26 Finger loops apply pressure to the underlying surface. They should be as wide as possible without limiting adjacent joint mobility. (From Fess, E. E., Gettle, K. S., Philips C. A., et al. [2005]. Principles of fit. In E. E. Fess & C. A. Philips [Eds.], *Hand splinting: Principles and methods* [3rd ed., p. 274]. St. Louis, MO: Mosby.)

Optimal regrowth involves the use of continuous (or almost continuous) tension.[6]

Tissue that is newly healing can be negatively affected by mechanical stress. Tension of a wound site may "reduce the rate of repair, compromise tensile strength, and increase the final width of the scar."[14] Rather than simply removing an orthosis and returning the extremity to function, immobilization orthoses should be gradually weaned as the affected skin and tissue become more mobile.[6]

When working with a person who has infected tissues, caution must be taken to avoid mechanical stress from motion (as from a mobilization orthosis). Blood and interstitial fluids are forced into motion, and this pushes infection into deeper tissue and results in a more widespread infection and delay in healing. In the presence of infection, it is best to immobilize a joint with an orthosis for a few days and then remove the orthosis to maintain normal or partial range of motion.

👤 SELF-QUIZ 4.1ᵃ

Answer the following.

Part I
Match the following with the correct orthosis.
a. Based on the palmar surface of the hand and forearm
b. Based on the dorsal surface of the hand and forearm
c. Based on the thumb side of the hand and forearm
d. Based on the little finger side of the hand and forearm
  1. Ulnar gutter wrist immobilization orthosis
  2. Volar- or palmar-based flexion mobilization orthosis
  3. Dorsal MCP protection orthosis
  4. Palmar-based wrist immobilization orthosis
  5. Radial gutter extension mobilization orthosis

Part II
From the following diagram, label the creases of the hand.
1.
2.
3.
4.
5.

Continued

SELF-QUIZ 4.1ᵃ—cont'd

Part III
From the following diagram, label the arches of the hand.
1.
2.
3.

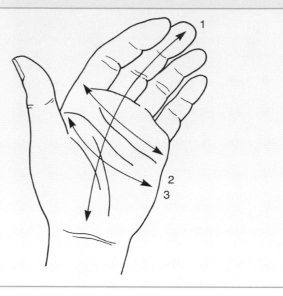

ᵃSee Appendix A for the answer key.

SELF-QUIZ 4.2ᵃ

For the following questions, circle either true (T) or false (F).
1. T F The forearm trough should be two-thirds the circumference of the forearm.
2. T F Short, narrow orthoses apply less pressure to the skin's surface than long, wide orthoses and are therefore better.
3. T F An orthosis should be approximately two-thirds the length of the forearm.
4. T F Avoidance of pressure over a bony prominence is preferable to unequal pressure.
5. T F A person uses a spherical grasp when holding a soda can.
6. T F An orthotic design must accommodate padding thickness.
7. T F In joints with flexion contractures, the skin on the dorsum of the joint shortens and exerts tension.
8. T F In the orthotic provision for persons with infection, caution is taken to avoid mechanical stress from motion such as mobilization orthoses.
9. T F Contour of an orthosis increases its strength.
10. T F Shear force results from forces pressing inwardly on an object.

ᵃSee Appendix A for the answer key.

SUMMARY

A therapist's knowledge of anatomical and biomechanical principles is important during the entire orthotic process. One must be familiar with terminology to interpret medical reports, therapy prescriptions, and professional literature. In addition, the therapist uses medical terminology to document evaluations and interventions. The application of biomechanical principles to orthotic design and construction results in better-fitting orthoses and thus contributes to adherence with therapeutic regimens. Ultimately, adherence to such principles impacts therapeutic outcomes.

REVIEW QUESTIONS

1. In regard to orthotic fabrication, what do the following terms refer to: *palmar, dorsal,* and *radial* (or *ulnar*)?
2. What are the three arches of the hand?
3. When therapists fabricate an orthosis for the hand, why is support for the hand's arches important?
4. What is the significance of the distal palmar crease when fabricating a hand orthosis?
5. If an orthosis' edge does not extend beyond the thenar crease toward the thumb, what thumb motions are possible?
6. What is an example of each of the following prehensile or grasp patterns: fingertip prehension, palmar prehension, lateral prehension, cylindrical grasp, spherical grasp, hook grasp, and intrinsic plus grasp?
7. How can a therapist determine the correct length of a forearm orthosis?
8. What is the correct width for an orthosis that has a forearm or thumb trough?
9. What precautions should a therapist take when using padding in an orthosis?

10. What are two methods a therapist can use to prevent the edges of an orthosis from causing a pressure sore?
11. Why is it important to consider contour when fabricating an orthosis?

12. How do skin and soft-tissue mechanics change in the presence of scar tissue, material application, edema, contractures, wounds, and infection?

REFERENCES

1. Agency for Health Care Policy and Research: *Pressure ulcers in adults: prediction and prevention (No. 92–0047)*, Rockville, MD, 1992, US Department of Health and Human Services.
2. Andrews KL, Bouvette KA: Anatomy for management and fitting of prosthetics and orthotics, *Phys Med Rehab: State of the Art Rev* 10(3):489–507, 1996.
3. Aulicino PL: Clinical examination of the hand. In Hunter JM, Mackin EJ, Callahan AD, editors: *Rehabilitation of the hand: surgery and therapy*, ed 4, St. Louis, 1995, Mosby.
4. Barr NR, Swan D: *The hand*, Butterworth, 1998, Boston.
5. Belkin J, English CB: Hand splinting: principles, practice, and decision making. In Pedretti LW, editor: *Occupational therapy: practice skills for physical dysfunction*, ed 4, St. Louis, 1996, Mosby.
6. Bell-Krotoski JA, Breger-Lee DE, Beach RB: Biomechanics and evaluation of the hand. In Hunter JM, Mackin EJ, Callahan AD, editors: *Rehabilitation of the hand: surgery and therapy*, ed 4, St. Louis, 1995, Mosby.
7. Bowers WH, Tribuzi SM: Functional anatomy. In Stanely BG, Tribuzi SM, editors: *Concepts in hand rehabilitation*, Philadelphia, 1992, FA Davis.
8. Buck WR: *Human gross anatomy lecture guide*, Erie, PA, 1995, Lake Erie College of Osteopathic Medicine.
9. Cailliet R: *Hand pain and impairment*, ed 4, Philadelphia, 1994, FA Davis.
10. Cailliet R: *Shoulder pain*, ed 2, Philadelphia, 1981, FA Davis.
11. Cannon NM, Foltz RW, Koepfer JM, et al.: *Manual of hand splinting*, New York, 1985, Churchill Livingstone.
12. Chase RA: Anatomy and kinesiology of the hand. In Hunter JM, Schneider LH, Mackin EJ, editors: *Rehabilitation of the hand: surgery and therapy*, ed 3, St. Louis, 1990, Mosby.
13. Clarkson HM, Gilewich GB: *Musculoskeletal assessment: joint range of motion and manual muscle strength*, Baltimore, 1989, Williams & Wilkins.
14. Evans RB, McAuliffe JA: Wound classification and management. In Mackin EJ, Callahan AD, Skirven TM, editors: *Rehabilitation of the hand and upper extremity*, ed 5, St. Louis, 2002, Mosby.
15. Fess EE: Splints: mechanics versus convention, *J Hand Ther* 9(1):124–130, 1995.
16. Fess EE, Gettle KS, Philips CA, et al.: *Hand and upper extremity splinting: principles and methods*, ed 3, St. Louis, 2005, Elsevier Mosby.
17. Kapandji IA: *The physiology of the joints*, London, 1970, E&S Livingstone.
18. Kleinert HE, Schepel S, Gill T: Flexor tendon injuries, *Surg Clin North Am* 61(2):267–286, 1981.
19. Long C, Conrad PW, Hall EA, et al.: Intrinsic-extrinsic muscle control of the hand in power grip and precision handling: an electromyographic study, *J Bone Joint Surg Am* 52(5):853–867, 1970.
20. Malick MH: *Manual on static hand splinting*, Pittsburgh, 1972, Hamarville Rehabilitation Center.
21. McGee P, Rivard A: Foundations of orthotic intervention. In Skirven TM, Osterman AL, Fedorczyk JM, et al.: *Rehabilitation of the hand and upper extremity*, ed 6, St. Louis, 2011, Mosby, pp 1577–1578.
22. Pedretti LW: Hand splinting. In Pedretti LW, Zoltan B, editors: *Occupational therapy: practice skills for physical dysfunction*, ed 3, St. Louis, 1990, Mosby, pp 18–39.
23. Pratt NE: *Clinical musculoskeletal anatomy*, Philadelphia, 1991, Lippincott.
24. Schultz-Johnson K: *Personal communication*, March 3, 1999.
25. Smith LK, Weiss EL, Lehmkuhl LD: *Brunnstrom's clinical kinesiology*, ed 5, Philadelphia, 1996, FA Davis.
26. Villeco JP, Mackin EJ, Hunter JM: Edema: therapist's management. In Mackin EJ, Callahan AD, Skirven TM, et al.: *Rehabilitation of the hand and upper extremities*, ed 5, St. Louis, 2002, Mosby, pp 183–193.
27. Wilton JC: *Hand splinting principles of design and fabrication*, Philadelphia, 1997, WB Saunders.
28. Wu PBJ: Functional anatomy of the upper extremity, *Phys Med Rehab: State Art Rev* 10(3):587–600, 1996.
29. Yamada H: *Strength of biological materials*, Baltimore, 1970, Williams & Wilkins.

Clinical Examination for Orthotic Intervention

Brenda M. Coppard

CHAPTER OBJECTIVES

1. List components of a thorough clinical examination as related to orthotic intervention.
2. Describe components of a history, an observation, and palpation.
3. Describe the resting hand posture.
4. Relate how skin, vein, bone, joint, muscle, tendon, and nerve assessments are relevant to orthotic intervention.
5. Identify specific assessments that can be used in a clinical examination before orthotic intervention.
6. Explain the three phases of wound healing.
7. Recognize the signs of abnormal illness behavior.
8. Explain how a therapist assesses a person's knowledge of orthotic precautions and wear and care instructions.

KEY TERMS

protocols	responsiveness	verbal analog scale (VeAS)
reliability	validity	visual analog scale (ViAS)

Mauri is a therapist who recently switched practice from pediatrics to an outpatient rehabilitation clinic. During his first week, he receives a referral for Blanche, an 82-year-old woman with a flare-up of rheumatoid arthritis. Before scheduling an appointment with, Mauri conceptualizes his screening and assessment plan.

CLINICAL EXAMINATION

A thoughtfully selected battery of clinical assessments is crucial to therapists' and physicians' intervention plans. A thorough, organized, and clearly documented examination is the basis for the development of an intervention plan. In today's health care system, therapists complete examinations that are time and cost efficient. This chapter addresses components of the assessment process in relation to orthotic provision.

Time-efficient, informal assessments may indicate the level of hand and upper extremity function initially observed by the therapist.[35] The results may prompt a therapist to select more sophisticated testing procedures, as indicated by the person's condition.[27] Generally, initial and discharge evaluations are most comprehensive in scope, whereas regular reassessments are usually more focused.

Reassessments typically occur at consistent intervals of time. For example, if Jose is evaluated at his Monday appointment, the therapist may reevaluate Jose every Monday or every other Monday thereafter. On some occasions a case manager may request the therapist to reevaluate a client. However, the time span between assessments is based on the person's condition and progress. For example, a person with a peripheral nerve injury may be reevaluated once every 3 weeks because of the slow nature of nerve healing. Another person being rehabilitated after a burn injury may be reevaluated every week because this condition changes more quickly, thereby affecting functional ability.

The assessment process for the upper extremity incorporates data from conducting a medical history, an interview, observation, palpation, and a selection of tests that are objective, valid, and reliable. Form 5.1 is a check-off sheet that therapists can use when evaluating a person with upper extremity dysfunction. Ancillary tools (such as radiographs, computerized tomography [CT] scans, magnetic resonance imaging [MRI] scans, electrodiagnostics, and laboratory tests) assist in confirming the diagnosis and provide the therapist with a broader context of the person's condition(s).[63]

History

Beginning with a medical history, the therapist gathers data from various sources. Depending on the setting, the therapist may have access to the person's medical chart, surgical or radiological reports, and the physician's referral or prescription. The person's age, gender, and diagnosis are typically easy to obtain from such sources. Client age is important because some congenital anomalies and diagnoses are unique to certain age groups. Age may also affect the prognosis or length of recovery. Some problems are unique to gender.

From available sources the therapist seeks out the person's past medical history, the dates of occurrences, current medical status, and treatment. The history includes invasive and noninvasive treatments. Conditions such as diabetes, epilepsy, kidney or liver dysfunction, arthritis, and gout should be reported because they can directly or indirectly influence rehabilitation (including orthotic intervention).[20] The therapist determines whether the current upper extremity problem is the result of neurological or orthopedic origin, or a combination of both. For example, Ken fell and sustained a traumatic brain injury and experienced upper extremity fractures. Some conditions are solely orthopedic in nature, resulting from trauma affecting soft tissue (i.e., tendon laceration, burn). The nature of dysfunction helps the therapist determine the orthotic approach.

With postoperative presentations, therapists must know the anatomical structures involved and the surgical procedures performed. Be aware that some physicians may prefer to follow conventional rehabilitative programs for certain diagnostic populations. Other physicians may prefer to follow rehabilitative programs that they developed for specific postoperative diagnostic populations. Whether standardized or nonstandardized, these programs are known as **protocols**. Protocols delineate which types of orthoses, exercises, and therapeutic interventions are appropriate in rehabilitation programs. Protocols often indicate the timing of interventions.

Interview

At the beginning of the interview, complete introductions, explain what occupational therapy is, and describe the purpose of evaluation and intervention. The goal of the interview is for the therapist to determine the impact of the condition on the person's function, family, economic status, and social/emotional well-being. Most important, the therapist asks what a person's goals are.[63] The therapist collects the person's history at the time of the initial evaluation. In addition, the therapist creates a teaching/learning environment compatible with the client's learning style. For example, a therapist informs the client that she should feel comfortable about asking any questions concerning therapy, evaluation, or intervention.

Therapists may obtain cohistories from family, parents, friends, and caretakers of children and persons who are unable to communicate or who have cognitive impairments and are unreliable or questionable self-reporters. The therapist obtains the following information by asking the person a variety of questions:

- Age
- Date of injury
- Nature of injury
- Hand dominance
- Goals
- Avocation interests
- Subjective complaints

- Support systems
- Vocation
- Functional abilities
- Family composition
- Social history
- Interventions to date
- Family/caregiver support

Therapists ask about general health and about prior orthopedic, neurological, psychological, or cardiopulmonary conditions.[20] Habits and conditions such as smoking,[51,64] alcohol or drug use, prescriptions and over-the-counter medications, stress,[20] obesity,[88] and depression[74] may influence rehabilitation.[58] The therapist asks the client about any previous upper extremity conditions and dates of onset to assess the current condition. The therapist asks about prior interventions and their results. The therapist determines the client's insight into the condition by asking the client to describe what he or she understands about the condition or diagnosis.

After background information is gleaned, the client is asked open-ended questions about the present signs and symptoms. The therapist asks probing questions about the current condition to gain insight about the client's level of irritability.[63] If a client reports minimal pain at rest, transient pain upon movement, and symptoms that are not easily provoked, the person is said to have low irritability. If pain is present upon resting, pain increases with movement, and decreased mobility is noted, the person has a highly irritable condition. Determining the irritability level determines how aggressively the surgeon and therapist may perform evaluations and interventions.

Observation

Observations are noted immediately when the person walks into a clinic or during the first meeting between the therapist and client. For example, the therapist observes how the person carries the upper extremity, looking for reduced reciprocal arm swing, guarding postures, and involuntary movements, such as tremors or tics.[68] The therapist notes spontaneous usage of involved upper extremity. Facial tics may be a sign of a neurological or psychological problem. Further information is gleaned from observing facial movements, speech patterns, and affect. For example, if there is a facial droop, the therapist may suspect that the client has Bell palsy or has had a stroke. The therapist always observes the person's ability to answer questions and follow instructions.

A general inspection of the person's upper quarter (including the neck, shoulder, elbow, forearm, wrist, and hand) and joint attitude is noted. The therapist notes the posture of the affected extremity and looks for any postural asymmetry and guarded or protective positioning. When clients hold a painful extremity with their other extremity, it is considered a guarded position. Clients often guard to avoid pain from touching, moving, or bumping into objects. A normal hand at rest assumes a posture of 10 to 20 degrees of wrist extension, 10 degrees of ulnar deviation, slight flexion and abduction of the thumb, and approximately 15 to 20 degrees of flexion of the metacarpophalangeal (MCP) joints. The fingers in a resting posture exhibit a greater composite flexion to the radial side of the hand (scaphoid bone)[63] (Fig. 5.1). The thumbnail usually lies perpendicular to the index finger. Observation of hand postures influences planning for orthotic provision because a person's hand often deviates from the normal resting posture in the presence of injury or disease.

A variety of presentations observed by the therapist contribute to the overall clinical picture of the person. The following are noteworthy observational points[63]:

- Position of hand in relationship to the body: protective or guarding posture
- Diminished or absent reciprocal arm swing
- Quality of movement
- Hand arches and creases
- Muscle atrophy
- Contractures
- Nails: ridged or smooth
- Edema, hematoma (blood clot), ecchymosis (bruise)
- Finger pads: thin or smooth (loss of rugal folds, fingerprint lines)
- Lesions: scars, abrasions, burns, wounds
- Abnormal web spaces
- Heberden or Bouchard nodes
- Neurological deficit postures: clawhand, wristdrop, simian hand
- Color: pale, red, blue
- Grafts or sutures

- External devices: percutaneous pins, external fixator, orthoses, slings, braces
- Deformities: boutonnière, mallet finger, intrinsic minus hand, swan neck
- Pilomotor signs: appearance of "goose pimples" or hair standing on end
- Joint deviation or abnormal rotation

Palpation

After a general inspection of the client, the therapist palpates the affected areas when appropriate. A therapist palpates areas in which the person describes symptoms, including any area that is swollen or abnormal.[68] Muscle bulk is palpated on each extremity to compare proximal and distal muscles and to compare right and left. Muscle tone is best assessed through passive range of motion (PROM). When assessing tone, the therapist coaches the client to relax the muscles so that the most accurate results are obtained. The client's skin is examined. In the presence of ulcers, gangrene, inflammation, or neural or vascular impairment, skin temperature may change and can be felt during palpation.[58] In the presence of infection, draining wounds, or sutured sites, therapists wear sterile gloves and follow universal precautions.

Assessments

Assessment selection is a critical step in formulating appropriate interventions. There are more than 100 assessments in the musculoskeletal literature.[73] Time efficiency has become a

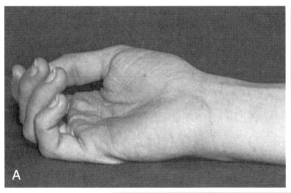
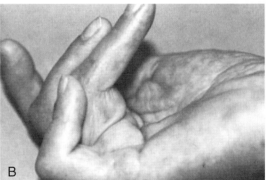
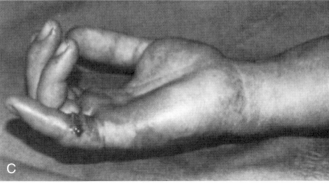

Fig. 5.1 Resting posture of the hand. A, Normal resting posture. Note that the fingers are progressively more flexed from the radial aspect to the ulnar aspect of the hand. B, This normal hand posture is lost because of contractures of the digits as a result of Dupuytren disease. C, Loss of the normal hand posture is due to a laceration of the flexor tendons of the fifth digit. (From Hunter, J. M., Mackin, E. J., & Callahan, A.D. [Eds.]. [1995]. *Rehabilitation of the hand: Surgery and therapy* [4th ed., p. 55]. St. Louis, MO: Mosby.)

contemporary priority in choosing assessments. For example, in 2015 hand therapists who were members of the American Society of Hand Therapists were surveyed about sensorimotor interventions and assessments for the hand and wrist. Of the 22% who responded, 79% of the therapists believed that occupation-based formal assessments were important; however, they reported not using them as much as they wanted due to time constraints in practice.[35] Perhaps more important than time efficiency are several factors that must be considered when selecting an assessment, including content, methodology, and clinical utility.[73] To critically choose appropriate assessment tools used for practice, one must understand the tool's psychometric development.

Content of an assessment is what the tool attempts to measure. Content is separated into three categories: type, scale, and interpretation. The type of content focuses on data gathered by the clinician or data reported by the client. The scale of the content refers to the measurements or questions that constitute the tool and how they are measured. Content interpretation addresses how scores or measures pertain to "excellent" or "poor" outcomes.[73]

Methodology of the tool relates to validity, reliability, and responsiveness. **Validity** is the extent to which the assessment measures what it intends to measure. Table 5.1 lists and defines the various types of validity. **Reliability** is the consistency of the assessment. Table 5.2 lists and defines the types of reliability. **Responsiveness** refers to the assessment's sensitivity to measuring change or differences in status.[73]

Clinical utility refers to the degree the tool is easy to administer and the degree of ease the client experiences in completing the assessment. Utility is a subjective component addressing the degree to which the tool is acceptable to the client and the degree to which the tool is feasible to the therapist. Factors that impact clinical utility include training for competent administration, cost and administration, and documentation and interpretation time.[73]

Assessment tools are categorized in several ways. There are standardized and nonstandardized (informal) assessment tools. Some assessments are norm based, whereas others are criterion based. Bear-Lehman and Abreu[3] suggest that evaluation is a quantitative and qualitative process. Thus therapists who select assessments that solely produce precise, objective, and quantitative measurement decrease subjective judgments and increase their ability to obtain reproducible findings. However, therapists are cautioned to reject the tendency to neglect important information about their clients that may not be quantifiable.[3] Qualitative information—such as attitude, pain response, coping mechanisms, and locus of control (center of responsibility for one's behavior)—influence the evaluation process. "The selection of the hand assessment tools to be used, the art of human interaction between the therapist and the client, the art of evaluating the client's hand as a part, but also as an integrated whole, are part of the subjective processes involved in hand assessment."[3] Even objective evaluation tools require the comprehension and motivation of the client.

Unfortunately, there is no universally accepted upper extremity assessment tool or battery. Depending on the setting, a battery of assessments may be developed ad hoc by a facility or department practitioners. In other settings, therapists use clinical reasoning to determine what battery of assessments will be used for each person. A theoretical perspective and a diagnostic population can influence the evaluation selection.[3] For example, one facility's assessment reflects a biomechanical perspective (e.g., goniometry, dynamometry, manual muscle testing [MMT]), whereas another facility's assessment reflects a sensorimotor perspective (e.g., Hand Active Sensation Test, stereognosis, Arm Dystonia Disability Scale).[78]

The sections that follow explore common assessments performed as part of an upper extremity battery of evaluations. There is a gamut of assessments for conditions not presented in this text.[46]

TABLE 5.1 Definitions of Types of Validity

Type of Validity	Definition
Construct validity	The degree to which a theoretical construct is measured by the tool
Content validity	The degree to which the items in a tool reflect the content domain being measured
Face validity	Determination if a tool appears to be measuring what it is intended to measure
Criterion validity	The degree to which a tool correlates with a gold standard or criterion test (It can be assessed as concurrent or predictive validity.)
Concurrent validity	The degree to which the scores from a tool correlate with a criterion test when both tools are administered relatively at the same time

TABLE 5.2 Definitions of Types of Reliability

Type of Reliability	Definition
Interrater reliability	The degree to which two raters can obtain the same ratings for a given variable
Test/retest reliability	The degree to which a test is stable based on repeated administrations of the test to the same individuals over a specified time interval
Internal consistency	The degree to which each item of a test measures the same trait
Intrarater reliability	The degree to which one rater can reproduce the same score in administering the tool on multiple occasions to the same individual

Pain

Several options for evaluating pain exist, including interview questions, rating scales, body diagrams, and questionnaires. Box 5.1 lists questions related to pain that can be asked of the client.[25] Therapists often use a combination of pain measures to obtain an accurate representation of the client's pain.[39]

The **verbal analog scale (VeAS)** is used to determine the person's perception of pain intensity. The client rates pain on a scale from 0 to 10 (0 refers to no pain, and 10 refers to the worst pain ever experienced). Reliability scores for retesting under the VeAS are moderate to high, ranging from 0.67 to 0.96.[29,34] When correlated with the **visual analog scale (ViAS)**, the VeAS had a reliability score of 0.79 to 0.95.[29,34] Finch and colleagues[29] reported that a three-point change in score is necessary to establish a true pain intensity change. Thus the VeAS may be limited to detecting small changes, and clients with cognitive deficits may have trouble following instructions to complete the VeAS.[29,30]

A ViAS is also used to rate pain intensity. A client refers to a 10-cm horizontal line, with the left side of the line representing "no pain" and the right side representing "pain as bad as it could be." The client indicates pain level by marking a slash on the line, which represents the pain experienced. The distance from no pain to the slash is measured and recorded in centimeters (Fig. 5.2). The ViAS "may have a high failure rate because patients may have difficulty interpreting the instructions."[87] Some errors occur due to changes in length of the line resulting from photocopying.[39] The VeAS and ViAS are unidimensional assessments of pain (i.e., intensity).[39] Although test-retest is not applicable to self-reported measures, researchers demonstrated a high range of test-retest reliability (intraclass correlation coefficient [ICC] = 0.71 to 0.99).[22,29,34] When compared with the VeAS, concurrent validity measures ranged from 0.71 to 0.78.[22]

A body diagram consists of outlines of a body with front and back views (Fig. 5.3). The client is asked to shade or color in the location of pain that corresponds to the painful body part. Colored pencils corresponding to a legend can be used to represent different intensities or types of pain, such as numbness, pins and needles, burning, aching, throbbing, and superficial.

Self-report questionnaires are commonly used. Questionnaires such as the Short Form-36 (SF-36), Disabilities of the Arm, Shoulder, and Hand (DASH), and disease- or condition-specific questionnaires exist.[25]

Therapists may use a more formal pain assessment, such as the McGill Pain Questionnaire (MPQ)[26] or the Schultz Pain Assessment.[87] Although formal assessments usually take more time to administer than screening tools, they comprehensively assess many aspects of pain and may provide important information related to the person's diagnosis, intervention needs, and prognosis.[60]

Melzack[49] developed the MPQ, which is widely used in clinical practice and for research purposes. The MPQ consists of a pain rating index, total number of word descriptors, and a present pain index. In its original version the MPQ required 10 to 15 minutes to administer. The MPQ is a valid and reliable assessment tool. High internal consistency within the MPQ exists with correlations of 0.89 to 0.90.[49] Test-retest reliability scores for the MPQ are reported as 70.3%.[49]

BOX 5.1   Assessment Questions Relating to Pain[a]

Location and Nature of Pain
- Where do you feel uncomfortable (pain)?
- Does your discomfort (pain) feel deep or superficial?
- Is your problem (pain) constant or intermittent? If constant, does it vary in intensity?
- How long does your discomfort (pain) last?
- What is the frequency of your discomfort (pain)?
- How long have you had this problem (pain)?
- Are you experiencing discomfort (pain) right now?

Pain Manifestations
- How would you describe your discomfort (pain): throbbing, aching/sharp, dull, electrical, and so on?
- Does the discomfort (pain) move or spread to other areas?
- Does movement aggravate the discomfort (pain)?
- Do certain positions aggravate the discomfort (pain)? If yes, can you show me the movement or postures that cause the discomfort (pain)?
- Do you have stiffness with your discomfort (pain)?
- Do you have discomfort (pain) at rest?
- Do you have discomfort (pain) during the morning or night?
- Does the discomfort (pain) wake you from sleep?
- Do you have discomfort (pain) during particular activities?
- Do you experience discomfort (pain) after performing particular activities?
- What makes your discomfort (pain) worse?
- What helps relieve your discomfort (pain)?
- What have you tried to reduce your discomfort (pain)?
- What worked to reduce your discomfort (pain)?

[a]Therapists working with persons experiencing chronic pain may find that focusing on pain and repeating the word *pain* over and over is not beneficial. Therapists may select questions according to their judgment and substitute alternative words for pain when necessary.

The visual analog scale (ViAS)

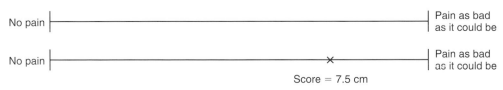

No pain |———————————————————————————| Pain as bad as it could be

No pain |—————————————————————×———| Pain as bad as it could be

Score = 7.5 cm

Fig. 5.2 The visual analog scale (ViAS) and an example of a completed ViAS with a score of 7.5.

For assessment of pediatric pain, self-reporting measures are considered the gold standard.[55] A therapist determines the child's concepts of quantification, classification, and matching before administering simple pain intensity scales.[13] Nonverbal scales using facial expressions and the ViAS are commonly used. Children's ability to report pain is affected by their stage in child development. Table 5.3 outlines ages and recommendations associated with the various types of reporting in children.

Skin

A thorough examination of the surface condition and contour of the extremity may define possible pathological conditions, which may influence orthotic design. During the examination the therapist observes and documents the skin's color, temperature, and texture. The therapist observes the skin for muscle atrophy, scarring, edema, hair patterns, sweat patterns, and abnormal masses. Clients with fragile skin (especially persons who are older, who have been taking steroids for a long time, or who have diabetes) require careful monitoring. For these persons the therapist carefully considers the orthotic material to prevent harm to the already fragile skin (see Chapter 16).

Regarding skin, most adult clients are aware if they have skin allergies. Some are allergic to bandages, adhesive, and latex (all of which can be used in the orthotic process). To avoid skin reactions, the therapist asks each client to disclose any types of allergy before choosing orthotic materials. When persons are unsure of skin allergies, the therapist should be aware that thermoplastic material, padding, and strapping supplies may create an allergic reaction. Therapists educate persons to monitor for any rashes or other skin reactions that develop from wearing an orthosis. The client experiencing a reaction should generally discontinue wearing the orthosis and report immediately to the therapist.

Scars

Scarring often results after burns, trauma, and surgical procedures. Scars have the potential for devastating impacts on function. Numerous scales exist to measure scars and scarring: Patient and Observer Scar Assessment Scale, Manchester Scar Scale, Modified Vancouver Scar Scale, Stony Brook Scar Evaluation Scale, and Patient Scar Assessment Questionnaire.[24,56] Most of these subjective scar assessment scales consider factors such as scar height or thickness, surface area, pliability, texture, pigmentation, and vascularity. It should be noted that these scar assessments are limited in use for studying large scars and for assessing the function effects of scars.[24,56]

Veins and Lymphatics

Normally the veins on the dorsum of the hand are easy to see and palpate. They are cordlike structures. Any tenderness, pain, redness, or firmness along the course of veins is noted.[58] Venous thrombosis, subcutaneous fibrosis, or lymphatic obstruction causes edema.[53]

Wounds

An assessment of wounds generally includes the size, depth, color, drainage (exudate), and odor. The therapist measures wound or incision size (usually in centimeters) and assesses discharge from wounds for color, amount, and odor. If there is concern about the discharge being a sign of infection, a wound culture is obtained by the medical staff to identify the source of infection, and appropriate medication is prescribed. Such warning signs of potential infection include yellow or green drainage, foul odor, and increased temperature of the skin surface.[40]

Wounds are classified by color: black, yellow, or red.[16] A black wound consists of dark, thick eschar, which impedes epithelialization. A yellow wound ranges in color from ivory to green-yellow (e.g., colonization with *Pseudomonas*). Typically, yellow wounds are covered with purulent discharge. A red wound indicates the presence of granulation tissue and is normal. Red wounds should be protected from mechanical forces, such as tapes, dressings, whirlpool agitation, and so on.[81]

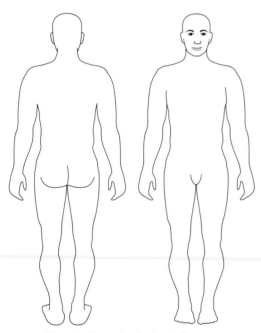

Fig. 5.3 Example of a body diagram.

TABLE 5.3	Children's Report of Pain
Age	**Report**
2 years	Presence and location of pain
3 to 4 years	Presence, location, and intensity of pain
	3 years old: Use a three-level pain intensity scale
	4 years old: Use a four- to five-item scale
5 years	Begin to use pain rating scales
8 years	Rate quality of pain

Data from O'Rourke, D. (2004). The measurement of pain in infants, children, and adolescents: from policy to practice. *Physical Therapy, 84,* 560–570.

Many wounds consist of a variety of colors.[16] Intervention focuses on treating the most serious color initially. For example, in the presence of eschar (common after thermal and crush injuries) a wound takes on a white or yellow-white color. Part of the intervention regimen for eschar is mechanical, chemical, or surgical debridement, which usually must be done before orthotic prescription. Debridement may result in a yellow wound. The yellow wound is managed by cleansing and dressing techniques to assist in the removal of debris. Once the desired red wound bed is achieved, it is protected by dressings.[83]

Because open wounds threaten exposure to the person's body fluids, the therapist follows universal precautions. The following precautions were derived from the Centers for Disease Control and Prevention (CDC)[65]:

- Wear gloves for all procedures that may involve contact with body fluids.
- Change gloves after contact with each person.
- Wear masks for procedures that may produce aerosols or splashing.
- Wear protective eyewear or face shields for procedures generating droplets or splashing.
- Wear gowns or aprons for procedures that may produce splashing or contamination of clothing.
- Wash hands immediately after removal of gloves and after contact with each person.
- Replace torn gloves immediately.
- Replace gloves after punctures, and discard the instrument causing the puncture.
- Cleanse areas of skin with soap and water immediately if contaminated with blood or body fluids.
- Make available mouthpieces, resuscitation bags, and other ventilatory devices for resuscitation to reduce the need for mouth-to-mouth resuscitation techniques.
- Take extra care when using sharps (especially needles and scalpels).
- Place all used disposable sharps in puncture-resistant containers.

Many upper extremity injuries result in wounds, whether from trauma or surgery. Therefore therapists must know the stages of wound healing. The healing of wounds is a cellular process.[81] Experts identified three overlapping stages,[69,70,81] which consist of the (1) inflammatory or epithelialization, (2) proliferative or fibroblastic, and (3) maturation and remodeling phases.[69,70,81]

The first stage of wound healing is the inflammatory (exudative) phase,[69,70,72,81] which begins immediately after trauma and lasts 3 to 6 days in a clean wound. Vasoconstriction occurs during the first 5 to 10 minutes, leading to platelet adhesion of the damaged vessel wall and resulting in clot formation. This activity stimulates fibroblast proliferation. During the inflammatory phase for a repaired tendon, cells proliferate on the outer edge of the tendon bundles during the first 4 days.[71] By day 7, these cells migrate into the substance of the tendon. In addition, there is vascular proliferation within the tendon, which provides the basis for intrinsic tendon healing.[18] Extrinsic repair of the tendon occurs when the adjacent tissues provide collagen-producing fibroblasts and blood vessels.[45] Fibrovascular tissue that infiltrates from tissues surrounding the tendon can become future adhesions. Adhesions prevent tendon excursion if allowed to mature with immobilization.[71]

The second stage of wound healing is the fibroblastic (reparative) phase, which begins 2 to 3 days after the injury and lasts approximately 2 to 6 weeks.[69,70,72,81] During this stage, epithelial cells migrate to the wound bed. Fibroblasts begin to multiply 24 to 36 hours after the injury. The fibroblasts initiate the process of collagen synthesis.[81] The fibers link closely and increase tensile strength. A balanced interplay between collagen synthesis and its remodeling and reorganization prevents hypertrophic scarring. During tendon healing the proliferative phase begins by day 7 and is marked by collagen synthesis.[18] In a tendon repair where there is no gap between the tendon ends, collagen appears to bridge the repair.[71] Collagen fibers and fibroblasts are initially oriented perpendicularly to the axis of the tendon. However, by day 10 the new collagen fibers begin to align parallel to the longitudinal collagen bundles of the tendon ends.[45]

The final stage is the maturation (remodeling) phase. This phase is seen typically after day 21 and can last up to 1 or 2 years after the injury.[69–71,81] During the maturation stage the tensile strength continually increases. Initially the scar may appear red, raised, and thick, but with maturation a normal scar softens and becomes more pliable. The maturation phase for healing tendons is lengthier than the time needed for skin or muscle because the blood supply to the tendons is much less.[71] Tendon strength increases in a predictable fashion.[71] Smith[71] points out that in 1941 Mason and Allen first described how tensile strength of a repaired tendon progresses. From 3 to 12 weeks after tendon repair, mobilized tendons appear to be twice as strong as immobilized tendons. At 12 weeks, immobilized tendons have approximately 20% of normal tendon strength. In comparison, mobilized tendons at 12 weeks have 50% of normal tendon strength.

Bone

When assessing a person who has a skeletal injury, the therapist reviews the surgery and radiology reports. The therapist places importance on knowing the stability level of the fracture reduction, the method the physician used to maintain good alignment, the amount of time since the fracture's repair, and fixation devices present in the upper extremity. A physician may request that a therapist fabricate an orthotic after the fracture heals. On occasion the therapist may fabricate a custom orthosis or use a commercial fracture brace to stabilize the fracture before healing is complete. For example, for a person with a humeral fracture a commercially available humeral cuff may be prescribed.

The rationale for using a commercially fabricated fracture brace rather than fabricating a custom orthosis is based on time, client comfort, ease of application, and cost. Custom fabrication of fracture braces can be challenging, because the client is typically in pain and the custom orthosis involves the use of large pieces of thermoplastic material, which can be difficult to control and often require more than one person to apply. A commercial fracture brace saves the therapist's time and therefore minimizes expense. A commercial brace reduces donning and doffing for fitting, which may be uncomfortable for the client. Indications for fabricating a custom fracture brace include bracing extremely small or large extremities.

Joint and Ligament

Joint stability is important to assess and is evaluated by carefully applying a manual stress to any specific ligament. Each digital articulation achieves its stability through the collateral ligaments and a dense palmar plate.[9] The therapist carefully assesses the continuity, length, and glide of these ligaments. Joint play or accessory motion of a joint is assessed by grading the elicited symptoms upon passive movement. The grading system is as follows[82]:

- 0 = Ankylosis
- 1 = Extremely hypomobile
- 2 = Slightly hypomobile
- 3 = Normal
- 4 = Slightly hypermobile
- 5 = Extremely hypermobile
- 6 = Unstable

Unstable joints, subluxations, dislocations, and limited PROM directly affect orthotic provision. Lateral stress on finger joints should be avoided. The person may wear an orthosis to prevent unequal stress on the collateral ligaments.[11]

Muscle and Tendon

Tensile strength is the amount of long-axis force a muscle or tendon can withstand.[28] When a tendon is damaged or undergoes surgical repair, tensile strength directly affects the amount of force an orthosis exerts. Tensile strength mandates which exercises or activities a person can safely perform.

Proximal musculature affects distal musculature tension in persons experiencing spasticity. For example, wrist position influences the amount of tension placed on finger musculature. When the therapist attempts to increase wrist extension in the presence of spasticity, the wrist, hand, and fingers must be incorporated into the orthotic design. If the orthotic design addresses only wrist extension, the result may be increased finger flexion. Conversely, if the orthotic design addresses only the fingers, the wrist may move into greater flexion.

Nerve

Sensory evaluations determine areas of diminished or absent sensibility. Conventional tests for protective sensibility include the sharp/dull and hot/cold assessments. Discriminatory sensibilities include assessment for stereognosis, proprioception, kinesthesia, tactile location, and light touch. Two-point discrimination testing is recommended as a quick screening for sensibility[10] (Fig. 5.4). Two-point discrimination testing is most accurate on the fingertips.[81] In addition, the American Society for Surgery of the Hand[2] recommends static and moving two-point discrimination tests. The Semmes-Weinstein Monofilament Test results in detailed mapping of the level of functional sensibility, particularly during rehabilitation of peripheral nerve injury (Fig. 5.5). This mapping is useful to physicians, therapists, clients, case managers, and employers.[76] The Semmes-Weinstein Monofilament Test is the most reliable sensation test available and is often used as the comparison for concurrent validity studies.[17]

Therapists searching for objective sensory assessment data should be aware that "tests that were considered objective in the past can be demonstrated to be subjective in application dependent on the technique of the examiner."[5,6] For example, when administering the Semmes-Weinstein Monofilament Test, if the stimulus is applied too quickly, "the force can result in an overshoot beyond the desired stimulus"[6] and affect the test results. In addition, even when the Semmes-Weinstein Monofilament Test is administered with excellent technique, the cooperation and comprehension of the client are required.

Various screen tests assist the therapist in gathering information about suspected peripheral nerve issues (Table 5.4). When peripheral nerve injuries have occurred or are suspected, a Tinel test can be conducted. A Tinel test can be performed in two ways. The first method involves gently tapping over the suspected entrapment site to help determine whether entrapment is present. The second method consists of tapping the nerve distal to proximal. The location where the paresthesias are felt is considered the level to which a nerve has regenerated after Wallerian degeneration (i.e., degeneration of the axon terminal) has occurred. A person has a positive Tinel sign if tingling or shooting sensations in one of two areas occurs (1) at the site of tapping or (2) in a direction distal from the tapped area.[58] If the person experiences paresthesia or hyperparesthesia in a direction proximal to the tapped area, the Tinel test is negative.

A Phalen sign is present if a person feels similar symptoms to a positive Tinel test while resting elbows on the table and flexing the wrists for 15 to 60 seconds.[66] Phalen sign may indicate a median nerve problem. Tinel and Phalen signs can be positive in normal subjects.[68]

A Froment sign is a positive test outcome when a client is asked to forcibly hold a piece of paper between the thumb and the radial side of the index finger—so that the person is "pulling the paper" in opposite direction. A positive Froment sign is noted in the thumb's position of flexion at the interphalangeal (IP) joint. Similar to the Froment sign is the Jeanne sign. The Jeanne sign is positive when the client is asked to pinch the tips of the index and thumb and the position of the thumb presents with IP flexion and MP joint hyperextension. Comparisons to both hands is important to conduct (see Chapter 14).

Cervical nerve problems are ruled out before a diagnosis of peripheral nerve injury is made.[48] For example, a person may have signs similar to carpal tunnel syndrome in conjunction with complaints of neck pain. In the absence of a cervical nerve screen, the person may be misdiagnosed with carpal tunnel syndrome when the cause of the problems is

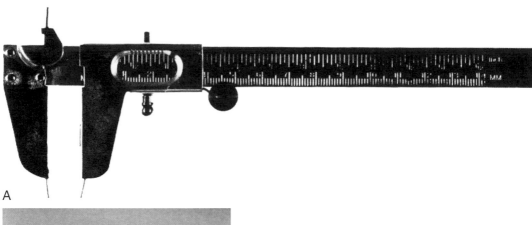

A

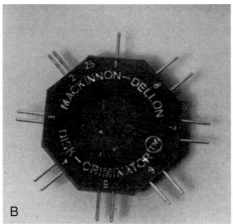

B

Fig. 5.4 The recommended instruments for testing two-point discrimination include the Boley gauge (A) and the Disk-Criminator (B). (From Hunter, J. M., Mackin, E. J., & Callahan, A.D. [Eds.]. [1995]. *Rehabilitation of the hand: Surgery and therapy* [4th ed., p. 146]. St. Louis, MO: Mosby.)

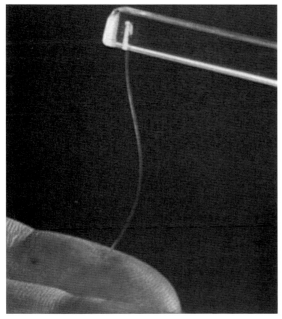

Fig. 5.5 The monofilament collapses when a force dependent on filament diameter and length is reached, controlling the magnitude of the applied touch pressure. (From Hunter, J. M., Mackin, E. J., & Callahan, A.D. [Eds.]. [1995]. *Rehabilitation of the hand: Surgery and therapy* [4th ed., p. 76]. St. Louis, MO: Mosby.)

TABLE 5.4 Screen Tests for Suspected Nerve Conditions

Name of Screen Test	Test Position	Positive Test Outcome
Tinel sign	1. Gently tapping over the suspected entrapment site 2. Tapping the nerve pathway distal to proximal	Tingling, numbness, paresthesia distal to area tapped
Phalen sign	With the client resting elbows on the table and flexing the wrists for 15 to 60 seconds	Tingling, numbness, paresthesias in thumb, index and radial side of middle finger (median nerve)
Froment sign	With the client forcibly holding a piece of paper between the thumb and the radial side of the index finger—so that the person is pulling the paper in opposite directions	Thumb IP flexion
Jeanne sign	With the client pinching the tips of the index and thumb	Thumb IP flexion with MCP hyperextension

IP, Interphalangeal; *MCP,* metacarpophalangeal.

actually cervical nerve involvement. In the absence of electrical studies, some physicians mistakenly make the diagnosis of peripheral nerve compression.

During the fitting process, hand orthoses may cause pressure and friction on vulnerable areas with impaired sensibility. If a person has decreased sensibility, the therapist uses an orthotic design with long, well-molded components. The reason for using such an orthosis is to distribute the forces of the orthosis over as much surface area as possible, thereby decreasing the potential for pressure areas.

When an orthosis is placed across the wrist, the superficial branch of the radial nerve is at risk for compression. If the radial edge of the forearm orthosis stops beyond the midlateral forearm near the dorsum of the thumb, the superficial branch of the radial nerve can be compressed.[11] During the evaluation of orthotic fit, therapists should be aware of the signs of compression of the superficial branch of the radial nerve. Orthoses that cause compression require adjustments to decrease the pressure near the dorsum of the thumb.

Vascular Status

To understand the vascular status of a diseased or injured hand, the therapist monitors the skin's color (i.e., red, pale, or cyanotic) and temperature and checks for edema. The therapist clearly defines areas of questionable tissue viability and adapts orthoses to prevent obstruction of arterial and venous circulation. To assess radial and ulnar artery patency, the therapist uses an Allen test. The Allen test is performed by having the client open and close the hand to exsanguinate it while the therapist occludes the radial and ulnar arteries by applying pressure on them at the wrist. The client opens the hand until it appears white and blanched. The therapist then releases the pressure on either the radial or ulnar artery, looking for revascularization evidenced by a change in color from white to pink of the hand. If the hand does not flush with the pink color, the artery is occluded[63] (Fig. 5.6).

A therapist can take circumferential measurements proximal and distal to the location of orthotic application. Then, after applying the orthosis to the extremity, the therapist measures the same areas and compares them with the previous measurements. An increase in measurements taken while the orthosis is on indicates that the orthosis is exerting too much force on the underlying tissues. This situation poses a risk for circulation. When fluctuating edema is present, the therapist should make the orthotic design larger. A well-fitting circumferential orthosis, sometimes in conjunction with a pressure garment, can control or eliminate fluctuating edema. In addition, fluctuating edema may signal poor compliance with elevation. A sling and education about its use may assist in edema control.

The therapist can also use the Fingernail Blanch Test to assess circulation.[63] Long-lasting blanched areas of the fingertips indicate restricted circulation.

When a therapist applies an orthosis to the upper extremity, the skin should maintain its natural color. Red or purple areas indicate obstructed venous circulation. Dusty or white areas indicate obstructed arterial circulation. Orthoses causing circulation problems must be modified or discontinued.

Range of Motion and Strength

The therapist records active and passive motions when no contraindications are present (Fig. 5.7) and takes measurements on both extremities for a baseline data comparison. The therapist records total active motion (TAM) and total passive motion (TPM).[63] Grasp and pinch strengths are completed and documented only when no contraindications are present (Figs 5.8 and 5.9). MMT assesses muscle strength but should be done only when there are no contraindications. For example, if a person with rheumatoid arthritis in an exacerbated state is being evaluated, MMT should be avoided to prevent further exacerbation of pain and swelling.

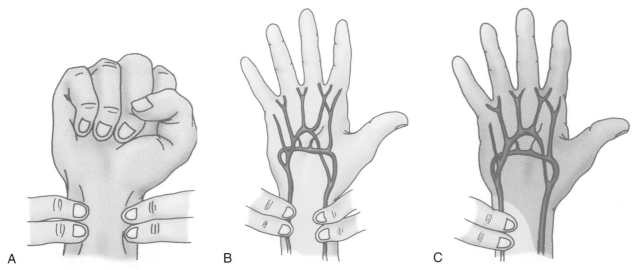

Fig. 5.6 The Allen test for arterial patency. (From Skirven, T. M., Osterman, A. L., Fedorczyk, J. M., et al. [Eds.]. [2011]. *Rehabilitation of the hand and upper extremity* [6th ed., p. 69]. St. Louis, MO: Mosby.)

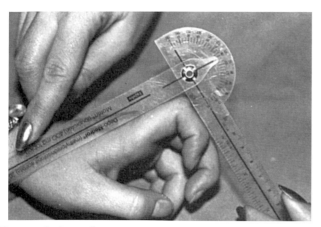

Fig. 5.7 Goniometric measurements of active and passive motion are taken regularly when no contraindications are present. (From Hunter, J. M., Mackin, E. J., & Callahan, A.D. [Eds.]. [1996]. *Rehabilitation of the hand: Surgery and therapy* [4th ed., p. 34]. St. Louis, MO: Mosby.)

Coordination and Dexterity

Hand coordination and dexterity are needed for many functional performance tasks, and it is important to evaluate them. Many standardized tests for coordination and dexterity exist, including the Nine Hole Peg Test (Fig. 5.10), Minnesota Rate of Manipulation Test (MRMT), Crawford Small Parts Dexterity Test, Purdue Pegboard Test, Rosenbusch Test of Dexterity, and Valpar Component Work Samples (VCWS) tests. Most dexterity tests are based on time measurements, and normative data are available for these tests. In particular, the VCWS uses a methods time measurement (MTM). MTM is a method of analyzing work tasks to determine how long a trained worker requires to complete a certain task at a rate that can be sustained for an 8-hour workday.

The Sequential Occupational Dexterity Assessment (SODA) was developed in the Netherlands.[79] The SODA is a test to measure hand dexterity and the client's perception of difficulty and pain while performing four unilateral and eight

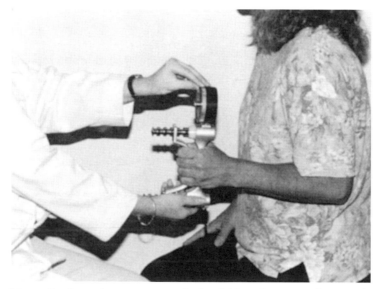

Fig. 5.8 Therapists use the Jamar dynamometer to obtain reliable and accurate grip strength measurements. (From Tubiana, R., Thomine, J. M., & Mackin, E. [1996]. *Examination of the hand and wrist* [p. 344.]. St. Louis, MO: Mosby.)

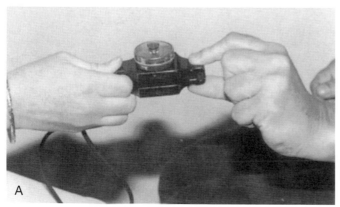
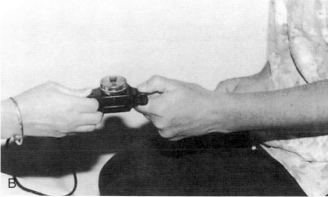

Fig. 5.9 The pinch meter measures pulp pinch (A) and lateral pinch (B). (From Tubiana, R., Thomine, J. M., & Mackin, E. [1996]. *Examination of the hand and wrist* [p. 344.]. St. Louis, MO: Mosby.)

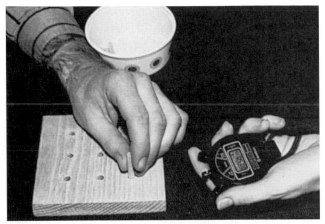

Fig. 5.10 The Nine Hole Peg Test is a quick test for coordination. (From Hunter, J. M., Mackin, E. J., & Callahan, A.D. [Eds.]. [1996]. *Rehabilitation of the hand: Surgery and therapy* [4th ed., p. 1158]. St. Louis, MO: Mosby.)

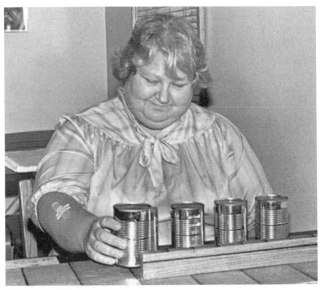

Fig. 5.11 The Jebsen-Taylor Hand Test assesses the ability to perform prehension tasks. (From Hunter, J. M., Mackin, E. J., & Callahan, A.D. [Eds.]. [1996]. *Rehabilitation of the hand: Surgery and therapy* [4th ed., p. 98]. St. Louis, MO: Mosby.)

bilateral activity of daily living (ADL) tasks.[47] The authors of a study conducted on 62 clients with rheumatoid arthritis concluded that "The SODA is also valid and reliable for assessing disability in a clinical situation that cannot be generalized to the home."[47] More research is needed to test such findings.

Function

Function is assessed by observation, interview, task performance, and standardized testing. Close observation during the interview and orthotic fabrication gives the therapist information regarding the person's views of the injury and impairment. The therapist observes the person for protected or guarded positioning, abnormal hand movements, muscle substitutions, spontaneous movement and pain involvement during functional tasks. During evaluation the person's willingness for the therapist to touch and move the affected extremity is noted.

During the initial interview the therapist questions the person about the status of ADLs, instrumental activities of daily living (IADLs), and avocational and vocational activities. The therapist notes problem areas. Having clients perform tasks as part of an evaluation may result in more detailed information, particularly when self-reporting accuracy is questioned by the therapist.

The therapist may use standardized hand function assessments. The Jebsen-Taylor Hand Function Test results in objective measurements of standardized tasks with norms the therapist uses for comparison (Fig. 5.11).[38] The Dellon modification of the Moberg Pick-up Test evaluates hand function when the person grasps common objects (Fig. 5.12).[50] Similar objects in the test require the person to have sensory discrimination and prehensile abilities.[10]

Other outcome and occupation-based assessments recommended for assessment of upper extremity injuries or conditions include the Canadian Occupational Performance Measure (COPM), the DASH, the SF-36, the Patient Specific Functional Scale, Handwriting Assessment Battery (HAB), and Manual Ability Measure (MAM).[35,41,75,86]

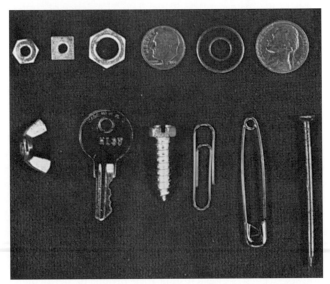

Fig. 5.12 Items used in the Dellon modification of the Moberg Pick-up Test. (From Hunter, J. M., Mackin, E. J., & Callahan, A.D. [Eds.]. [1996]. *Rehabilitation of the hand: Surgery and therapy* [4th ed., p. 608]. St. Louis, MO: Mosby.)

The COPM is a client-centered outcome measure used to assess self-care, productivity, and leisure.[43] Clients rate their performance and satisfaction with performance on a 1- to 10-point scale. The result is a weighted individualized client goal plan.[42] The COPM is a top-down assessment, which is completed before administration of tests to evaluate performance components. Test-retest reliability was reported as ICC = 0.63 for performance and ICC = 0.84 for satisfaction—as cited in Case-Smith, "Validity was estimated by correlating COPM change scores with changes in overall function as rated by caregivers (r = 0.55, r = 0.56), therapist (r = 0.30, r = 0.33), and clients (r = 0.26, r = 0.53)."[12,62] The COPM may take more time to administer than other tools. In addition, therapists administering the COPM should be trained in its administration, scoring, and interpretation.

The DASH is a standardized questionnaire rating disability and symptoms related to upper extremity conditions.[19] The measure is available as a QuickDASH (11 items) as well as a longer version, DASH (30 items). The DASH includes 30 predetermined questions that explore function within performance areas. The client rates current ability to complete particular skills, such as opening a jar or turning a key, on a scale of 1 (no difficulty) to 5 (unable). Beaton and colleagues[4] studied reliability and validity of the DASH. Excellent test-retest reliability was reported (ICC = 0.96) in a study of 86 clients. Concurrent validity was established with correlations with other pain and function measures (r > 0.69). Internal consistency is reported at <0.95, indicating no item redundancy.[32] The full DASH, due to its greater precision, is recommended when therapists wish to monitor pain and function.[19]

The SF-36 measures eight aspects of health that contribute to quality of life.[85] The SF-36 "yields an eight scale profile of functional health and well-being scores, as well as psychometrically based physical and mental health summary measures and a preference based health utility index."[85] Reliability scores range from r = 0.43 to r = 0.96.[8] Evidence of content, concurrent, criterion, construct, and predictive evidence of validity have been established.[84] The tool has been translated for use in more than 60 countries and languages.

The Patient Specific Functional Scale (PSFS) is a self-report measure that was developed to elicit and record functional issues that are important to the client.[77,89] The instrument takes 4 minutes to complete and is easy to administer.[59] Clients identify three activities they have difficulty in performing. Then clients rate their current lives of difficulty associated with each of the three activities. The scoring uses an 11-point scale from 0 (unable to perform the activity) to 10 (able to perform at the same level as before the injury/problem). The PSFS is available in several languages[44,59] and appears to have good ability to detect clinical change in clients with a variety of musculoskeletal diagnoses.[1,15,31,36,77]

The HAB consists of three sections with items from eight subtests.[23] Each subtest results in a profile of performance related to pen control and manipulation, writing speed, and legibility. Administration of the HAB requires approximately 20 minutes and another 15 minutes to score. Although the HAB demonstrates excellent interrater reliability, further testing is needed.

The MAM is available in two versions: MAM-16 (16 items) and MAM-36 (36 items).[13,14,57] The MAM is occupation based in that the assessment items are everyday tasks, such as eating a sandwich, cutting meat, and wringing a towel. Clients use a 4-point ordinal rating scale that asks how easy or hard it is to perform such tasks (1 = cannot do, 2 = very hard, 3 = a little hard, 4 = easy). Administration takes approximately 15 minutes. The MAM-36 is appropriate to use with clients who have neurological and musculoskeletal disorders.[13] Research indicates that MAM-36 outcomes positively correlate with improvements in task performance speeds and grip strength.[14]

Therapists are interested in determining if any changes in function are made during intervention. Decisions to continue therapy (with implications for reimbursement) include if the client is progressing. Thus the assessments chosen must be sensitive to note the changes over time. For example, in a study of three patient report outcome (PRO) measures in persons with hand fractures, the ability to describe functional limitations in a client cohort were found.[86] The DASH and Michigan Hand Outcomes Questionnaire (MHQ) were each able to articulate the functional limitations in the cohort of patients with hand fractures during a 2-month time frame.

Work

Evaluations of paid and unpaid work entail assessment of the work to be done and how the work is performed.[52] It is estimated that 36% of all functional capacity evaluations (FCEs) are conducted because of upper extremity and hand injuries.[52] Some facilities use a specific type of FCE system, such as the Blankenship System or the Key Method. Standardized testing includes the Work Evaluations Systems Technologies II (WEST II), the EPIC Lift Capacity (ELC), the Bennett Hand Tool Dexterity Test, the Purdue Pegboard, the MRMT, and the VCWS. Commercially available computerized tests can be administered in work evaluations. Isometric, isoinertial, and isokinetic tests can be performed on equipment tools manufactured by Cybex, Biodex, and Baltimore Therapeutic Equipment (BTE). FCEs frequently assess abnormal illness behavior and often include observation, psychometric testing, and physical or functional testing. New and experienced therapists should have specialized training in administering and interpreting FCEs because of the standardized nature of the examination and the legal implications of these assessments.[41]

Other Considerations

The person's motivation, health literacy, ability to understand and carry out instructions, and adherence may affect the type of orthosis the therapist chooses and how client education is provided. The tools available to assess health literacy are plentiful.[54,67,90] The Health Literacy Tool Shed[37] (http://health-literacy.bu.edu) is an example of one website that contains health literacy tools, measures, instruments, and items. Other resources online exist.

The therapist considers a person's vocational and avocational interests when designing an orthosis. Some persons wear more than one orthosis throughout the day to allow for completion of various activities. Particularly for athletes, orthotic designs are impacted by sport regulations and team physicians.[61] Athletes may wear one orthosis during play and a different orthosis when not playing. In addition, some persons wear one orthotic design during the day and a different design at night.

Related to client motivation during rehabilitation may be the presence or absence of a third-party payment source. Whenever possible, the therapist discusses payment issues with the client before completing the initial visit. If a third party is paying for the client's services, the therapist first determines whether that source intends to pay for any orthotic fabrication services. At times, some clients are very motivated to adhere to the rehabilitation program if they self-pay for the services. In other cases, when third-party reimbursement is quite good and the client is temporarily on a medical leave from work, the client may be less motivated and perhaps show signs of abnormal illness behavior. Terms such as *malingering, secondary gain, hypochondriasis, hysterical neurosis, conversion, somatization disorder, functional overlay,* and *nonorganic pain* have been used to describe abnormal illness behaviors.[52] With clients who appear to have obvious psychological issues, the therapist contacts the client's physician for a possible referral to appropriate psychological professionals. Gatchel and colleagues[33] reported the following red flags, which can assist the therapist in identifying such abnormal behaviors[7]:

- Client agitates other clients with disruptive behaviors.
- Client has no future work plan or changes to previous work plan.
- Client is applying for or receiving Social Security or long-term disability.
- Client opposes psychological services and refuses to answer questions or fill out forms.
- Client has obvious psychosis.
- Client has significant cognitive or neuropsychological deficits.
- Client expresses excessive anger at persons involved in case.
- Client is a substance abuser.
- Client's family is resistant to his or her recovery or return to work.
- Client has young children at home or has a short-term work history for primarily financial reasons.
- Client perpetually complains about the facility, staff, and program rather than being willing to deal with related physical and psychological issues.
- Client is chronically late to therapy and is noncompliant with excuses that do not check out.
- Client focuses on pain complaints in counseling sessions rather than dealing with psychological issues.

POST–ORTHOTIC PROVISION EVALUATION AND FOLLOW-UP

After the client has undergone the assessment process, intervention may include the provision of an orthosis. After the orthosis is fabricated, the therapist engages in an evaluation process of the orthosis. The orthotic evaluation includes determining orthotic precautions that must be relayed to the client via education. The therapist must ensure that the client understands the importance of the wearing regimen. The client must know how to care for the orthosis and identify any warning signs that follow-up care is needed from the therapist.

ORTHOTIC PRECAUTIONS

During the orthotic assessment, the therapist is aware of orthotic precautions. An ill-fitting orthosis can harm a person. Several precautions are outlined in Form 5.2, which a therapist uses as a check-off sheet. The therapist must not only educate a client about appropriate precautions but evaluate the client's understanding of them (i.e., health literacy—see Chapter 6). The client's understanding can be assessed by having him or her repeat important precautions to follow or by role-playing (e.g., "If this happens, what will you do?"). In follow-up visits the client can be questioned again to determine whether precautions are understood. Form 5.3 lists orthotic fabrication hints to follow. Adherence to the hints assists in avoiding situations that result in clients experiencing problems with their orthoses.

Pressure Areas

After fabricating an orthosis, the therapist does not allow the person to leave until the orthosis has been evaluated for problem areas. A general guideline is to have the person wear the orthosis at least 20 to 30 minutes after fabrication. Red areas should not be present 20 minutes after removal of the orthosis. Orthoses often require some adjustment. After receiving assurance that no pressure areas are present, the therapist instructs the person to remove the orthosis and to call if any problems arise. Persons with fragile skin are at high risk of developing pressure areas. The therapist provides the person with thorough written and verbal instructions on the wear and care of the orthosis. The instructions should include a phone number for emergencies. During follow-up visits, the therapist makes inquiries about the orthotic fit to determine whether adjustments are necessary in the design or wearing schedule.

Edema

The therapist completes an evaluation for excessive tightness of the orthosis or straps. Often edema is caused by inappropriate strapping, especially at the wrist or over the MCP joints. Strapping systems are evaluated and modified if they are contributing to increased edema. If the orthosis is too narrow, it may also inadvertently contribute to increased edema. Persons can usually wear orthoses over pressure garments if necessary. However, therapists must monitor circulation closely.

The therapist assesses edema by taking circumferential or volumetric measurements (Fig. 5.13).[80] When taking volumetric measurements, the therapist administers the test according to the testing protocol and then compares the involved extremity measurement with that of the uninvolved extremity. If edema fluctuates throughout the day, it is best to fabricate the orthosis when edema is present to ensure that the orthosis accommodates the edema fluctuation. When edema is minimal but changes during the day, the orthotic design must be wider to accommodate the fluctuating edema.[11]

Orthotic Regimen

Upon provision of an orthosis, the therapist determines a wearing schedule for the client. Most diagnoses allow persons to remove the orthoses for some type of exercise and hygiene. The therapist provides a written orthotic schedule and reviews the schedule with the person, nurse, and/or caregiver

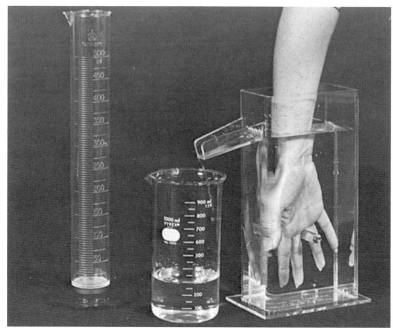

Fig. 5.13 The volumeter measures composite hand mass via water displacement. (From Hunter, J. M., Mackin, E. J., & Callahan, A.D. [Eds.]. [1996]. *Rehabilitation of the hand: Surgery and therapy* [4th ed., p. 63]. St. Louis, MO: Mosby.)

responsible for putting on and taking off the orthosis. If the person is confused, the therapist is responsible for instructing the appropriate caregiver regarding proper orthotic wear and care. The therapist must evaluate the client's or caregiver's understanding of the wearing schedule.

Clients wearing mobilizing (dynamic) orthoses follow several general precautions. Therapists must be cautious when instructing clients who must wear mobilizing (dynamic) orthoses during sleep. Because of moving parts on mobilization orthoses, people can accidentally scratch, poke, or cut themselves. Therefore, therapists must design orthoses with no sharp edges and must consider the possibility of using elastic traction (see Chapter 13).

Typically persons wear mobilizing (dynamic) orthoses for a few minutes out of each hour and gradually work up to longer time periods. As with all orthoses, a therapist never fabricates a mobilizing (dynamic) orthosis without checking its effect on the person. The therapist considers the diagnosis and appropriately schedules orthotic wearing. Often, but not always, an orthotic regimen allows for times of rest, exercise, hygiene, and skin relief. The therapist considers the client's daily activity schedule when designing the orthotic regimen. However, intervention goals must sometimes supersede the desire for the client to perform activities. In addition, the therapist uses clinical judgment to determine and adjust the orthotic wearing schedule and reevaluates the orthosis consistently to alter the intervention plan as necessary.

ADHERENCE

Based on the initial interview and statements from conversations, the therapist determines whether adherence with the wearing schedule and rehabilitation program is a problem. (Chapter 6 contains strategies to help persons with adherence and acceptance.) If the hand (or wrist, elbow, shoulder, etc.) demonstrates that the orthosis is not achieving its goal, the therapist must check that the orthosis is well designed and fits properly and then determine whether the orthosis is being worn. If the therapist is certain about the design and fit, adherence is probably poor. Clients returning for follow-up visits must bring their orthoses. The therapist can generally determine whether a client is wearing the orthosis by looking for signs of normal wear. Signs include dirty areas or scratches in the plastic, soiled straps, and nappy straps (caused by pulling the strap off the Velcro hook).

ORTHOTIC CARE

Therapists are responsible for educating persons about orthotic care. An evaluation of a person's understanding of orthotic care is completed before the client leaves the clinic or is discharged. Assessment is accomplished by asking the client to repeat instructions or demonstrate orthotic care. To keep the orthosis clean, washing the hand with warm water and a mild soap and cleansing the orthosis with rubbing alcohol are effective. The person or caregiver thoroughly dries the hand and orthosis before reapplication. Chlorine occasionally removes ink marks on the orthosis. Rubbing alcohol, chlorine bleach, and hydrogen peroxide are good disinfectants to use on the orthosis for infection control.

Persons should be aware that heat may melt their orthoses and should be careful not to leave their orthoses in hot cars, on sunny windowsills, or on radiators. Therapists discourage persons from making self-adjustments, including the heating of orthoses in microwave ovens (which may cause orthoses to soften, fold in on themselves, and adhere). If the person successfully softens the plastic, a burn could result from the application of hot plastic to the skin. However, clients are encouraged to make suggestions to improve an orthosis. Some therapists tend to ignore the client's ideas. Not only does this send a negative message to the client, but clients often have wonderful ideas that are too beneficial to discount.

👤 SELF-QUIZ 5.1ᵃ

For the following questions, circle either true (T) or false (F).

1. T F All physicians follow the same protocol for postoperative conditions.
2. T F Motivation may affect the person's adherence to wearing an orthosis, and thus determining the person's motivational level is an important task for the therapist.
3. T F The resting hand posture is 10 to 20 degrees of wrist extension, 10 degrees of ulnar deviation, 15 to 20 degrees of metacarpophalangeal (MCP) flexion, and partial flexion and abduction of the thumb.
4. T F Proximal musculature never affects distal musculature.
5. T F Therapists should encourage persons to carry their affected extremities in guarded or protective positions to ensure that no further harm is done to the injury.
6. T F A general guideline for evaluating orthotic fit is to have the person wear the orthosis for 20 minutes and then remove the orthosis. If no reddened areas are present after 20 minutes of orthosis removal, no adjustments are necessary.
7. T F All orthoses require 24 hours of wearing to be most effective.
8. T F Every person should receive an orthotic wearing schedule in written and verbal forms.
9. T F For infection control purposes, persons and therapists should use extremely hot water to clean orthoses.
10. T F Strength of a healing tendon is stronger when the tendon is immobilized rather than mobilized.
11. T F A red wound is a healthy wound.
12. T F A score of 10 on a verbal analog scale (VeAS) indicates that pain does not need to be addressed in the intervention plan.
13. T F Strapping, padding, and thermoplastic materials may cause a skin allergic reaction in some persons.
14. T F Assessments of function include the Nine Hole Peg Test and the Semmes-Weinstein Monofilament Test.

ᵃSee Appendix A for the answer key.

SUMMARY

Evaluation before orthotic provision is an integral part of the orthotic provision process. The evaluation process includes report reading, observation, interview, palpation, and formal and informal assessments. Evaluation before, during, and after orthotic provision results in the therapist's ability to understand how the orthosis affects function and how function affects the orthosis. A thorough evaluation process ultimately results in client satisfaction.

REVIEW QUESTIONS

1. What are components of a thorough hand examination before orthotic fabrication?
2. What is the posture of a resting hand?
3. What information should a therapist obtain about the person's history?
4. What sources can therapists use to obtain information about persons and their conditions?
5. What should a therapist be noting when palpating a client?
6. What observations should be made when a client first enters a clinic?
7. What types of formal upper extremity assessments for function are available?
8. What procedure can a therapist use when assessing whether a newly fabricated orthosis fits well on a person?
9. What precautions should a therapist keep in mind when designing and fabricating an orthosis?
10. How can a therapist evaluate a client's understanding of an orthotic wearing schedule?
11. What safeguard can a therapist employ to avoid skin reactions from orthotic materials?

REFERENCES

1. Adams Z, Newington L, Blakeway M: Evaluation of outcomes for patients attending a rehabilitation group after complex hand injury, *Hand Therapy* 17(30):68–782, 2012.
2. American Society for Surgery of the Hand: *The hand*, New York, 1983, Churchill Livingstone.
3. Bear-Lehman J, Abreu BC: Evaluating the hand: issues in reliability and validity, *Phys Ther* 69(12):1025–1031, 1989.
4. Beaton DE, Katz JN, Fossel AH, et al.: Measuring the whole or the parts? Validity, reliability, and responsiveness of the Disabilities of the Arm, Shoulder and Hand outcome measure in different regions of the upper extremity, *J Hand Ther* 14(2):128–146, 2001.

5. Bell-Krotoski JA: Sensibility testing: history, instrumentation, and clinical procedures. In Skirven TM, Osterman AL, Fedorczyk JM, et al.: *Rehabilitation of the hand: surgery and therapy*, ed 6, St. Louis, 2011, Mosby.

6. Bell-Krotoski JA, Buford WL: The force/time relationship of clinically used sensory testing instruments, *J Hand Ther* 10(4):297–309, 1997.

7. Blankenship KL: *The Blankenship system: functional capacity evaluation, The procedure manual*, Macon, GA, 1989, Blankenship Corporation, Panaprint.

8. Brazier JE, Harper R, Jones N, et al.: Validating the SF-36 Health Survey Questionnaire: new outcome measure for primary care, *Br Med J* 305:160–164, 1992.

9. Cailliet R: *Hand pain and impairment*, ed 4, Philadelphia, 1994, FA Davis.

10. Callahan AD: Sensibility testing: clinical methods. In Hunter JM, Schneider LH, Macklin EJ, et al.: *Rehabilitation of the hand: surgery and therapy*, ed 3, St. Louis, 1990, Mosby.

11. Cannon NM, Foltz RW, Koepfer JM, et al.: *Manual of hand splinting*, New York, 1985, Churchill Livingstone.

12. Case-Smith J: Outcomes in hand rehabilitation using occupational therapy services, *Am J Occup Ther* 57:499–506, 2003.

13. Chen C, Bode K: Psychometric validation of Manual Ability Measure (MAM-36) in patients with neurologic and musculoskeletal disorders, *Arch Phys Med Rehabil* 91(3):414–420, 2010.

14. Chen CC, Palmon O, Amini D: Responsiveness of the Manual Ability Measures-36 (MAM-36): changes in hand function using self-reported and clinician-reported assessments, *Am J Occup Ther* 68:187–193, 2014.

15. Cleland JA, Fritz JM, Whitman JM, Palmer JA: The reliability and construct validity of the neck disability index and Patient Specific Functional Scale in patients with cervical radiculopathy, *Spine* 31(5):598–602, 2006.

16. Cuzzell JZ: The new RYB color code: next time you assess an open wound, remember to protect red, cleanse yellow and debride black, *Am J Nurs* 88(10):1342–1346, 1988.

17. Dannenbaum RM, Michaelsen SM, Desrosiers J, et al.: Development and validation of two new sensory tests of the hand for patients with stroke, *Clin Rehabil* 16(6):630–639, 2002.

18. de Klerk AJ, Jouck LM: Primary tendon healing: an experimental study, *S Afr Med J* 62(9):276–281, 1982.

19. Disabilities of the Arm, Shoulder and Hand (nd). Retrieved from http://dash.iwh.on.ca/.

20. Ebrecht M, Hextall J, Kirtley LG, et al.: Perceived stress and cortisol levels predict speed of wound healing in healthy male adults, *Psychoneuroendocrinology* 29(6):798–809, 2004.

21. Ellem D: Assessment of the wrist, hand and finger complex, *J Man Manip Ther* 3(1):9–14, 1995.

22. Enebo BA: Outcome measures for low back pain: pain inventories and functional disability questionnaires, *J Chiropractic Technique* 10:68–74, 1998.

23. Faddy K, McCluskey A, Lannin NA: Interrater reliability of a new handwriting assessment battery for adults, *Am J Occup Ther* 62(5):595–599, 2008.

24. Fearmonti R, Bond J, Erdmann D: Levinson: a review of scar scales and scar measuring devices, *Open Access J Plast Surg* 10:354–363, 2010.

25. Fedorczyk JM: Pain management: principles of therapist's intervention. In Skirven TM, Osterman AL, Fedorczyk JM, et al.: *Rehabilitation of the hand: surgery and therapy*, ed 6, St. Louis, 2011, Mosby.

26. Fedorczyk JM, Michlovitz SL: Pain control: putting modalities in perspectives. In Hunter JM, Mackin EJ, Callahan AD, editors: *Rehabilitation of the hand: surgery and therapy*, St. Louis, 1999, Mosby.

27. Fess EE: Documentation: Essential elements of an upper extremity assessment battery. In Hunter JM, Mackin EJ, Callahan AD, editors: *Rehabilitation of the hand*, ed 4, St. Louis, 1995, Mosby.

28. Fess EE, Gettle KS, Philips CA, et al.: *Hand and upper extremity splinting: principles and methods*, ed 3, St. Louis, 2005, Elsevier Mosby.

29. Finch E, Brooks D, Stratford PW, et al.: *Physical rehabilitation outcome measures: a guide to enhanced clinical decision making*, ed 2, Baltimore, 2002, Lippincott, Williams & Wilkins.

30. Flaherty SA: Pain measurement tools for clinical practice and research, *AANA Journal* 64:133–140, 1996.

31. Gabel CP, What is the optimum tool for assessing the upper limb. A comparison of 10 different outcomes tools, *J Hand Ther* 29:356, 2016.

32. Gabel CP, Cuesta A: The Dash and Quick-Dash: Based on consensus findings for internal consistency and factor structure—Are they suitable and valid outcome measures for the upper limb? *J Hand Ther* 29:357–358, 2016.

33. Gatchel R, Mayer T, Capra P, et al.: Million behavioral health inventory: its utility in predicting physical function in patients with low back pain, *Arch Phys Med Rehabil* 67(12):879–882, 1996.

34. Good M, Stiller C, Zauszniewski JA, et al.: Sensation and distress of pain scales: reliability, validity, and sensitivity, *J Nurs Meas* 9(3):219–238, 2001.

35. Grice KO: The use of occupation-based assessments and intervention in the hand therapy setting—A survey, *J Hand Ther* 28(3):300–306, 2015.

36. Gross DP, Battié MC, Asante AK: The patient-specific functional scale: validity of workers' compensation claimants, *Arch Phys Med Rehabil* 89:1294–1299, 2008.

37. Health Literacy Tool Shed: http://healthliteracy.bu.edu.

38. Jebsen RH, Taylor N, Trieschmann RB, et al.: An objective and standardized test of hand function, *Arch Phys Med Rehabil* 50(6):311–319, 1969.

39. Kahl C, Cleland JA: Visual analogue scale, numeric pain rating scale and the McGill Pain Questionnaire: an overview of psychometric properties, *Phys Ther Rev* 10:123–128, 2005.

40. Klein LJ: Evaluation of the hand. In Cooper C, editor: *Fundamentals of hand therapy*, ed 2, St. Louis, 2014, Elsevier, pp 67–86.

41. Langer D, Luria S, Maeir A, Erez A: Occupation-based assessments and treatments of trigger finger: a survey of occupational therapists from Israel and the United States, *Occup Ther Int* 21:143–155, 2014.

42. Law M, Baptiste S, Carswell A, et al.: *Canadian occupational performance measures*, ed 3, Ottawa, Ontario, 1998, CAOT.

43. Law M, Baptiste S, McColl M, et al.: The Canadian occupational performance measure: an outcome measure for occupational therapy, *Can J Occup Ther* 57(2):82–87, 1990.

44. Lehtola V, Kaksonen A, Luomajoki H, Leinonen V, Gibbons S, Airaksinen O: Content validity and responsiveness of a finnish version of the patient-specific functional scale, *Eur J Physiother* 15:134–138, 2013.

45. Lindsay WK: Cellular biology of flexor tendon healing. In Hunter JM, Schneider LH, Mackin EJ, editors: *Tendon surgery in the hand*, St. Louis, 1987, Mosby.

46. MacDermid JC: Outcome measurement in upper extremity practice. In Skirven TM, Osterman AL, Fedorczyk JM, et al.: *Rehabilitation of the hand: surgery and therapy*, ed 6, St. Louis, 2011, Mosby.
47. Massy-Westropp N, Krishnan J, Ahern M: Comparing the AUSCAN osteoarthritis hand index, Michigan hand outcomes questionnaire, and sequential occupational dexterity assessment for patients with rheumatoid arthritis, *J Rheumatol* 31(10):1996–2001, 2004.
48. McClure P: Upper quarter screen. In Skirven TM, Osterman AL, Fedorczyk JM, et al.: *Rehabilitation of the hand: surgery and therapy*, ed 6, St. Louis, 2011, Mosby.
49. Melzack R: The McGill pain questionnaire: major properties and scoring methods, *Pain* 1:277–299, 1975.
50. Moberg E: Objective methods for determining the functional value of sensibility in the hand, *J Bone Joint Surg Br* 40:454–476, 1958.
51. Mosely LH, Finseth F: Cigarette smoking: impairment of digital blood flow and wound healing in the hand, *Hand* 9:97–101, 1977.
52. Mueller BA, Adams ED, Isaac CA: Work activities. In Van Deusen J, Brunt D, editors: *Assessment in occupational therapy and physical therapy*, Philadelphia, 1997, WB Saunders.
53. Neviaser RJ: Closed tendon sheath irrigation for pyogenic flexor tenosynovitis, *J Hand Surg* 3:462–466, 1978.
54. O'Hara J, Hawkins M, Batterham R, Dodson S, Osborne RH, Beauchamp A: Conceptualization and development of the Conversational Health Literacy Assessment Tool (CHAT), *BMC Health Serv Res* 18:199, 2018.
55. O'Rourke D: The measurement of pain in infants, children, and adolescents: from policy to practice, *Phys Ther* 84:560–570, 2004.
56. Packham TL, Mehta S, Iacob S, Patel V, Cooper M: Psychometric properties of assessments of scars and scarring: a systematic review, *J Hand Ther* 29:369–370, 2016.
57. Rallon CR, Chen CC: Relationship between performance based and self-reported assessment of hand function, *Am J Occup Ther* 62(5):574–579, 2008.
58. Ramadan AM: Hand Analysis. In Van Deusen J, Brunt D, editors: *Assessment in occupational therapy and physical therapy*, Philadelphia, 1997, WB Saunders.
59. Rosengren J, Brodin N: Validity and reliability of the Swedish version of the Patient Specific Functional Scale in patients treated surgically for carpometacarpal joint osteoarthritis, *J Hand Ther* 26:53–61, 2013.
60. Ross RG, LaStayo PC: Clinical assessment of pain. In Van Deusen J, Brunt D, editors: *Assessment in occupational therapy and physical therapy*, Philadelphia, 1997, WB Saunders.
61. Russell CR: Therapy challenges for athletes: splinting options, *Clin Sports Med* 43:181–191, 2015.
62. Sanford J, Law M, Swanson L, et al.: *Assessing clinically important change on an outcome of rehabilitation in older adults*, San Francisco, 1994, Paper presented at the Conference of the American Society of Aging.
63. Seftchick JL, Detullio LM, Fedorczyk JM, et al.: Clinical examination of the hand. In Skirven TM, Osterman AL, Fedorczyk JM, et al.: *Rehabilitation of the hand: surgery and therapy*, ed 6, St. Louis, 2011, Mosby.
64. Siana JE, Rex S, Gottrup F: The effect of cigarette smoking on wound healing, *Scand J Plast Reconstr SurgHand Surg* 23(3):207–209, 1989.
65. Singer DI, Moore JH, Byron PM: Management of skin grafts and flaps. In Hunter JM, Mackin EJ, Callahan AD, editors: *Rehabilitation of the hand: surgery and therapy*, ed 4, St. Louis, 1995, Mosby.
66. Skirven TM, Osterman AL: Clinical examination of the wrist. In Skirven TM, Osterman AL, Fedorczyk JM, et al.: *Rehabilitation of the hand: surgery and therapy*, ed 6, St. Louis, 2011, Mosby.
67. Smith DL, Gutman SA: Health literacy in occupational therapy practice and research, *Am J Occup Ther* 65(4):367–369, 2011.
68. Smith GN, Bruner AT: The neurologic examination of the upper extremity, physical medicine and rehabilitation, *State of the Art Reviews* 12(2):225–241, 1998.
69. Smith KL: Wound care for the hand patient. In Hunter JM, Schneider LH, Macklin EJ, et al.: *Rehabilitation of the hand: surgery and therapy*, ed 3, St. Louis, 1990, Mosby.
70. Smith KL: Wound care for the hand patient. In Hunter JM, Mackin EJ, Callahan AD, editors: *Rehabilitation of the hand: surgery and therapy*, ed 4, St. Louis, 1995, Mosby.
71. Smith KL: Wound healing. In Stanley BG, Tribuzi SM, editors: *Concepts in hand rehabilitation*, Philadelphia, 1992, FA Davis.
72. Staley MJ, Richard RL, Falkel JE: Burns. In O'Sullivan SB, Schmidtz TJ, editors: *Physical rehabilitation: assessment and treatment*, ed 3, Philadelphia, 1988, FA Davis.
73. Suk M, Hanson B, Norvell D, et al.: *Musculo-skeletal outcome measures and instruments*, Switzerland, 2005, AO Publishing.
74. Tarrier N, Gregg L, Edwards J, et al.: The influence of pre-existing psychiatric illness on recovery in burn injury patients: the impact of psychosis and depression, *Burns* 31:45–49, 2005.
75. The Canadian Occupational Performance Measure (nd). Retrieved from http://www.thecopm.ca/about/
76. Tomancik L: *Directions for using Semmes-Weinstein monofilaments*, San Jose, CA, 1987, North Coast Medical.
77. Valdes IK, Algar LA, Connors B, et al.: The use of patient-centered outcome measures by hand therapists: a practice survey, *J Hand Ther* 29:356–384, 2014.
78. Valdes K, Naughton N, Algar L: Sensorimotor interventions and assessments for the hand and wrist: a scoping reviewing, *J Hand Ther* 27:272–286, 2014.
79. Van Lankveld W, van't Pad Bosch P, Bakker J, et al.: Sequential occupational dexterity assessment (SODA): a new test to measure hand disability, *J Hand Ther* 9(1):27–32, 1996.
80. Villeco JP: Edema: therapist's management. In Skirven TM, Osterman AL, Fedorczyk JM, et al.: *Rehabilitation of the hand: surgery and therapy*, ed 6, St. Louis, 2011, Mosby.
81. Von Der Heyde RL: Evans RB: Wound classification and management. In Skirven TM, Osterman AL, Fedorczyk JM, et al.: *Rehabilitation of the hand: surgery and therapy*, ed 6, St. Louis, 2011, Mosby.
82. Wadsworth CT: Wrist and hand examination and interpretation, *J Orthop Sports Phys Ther* 5(3):108–120, 1983.
83. Walsh M, Muntzer E: Wound management. In Stanley BG, Tribuzzi SM, editors: *Concepts in hand rehabilitation*, Philadelphia, 1992, FA Davis.
84. Ware JE: SF-36 health survey update. In ed 3, Maruish ME, editor: *The use of psychological testing for treatment planning and outcomes assessment*, vol. 3. Mahwah, NJ, 2004, Lawrence Erlbaum Associates, pp 693–718.
85. Ware JE, Snow KK, Kosinski M, et al.: *SF-36 health survey: manual and interpretation guide*, Lincoln, RI, 2000, Quality-Metric, Inc.

86. Weinstock-Zlotnick G, Page C, Ghomrawi HMK, Wolff AL: Responsiveness of three patient report outcome (PRO) measures in patients with hand fractures: a preliminary cohort study, *J Hand Ther* 28:403–411, 2016.

87. Weiss S, Falkenstein N: *Hand rehabilitation: a quick reference guide and review*, ed 2, St. Louis, 2005, Mosby.

88. Wilson JA, Clark JJ: Obesity: impediment to postsurgical wound healing, *Adv Skin Wound Care* 17:426–435, 2004.

89. Wright HH, O'Brien V, Valdes K: Relationship of the Patient-Specific Functional Scale to commonly used clinical measures in hand osteoarthritis, *J Hand Ther* 30:538–545, 2017.

90. Ylitalo KR, Meyer MRU, Lanning BA, During C, Laschober R, Griggs JO: Simple screening tools to identify limited health literacy in a low-income patient population, *Medicine* 97(10):e0110, 2018.

APPENDIX 5.1 FORMS

Form 5.1 Hand Evaluation Check-Off Sheet

Person's History: Interviews, Chart Review, and Reports:
• Age • Vocation • Date of injury and surgery • Method of injury • Hand dominance • Treatment rendered to date (surgery, therapy, and so on) • Medication • Previous injury • General health • Avocational interests • Family composition • Subjective complaints • Support systems • Activity of daily living (ADL) responsibilities before and after injury • Impact of injury on family, economic status, and social well-being • Reimbursement • Motivation
Observation:
• Walking, posture • Facial movements • Speech patterns • Affect • Hand posture • Cognition
Palpation:
• Muscle tone • Muscle symmetry • Scar density/excursion • Tendon nodules • Masses (ganglia, fistulas)
Assessments for:
• Pain • Skin and allergies • Wound healing/wound status • Bone • Joint and ligament • Muscle and tendon • Nerve/sensation • Vascular status • Skin turgor and trophic status • Range of motion • Strength • Coordination and dexterity • Function • Reimbursement source • Vocation
Follow-Up Considerations:
• Orthosis fit • Compliance

Form 5.2 Orthotic Precaution Check-Off Sheet

- Account for bony prominences such as the following:
  - Metacarpophalangeal (MCP), proximal interphalangeal (PIP), and distal interphalangeal (DIP) joints
  - Pisiform bone
  - Radial and ulnar styloids
  - Lateral and medial epicondyles of the elbow
- Identify fragile skin, and select the orthotic material carefully. Monitor the temperature of the thermoplastic material closely before applying the material to the fragile skin.
- Identify skin areas having impaired sensation. The orthotic design should not impinge on these sites.
- If fluctuating edema is a problem, consider pressure garment wear in conjunction with an orthosis.
- Do not compress the superficial branch of the radial nerve. If the radial edge of a forearm orthosis impinges beyond the middle of the forearm near the dorsal side of the thumb, the branch of the radial nerve may be compressed.

Form 5.3 Hints for Orthotic Provision

- Give the person oral and written instrctions regarding the following:
  - Wearing schedule
  - Care of the orthosis
  - Purpose of the orthosis
  - Responsibility in therapy program
  - Phone number of contact person if problems arise
  - Actions to take if skin reactions such as the following occur: rashes, numbness, reddened areas, pain increase because of orthotic application
- Evaluate the orthosis after the person wears it at least 20 to 30 minutes and make necessary adjustments.
- Position all joints incorporated into the orthosis at the correct therapeutic angle(s).
- Design the orthosis to account for bony prominences such as the following:
  - Metacarpophalangeal (MCP), proximal interphalangeal (PIP), and distal interphalangeal (DIP) joints
  - Pisiform
  - Radial and ulnar styloids
  - Lateral and medial epicondyles of the elbow
- If fluctuating edema is a problem, make certain the orthotic design can accommodate the problem by using a wider design. Consider a pressure garment to wear under the orthosis.
- Make certain the orthotic design does not mobilize or immobilize unnecessary joint(s).
- Make certain the orthosis does not impede or restrict motions of joints adjacent to the orthosis.
- Make certain the orthosis supports the arches of the hand.
- Take into consideration the creases of the hand for allowing immobilization or mobilization, depending on the purpose of the orthosis.
- Make certain the orthosis does not restrict circulation.
- Make certain application and removal of the orthosis are easy.
- Secure the orthosis to the person's extremity using a well-designed strapping mechanism.
- Make certain the appropriate edges of the orthosis are flared or rolled.

Clinical Reasoning for Orthotic Intervention

Helene L. Lohman
Linda S. Scheirton

CHAPTER OBJECTIVES

1. Describe clinical reasoning approaches and their application to orthotic intervention.
2. Identify essential components of an orthotic referral.
3. Discuss reasons for the importance of communication with the physician about an orthotic referral.
4. Discuss diagnostic implications for orthotic provision.
5. List helpful hints regarding the hand evaluation for orthotic provision.
6. Explain factors the therapist considers when selecting an orthotic intervention approach and design.
7. Describe what therapists problem solve during orthotic fabrication.
8. Describe areas that require monitoring after orthotic fabrication is completed.
9. Describe the reflection process of the therapist before, during, and after orthotic fabrication.
10. Discuss important considerations concerning an orthotic-wearing schedule.
11. Identify conditions that determine orthotic discontinuation.
12. Identify patient safety issues related to orthotic intervention errors.
13. Discuss factors that affect orthotic cost and payment.
14. Discuss how the Health Insurance Portability and Accountability Act (HIPAA) regulations influence orthotic provision in a clinic.
15. Discuss documentation of orthotic intervention.

KEY TERMS

adherence
client safety
clinical reasoning

documentation
Health Insurance Portability and
Accountability Act (HIPAA)

intervention process
orthotic intervention error

Ali works in an acute care hospital, where she follows patients in both inpatient and outpatient care. She enjoys her job because she sees a variety of diagnoses and is constantly challenged to apply clinical reasoning to novel situations. On Friday, Ali has a walk-in client with an order for an orthosis and therapy following a Dupuytren contracture release. The order was not specific as to which orthotic type, and Ali noticed that the patient had an open wound. Although in school she was educated about wound care, she did not have experience with open wounds in practice. Ali did not have much time to think about the orthosis because she had a tight schedule that day. Ali thought, "I have made other orthoses, and although I don't know exactly what to do with this diagnosis, I can figure it out because I am familiar with basic orthotic fabrication skills. I will quickly call the physician's office to find out her preferences with wound care." Ali thoughtfully considered factors such as the location of the surgery, infection precautions, objectives for the orthosis, and the client's occupational needs. Ali consulted books and

quickly called a therapist who informally mentored her. She then successfully fabricated an appropriate orthosis while following wound-care precautions.

In clinical practice there is no simple design or type of orthosis that applies to all diagnoses. Orthotic design and wearing protocols vary because each injury is unique. **Clinical reasoning** about which orthosis to fabricate involves considering the physician's referral, the surgical and rehabilitation protocol, and the therapist's conceptual model. Clinical reasoning also involves the assessment of the client's needs based on objective and subjective data gathered during the evaluation process and knowledge about the payment source.

Instructors often teach students only one way to do something when there may be multiple ways to achieve a goal. For example, this book emphasizes the typical methods that generalist clinicians use to fabricate common orthoses. Learning a foundation for orthotic fabrication is important. In clinical

---

Note: This chapter includes content from previous contributions from Sally E. Poole, MA, OTR, CHT, and Joan L. Sullivan, MA, OTR, CHT.

practice, however, the therapist should use a problem-solving approach and apply clinical reasoning to address the needs of each client who requires an orthosis. Clinical reasoning may include integration of knowledge of biomechanics, anatomy, kinesiology, psychology, conceptual models, and pathology. Clinical reasoning also involves orthotic intervention protocols and techniques, clinical experience, and awareness of the client's motivation, adherence, and lifestyle (occupational) needs.

This chapter first overviews clinical reasoning models and then addresses approaches to clinical reasoning from the moment the therapist obtains an orthotic referral until the client's discharge. This chapter also presents prime questions to facilitate the clinical reasoning process that therapists undertake during intervention planning throughout the course of therapy.

CLINICAL REASONING MODELS

Clinical reasoning helps therapists approach the complexities of clinical practice. Clinical reasoning involves professional thinking during evaluation and intervention.[38] Professional thinking is the ability to distinctly and critically analyze the reasons for whatever actions therapists make and to reflect on the decisions afterward.[40] Skilled therapists reflect throughout the entire orthotic **intervention process** (reflection in action), not solely after the orthosis is completed.[45] Clinical reasoning also entails understanding the meaning a disability, such as a hand injury, has from the client's perspective.[33]

With clinical reasoning, therapists consider available evidence in the literature to critically reflect on whether orthoses can help their clients. Based on a review of various studies,[7] therapists consider client characteristics and outcomes with orthotic intervention. Therapists analyze how clients that they are following relate to those discussed in the studies.

Various approaches to clinical reasoning are depicted in the literature. Facione discussed an "argument and heuristic analysis model of decision making" for critical thinking.[18] System 1 involves automatic quick reactive thinking, and System 2 involves logical reflective thinking. Both types of critical thinking can be used with orthotic fabrication. Therapists apply System 1 to think quickly as the working time with thermoplastic materials is very short. Yet to appropriately fabricate orthoses, therapists must use System 2 to logically and reflectively consider factors such as which orthosis to provide, length of provision, wearing schedule, and principles of fabrication.

One clinical reasoning model in occupational therapy literature includes interactive, narrative, pragmatic, conditional, and procedural reasoning. Although each of these approaches is distinctive, experienced therapists often shift from one type of thinking to another to critically analyze complex clinical problems,[21] such as with orthotic intervention.

Interactive reasoning involves getting to know the client as a human being to understand the impact that the hand condition has on the client's life.[21] Understanding this impact can help identify the proper orthosis to fabricate. For example, for a client who is very sensitive about appearance after a hand injury, the therapist may select a skin-tone thermoplastic material that blends with the skin and attracts less attention than a white thermoplastic material.

With narrative reasoning the therapist reflects on the client's occupational story (or life history), taking into consideration activities, habits, and roles.[38] For assessment and intervention, the therapist first takes a top-down approach[52] by considering the roles that the client had before the hand condition and the meaning of occupations in the client's life. The therapist also considers the client's future and the impact that the therapist and the client can have on it.[21] For example, through discussion or a formal assessment interview, a therapist learns that continuation of work activities is important to a client with carpal tunnel syndrome. Therefore, the therapist fabricates a wrist immobilization orthosis to position the wrist in neutral and has the client practice typing on a computer while wearing the orthosis.

With pragmatic reasoning the therapist considers practical factors, such as payment, public policy regulations, documentation, availability of equipment, and the expected discharge environment. Pragmatic reasoning includes considerations of the therapist's values, knowledge, and skills.[38,44] For example, a therapist may need to review the literature and research evidence if the therapist is unknowledgeable about a diagnosis that requires an orthosis. If a therapist does not have the expertise to fabricate an orthosis for a client with a complicated injury, the therapist might consider referring the client to another therapist who has the expertise.

In addition, a therapist may need to make ethical decisions, such as whether to fabricate an orthosis for a terminally ill 98-year-old client. This ethical decision involves the therapist's values about age and terminal conditions. In today's ever-changing health care environment, there is a trend toward cost containment. Budgetary shortages may require therapists to ration clinical services. Prospective payment systems for reimbursing the costs of rehabilitation, such as in skilled nursing facilities (SNFs), are a reality. Therapists fabricate orthoses quickly and efficiently to save costs. The information provided throughout this book may assist with pragmatic reasoning.

With conditional reasoning the therapist reflects on the client's "whole condition" by considering the client's life before the injury, the disease or trauma, current status, and possible future life status.[34] Reflection is multidimensional and includes the condition that requires orthotic intervention, the meaning of having the condition or dysfunction, and the social and physical environments in which the client lives.[22] The therapist then envisions how the client's condition might change as a result of orthotic provision and therapy. Finally, the therapist realizes that success or failure of the intervention ultimately depends on the client's adherence to the orthotic requirements.[21,38] Evaluation and intervention with this clinical reasoning model begin with a top-down approach, considering the meaning of having an injury in the context of a client's life.

Procedural reasoning involves finding the best orthotic intervention approach to improve functional performance, taking into consideration the client's diagnostically related performance areas, components, and contexts.[20,21,38] Much of the material in this chapter, which summarizes the intervention process from referral to discontinuation of an orthosis, can be used with procedural reasoning. To demonstrate clinical reasoning, Table 6.1 summarizes each approach and includes questions for the therapist to either ask the client or reflect on during orthotic provision and fabrication. As stated at the beginning of this discussion, each approach is explained separately. However, experienced therapists combine these approaches, moving easily from one to another.[34]

CLINICAL REASONING THROUGHOUT THE INTERVENTION PROCESS

The following information assists with pragmatic and procedural reasoning.

Essentials of Orthotic Referral

The first step in the problem-solving process is consideration of the orthotic referral. The ideal situation is to receive the orthotic referral from the physician's office early to allow

ample time for preparation. However, the first time the therapist sees the referral is often when the client arrives for the appointment. In these situations, the therapist makes quick clinical decisions. Aside from client demographics, Fess and colleagues[19] suggested that therapists also need to determine the following information:

- Diagnosis
- Date of the condition's onset
- Medical or surgical management
- Purpose of the orthosis
- Type of orthosis (immobilization, mobilization, restriction, torque transmission)
- Anatomical parts the orthosis should immobilize or mobilize
- Precautions and other instructions
- Duration of orthotic intervention
- Wearing schedule

In addition to this list, therapists should take into account occupational considerations.

TABLE 6.1 Clinical Reasoning Approaches[a]

Summary of Approach	Key Questions for Orthotic Provision
Interactive Reasoning	
Getting to know the person through understanding the impact the hand condition has had on the person's life. The focus of this approach is the person's perspective.	Questions directed to person: • How are you coping with having a hand condition? • How has your hand condition impacted all areas of your life? • How will you go about following an orthotic schedule based on your lifestyle? • What type of support do you need to help you with your orthosis and hand injury?
Narrative Reasoning	
Consider the person's occupational story (or life history), taking into consideration activities, habits, and roles. The focus of this approach is the person's perspective.	Questions directed to person: • How have you dealt with difficult situations in your life? • What was your typical daily routine before and after the injury? • How do you deal with changes in your schedule? • What roles (such as parent, friend, professional, hobbyist, volunteer) do you have in your life? • What activities have interested you throughout your life? • What activities are difficult for you to perform? • What activities would you like to continue after therapy is over?
Pragmatic Reasoning	
Consider practical factors, such as payment, documentation, equipment availability, and the expected discharge environment. Also consider the therapist's values, knowledge, and skills.	Questions directed to therapist for self-reflection: • Do I have adequate skills to fabricate this orthosis? • Where can I get more information to best fabricate the orthosis? • Are there any ethical issues that I will need to address with the provision of this orthosis? • How long will I be working with this person? • What is the payment source for orthotic coverage? • If it is a managed care source, have I received proper preauthorization and precertification? • Have I clearly communicated the need for this orthosis with all appropriate medical personnel, such as case managers? • Have I documented succinctly with adequate detail? • Is my documentation functionally based? • Am I basing the orthotic protocol on evidence-based practice? • Have I considered the legal aspects of documentation? • What are the proper supplies to fabricate this orthosis? • Are there ways I can be more timely and cost-effective in fabricating this orthosis? • What is the person's discharge environment, and how will that impact orthotic provision?

Continued

TABLE 6.1   Clinical Reasoning Approaches[a]—cont'd

Summary of Approach	Key Questions for Orthotic Provision
Conditional Reasoning Reflect on the person's whole condition, taking into consideration the person's life before the condition happened, current status, and possible future status. Consider the condition and meaning of having it, social and physical environments, and cooperation of the person.	Questions directed to the person: • What is your medical history? • What is your social history? Questions directed to the therapist for self-reflection: • What is the person's current medical and functional status? • How will orthotic provision impact the person's functional status? • Will the orthosis provided assist the client in carrying out valued occupations for activities of daily living (ADLs), work, and leisure? • What is the person's expected discharge environment, and how can this orthosis help with the person's discharge plans? • Does the person have adequate resources to attend therapy or follow through with a home program? • Describe the person's level of adherence. • If the person is not adherent with orthotic wear, how will that be addressed?
Procedural Reasoning Problem-solving the best orthotic approach, taking into consideration the person's diagnostically related performance areas, components, and contexts.	Questions directed to therapist: • What in the person's medical history warrants an orthosis? • What conceptual model will I use to approach orthotic fabrication? • What problems have I identified from the evaluation that will need to be addressed with orthotic provision? • What problems could occur if the hand is or is not provided an orthosis? • What is the person's rehabilitation potential as a result of getting an orthosis? • Am I basing the orthotic protocol on evidence-based practice? • Am I basing the orthotic protocol on functional outcomes? • What is the purpose of this orthosis (prevention, immobilization, protection, correction of deformity, control/modify scar formation, substitution, exercise)? • Will a fabricated or prefabricated orthosis best meet the person's needs? • What will be my orthotic approach (immobilization, mobilization, restriction, torque transmission)? • How many joints will be included in the orthosis? • What precautions will I follow? • What precautions should the person follow? • Have I developed an appropriate home program? • How is the person's function progressing as a result of the orthotic regimen? • Do I need to make adjustments with the orthotic protocol? • What would I do differently to fabricate this orthosis next time?

[a]Examples are inclusive, not exclusive.

Therapist/Physician Communication About Orthotic Referral

A problem that many therapists encounter is an incomplete orthotic referral that lacks a clear diagnosis. Even an experienced therapist becomes frustrated upon receiving a referral that states "Provide orthosis." A proper referral would answer these questions for the therapist:

• Orthosis for what purpose?
• For what body part(s)?
• For how long?

An open line of communication between the physician and the therapist is essential for good orthotic selection and fabrication. Most physicians welcome calls from the therapist when calls are specific. If the physician's referral does not contain the pertinent information, the therapist is responsible for requesting this information (Box 6.1). The therapist prepares a list of questions before calling; and if the physician is not available, the therapist conveys the list to the physician's administrative assistant, nurse, or physician assistant and agrees on a specific time to call again. Sometimes the contact staff member at the physician office can read the chart notes or fax an operative report to the therapist. With electronic medical records, radiographic reports, operative reports, and any other relevant reports are accessible for review. The therapist must never rely solely on the client's perception of the diagnosis and orthotic requirements.

In some cases, the physician expects the therapist to have the clinical reasoning skills to select the appropriate orthosis for the specific clinical diagnosis. Sometimes a therapist receives a physician's order for an inappropriate orthosis, a nontherapeutic wearing schedule, or a less than optimal material. The therapist is responsible for always scrutinizing each physician referral. If the

BOX 6.1 Examples of Incomplete and Complete Orthotic Referrals

Incomplete Referral	Complete Referral
• From the Office of Dr. S. • Name: Mrs. P. MR. Number: 415672 Age: 51 Diagnosis: de Quervain tenosynovitis • Date: August 12th • Fabricate a left hand orthosis • Dr. S.	• From the Office of Dr. S. • Date: August 12th • Name: Mrs. P. MR. Number: 415672 Age: 51 Diagnosis: de Quervain tenosynovitis • Fabricate a volar-based thumb immobilization orthosis L UE with the wrist in 15 degrees dorsiflexion, the thumb CMC joint in 40 degrees palmar abduction, and the MCP joint in 10 degrees flexion. • Dr. S.

CMC, Carpometacarpal; L, left; MCP, metacarpophalangeal; UE, upper extremity.

referral is inappropriate, the therapist should apply clinical reasoning skills to determine the appropriate orthotic intervention approach. The therapist makes successful independent decisions with a knowledge base about the fundamentals of orthotic intervention and with the ability to locate additional information. Then the therapist calls the physician's office and diplomatically explains the problem with the referral and suggests a better orthotic intervention approach and rationale.

Diagnostic Implications for Orthotic Provision

The therapist identifies the client's diagnosis after reviewing the orthotic order. Often, the therapist can begin the clinical reasoning process by using a categorical orthotic intervention approach according to the diagnosis. The first category involves chronic conditions, such as hemiplegia. In such situations an objective of the orthotic provision may be to prevent contracture. The second category involves a traumatic or acute condition that may encompass surgical or nonsurgical intervention. For example, the client may have tendinosis and require a nonsurgical orthotic intervention for the affected extremity.

Regardless of whether the condition is acute or chronic, it is important that the therapist have an adequate knowledge of diagnostic protocols. By knowing protocols, therapists are aware of precautions for orthotic intervention. For example, for a client with carpal tunnel syndrome, the therapist knows to place the wrist in a neutral position. If the therapist placed the wrist in a functional position of 30 degrees extension, it could cause more pain by putting too much pressure on the median nerve. Therapists should keep abreast of current intervention trends through review of evidence in literature, continuing education, and communication with physicians. In all cases the orthotic provision

approach is individually tailored to each client, beginning with categorization by diagnosis and then adapting the approach according to the client's performance, cognition, and occupational needs.

Factors Influencing the Orthotic Approach

The following sections offer specific hints that elaborate on areas of the orthotic evaluation the therapist can use with clinical reasoning. (See Chapter 5 for essential components to include in a thorough hand evaluation.)

Age

The client's age is important for many reasons. Barring other problems, most children, adolescents, and adults can wear orthoses according to the respective protocol. An infant or toddler, however, can usually get out of any orthosis at any time or place. Extraordinary and creative methods are often necessary to keep orthoses on these youngsters.[3] Older clients, especially those with diminished functional and cognitive capacities, may require careful monitoring by the caregiver to ensure a proper fit and adherence with the wearing schedule. For more information about working with older adults refer to Chapter 16 and for pediatrics refer to Chapter 17.

Occupation

From the interview with the client, family, and caregiver (and from medical record review), the therapist surmises the impact that an orthosis may have on occupational function, economic status, and social well-being. The therapist carefully considers the meaning that the upper extremity condition has for the client, how the client has dealt with medical conditions in the past, how the client's condition may change because of the orthotic provision, and the client's social environment. Thus, when choosing the orthotic design and material, the therapist considers the client's lifestyle needs. The following are some specific questions to reflect on when determining lifestyle needs:

- What valued occupations, such as work or sports, will the client engage in while wearing the orthosis?
- Do special considerations exist because of rules and regulations for work or sports?
- In what type of environment will the client wear the orthosis? For example, will the orthosis be used in extreme temperatures? Will the orthosis get wet?
- Will the orthosis impede a hand function necessary to the client's job or home activities?
- What is the client's normal schedule, and how will wearing an orthosis impact that schedule?

If a physician refers a client for a wrist immobilization orthosis because of wrist strain, the therapist might contemplate the following question: Is the client a construction worker who does heavy manual work or a computer operator who does light, repetitive work? A construction worker may require an orthosis of stronger material with extremely secure strapping. The computer operator may benefit from lighter, thinner thermoplastic material with wide soft straps. In some situations, the client may best benefit from a prefabricated orthosis.

The therapist determines the client's activity status, including when the client is wearing an orthosis that does not allow for function or movement (such as a positioning orthosis). If the client must return to work immediately, albeit in a limited capacity, the orthosis must always be secure. Proper instructions regarding appropriate care of the limb and the orthosis are necessary. This care may involve elevation of the affected extremity, wound management, and periodic range of motion (ROM) exercises while the client is working.

When the client plans to continue in a sports program (professional, school, or community-based), the therapist checks the rules and regulations governing that sport. Rules and regulations usually prevent athletes from wearing hard thermoplastic material during participation in the sport unless the orthotic design includes exterior and interior padding. Therapists need to communicate with the coach or referee to determine appropriateness of an orthosis[63] and perhaps consider alternative interventions, such as applying Kinesio tape to the area.

Expected Environment

The therapist must consider the client's discharge environment. Some clients return to their own homes and have families and friends who can lend assistance if necessary. For those clients returning to inpatient units or nursing homes, therapists consider instructing the staff in the care and use of the orthoses. If clients return to psychiatric units or prison wards, consider whether supervision is necessary so that orthoses are not used as weapons to harm themselves or others.

Activities of Daily Living Responsibilities

The therapist considers the following question: Is the client able to successfully complete all activities of daily living (ADLs) and instrumental activities of daily living (IADLs) if an orthosis needs to be worn? For example, the therapist may consider how a client can successfully prepare a meal wearing an orthosis that immobilizes one extremity. In that case, the therapist may address one-handed meal-preparation techniques.

Client Adherence and Motivation

Orthotic provision requires adherence on many levels, including attending therapy sessions, following wearing schedules and home programs, and adhering to safety expectations.[39] The terminologies of adherence and compliance are often discussed interchangeably, but there are differences with the definitions. Compliance can be perceived as follow-through with intervention instructions. **Adherence** can be perceived as more client centered as the client collaborates with the intervention. Adherence is currently the more utilized term.[31] The World Health Organization (WHO) defines adherence as "numerous health-related behaviours"[62] and discusses five dimensions of adherence related to factors and interventions that include "(1) social economic, (2) health system and health care team, (3) therapy, (4) condition, and (5) patient."[62]

Other considerations affecting adherence with intervention regimens include external factors, such as socioeconomic status and family support. Internal factors such as the client's perception of the severity of the condition are also considered. Knowledge, beliefs, and attitudes about the condition can influence adherence.[8,24]

There is a limited amount of research investigating how adherence relates to clients with hand injuries[23,29] or with orthotic provision. A systematic review[39] considered adherence with orthotic wear in adults. Six studies met the selection criteria for a total of 490 subjects. The author concluded that there was "no consistent correlation [with adherence to orthotic wear] to age or gender" or to "socioeconomic and condition related factors."[39] However, the author found some evidence supporting the importance of intervention factors (such as the comfort of the orthosis) and impact of the orthosis on lifestyle and occupations.

Another factor addressed in research is the psychosocial construct of locus of control, which proposes a relationship between a client's perception of control over intervention outcomes and the likelihood that the client will adhere to intervention. This perception of control can be internally or externally based.[8] For example, an internally motivated client would follow an orthotic schedule based on self-motivation. An externally motivated client may need encouragement from the therapist or caregiver to follow an orthotic-wearing schedule. Often not discussed with adherence are organizational variables and clinic environment issues, such as transportation problems, interference with daily schedule, wait time, inconsistent therapists, and clinic location.[29]

The therapist can positively influence the client's adherence and motivation to wear an orthosis. Establishing goals together may encourage the client to follow through with the intervention. Perhaps completing an occupation-focused assessment, such as the Canadian Occupational Performance Measure (COPM), can encourage the client to wear the orthosis.[30] If the goals determined by the COPM are improvement of hand function, the therapist discusses how the orthosis will meet these goals. Furthermore, it is important for the therapist to examine intervention goals in relation to the client's goals because there might be disparity between them.[29] Sometimes the client will have input about the orthotic design, which should be considered seriously by the therapist. Therapists should convey to clients that success with rehabilitation and orthoses involves shared responsibility. To attain the therapeutic goal, the therapist must always reiterate the client's responsibilities in the intervention plan.

In addition, the therapist should perceive the client as an individual with a lifestyle beyond the clinic, not just as a client with an injury. Paramount to adherence is education about the medical necessity of wearing the orthoses. The therapist should consider the client's perspectives on the impact of the orthoses on lifestyle. Education should be repetitive throughout the time the client wears the orthosis.[23,48] When the therapist and the physician communicate clearly about the type of orthosis necessary, the client receives consistent information regarding the rationale for wearing the orthosis. Demonstrating how the orthosis works and explaining the goal of the orthosis enhances client adherence.

BOX 6.2   Examples of Factors That May Influence Adherence With Orthotic Wear

Organizational/Clinic Environment
- Time involved with orthotic wear
- Interference with life tasks
- Inconsistent therapists
- Transportation issues
- Long wait time for therapy
- Inconvenient clinic location
- Noisy clinic with little privacy

Client
- Belief in the efficacy of wearing an orthosis
- Belief in one's ability to follow through with the orthosis-wearing schedule
- Poor social support

Intervention
- Orthosis is uncomfortable
- Orthosis is cumbersome
- Orthosis is poorly made

Therapeutic Relationship and Communication
- Inconsistent communication between therapists and physicians concerning the orthosis
- Poor understanding, difficulty reading, or being forgetful about instructions on orthotic wear and care

Adapted from Kirwan, T., Tooth, L., & Harkin, C. (2002). Compliance with hand therapy programs: Therapists' and patients' perceptions. *Journal of Hand Therapy, 15*(1), 31–40.

BOX 6.3   Questions for Follow-up Telephone Calls or Email Communication Regarding Clients With Orthoses

The following open- and closed-ended questions may assist the therapist in eliciting pertinent information from clients about orthotic adherence, fit, and follow-up. Closed-ended questions usually elicit a brief response, often a yes or no.
- Have you been wearing your orthosis according to the schedule I gave you? If no, why aren't you wearing your orthosis?
- Have you noticed any reddened or painful areas after removing your orthosis? If so, where?
- Is the orthosis easy to put on and take off?
- Are there any tasks you want to do but cannot do when wearing your orthosis?
- Do you have any concerns about your orthotic-wearing schedule or care?
- Are there any broken or faulty components on your orthosis?
- Do you have any questions for me?
- Do you know how to reach me?
- Have you noticed any increased swelling or pain since you've been wearing the orthosis?

Open-ended questions elicit a qualitative response that may give the therapist more information.
- Will you tell me about a typical day and when you put your orthosis on and take it off?
- What concerns, if any, might you have about your orthotic wear and care schedule?
- What precautions have you been taking in regard to monitoring your orthotic wear?
- How is the orthosis affecting your activities at home and at work?
- Are there any areas to improve with our clinic management that would help with your follow-through with orthotic wear?
- Can you tell me how you would contact me if you need to do so?
- Do you have any questions for me?

Adherence involves both therapist and client (Box 6.2).[29] Rather than labeling clients as noncompliant or uncooperative, therapists must make serious attempts to help clients better cope with their injury. The therapist should be an empathetic listener as the client learns to adjust to the diagnosis and to the orthosis. The therapist can ask questions of the client to assist in eliciting pertinent information about orthotic adherence, fit, and follow-up (Box 6.3).

Others can also have an impact on client adherence. Sometimes a peer wearing an orthosis can be a positive role model to help a client who is not adhering to the intervention plan. A supportive spouse or caregiver encourages adherence. Furthermore, physician support influences adherence. Sometimes a client may need more structured psychosocial support from mental health personnel.

Selection of an appropriate design may alleviate a client's difficulty in adjusting to an injury and wearing an orthosis. Therapists should ask themselves many questions as they consider the best design. (See the questions listed in the section on procedural reasoning in Table 6.1.)

In addition to orthotic design, material selection (e.g., soft versus hard) may influence satisfaction with an orthosis.[10] People with rheumatoid arthritis who wear a soft prefabricated orthosis consider comfort and ease of use when involved in activities, which are important factors for orthotic satisfaction.[49] (See the discussion of advantages and disadvantages of prefabricated soft orthoses in Chapter 3.)

Making the orthosis aesthetically pleasing helps with adherence. A client is less likely to wear an orthosis that is messy or sloppy. This is especially true of children and adolescents for whom personal appearance is often an important issue. Therapists need to think of an orthosis as a representation of their work, because other people will see it in public and may inquire about it.

Thermoplastic and strapping materials are now available in a variety of colors and sometimes imprinted with patterns. Clients, both children and adults, who are coping successfully with the injury may want to have fun with the orthosis and select one or more colors. However, a client who is having a difficult time adjusting to the injury may not want to wear an orthosis in public at all, let alone an orthosis with a color that draws more attention.

Finally, fabrication of a correctly fitting orthosis on the first attempt eases a client's anxiety. The therapist is responsible for listening to the client's complaints and adjusting the orthosis. A therapist's attitude about orthotic adjustments makes a difference. If the therapist seems relaxed, the client may consider adjustment time a normal part of the orthotic fabrication process. Encouraging effective communication with the client facilitates understanding and satisfaction about orthotic provision.

Cognitive Status

Besides adherence, the client's cognitive status is a consideration that can influence orthotic provision. When a client is unable to attend to the therapy program and follow the orthotic intervention regimen because of cognitive status, the therapist must educate the family, caregiver, or staff members. Education includes medical reasons for the orthotic provision, wearing schedule, home program, precautions, and cleaning. Education leads to better cooperation. Sometimes the therapist selects designs and techniques to maximize the client's independence. For example, instructions are written directly on the orthosis. Symbols, such as suns and moons to represent the time of day, can be used in written instructions of wearing schedules.[46] Simple communication strategies (such as showing the client a sheet with a smiley face, neutral face, or frowning face) can be used to determine how the client feels about orthotic comfort.

Health Literacy

An important consideration in today's health care environment is health literacy. Health literacy, or the ability to "obtain, process, and understand health information,"[56] influences communication between the therapist and the client. Older adults, people from lower economic groups, minorities, people with limited English speaking and reading abilities, people with chronic conditions, and people experiencing stress are at risk for low health literacy.[35] Consider the stress a client may feel following a traumatic hand injury and not being able to work.

Therapists who are aware of the health literacy requirements of their clients focus orthotic education in a manner that is understandable, resulting in better adherence to the intervention plan. Simply asking clients about their reading abilities is one way to open the conversation about health literacy[35] and orthotic education. Additionally, asking clients about their learning styles,[57] such as preferring demonstration, visual information, written information, or a combination, helps focus the format and approach to orthotic education. When providing educational handouts or home programs, therapists must be careful to simplify language and not use medical language. For example, some people in the public may not be familiar with the word *orthosis,* or even splint. So, the therapist should use words that are familiar to the person. Handouts are easier to understand when pictures and graphics accompany narrative.[57] For example, the therapist includes a picture of the correct way to secure straps when donning the orthosis in a patient education handout. Another useful health literacy technique is called "teach back," in which the therapist asks the client to demonstrate any therapeutic activities that have been taught. From the demonstrations, therapists become aware if the education needs to change or be simplified. For example, therapists ask clients to show them how they will put on the orthosis. Sometimes chunking the education in manageable segments or starting with the most important learning concept will increase retention.[35] For example, presenting safety precautions about the orthosis first may help the client's learning and retention.

ORTHOTIC INTERVENTION APPROACH AND DESIGN CONSIDERATIONS

The five approaches to orthotic design are dorsal, palmar, radial, ulnar, and circumferential. The therapist must determine the type of orthosis to fabricate, such as a mobilization orthosis or immobilization orthosis. Understanding the purpose of the orthosis clarifies these decisions. For example, when working with a client who has a radial nerve injury, the therapist may choose to fabricate a dorsal torque transmission orthosis (wrist flexion: index-small finger metacarpophalangeal [MCP] extension/index-small finger MCP flexion, wrist extension torque transmission orthosis)[2] to substitute for the loss of motor function in the wrist and MCP extensors. Based on clinical reasoning, the therapist may also choose to fabricate a palmar-based wrist extension immobilization orthosis once the client regains function of the MCP extensors. The wrist orthosis allows the client to engage in functional activities.

In addition to the information that the therapist obtains from a thorough evaluation, other factors dictate orthosis choice. To determine the most efficient and effective orthosis choice, the therapist must consider the physician's orders, the diagnosis, the therapist's judgment, the payment source, and the client's function.

Physician's Orders

Physicians often predetermine the orthotic-application approach based on their training, surgical technique, and evidence in the literature. As discussed, sometimes the therapist may apply clinical reasoning to determine a different orthotic design or material than what was ordered. In that case, the therapist calls the physician.

Diagnosis

Frequently the diagnosis mandates the approach to orthotic design. The diagnosis determines the number of joints that the therapist must involve. The least number of joints possible should be restricted while allowing the orthosis to accomplish its purpose. Diagnosis also determines positioning and whether the orthosis should be of the mobilization or immobilization type. For example, using one early mobilization protocol for a flexor tendon repair, the therapist places the orthosis on the dorsum of the forearm and hand to protect the tendon and to allow for rubber band traction. The wrist and MCP joints should be in a flexed position. (Alternatively, some physicians now prefer a neutral wrist position to block extension.) These orthoses protect the repair and allow early tendon glide. In this example the repaired structures and the need to begin tendon gliding guide the approach. (See

Chapter 13 for more information on mobilization orthotic fabrication with tendon repairs.)

Therapist's Judgment

The therapist determines the orthotic design and type based on knowledge and experience. For example, after a carpal tunnel release, the therapist can place a wrist immobilization orthosis dorsally or volarly directly over the surgical site. As an advocate of early scar management, the therapist chooses a palmar orthosis and adds silicone elastomer or Otoform to the orthosis.

Client's Function

The client's primary task responsibilities may influence the type of orthosis. A construction worker's wrist has different demands placed on it than the wrist of a computer operator with the same diagnosis. Not only does the therapist choose different materials for each client, but the design approach may be different. A thumb-hole volar wrist immobilization orthosis decreases the risk of the orthosis migrating up the arm during the construction worker's activities, because it tightly conforms to the hand. The computer operator may prefer a dorsal wrist immobilization orthosis to allow adequate sensory feedback and unimpeded flexibility of the digits during keyboard use. (See Chapter 7 for patterns of wrist orthoses.)

Table 6.2 outlines a variety of positioning choices for orthotic design. However, therapists should not view these suggestions as strict rules. For example, a skin condition (such as eczema) may necessitate that a mobilization extension orthosis be volarly based rather than dorsally based.

CLINICAL REASONING CONSIDERATIONS FOR DESIGNING AND PLANNING THE ORTHOSIS

The orthotic designing and planning process involves many clinical decisions about materials and techniques the therapist can use. (Refer to chapters throughout this book for more specific information about materials and techniques.) Initial considerations are often related to infection control procedures.

Infection Control Procedures

The therapist considers whether dressing changes are necessary and consults with the physician's office for any guidance. If so, the therapist follows universal precautions and maintains a sterile environment. The therapist should be aware that skin maceration under an orthosis can occur more easily in the presence of a draining wound. With skin maceration the therapist first carefully applies a dressing to absorb the fluid. Orthotic fabrication should take place over the dressing, and the therapist should instruct the client in how to apply new dressings at appropriate intervals.[47] Before the application of the thermoplastic material, the therapist can place a stockinette over the client's bandages to prevent the thermoplastic material from sticking to the bandages.

If the client has a draining or infected wound, the therapist does not use regular strapping material to hold the orthosis in place to absorb bacteria. Instead, the therapist uses gauze bandages that are replaced at each dressing change. If a client is unwilling or unable to change a dressing, the therapist can instruct a family member or friend to do so. If assistance is not possible, the client may need to visit the therapist more frequently.

Time Allotment for Orthotic Fabrication and Client and Nursing or Caregiver Education

The therapist considers the time required for orthotic fabrication and education. Fabrication time varies according to the complexity of the orthosis and the client's ability to comply with the fabrication process. For example, squirmy babies and people with spasticity are more difficult to fabricate an orthosis for and require more time. In these cases, it may be beneficial to have an additional staff member or a caregiver help position the client.

Orthotic fabrication time is also dependent on the therapist's experience. If possible, a beginning therapist should schedule a large block of time for orthotic fabrication. As therapists gain clinical experience, they require less time to fabricate orthoses. With any orthotic application, the therapist should allow enough time for educating the client, family, and caregiver about the wear schedule, precautions, and their responsibility in the rehabilitation process. As discussed, education helps with adherence.

TABLE 6.2 Common Positioning Choices in Orthotic Design				
Orthosis	**Volar**	**Dorsal**	**Radial**	**Ulnar**
Hand immobilization hand orthosis	X	X	—	—
Wrist immobilization orthosis	X	X	—	X
Thumb orthosis	X	X	X	—
Ulnar nerve orthosis (anticlaw)	—	X	—	X
Radial nerve orthosis	—	X	—	—
Median nerve orthosis (thumb CMC palmar abduction mobilization orthosis)	X	X	X	—
Elbow positioning orthosis	X	X	—	—
Mobilization hand extension orthosis	—	X	—	—
Mobilization hand flexion orthosis	X	—	—	—

CMC, Carpometacarpal.

Batteson[6] found that in an institutional setting, a nurse training program (developed by the occupational therapist) that addressed orthotic fabrication was very helpful in increasing adherence with an orthotic-wearing schedule. This program included orthotic rationale, common orthotic care questions, and familiarization with thermoplastic materials. A nurse liaison was identified to deal specifically with the client's orthosis concerns. In addition, an orthotic resource file developed by the therapist was made available to the nurses. A similar system could be created on the computer.

POSTFABRICATION MONITORING

The therapist uses clinical reasoning skills to thoroughly evaluate and monitor the fabricated orthosis. In particular, the therapist must be aware of pressure areas and edema.

Monitoring Pressure

Regardless of its purpose or design, the orthosis requires monitoring to determine effects on the skin. A client wearing an orthosis is superimposing a hard lever system on an existing lever system that is covered by skin, a living tissue that requires an adequate blood supply. The therapist must therefore follow mechanical principles during orthotic fabrication to avoid excessive pressure on the skin. With fabrication, therapists weigh the pros and cons of the amount of orthotic coverage. With minimal coverage from an orthosis, there is increased mobility. Increased coverage by an orthosis allows for more protection and better pressure distribution. To reduce pressure, the therapist designs an orthosis that covers a larger surface area.[19] Warning signs of an ill-fitting orthosis are red marks, indentations, and ulcerations on the skin.

A well-fitting orthosis, after its removal, may leave a red area on the client's skin. This normal response to the pressure of the orthosis disappears within seconds. When an orthosis exerts too much pressure on one area (usually occurs over a bony prominence) the redness may last longer. For clients of color, in whom redness is not easily visible, the therapist may lightly touch the skin to determine the presence of hot spots or warmer skin. Another way to check skin temperature is with a thermometer. With any orthosis the therapist checks the skin after 20 to 30 minutes of wearing time before the client leaves the clinic. If red areas are present after 20 to 30 minutes of wearing the orthosis, adjustments need to be made.

A client with intact sensibility who has an ill-fitting orthosis usually requests an adjustment or simply discards the orthosis because it is not comfortable. For a condition in which sensation is absent, vigorous orthotic monitoring is critical.[9,19] The therapist teaches the client and the family to remove the orthosis every 1 to 2 hours to check the skin to avoid skin breakdown.

Monitoring for Skin Maceration

Wet, white, macerated skin can occur when the skin under an orthosis holds too much moisture. Skin maceration occurs for many reasons, such as a child drooling on an orthosis. When this happens to a client with intact skin who has simply forgotten to remove the orthosis, the therapist can easily correct the problem by washing and drying the area. Educating the client about proper care of the hand and providing a polypropylene stockinette to absorb moisture should resolve this situation.

Monitoring Edema

A therapist frequently needs to fabricate an orthosis for an edematous extremity. Edema is often present after surgery, in the presence of infection, with severe trauma (e.g., from a burn), or with vascular or lymphatic compromise. A well-designed, well-fitting orthosis can reduce edema and prevent the sequelae of tissue damage and joint contracture. A poorly designed or ill-fitting orthosis can contribute to the damaging results of persistent edema. Generally, the design and fit principles already discussed in this text apply.

The therapist considers the method used to hold the orthosis in place. Soft, wide straps accommodate increases in edema and are better able to distribute pressure than rigid, nonyielding Velcro straps.[11] When too tight, strapping can contribute to pitting edema as a result of hampered lymphatic flow.[13] For severe edema the therapist may gently apply a wide elastic wrap to keep the orthosis in place. The continuous contact of the wrap helps reduce edema.[13] Therapists should be cautioned that straps applied at intervals may further restrict circulation and cause "windowpane" edema distally and between the straps. When using Ace wraps or compressive gauze, the therapist must apply them in a spiral pattern and use gradient distal-to-proximal pressure. The therapist must properly monitor the orthosis and wrap to ensure that the wrap does not roll or bunch.[31] Pressure created by rolling or bunching could cause constriction and further edema and stiffness.

If the lymphatic system is not damaged, edema reduction usually begins relatively quickly with appropriate wound healing (i.e., no infection), proper elevation, and gentle active exercises as permitted. As edema resolves, the therapist remolds the orthosis to fit the new configuration of the extremity. The therapist asks the client with severe edema to return to the clinic daily for monitoring and intervention. When the edema appears to be within the normal postoperative range, the therapist asks the client to return to the clinic in 3 to 5 days for an orthotic check. Helping the client understand the frequency and purpose of the orthotic adjustments is also important. Again, education is an important part of the edema-reduction regimen.[32]

Monitoring Physical and Functional Status

When a client's physical or functional status changes, an orthotic adjustment is often necessary. If a client is receiving intervention for a specific injury and it is effective, the orthosis requires adjustments in conjunction with improvement. For example, if a client has a median nerve injury in which the thumb has an adduction contracture, the therapist fabricates a thumb carpometacarpal (CMC) palmar abduction mobilization orthosis[2] to gradually widen the tight web space. As intervention progresses and thumb motions increase, the therapist adjusts the orthosis to accommodate the gains in motion.[42]

EVALUATION AND ADJUSTMENT OF ORTHOSES

After fabricating the orthosis, the therapist carefully evaluates the design to determine fit and necessary adjustments. The therapist looks carefully at the orthosis when the client is and is not wearing it and considers whether the orthosis serves its purpose. The orthosis should be functional for the client and should accomplish the goals for which it was intended. It should also have a design that uses correct biomechanical principles and should be cosmetically appealing. (Refer to specific chapters in this book for hints and orthosis-evaluation forms.)

Therapists learn from self-reflection before, during, and after each orthosis is made. Reflection helps fine-tune critical thinking skills. The following are reflective questions that the therapist can consider after orthotic fabrication:

- Did the orthosis accomplish the purpose for which it was intended?
- Is it correctly fitted according to biomechanical principles?
- Did I select the best materials for the orthosis?
- Did I take into consideration fluctuating edema?
- Is it cosmetically appealing?
- Is it comfortable for the client and free of pressure areas?
- Have I addressed how orthotic intervention impacts the client's valued occupations?
- Have I addressed functional considerations?
- What would I do differently if I were to refabricate this orthosis?
- Did I properly educate the client/caregiver about the orthosis?

If major adjustments are required, the therapist should avoid using a heat gun except to smooth the orthotic edges. If the therapist has selected the appropriate simple orthotic design and has used a thermoplastic product that is easily reheatable and remoldable, the water-immersion method is the best way to adjust the orthosis. Years of experience demonstrate that reheating the entire orthosis in water and reshaping it is more efficient than spot heating. The activity of the therapist reheating and adjusting one spot often affects the adjacent area, thereby producing another area requiring adjustment. This cycle may not end until the orthosis is useless. When possible, the therapist should use an orthosis product that is reheatable in water and easily reshapable to obtain a proper fit for the client.

ORTHOTIC-WEARING SCHEDULE FACTORS

Development of an orthotic-wearing schedule for a client is sometimes extremely frustrating for a novice therapist, because there are no magic numbers or formulas for each type of orthosis or diagnostic population. The therapist tailors and customizes the wearing schedule to the individual and exercises clinical judgment. Only general guidelines for orthotic-wearing schedules exist.

In the case of joint limitation, the therapist increases the wearing frequency and time as much as the client can tolerate. Alternatively, the therapist adjusts the intervention plan to try a different orthosis. If motion is increasing steadily, the therapist may decrease the orthotic-wearing time, allowing the client to engage in function by using the limited joint or joints. If the orthosis improves function or the extremity requires protection, the client wears the orthosis when necessary. The following are questions to consider when determining a wearing schedule:

- What is the purpose of the orthosis?
- Does the therapist anticipate that the client will be compliant with an orthotic-wearing schedule?
- Does the client have any medical contraindications or precautions for removing the orthosis?
- Which variables may affect the client's tolerance of the orthosis?
- Does the client need assistance to apply or remove the orthosis?
- Is the orthosis for day or night use, or both?
- Does the client need to apply or remove the orthosis for functional activities?
- How often does the client need to perform exercise and hygiene tasks?

Answers to these questions should guide the development of a wearing schedule. The therapist should keep in mind that the wearing schedule may require adjustment as the client's condition progresses. In any situation the therapist should discuss the wearing schedule with the client and caregiver (Box 6.4).

BOX 6.4 Sample Wearing Schedule

Person's name:
Name of orthosis:
The purpose of this orthosis is to maintain the hand in a functional position.
Prescribed wearing schedule:
8 a.m. to 12 p.m. On[a]
12 p.m. to 2 p.m. Off Provide PROM
2 p.m. to 6 p.m. On
6 p.m. to 8 p.m. Off Provide PROM
8 p.m. to 12 p.m. On
12 a.m. to 2 a.m. Off Provide PROM
2 a.m. to 6 a.m. On
6 a.m. to 8 a.m. Off Provide PROM
Wear the orthosis on the right upper extremity. Please contact J. Smith at [phone number] in the Occupational Therapy Department if any of the following occur:
- Pink or reddened areas
- Complaints of increased pain because of the orthosis
- Increased swelling with orthotic wear
- Skin rash
- Complaints of decreased sensation because of the orthosis

PROM, Passive range of motion.
[a]Skin check to be performed.

DISCONTINUATION OF AN ORTHOSIS

No distinct rules exist concerning discontinuation of an orthosis. Frequently the physician makes the decision to discontinue an orthosis. Other times the physician defers to the clinical judgment of the therapist to determine when an orthosis is no longer beneficial. Specific protocols, such as for a flexor tendon repair, indicate when an orthosis is discontinued. In such cases the therapist should contact the physician for a discharge order. Sometimes physicians order an orthosis to be discontinued "cold turkey." If the therapist clinically reasons that the client would benefit from being weaned off the orthosis, the physician should be contacted. The therapist should communicate the rationale for the weaning and ask for approval. The following are questions to consider when making the clinical decision to discontinue an orthosis:

- Have the client and the caregivers been compliant with the orthotic-wearing schedule? If not, why?
- What are the original objectives for orthotic provision, and has the client accomplished them?
- Will the same objectives be compromised or accomplished without an orthosis?

Adherence of the person and the caregiver is essential for success with an orthotic-wearing regimen. If the client is not wearing the orthosis, the therapist first uses clinical reasoning to identify the reasons for nonadherence. For example, the nonadherence of an older client in an institutional setting could be the result of one or more of the following factors:

- Poor communication among the staff about the wearing schedule
- Poor staff follow-through with the wearing schedule
- The older adult's lack of understanding about the orthosis' purpose
- Discomfort of the orthosis
- The older adult's fear of hidden costs associated with the orthosis
- The older adult's dislike of the orthosis' cosmetic appearance

Reasons for nonadherence could be beyond this list, and it would be up to the therapist to ascertain the problem. After identifying the reason or reasons for nonadherence, the therapist can work on possible solutions.

An important factor in determining when to discontinue the orthosis is a careful review of the orthosis' objectives. For example, a therapist fabricates a mobilization orthosis for a client who has a proximal interphalangeal (PIP) soft-tissue flexion contracture of the middle finger. The objective is mobilization of the PIP joint to help correct the flexion deformity. Gradually the orthosis facilitates lengthening of the restricting structures, and extension is restored. By monitoring ROM and evaluating the orthosis' line of pull, the therapist determines that the orthosis has maximally helped the client and that the original intervention objectives were accomplished. At that time the therapist calls the physician for an order to discontinue the orthosis.

Therapists must consider whether accomplishment of the objectives is possible without the orthosis. Timely discontinuation of any orthosis is important. Therapists should keep in mind that inappropriately provided or poorly fabricated orthoses can restrict movement, make postural compromises by causing atrophy in one muscle group and overuse in another, and injure other parts of the anatomy. In addition, preventing the client's dependence on an orthosis is important. When the client has the functional capabilities, therapists should adjust the orthotic-wearing schedule to gradually wean the client away from the orthosis.[41]

COST AND PAYMENT ISSUES

Two issues exist regarding the cost of orthoses. First, how does the therapist arrive at the price of an orthosis? Second, how does the therapist receive payment for an orthosis? To calculate the price of an orthosis, the therapist totals the direct and indirect costs (Box 6.5). Direct costs include items such as the thermoplastic material, strapping material, stockinette, rivets, shipping costs, tax, and so on. A hospital or clinic purchases supplies at wholesale cost. However, a percentage markup may appear on the cost. (This assists with replenishing the inventory.) Indirect costs include nondisposable supplies (such as scissors and fry pans), the time required for the average therapist to make the orthosis, and overhead costs (such as rent and electricity).

BOX 6.5 Hints for Determining Direct and Indirect Costs

Direct Costs	Indirect Costs
<ul><li>Thermoplastic material</li><li>Know cost of sheet</li><li>Estimate how much of the sheet you used</li><li>Determine cost (¼ sheet used)</li><li>Strapping</li><li>Know cost per inch</li><li>Charge for number of inches used</li><li>Padding</li><li>Know cost per square inch</li><li>Charge for number of square inches used</li><li>Chemicals (cold spray, glue, solvent, and so on)</li><li>Usually a small set amount is charged whenever chemicals are used</li><li>Other materials (finger loops, outrigger kit, D-rings, and so on)</li><li>Charge the purchase amount</li><li>Time</li><li>Know cost per unit of time</li><li>Charge for number of units used to make the orthosis</li></ul>	<ul><li>Lighting, space, fry pan, hydrocollator, scissors, heat gun, shipping, handling, and storage charges for materials</li><li>Indirect costs are usually figured in a percentage markup of the direct costs of an orthosis (for example, a 10% markup cost)</li></ul>

Because of tighter control of health-care dollars, many therapists are finding that payment for orthoses is becoming increasingly difficult. It is important that when necessary the therapist take an active role in the outcome of a payment policy of an insurance plan regarding the orthosis. This may help obtain payment for the orthosis. For example, the therapist communicates with the case manager the purpose of the orthosis.

The therapist must remember, however, that the plan belongs to the client, not to the therapist. If an insurance plan reimburses costs partially or not at all, the therapist should inform the client of the responsibility for paying the balance of the cost. Some facilities make accommodations for people who are uninsured or underinsured and need orthotic provision, or there might be a pro bono clinic available in the area. In addition, the therapist should provide specific documentation to insurance companies about the affected extremity and the type of orthosis and purpose of the orthosis.[17]

It is important that therapists know how to effectively navigate the system to receive payment for orthotic fabrication. If an orthosis is ordered, it needs to be made. If the client declines the orthosis for any reason, appropriate documentation and communication with the referring physician is highly recommended. The therapist and the client should work out financial aspects with the facility and communicate with the appropriate clients, such as billing personnel. If the therapist works in a private clinic, billing and payment may be more challenging and require diligence to understand the variable nuances of the individual payer sources. Payment is always determined by the payer source. Generally, when billing, insurance companies expect a line item bill detailing all charges applied, including therapy codes, such as Current Procedural Terminology (CPT) codes[12] and supply charges. CPT codes are numeric codes covering tasks and services for payment.

For outpatient services, coding systems such as CPT codes are used for payment of orthotics. With Medicare Part B (outpatient therapy) therapists currently access Level I and Level II codes of the Healthcare Common Procedure Coding System (HCPCS) codes,[12] and the term *orthotics* is used with billing—not *splinting*. For Level I codes, therapists currently utilize the Medicare Physician Fee Schedule (MPFS) to determine the proper CPT codes. Different pricing exists for the MPFS between states. Level II HCPCS codes address products and supplies, including orthotics.[12] There are specific guidelines for filing a claim depending on the setting where the services are provided, such as for hospital outpatient, SNF Part B, in private practice, or in a physician's office practice. Billing is site specific, depending on what population is served with respect to individual insurance scenarios. Additionally, as payment is often linked closely with changes in public policy, therapists must keep abreast of these changes.

For some clients with upper extremity problems that occurred on the job, rehabilitation is reimbursed from the workers' compensation system. Therapists must keep in mind that in every state workers' compensation laws are interpreted differently. Therefore, it is important to be familiar with the state guidelines. Most state workers' compensation plans cover medical costs related to the injury, such as medical care (including receiving an orthosis), vocational rehabilitation, and temporary disability. (The amount varies from state to state.[4]) Many states have adopted a managed care system. With case managers the therapist should provide consistent and clear communication about the client's progress.

Some insurance companies simply refuse to pay for orthoses, and others ask for so much documentation that more time is required to prepare the bill than to make the orthosis. For example, some insurance companies ask therapists for original invoices for the purchase of thermoplastic and strapping materials. Developing outcome studies or finding evidence in the literature may help obtain payment from insurers. Giving these outcomes to insurers will increase their understanding of the importance of orthotic intervention in its relation to function. The American Society of Hand Therapists[2] published *Splint Classification Systems,* a book about naming and designing orthoses. This book helps terminology become more uniform.[2]

Policy Regulations: The Health Insurance Portability and Accountability Act

This broad health legislation enacted in 1996 covers many areas with Title II, or Administrative Simplification, influencing therapy practice. Title II includes three main parts: Transaction Rule, Privacy Rule, and Security Rule. The first part, Transaction Rule, affects billing procedures. It mandates uniform national requirements for formats and codes for electronic transmission.[61]

Privacy Rule is another major component of Administrative Simplification and directly influences clinical practice. Privacy rules involve protection of client-identifying or confidential information and client rights about their health information. These rules regulate how protected health information (PHI) or any client-identifying information is presented in written, verbal, or electronic format.[53] Therapists should obtain the client's consent before using PHI for intervention, payment, or health care operations. However, if a client objects or fails to provide consent, therapists are permitted to use PHI for intervention, payment, or health care operations without the client's consent. In most other circumstances, with very few exceptions, therapists may not disclose PHI without the client's written authorization to do so.[54]

Numerous privacy rights with respect to the client's health information are written into the regulations. For example, clients have a right to request to see their medical record. See Box 6.6 for a listing of client protections. Therapy clinics should have policies in place to protect the privacy of client information. Requiring working charts to be kept in a locked cabinet with the documents shredded after intervention completion is an example of an internal policy protecting privacy.[15] Other guidelines for protecting client privacy apply to use of electronic health records (EHRs). Some areas of client

---

BOX 6.6 Client Protections

The following are key client protections with a brief description:

- Access to medical records: See or obtain copies of medical records, and ask for corrections of errors.
- Notice of privacy practice: Covered providers must provide information on how personal medical information will be used and patient rights under HIPAA regulations.
- Limits on use of personal medical information: Sets guidelines on minimal standards of health care information sharing.
- Prohibition on marketing: Sets guidelines on disclosing of client information for marketing purposes.
- Stronger state laws: State laws that are stronger than HIPAA are followed.
- Confidential communications: Clients can request that confidentiality be kept (e.g., asking the therapist to call his or her work instead of home).
- Complaints: Clients have a right to file a formal complaint.

HIPAA, Health Insurance Portability and Accountability Act.

---

information are excluded from the law, such as allowing clients to sign in for intervention, calling out a client's name to go into the orthotic fabrication room, or sharing information with another health professional about the orthosis.[15,51] However, reasonable efforts to avoid these types of disclosures should be taken. For instance, instead of calling out, "Mr. Edward Jones, the therapist will see you now to customize your resting hand orthosis," a better approach would be, "Edward, the therapist will see you now."

Incidental disclosures (information that is heard with reasonable efforts to not be overheard) or sharing information that is limited are not considered in violation of the **Health Insurance Portability and Accountability Act (HIPAA) law.**[51] An example of an incidental disclosure is an occupational therapist discussing information about an orthosis bill with the secretary in the waiting room. These disclosures are not considered liable under the law as long as there are no other reasonable options (i.e., no other area for individual privacy to discuss the bill).[50] Because therapy often takes place in an open area with several people involved in conversations, some of which potentially involve sharing of PHI, it needs to be clear in the consent form about the clinic setup.[37,38] Therapists working in clinics with an open area can employ simple strategies to allow more privacy, such as partitioning off a private area or using a private room available for intervention, communicating with lower voices, and being careful with leaving sensitive messages on answering machines.[64] As York states, "creating a culture of privacy and maintaining good rapport with patients will go a long way to preventing HIPAA complaints as well as other types of legal problems."[64]

The third main part of Administrative Simplification, the Security Rule, involves the policies and procedures that a facility has in place to protect the PHI through "administrative, technical and physical safeguards."[61] The Security Rule mainly focuses on "electronic protected health information,"[61] such as who has access to computer data in a clinic. The simplification provisions include national identifiers for health care providers and practitioners.[55] Finally, therapists must keep abreast of their state privacy laws. If they are stricter, they take priority over the HIPAA regulations.[64]

Documentation

Orthotic application must be well documented. **Documentation** assists in third-party payment and communication with other health care providers, helps ascertain the medical-legal necessity, and demonstrates the efficacy of the intervention. This section provides an overview of general documentation principles to be used with orthotics whether documentation is in written or in electronic format.

Orthotic documentation should be specific and should include several elements, such as the onset of the medical condition that warrants an orthosis; the medical necessity for the orthosis; the level of function before the orthosis; the client's rehabilitation potential with the orthosis; and type, purpose, and anatomical location of the orthosis. Therapists should also document that they have communicated with the client an oral and written wearing schedule and have had discussions about precautions. Any input that the client provides to the intervention plan, such as mutual goal setting, should be documented.

Orthotic documentation, including goal setting, should be related to function. It is not sufficient to document that a client's ROM has improved to a certain level because of wearing an orthosis. The therapist should specifically document how the improved ROM has helped the client perform specific functional activities. For example, the therapist may document that because of improved wrist motion from wearing an orthosis, the client is able to work on a computer. As with any documentation, the therapist should consider legal implications. Documentation should be thorough, complete, and objective. The therapist should always remember, "If it wasn't documented, it didn't happen." For example, the therapist should document the specific measurements by which the hand is positioned, the diagnosis and type of orthosis fabricated and any client communication. Also, for example, if the client has a reddened area because of wearing an orthosis, the specific location and size of the reddened area as well as any orthotic adjustments made should be documented. Any communication or advice about the orthosis from the physician should be documented with the time and date of the call.[16]

Documentation for follow-up visits should include the date and time that the client is supposed to return and a notation that the date and time have been discussed with the client. This helps protect the therapist if there are claims of negligence with follow-up care.[16] Documentation for follow-up visits should also include any changes in the orthotic design and wearing schedule. In addition, the therapist should note whether problems with adherence are apparent. Documenting evidence of adherence includes documenting instructions provided and objective client's or caregiver's behavior that contradicts instructions. For example, the therapist might document that the client stated that he or she did not follow the orthotic-wearing schedule. Documenting dates and times that the orthotic-wearing schedule is not being followed for a client in a SNF is an example of specific documentation. If this happens, the therapist may further educate the caregivers and note when and what type of education was completed. If the caregivers still do not properly follow the schedule, the therapist should come up with another plan and involve the caregivers in the decision-making process to ensure adherence.

Another objective observation for a client followed in any setting is notation of signs of wear, such as scratching, light soil, or strap wear. With documentation, it is inappropriate to criticize other health care professionals, such as documenting that contractures developed because the nursing staff did not apply an orthosis.[16]

The therapist should perform orthotic reassessments regularly until completion of the client's weaning from the orthosis or discharge from services. Documentation after the reassessments should be timely and based on guidelines from the insurer.[16] Finally, the therapist should keep in mind that different facilities use different methods to document, and the therapist should be familiar with the routine method of the facility. (See Examples 6.1 and 6.2 for illustrations of a narrative and a SOAP note for an orthosis, respectively.)

ORTHOTIC INTERVENTION ERROR AND CLIENT SAFETY ISSUES

Orthotic intervention errors occur in occupational therapy.[43] Examples of these errors include fabricating the wrong type of orthosis for the condition or failure to follow through with the orthotic-wearing schedule. Either of these errors could cause client harm, such as severe pain or breakdown of the skin. Although many errors are the direct result of individual failure, most errors are caused by system problems. System errors may occur due to diagnostic error, equipment/product failure, or miscommunication of medical orders, to name a few.

Orthotic intervention errors can easily result from incorrect or inadequate communication. A physician, for example, may order a right-hand orthosis when it is meant for the left hand. If the therapist fails to question the physician order, an orthosis may be fabricated for the wrong site. Wrong patient, wrong site, or wrong procedure is one of the leading sentinel events reported to the Joint Commission on Accreditation of Healthcare Organizations (The Joint Commission).[27] According to data collected by The Joint Commission, team miscommunication is at the root of a great proportion of all errors made in health care.[28] Occupational therapists often lack assertiveness when communicating with physicians, and

this failure to adequately communicate can result in patient harm.[14]

Understanding the nature of hierarchical organizational structures and the need for coordination of care through "interdisciplinary care management" and "coordinated communication" are vital to **client safety**.[26] Occupational therapists need to participate in team training.[22] Team training allows therapists to have the knowledge, skill, and attitude competencies,[36] as well as assertiveness and adaptability capability to enhance communication, team effectiveness, and the culture of safety.[18]

To create this culture of safety, occupational therapists must also debunk or dispel the myth of performance perfection. To err is human! After all, health care delivery is a very complex system. In complex systems, errors are inevitable regardless of how well trained, well intentioned, or ultracareful the individual therapist may be. In the case of the therapist acting on the physician's wrong order, it would be unjust to simply require the last treating practitioner to be fully accountable for the error. In this situation, blaming and sanctioning would only encourage the therapist and/or physician to hide the error rather than disclose and report it.

Today's undisclosed near miss or minor error can become tomorrow's egregiously harmful error. Only by acknowledging error can health practitioners individually and collectively learn from that error and make individual and system practice changes to prevent errors in the future. Furthermore, truthful disclosure of error to clients by the therapist or a disclosure team is not only an ethical obligation but organizations (such as The Joint Commission, the University of Michigan Health System, and the Veterans Health Administration) and several states now mandate disclosure.[1,58]

Part of the disclosure process should be expressions of sympathy and a formal and authentic apology. There is an advocacy organization, The Sorry Works! Coalition,[59] that provides disclosure and apology educational programs to practitioners to assist them in communicating with clients who have been harmed by an error.[60] In the past, health care practitioners were actually cautioned by their malpractice insurance carriers not to apologize, because an apology might increase the chances of being sued.[5] Currently at least 36 states have enacted statutes that prevent some or all information given in an apology from being used if a client sues a practitioner.[25] Clients want to receive apologies and to be told the truth when an error occurs that causes them harm. Many health care organizations that have instituted disclosure programs now have evidence that disclosing errors can lower liability lawsuit expenses.

Ultimately, creating an environment where practitioners are encouraged and supported for promoting safety, reporting errors, and truthfully disclosing them to clients is everyone's goal. This practice safety goal should always be a guidepost for clinical reasoning when orthotic fabrication failures occur.

🔲 SELF-QUIZ 6.1[a]

For the following questions, circle either true (T) or false (F).

1. T F An infant can follow an orthotic-wearing program without extraordinary methods.
2. T F Determining a client's lifestyle needs for orthotic design and material is important.
3. T F Paramount to a client's cooperation is education about the medical necessity for wearing an orthosis.
4. T F If a client has a wound that requires dressing changes, the therapist should fabricate the orthosis over the dressing and instruct the client to apply new dressings at appropriate intervals.
5. T F The only sign of an ill-fitting orthosis is red marks.
6. T F A well-fitting orthosis, upon removal, may leave a red area on the client's skin.
7. T F In the presence of severe edema, the therapist should use circumferential straps.
8. T F The therapist should use a heat gun for all necessary adjustments.
9. T F If motion is decreased because of joint limitation, the therapist should decrease the frequency or time the client wears the orthosis.
10. T F When deciding to discontinue an orthosis, the therapist must consider the original objectives of the orthotic fabrication.
11. T F To calculate the cost of an orthosis, the therapist should consider the direct and indirect costs.
12. T F Payment is always determined by the payer source.
13. T F If a client develops a reddened area because of wearing an orthosis, the therapist should just document that fact and note specifics about location or size of the affected area.
14. T F Calling out a client's name in a waiting room to go back into the orthotic fabrication area is considered in violation of HIPAA.

[a]See Appendix A for the answer key.

REVIEW QUESTIONS

1. How would a therapist apply the various clinical reasoning models to orthotic provision?
2. What does an orthosis referral include?
3. How can the therapist facilitate communication with the physician's office about the orthosis referral?
4. Why is knowing the client's age important to the therapist when fabricating an orthosis?
5. Which lifestyle needs of the client must the therapist consider with orthotic provision?
6. How can the therapist enhance the adherence of a client wearing an orthosis?
7. What are the infection control procedures that a therapist should follow with orthotic provision?
8. What should therapists monitor when providing an orthosis for a client during the following conditions: pressure, edema, and physical status of a client?
9. What are the four directions of orthotic design?
10. What are some helpful hints for adjusting after orthotic fabrication?
11. What are the factors that the therapist should consider when establishing a client on an orthotic-wearing schedule?
12. What are the factors that a therapist should consider for orthosis discontinuation?
13. What are the cost and payment issues the therapist must keep in mind?
14. How might HIPAA influence communication with clients about orthoses in a clinical setting?
15. What documentation issues should the therapist be aware of with orthotic intervention?
16. What is the best way to morally manage an orthotic fabrication error that causes harm to a client?

REFERENCES

1. AHRQ (Agency for Healthcare Research and Quality: *PS Network (Patient Safety Network), Patient safety primer, disclosure of errors*, 2017. Retrieved from https://psnet.ahrq.gov/primers/primer/2/disclosure-of-errors.
2. American Society of Hand Therapists: *Splint Classification Systems*, Garner, NJ, 1992, The American Society of Hand Therapists.
3. Armstrong J: Splinting the pediatric patient. In Fess EE, Gettle KS, Philips CA, et al.: *Hand and upper extremity splinting: principles and methods*, ed 3, St. Louis, 2005, Elsevier Mosby, pp 480–516.
4. Bailey DM: Legislative and reimbursement influences on occupational therapy: changing opportunities. In Neistadt ME, Crepaeau EB, editors: *Willard & Spackman's occupational therapy*, ed 9, Philadelphia, 1998, Lippincott, pp 763–772.
5. Banja J: Does medical error disclosure violate the medical malpractice insurance cooperation clause? In Henriksen K,

Battles JB, Marks ES, et al.: *Advances in patient safety: from research to implementation (Volume 3: Implementation Issues)*, Rockville, MD, 2005, Agency for Healthcare Research and Quality.
6. Batteson R: A strategy to improve nurse/occupational therapist communication for managing clients with splints, *Br J Occup Ther* 60:451–454, 1997.
7. Benner P, Hughes RG, Sulphen M: Chapter 6: Clinical reasoning, decision making, and action: thinking critically and clinically. In Hughes RG, editor: *Patient safety and quality: an evidence-based handbook for nurses*, Rockville, MD, 2008, Agency for Healthcare Research and Quality.
8. Bower KA: Compliance as a patient education issue. In Woldum KM, Ryan-Morrell V, Towson MC, et al.: *Patient education: foundations of practice*, Rockville, MD, 1985, Aspen Publications, pp 45–111.
9. Brand PW, Hollister A: *Clinical mechanics of the hand*, ed 2, St. Louis, 1993, Mosby.

10. Callinan NJ, Mathiowetz V: Soft versus hard resting hand splints in rheumatoid arthritis: pain relief, preference, and compliance, *Am J Occup Ther* 50(5):347–353, 1996.

11. Cannon NM, Foltz RW, Koepfer JM, et al.: *Manual of Hand Splinting*, New York, 1985, Churchill Livingstone.

12. Centers for Medicare & Medicaid Services: *HCPCS—general information*, CMS.gov (website). Retrieved from https://www.cms.gov/MedHCPCSGenInfo/.

13. Colditz JC: Therapist's management of the still hand. In Mackin EJ, Callahan AD, Skirven TM, et al.: *Rehabilitation of the hand and upper extremity*, ed 5, St. Louis, 2002, Mosby, pp 1021–1049.

14. Cochran TM, Mu K, Lohman H, et al.: Physical therapists' perspectives on practice errors in geriatric, neurologic, or orthopedic settings, *Physiother Theory Pract* 25(1):1–13, 2009.

15. Costa DM, Whitehouse D: HIPAA and fieldwork, *OT Practice* 8(17):23–24, 2003.

16. Ekelman-Ranke BR: Documentation in the age of litigation, *OT Practice* 3(3):20–24, 1998.

17. Evans RB: *Personal communication*, February 7, 1995.

18. Facione NC, Facione PA: Critical thinking and clinical judgement. In Facione NC, Facione PA, editors: *Critical thinking and clinical reasoning in the health sciences: an international multidisciplinary teaching anthology*, Millbrae, CA, 2008, The California Academic Press.

19. Fess EE, Gettle KS, Philips CA, et al.: *Hand and upper extremity splinting: principles and methods*, ed 3, St. Louis, 2005, Elsevier Mosby.

20. Fleming MH: Conditional reasoning: creating meaningful experiences. In Mattingly C, Fleming MH, editors: *Clinical reasoning: forms of inquiry in a therapeutic practice*, Philadelphia, 1994, FA Davis, pp 197–235.

21. Fleming MH: The therapists with the three-track mind, *Am J Occup Ther* 45:1007–1014, 1991.

22. Gaston T, Short N, Ralyea C, Casterline G: Promoting patient safety: results of a TeamSTEPPS Initiative, *J Nurs Admin* 46(4):201–207, 2016.

23. Groth GN, Wilder DM, Young VL: The impact of compliance of rehabilitation of patients with mallet finger injuries, *J Hand Ther* 7(1):21–24, 1994.

24. Groth GN, Wulf MB: Compliance with hand rehabilitation: health beliefs and strategies, *J Hand Ther* 8(1):18–22, 1995.

25. Ho B, Liu E: Does sorry work? The impact of apology laws on medical malpractice, *J Risk Uncertain* 43:141–167, 2011.

26. Joint Commission on Accreditation of Health Care Organizations: *Patient safety: Essentials for healthcare*, ed 3, Oakbrook, IL, 2005, Joint Commission Resources.

27. Joint Commission: *Summary data of sentinel events reviewed by The Joint Commission, 2014–2017*, Retrieved from https://www.jointcommission.org/assets/1/18/Summary_4Q_2017.pdf.

28. Joint Commission: *Sentinel event data—Root causes by event type 2004-2015*, Retrieved from http://www.tsigconsulting.com/tolcam/wp-content/uploads/2015/04/TJC-Sentinel-Event-Root_Causes_by_Event_Type_2004-2014.pdf.

29. Kirwan T, Tooth L, Harkin C: Compliance with hand therapy programs: therapists' and patients' perceptions, *J Hand Ther* 15(1):31–40, 2002.

30. Law M, Baptiste S, Carswell A, et al.: *Canadian Occupational Performance Measure*, ed 3, Ottawa, ON, 1998, CAOT Publications.

31. Loue S, Sajatovic M: Adherence. *Encyclopedia of aging and public health*, ed 1, New York, Springer.

32. Mackin EJ, Callahan AD, Skirven TM, et al.: *Rehabilitation of the hand and upper extremity*, ed 5, St. Louis, 2002, Mosby.

33. Mattingly C: The narrative nature of clinical reasoning, *Am J Occup Ther* 45:998–1005, 1991.

34. Mattingly C, Fleming MH: *Clinical reasoning: forms of inquiry in a therapeutic practice*, Philadelphia, 1994, FA Davis.

35. McCune RL: Understanding health literacy, *Home Healthc Nurse* 32(10):617–618, 2014.

36. Mu K, Lohman H, Scheirton L, et al.: Improving client safety: strategies to prevent and reduce practice errors in occupational therapy, *Am J Occup Ther* 65(6):69–76, 2011.

37. Murer CG: Trends and issues: protecting patient privacy, *Rehab Management* 15(3):46–47, 2002.

38. Neistadt ME: Teaching clinical reasoning as a thinking frame, *Am J Occup Ther* 52:211–229, 1998.

39. O'Brien L: Adherence to therapeutic splint wear in adults with acute upper limb injuries: a systematic review, *Hand Ther* 15:3–10, 2010.

40. Parham D: Towards professionalism: the reflective therapist, *Am J Occup Ther* 41:555–560, 1987.

41. Pascarelli E, Quilter D: *Repetitive strain injury*, New York, 1994, John Wiley & Sons.

42. Reynolds CC: Preoperative and postoperative management of tendon transfers after radial nerve injury. In Hunter JM, Mackin EJ, Callahan AD, editors: *Rehabilitation of the hand*, ed 4, St. Louis, 1995, Mosby, pp 753–763.

43. Scheirton LS, Mu K, Lohman H: Occupational therapists' responses to practice errors in physical rehabilitation settings, *Am J Occup Ther* 57(3):307–314, 2003.

44. Schell BA, Cervero RM: Clinical reasoning in occupational therapy: an integrated review, *Am J Occup Ther* 47:605–610, 1993.

45. Schon DA: *Educating the reflective practitioner*, San Francisco, 1987, Jossey-Bass.

46. Schultz-Johnson K: *Personal communication*, March 1999.

47. Skotak CH, Stockdell SM: Wound management in hand therapy. In Cromwell FS, Bear-Lehman J, editors: *Hand rehabilitation in occupational therapy*, Binghamton, NY, 1988, Haworth Press, pp 17–35.

48. Southam MA, Dunbar JM: Integration of adherence problems. In Meichenbaum D, Turk DC, editors: *Facilitating treatment adherence*, New York, 1987, Plenum Publishing.

49. Stern EB, Ytterberg SR, Krug HE, et al.: Commercial wrist extensor orthoses: a descriptive study of use and preference in patients with rheumatoid arthritis, *Arthritis Care Res* 10(1):27–35, 1997.

50. Sullivan JM: *Personal communication*, October 12, 2004.

51. Sullivan JM: *The OT's guide to HIPAA: the impact of privacy laws on the practice of occupational therapy*, Minneapolis, MN, 2004, The American Occupational Therapy Association.

52. Trombly C: Anticipating the future: assessment of occupational function, *Am J Occup Ther* 47:253–257, 1993.

53. U.S. Department of Health & Human Services: *Fact sheet: protecting the privacy of patients' health information*. Retrieved from http://dlthede.net/informatics/chap20ehrissues/privacyfactsapril03.pdf.

54. U.S. Department of Health & Human Services: *What is the difference between "consent" and "authorization" under the HIPAA Privacy Rule?* Retrieved from https://www.hhs.gov/hipaa/for-professionals/faq/264/what-is-the-difference-between-consent-and-authorization/index.html.

55. U.S. Department of Health & Human Services: *HIPAA for professionals, 2017*. Retrieved from http://www.hhs.gov/ocr/privacy/hipaa/administrative/index.html.

56. U.S. Department of Health & Human Services: *National action plan to improve health literacy: summary*. Retrieved from https://health.gov/communication/HLAction-Plan/pdf/Health_Lit_Action_Plan_Summary.pdf, 2010.

57. U.S. Department of Health & Human Services: *Quick guide to health literacy: strategies*. Retrieved from https://health.gov/communication/literacy/quickguide/healthinfo.htm.

58. Veterans Health Administration (VHA): *Disclosure of adverse events to patients*. VHA Handbook 1004.08, Retrieved from: https://www.ethics.va.gov/Handbook1004-08.pdf, 2012.

59. Wojcieszak D: *Sorry Works*. Sorry works! Tool Kit Book, Bloomington, IN, 2015, AuthorHouse. Retrieved from http://sorryworks.net.

60. Wojcieszak D: Online disclosure learning courses for front-line staff. Retrieved from https://sorryworks.net/online-disclosure-training/.

61. Wilson HP: HIPAA: the big picture for home care and hospice, *Home Health Care Mang Pract* 16(2):127–137, 2004.

62. World Health Organization: *Adherence to long-term therapies: evidence for action*. Retrieved from http://www.who.int/entity/chp/knowledge/publications/adherence_full_report.pdf?ua=1.

63. Wright HH, Rettig A: Management of common sports injuries. In Mackin EJ, Callahan AD, Skirven TM, et al.: *Rehabilitation of the hand and upper extremity*, ed 5, St. Louis, 2005, Mosby, pp 2076–2109.

64. York AM: HIPAA smarts: top 10 privacy musts, *Rehab Management* 16(2):44–45, 2003.

APPENDIX 6.1 CASE STUDIES

Case Study 6.1[a]

Read the following scenario, and answer the questions based on information in this chapter.

Steven, a 46-year-old construction worker who has problems with alcohol consumption, awakened from a drinking binge after he fell asleep with his arm over the top of a chair to find that his right hand and wrist were limp. He showed his wife how he could no longer extend his wrist to do activities and stated, "Maybe I had a stroke." Hoping that his function would improve, he waited a few days and then decided to see his primary physician. Steven asserted to his physician that he thought he had a stroke and was concerned about his ability to do work. The physician examined Steven's arm and stated, "I can't say for certain whether it was a small stroke or a nerve injury. In the past with issues like this, I have referred patients to an occupational therapist at an outpatient therapy clinic." Occupational therapy was ordered for intervention and orthotic fabrication. The order was vague as to what type of orthosis.

You are a new therapist at the outpatient clinic. Initial evaluation reveals decreased sensation in the pathway of the radial nerve, absent wrist extension, metacarpophalangeal (MCP) finger extension, and thumb abduction and extension. Please refer to Chapter 13 for information on nerve injuries.

1. What injury do you assume Steven has sustained, and how did he sustain it?
2. How do you clarify the physician's order if you are unsure about it?
3. As a new therapist unsure about which one, where would you find the information about an appropriate orthosis for this patient?
4. After completion of the orthosis, you send Steven home with a home exercise program and instructions about orthotic wear. What type of education and orthotic-wearing schedule will you provide? Why?
5. Upon return to the clinic, Steven states that he does not like wearing the orthosis because, as he states, "It does not fit with my macho image, and it seems like it is taking forever to do any good." He reports minimal wear of the orthosis. How will you handle his nonadherence?

Case Study 6.2[a]

Read the following scenario, and answer the questions based on information in this chapter.

Marie, a 57-year-old woman, is employed as a department store clerk. She works part-time except for the winter holiday season. She has been in good health except for having diabetes, which is well regulated. Her job demands involve unloading boxes, stocking new merchandise, and operating a cash register. During the winter holiday season, Marie worked 40-hour weeks. In addition, she was busy at home decorating and baking. One week before Christmas she noted pain radiating up her dominant right forearm and around the radial styloid.

[a] See Appendix A for the answer key.

Marie complained to her employer of pain when moving the thumb and when turning her forearm up. Marie was seen by the company physician, who diagnosed her condition as de Quervain tenosynovitis. She was provided with a prefabricated thumb immobilization orthosis, which she did not wear due to it being uncomfortable and causing some chafing on the volar surface of the thumb interphalangeal (IP) joint. Two weeks later, when symptoms did not improve, the company physician ordered occupational therapy. The order read: "Fabricate an R thumb orthosis and provide a home exercise program." The following initial therapy note purposely displays flawed documentation.

10-13

Client was followed on 10-13 for fabrication of an orthosis and to provide a home exercise program. Client was wearing a prefabricated orthosis. Reddened areas were noted on the thumb. Client was instructed in a home exercise program, orthotic precautions, and a wearing schedule. It doesn't appear that the client will be compliant with wearing the orthosis.

Results of the evaluation are as follows:

ROM	All ROM was WNL except for the following:
	• Thumb:
	• DIP flexion, 0-50; MP flexion, 0-30; palmar abduction, 0-30
	• Radial abduction, 0-30; Opposition: to ring finger
	• Wrist:
	• Flexion, 0-50; extension, 0-40; ulnar deviation, 0-15; radial deviation, 0-15
	• FA: supination, 0-45
Strength	• Grasp strength: R UE, 35#s; L UE, 52#s
	• Pinch strength: Lateral, tip, and key pinch R UE, 5#s; L UE, 10#s
Edema evaluation	Edema noted around area of radial styloid. Circumferential measurement at that area: R UE, 10 cm; L UE, 9 cm.
Volometer reading	• R UE, 420; L UE, 380
Circulation	• WNL for Allen testing. Temperature: WNL
Sensory evaluation	• WNL to Semmes-Weinstein Monofilament Test

DIP, Distal interphalangeal; *FA,* forearm; *L,* left; *MP,* metacarpal; *R,* right; *ROM,* range of motion; *UE,* upper extremity; *WNL,* within normal limits.

Goals

• Long-term goal: Patient will follow provided orthotic-wearing schedule by discharge from therapy.
• Short-term goal: Patient will show decreased symptoms from de Quervain tenosynovitis.

To encourage clinical reasoning skills, answer the following questions about the case. See Chapter 8 for specifics about orthoses for de Quervain tenosynovitis.

1. List a minimum of five areas of the documentation that could be improved by being more specific or more complete.

2. Based on the interactive clinical reasoning approach, what are two questions that will facilitate an understanding of the impact that having de Quervain tenosynovitis and wearing an orthosis has on Marie's work and home life?

3. What are some concerns about adherence you may have based on Marie's history with her prefabricated orthosis? How will you approach any adherence concerns?

4. Considering that the referral came from work, what type of insurance might Marie have?

APPENDIX 6.2 EXAMPLES

Example 6.1

The following is an initial progress note (IPN) following orthotic fabrication. Although this note is an exemplar for written documentation, the same information should be included in electronic format.

February 24, 20___, 4:00 PM

This 42-year-old female was seen by an occupational therapist for fabrication of a right wrist immobilization orthosis on the dominant R UE. Client has a history of carpal tunnel syndrome since August 20, 20___. Client reports being independent in ADLs, work, and leisure tasks before condition developed. Client displays problems related to carpal tunnel syndrome, including decreased R grip strength, R hand swelling at end of day, pain, tingling, decreased sensation in the area of the median nerve, and a positive Phalen sign. (Refer to the summary report of the Semmes-Weinstein Monofilament Test.) Client displays problems with cooking meals and typing on computer at work. Client currently requires help from her daughter for such tasks as opening cans and jars and cutting food with a knife. Client is employed as a secretary, and job demands primarily involve computer work. At work, client tolerates 20 minutes of typing on computer before pain and tingling develop in the R hand. Client stated, "It is difficult for me to type on the computer and cook a meal." B UE AROM was WNL except for the following R UE motions:

- Thumb: Opposition to ring finger—unable to oppose little finger
- R finger TAMs (Normal = 250 to 265 degrees):
  - Index = 230 degrees
  - Middle = 230 degrees
  - Ring = 240 degrees
  - Little = 270 degrees
- R wrist:
  - Flexion = 0 to 50 degrees (Normal = 0 to 80 degrees)
  - Wrist extension (WNL)
  - Radial deviation = 0 to 15 degrees (Normal = 0 to 20 degrees)
  - Ulnar deviation (WNL)

Grip strength was tested with Jamar dynamometer. R grip strength = 30 pounds (10th percentile for age and gender) and L grip strength = 64 pounds (Normal = 75th percentile for age and gender). MMT results are as follows:

- R abductor pollicis = 3 (fair)/5, L = 5 (normal)/5
- R opponens pollicis = 3 (fair)/5, L = 5 (normal)/5

A R volar-based, neutral wrist immobilization orthosis was fabricated. Client presented with no pressure marks or rash after orthotic application. Client was evaluated for functional hand motions while wearing the orthosis. The orthosis did not restrict finger and thumb motions. Client received verbal and written instructions about orthotic-wearing schedule and a form to document wearing adherence. Client could independently don and doff her orthosis. Client received verbal and written instructions for a home exercise program, orthosis precautions, and ergonomic adaptations for home and work environments. Client's understanding of all instructions appeared to be good. Client will be followed two more times per physician order to monitor orthosis and program and ergonomic adaptations.

OT Goals

LTGs: Client will report a decrease in R hand pain and tingling to complete home and work activities independently by [date].

STGs:

- Client will independently complete computer tasks at work while wearing R wrist orthosis for 3 hours daily and taking hourly exercise breaks by [date].
- Client will independently cook a meal while wearing R wrist orthosis and report reduced pain by [date].
- Client will properly position B UEs during computer work activities and utilize ergonomic office equipment by [date].
- Client will comply with orthotic-wearing schedule 90% of the time as evidenced by the orthotic-wearing schedule adherence sheet by [date].

ADLs, Activities of daily living; *AROM,* active range of motion; *B,* bilateral *L,* left; *LTG,* long-term goal; *MMT,* manual muscle testing; *OT,* occupational therapy; *R,* right; *STG,* short-term goal; *TAM,* total active motion; *UE,* upper extremity; *WNL,* within normal limits.

Example 6.2

The following is an OT SOAP note. Although this note is an exemplar for written documentation, the same information can be included in electronic format.

February 24, 20___, 4:00 PM

S (subjective): "My right hand tingles and hurts all the time." Client also reports difficulty cooking meals and typing on the computer while at work.

O (objective): Client presents with an Hx of carpal tunnel symptoms in dominant, R, hand since August 20, 20___. Client reports being independent in ADLs, work, and leisure tasks before condition developed. Client displays a positive R Phalen sign with decreased sensation in the R median nerve distribution area. (Refer to Semmes-Weinstein Monofilament

Test summary sheet.) B UE AROM was WNL, except for the following motions:

R thumb opposition to ring finger—unable to oppose little finger

R finger TAMs (Normal = 250 to 265 degrees):

- Index = 230 degrees
- Middle = 230 degrees
- Ring = 240 degrees
- Little = 270 degrees
- R wrist: Flexion = 0 to 50 degrees (Normal = 0 to 80 degrees)
- Wrist extension (WNL)
- Radial deviation = 0 to 15 degrees (Normal = 0 to 20 degrees)
- Ulnar deviation (WNL)

Grip strength was tested with Jamar dynamometer. R grip strength = 30 pounds (10th percentile for age and gender). L grip strength = 64 pounds (75th percentile for age and gender). MMT results as follows:

- Abductor pollicis: R = 3 (fair)/5, L = 5 (normal)/5
- Opponens pollicis: R = 3 (fair)/5, L = 5 (normal)/5

Client displays problems related to carpal tunnel syndrome, including decreased R grip strength, R hand swelling at end of day, and problems with cooking meals and typing on computer at work. Client currently requires help from her daughter for such tasks as opening cans and jars and cutting food with a knife. At work, client tolerates 20 minutes of typing on computer before pain and tingling develop in the R hand.

A R volar-based, neutral wrist immobilization orthosis was fabricated. Client presented with no pressure marks or rash after orthotic application. Client was evaluated for functional hand motions while wearing the orthosis. The orthosis does not restrict finger and thumb motions. Client received verbal and written instructions about orthotic-wearing schedule and a form to document wearing adherence. Client was able to independently don and doff orthosis. Client received verbal and written instructions for a home exercise program, orthosis precautions, and ergonomic adaptations for home and work environments. Client's understanding of all instructions appeared to be good.

A (assessment): Client seems to have a good rehabilitation potential as she reports motivation to comply with OT intervention. Client is able to complete functional activities while wearing the R wrist immobilization orthosis. Symptoms may decrease with orthosis wear and with implementation of the home exercise program and ergonomic home and work adaptations.

P (plan): Client will be followed two more times per physician order to monitor orthosis and program and ergonomic adaptations.

OT Goals

LTGs: Client will report a decrease in R hand pain and tingling so as to complete home and work activities independently by [date].

STGs:

- Client will independently complete computer tasks at work while wearing R wrist orthosis for 3 hours daily and taking hourly exercise breaks by [date].
- Client will independently cook a meal while wearing R wrist orthosis and report reduced pain by [date].
- Client will properly position B UEs during computer work activities and utilize ergonomic office equipment by [date].
- Client will comply with orthotic-wearing schedule 90% of the time as evidenced by the orthotic-wearing schedule adherence sheet by [date].

(John Smith, OTR)

ADLs, Activities of daily living; *AROM,* active range of motion; *B,* bilateral; *Hx,* history; *L,* left; *LTG,* long-term goal; *OT,* occupational therapy; *OTR,* registered occupational therapist; *R,* right; *STG,* short-term goal; *TAM,* total active motion; *UE,* upper extremity; *WNL,* within normal limits.

UNIT TWO

Orthosis for Conditions and Populations

7

Orthoses for the Wrist

Helene L. Lohman

CHAPTER OBJECTIVES

1. Discuss diagnostic indications for wrist immobilization orthoses.
2. Identify major features of wrist immobilization orthoses.
3. Describe the fabrication process for a volar or dorsal wrist orthosis.
4. Relate hints for a proper fit for a wrist immobilization orthosis.
5. Review precautions for wrist immobilization orthotic intervention.
6. Use clinical reasoning to evaluate a problematic wrist immobilization orthosis.
7. Use clinical reasoning to evaluate proper fit of a fabricated wrist immobilization orthosis.
8. Apply knowledge about the application of wrist immobilization orthoses to case studies.
9. Explain the importance of evidence-based practice and how it informs wrist orthotic provision.
10. Describe the appropriate use of prefabricated wrist orthoses.

KEY TERMS

carpal tunnel syndrome (CTS)
circumferential
complex regional pain syndrome (CRPS)
dorsal

forearm trough
hypothenar bar
metacarpal bar
radial nerve injuries
rheumatoid arthritis (RA)

tendinopathy
tendinosis
ulnar
volar

You are dining with your good friend, Julia. She tells you she has been experiencing night pain in her right wrist, thumb, index, and middle fingers. You ask her to describe the pain, and she says it feels like pins and needles and sometimes her fingers become numb. Immediately you inquire what she has been doing lately. Julia is a student in a rigorous professional speech language therapy program. Besides much repetitive typing on the computer, she works part-time in a lawn and gardening business. That job involves repetitive pinching and wrist flexion with weeding as well as sustained grip and vibration when using an electric lawn mower. You suspect she might have carpal tunnel syndrome (CTS) and advise her to see her physician. A week later you see Julia again. She informs you that she was diagnosed with CTS and asks you what types of therapy could help alleviate the symptoms. You tell her that based on evidence, an effective intervention in early stages of CTS is to wear an orthosis that positions her wrist in neutral.

Maintaining the wrist in proper alignment is essential because the wrist is important to the health and balance of the entire hand. During functional activities the wrist is positioned in extension for grasp and prehension. Therefore the wrist extension immobilization type 0 orthosis[3] or the wrist cock-up orthosis is one the most common orthoses fabricated in clinical practice. Wrist immobilization orthoses usually maintain the wrist in either a neutral or a mildly extended position, depending on the protocol for a diagnostic condition and the person's intervention goals. A wrist immobilization orthosis positions the wrist while allowing full metacarpophalangeal (MCP) flexion and thumb mobility. Thus the person can continue to perform functional activities with the added support and proper positioning of the wrist that the orthosis provides. Positioning the wrist in 0 to 30 degrees of wrist extension in an orthosis promotes functional hand patterns for completing functional activities.[46,56]

Therapists fabricate wrist immobilization orthoses to provide volar; dorsal; ulnar; circumferential forearm, wrist, and hand; and occasionally radial support (Figs. 7.1–7.4). Therapists also use wrist immobilization orthoses as bases for mobilization and static progressive orthotic intervention (see Chapter 13). Although some wrist immobilization orthoses are commercially available, they cannot provide the exact fit of custom-made orthoses. However, commercially available

Note: This chapter includes content from previous contributions from Robert Gilmore, OTS.

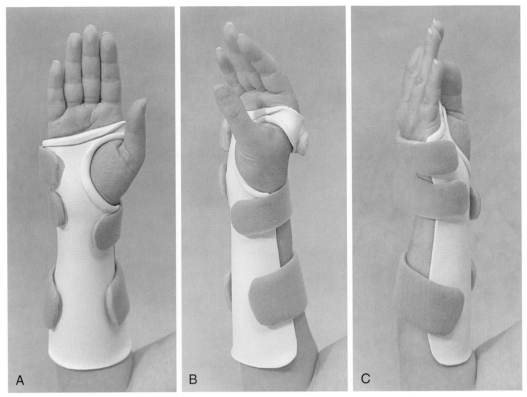

Fig. 7.1 A to C, A volar wrist immobilization orthosis.

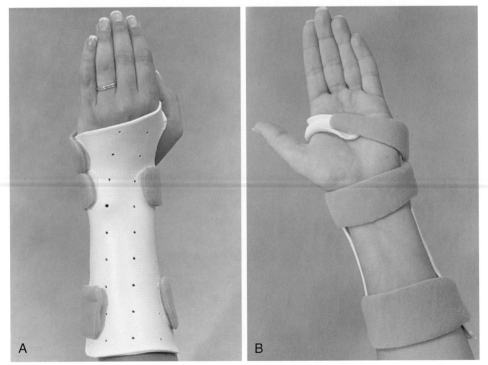

Fig. 7.2 A and B, A dorsal wrist immobilization orthosis.

or prefabricated orthoses made from soft material may be more comfortable in certain situations, especially in a work or sports setting. Commercially available orthoses are not as restrictive and allow more functional hand use.[71] Some people with rheumatoid arthritis (RA) may also prefer the comfort of a soft wrist orthosis due to its ability to reduce pain and provide stability during functional activities.[11,51,72]

This chapter gives an overview of wrist immobilization orthoses according to type, features, and diagnoses. The chapter addresses technical tips, troubleshooting tips, the use of prefabricated orthoses, the impact on occupations, and the application of a wrist mobilization and serial static approach. Interspersed throughout this chapter are discussions of evidence to understand current wrist orthosis provision.

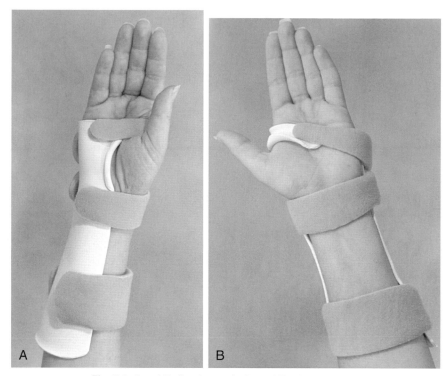

Fig. 7.3 A and B, An ulnar wrist immobilization orthosis.

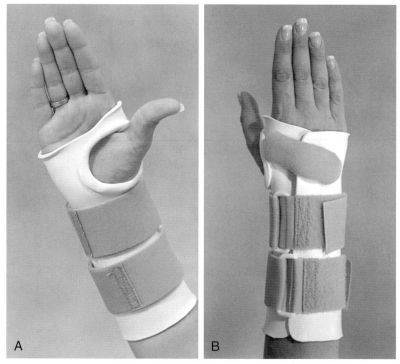

Fig. 7.4 A and B, A circumferential wrist immobilization orthosis.

VOLAR, DORSAL, ULNAR, CIRCUMFERENTIAL, AND DART THROWER'S WRIST ORTHOSES

In clinical practice the therapist must decide whether to fabricate a volar, dorsal, ulnar, or circumferential wrist immobilization orthosis. Each has advantages and disadvantages.[21]

Volar

The **volar** wrist immobilization orthosis (see Fig. 7.1) depends on a dorsal wrist strap to secure the wrist in the orthosis. An appropriate design furnishes adequate support for the weight of the wrist and hand. In cases in which the weight of the hand (flaccidity) must be held by the orthosis or in which the person is pulling against it (spasticity), the strap may not be adequate to hold the wrist in the orthosis. However, a well-designed volar wrist orthosis with a properly placed wide wrist strap will support a flaccid wrist.[64] The volar design is best suited for circumstances that require rest or immobilization of the wrist when the person still has muscle control of the wrist.[21]

A volar wrist orthosis' greatest disadvantage is interference with tactile sensibility on the palmar surface of the hand and the loss of the hand's ability to conform around objects.[64] In the presence of edema, one must use this design carefully because the dorsal strap can impede lymphatic and venous flow.[21] To address the presence of edema, a strap adaptation is made by circumferentially wrapping a continuous strap that is gently overlapping from distal to proximal until the whole hand/splint is covered.

Dorsal

Some therapists fabricate **dorsal** orthoses with a large palmar bar that supports the entire hand. This large palmar bar tends to distribute pressure well and is necessary for comfort and function. However, a large palmar bar does not free up the palmar surface as much for sensory input as a dorsal orthosis fabricated with a thinner palmar bar (see Fig. 7.2). Dorsal wrist orthoses designed with a standard strap configuration can be better tolerated by persons who have edematous hands because of the pressure distribution. Either the volar or the dorsal design may be used as a base for mobilization (dynamic) orthotic intervention. However, these designs can sometimes lead to orthotic migration and suboptimal orthotic performance.

Ulnar

The **ulnar** wrist orthosis is easy to don and doff and can be applied if the person warrants more protection on the ulnar side of the hand, such as with sports injuries (see Fig. 7.3). This ulnar orthotic design is sometimes used for a person who has **carpal tunnel syndrome (CTS)** or ulnar wrist pain.[42] It can also be used as a base for mobilization orthoses.

Circumferential

A **circumferential** orthosis is helpful to prevent migration, especially when used as a base for mobilization orthoses. Circumferential wrist orthoses also provide good forearm support, control edema, provide good pressure distribution, and eliminate edge pressure.[65] Some people may feel more confined in a circumferential orthosis. When fabricating a circumferential orthosis, the therapist is conscious of a possible pressure area over the distal ulna and checks that the fingers and thumb have full motion (see Fig. 7.4).[40] Among many circumferential orthosis design options are a bivalve design and a "zipper" orthosis. The bivalve design provides rigid immobilization and allows for easy adjustments when edema levels change, so a new orthosis does not need to be fabricated (Fig. 7.5A). A zipper orthosis is made from perforated thermoplastic material and can provide stabilization and support. Zipper orthoses work well with edema that does not change. Some zipper orthoses can get fully wet in water and they have no straps to get caught on items (Fig. 7.5B).

Dart Thrower's

Researchers defined a plane of wrist motion closely related to performance of activities of daily living (ADLs) called the dart-throwing motion. This motion occurs in the plane from "radial deviation and extension" to "ulnar deviation and flexion"[48,66] A hinged type of wrist orthosis called a dart orthosis is based on the defined plane of dart-thrower's motion. Dart orthoses aid the rehabilitative process by restricting the radiocarpal joint and scapholunate ligament movements. It is hypothesized that with the early protected motion provided by dart orthoses, they speed up functional wrist recovery after injuries to the ligaments of the proximal carpal row and the wrist.[9,66] Dart thrower's orthoses present a new intervention approach for some wrist conditions. However, further research is necessary to demonstrate their efficacy (Fig. 7.6).

FEATURES OF THE WRIST IMMOBILIZATION ORTHOSIS

Understanding the features of a wrist immobilization orthosis helps therapists design orthotic interventions appropriately. Whether fabricating a volar, dorsal, ulnar, or circumferential wrist orthosis, the therapist must be aware of certain features of the various components of the wrist immobilization orthosis—such as a forearm trough, metacarpal bar, and hypothenar bar (Figs. 7.7 and 7.8).[28] With a volar or dorsal immobilization orthosis the **forearm trough** should be two-thirds the length of the forearm and one-half the circumference of the forearm to allow for appropriate pressure distribution. It is sometimes necessary to notch or flare the area near the distal ulna on the forearm trough to avoid a pressure point.

The **hypothenar bar** helps to place the hand in a neutral resting position by preventing extreme ulnar deviation. The hypothenar bar should not inhibit MCP flexion of the ring and little fingers. The **metacarpal bar** supports the transverse metacarpal arch. When supporting the palmar surface of the hand, the metacarpal bar is sometimes called a *palmar bar*. With a volar wrist immobilization orthosis, the therapist positions this bar proximal to the distal palmar crease and distal and ulnar to the thenar crease to ensure full MCP flexion. On the ulnar side of the hand, it is especially important that the metacarpal bar be positioned proximal to the distal palmar crease to allow full little finger metacarpal flexion.

On the radial side it is important for the position of the metacarpal bar to be proximal to the distal palmar crease and distal to the thenar crease to allow adequate index and middle MCP flexion and thumb motions. On a dorsal wrist immobilization orthosis, the therapist positions this bar slightly proximal to the MCP heads on the dorsal surface of the hand when it winds around to the palmar surface. The same principles apply when positioning the metacarpal bar on the volar surface of the hand (proximal to the distal palmar crease, and distal and ulnar to the thenar crease).

The therapist should also carefully consider the application of straps to the wrist orthosis. Straps are applied at the level of the metacarpal bar, exactly at the wrist level, and at the

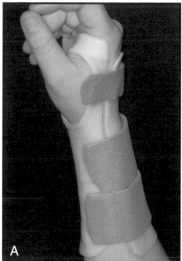
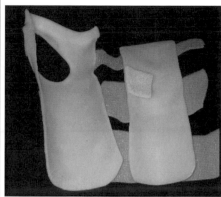
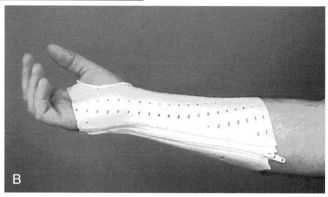

Fig. 7.5 A, A bivalve circumferential design. B, A "zipper" orthosis option for making a circumferential orthosis (Sammons Preston & Rolyan). (A courtesy Mojca Herman. B from Bednar, J. M., & Von Lersner-Benson, C. [2002]. Wrist reconstruction: Salvage procedures. In E. J. Mackin, A. D. Callahan, T. M. Shirven, et al. (Eds.), *Rehabilitation of the hand and upper extremity* [5th ed., p. 1200]. St. Louis, MO: Mosby.)

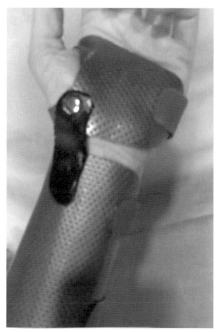

Fig. 7.6 A dart orthosis. Developed by Deborah A. Schwartz OTD, OTR/L CHT. (From Schwartz, D. A. [2016]. An alternative fabrication method of the dart thrower's motion orthosis [also known as the dart orthosis]. *Journal of Hand Therapy, 29*[3], 339–347.)

proximal end of the orthosis. The straps attach to the orthosis with pieces of self-adhesive Velcro hook. The therapist should note that the larger the piece of self-adhesive hook Velcro, the larger the interface between it and the thermoplastic material. This larger interface helps ensure that it remains in place and does not peel off (see Figs. 7.1 and 7.7). With the identification of potential pressure or shear problems, the therapist applies padding to the orthosis.

Diagnostic Indications

The clinical indications for a wrist immobilization orthosis vary according to the diagnosis. The therapist can apply the wrist immobilization orthosis for any upper extremity condition that requires the wrist to be in a static position. Application of this orthosis addresses a variety of goals, depending on the client's intervention needs. These goals include decreasing wrist pain or inflammation, providing support, enhancing digital function, preventing wrist deformity, minimizing pressure on the median nerve, and minimizing tension on involved structures.

In some cases, a wrist mobilization orthosis serial static approach is used to increase passive range of motion (PROM). Specific diagnostic conditions that may require a wrist immobilization orthosis can include, but are not limited to,

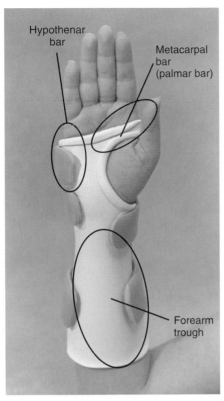

Fig. 7.7 A volar wrist immobilization orthosis with identified components.

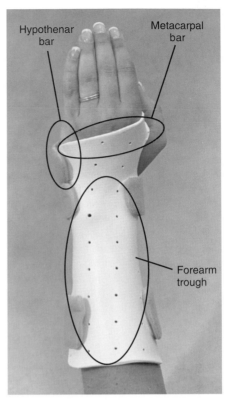

Fig. 7.8 A dorsal wrist immobilization orthosis with identified components.

tendinopathy, distal radius fracture, wrist sprain, radial nerve palsy, RA and wrist arthroplasty, and nerve compression at the wrist (CTS). Wrist orthoses for complex regional pain syndrome (CRPS) may be applied if the person is posturing in flexion, but application of orthoses for this condition is controversial because immobilization may increase the pain cycle.[23]

The specific wrist positioning depends on the diagnostic protocol, physician referral, and person's intervention goals. When the goal is functional hand use during orthotic wear, the therapist avoids extreme wrist flexion or extension because either position disrupts the normal functional position of the hand. Extreme positions can contribute to the development of CTS.[28,29] An exception to this rule is when the orthotic goal is to increase PROM. In that case an extreme position may be indicated. However, extreme positions may preclude function. The therapist must judge whether the trade-off is worth the loss of function.[65] Another consideration is choice of the thermoplastic material thickness. Generally, for most of the diagnoses discussed in this chapter, ⅛-inch thickness provides the proper amount of support. Thinner material (e.g., ¹⁄₁₆ inch) works well with skin that might be prone to breakdown. Thinner material may be useful when fabricating a wrist orthosis for CTS on an older adult with thinner skin, when fabricating an orthosis on a small hand (e.g., a child), or for someone with RA.

The therapist performs a thorough hand evaluation before fitting a person with a wrist immobilization orthosis and provides the person with a wearing schedule, instructions about orthotic maintenance and precautions, and an exercise program based on needs. Physicians and experienced therapists may have detailed guidelines for positioning and wearing schedules. Every hand and diagnosis is slightly different,

and thus orthotic positioning and wearing protocols vary. Table 7.1 lists suggested wearing schedules and positioning protocols of common hand conditions that may require wrist immobilization orthoses.

Wrist Orthotic Intervention for Carpal Tunnel Syndrome

CTS is a common and painful wrist and hand condition caused by increased compression of the median nerve as it passes through the very narrow carpal tunnel. To relieve pressure, wrist orthotic provision is typically part of conservative intervention, and research supports its use. According to recent evidence-based clinical guidelines for CTS from the American Academy of Orthopaedic Surgeons (AAOS), strong evidence supports wrist orthotic provision to improve patient outcomes, specifically with conservative management.[1] The AAOS report highlights two high-quality studies[31,44] with findings that full-time[31] or nighttime orthotic wear[44] as compared to no wear resulted in statistically significant change in reduction of pain and improvement in functional abilities. Quality measures for CTS recommend orthotic intervention for conservative management.[52] A recent Cochrane systematic review, however, suggests further research about the efficacy of wrist orthoses for CTS.[57]

Research has consistently suggested that for orthotic intervention with CTS the wrist should be positioned as close as possible to zero degrees (neutral) to avoid added pressure on the median nerve.[13,15,29,39,52] This neutral position may help with blood circulation.[53] Additionally, recent research for a newer approach to CTS orthotic provision includes MCP immobilization to rest the lumbricals in a neutral position.[7,12,13,30]

TABLE 7.1 Conditions That May Require a Wrist Immobilization Orthosis

Hand Condition	Suggested Wearing Schedule	Type of Orthosis and Wrist Position
Nerve Compression		
Carpal tunnel syndrome (CTS) (median nerve compression)	There is no consistent protocol for orthotic provision with CTS. Some therapists determine the wear schedule based on what activities are irritating for the person. For example, if activities during the day are irritating the person, the orthosis should be worn during the day. The AAOS recommends at minimum nighttime wear and day wear during aggravating activities.[2] Often during an acute flare-up the person wears the wrist immobilization orthosis continuously for 4 to 6 weeks with removal for hygiene and range of motion (ROM) exercises. The orthotic-wearing schedule gradually decreases.	Volar, dorsal, or ulnar gutter orthosis with the wrist in a neutral position. Current research suggests fabricating a volar wrist orthosis with an MCP block in neutral, especially if symptoms are not improving
Carpal tunnel release surgery	There is no consistent protocol for orthotic provision with carpal tunnel release surgery. Some physicians have the orthosis fabricated preoperatively, and some are fabricated immediately postoperatively. Some physicians do not prescribe orthoses at all. Others may recommend a wrist immobilization orthosis 1 week after surgery with the therapist providing instructions for an orthotic-wearing schedule (which includes orthotic application during sleep, during strenuous activities, and for support throughout the healing phase). Orthosis is weaned as soon as appropriate to prevent adhesion formation.	A volar orthosis with the wrist in neutral or slightly extended position.
Radial nerve palsy	Some physicians may suggest a wrist immobilization orthosis that maintains the wrist in a functional position and substitutes for the loss of the radial nerve by placing the wrist in extension. This static orthosis may be worn at night. Many other orthotic options for radial nerve palsy besides a static wrist orthosis are discussed in Chapter 14.	Volar or dorsal, approximately 30 degrees of wrist extension. For night splinting a resting hand orthosis is appropriate for positioning the MCPs in extension and thumb MP and IP in extension to use in conjunction with a day wrist orthosis (see Chapter 9).
Tendinopathy: Tenosynovitis/Tendinosis		
Any inflammation or degradation of the tendon and tendon sheath within the wrist	The person wears a wrist immobilization orthosis to avoid painful activity with removal for hygiene and ROM exercises followed by gradual weaning of the orthosis.	Volar or dorsal, 20 to 30 degrees of wrist extension.
Wrist synovitis	The person wears a wrist immobilization orthosis continuously during acute flare-ups with removal for hygiene and ROM exercises.	Volar, 0 to 15 degrees of extension.
Rheumatoid Arthritis		
Periods of swelling, wrist subluxation, and joint inflammation	The person continuously wears a wrist immobilization orthosis with established periods for ROM exercises and hygiene during the orthotic-wearing schedule. If MCP joints are developing an ulnar drift and IP joints are not involved, the therapist may fabricate a wrist orthosis that includes the MCP joints.	Volar in extension up to 30 degrees based on person's comfort level. During the early stage of the development of metacarpal ulnar drift, position close to neutral.
Wrist fractures	After the removal of the cast and healing of the fracture, the therapist fabricates a wrist immobilization orthosis. Usually the therapist discontinues the orthosis use as soon as possible to encourage functional movement. Sometimes the therapist may need to fabricate serial orthoses if the wrist does not have enough functional extension.	Dorsal, volar, or circumferential (if more support is needed) maximum passive extension the person can tolerate up to 30 degrees.
Wrist Sprain		
Any grade I or grade II tear of the ligament	The person wears a wrist immobilization orthosis continuously for 3 to 6 weeks. The physician may allow removal during bathing, depending on severity.	Choose approach as needed for function. Location of ligament may help dictate position. The orthosis should remove stress (tension from ligament).
Other		
Complex regional pain syndrome (CRPS)	The person wears a wrist immobilization orthosis during functional activities if activities are painful without the orthosis. Other reasons are to promote circulation and tissue nutrition and to regain a functional wrist position.	Volar, in extension as person tolerates. A circumferential wrist orthosis might also be used as it helps avoid pressure on the edges and problems with edema.

AAOS, American Academy of Orthopaedic Surgeons; *IP,* interphalangeal; *MCP,* metacarpophalangeal.

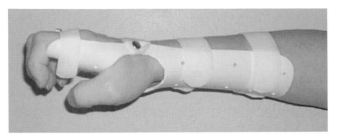

Fig. 7.9 A fabricated wrist immobilization (lumbrical positioning) orthosis with the wrist and metacarpophalangeals in a neutral position. (From Brininger, T. L., Rogers, J. C., Holm, M. B., et al. [2007]. Efficacy of fabricated customized splint and tendon and nerve gliding exercises for the treatment of carpal tunnel syndrome: A randomized controlled trial. *Archives of Physical Medicine and Rehabilitation, 88*[11], 1429–1436.)

One must be careful when applying prefabricated wrist orthoses for CTS because some orthoses place the wrist in a functional position of 20 to 30 degrees of extension.[52,54,80] Therefore, if it is possible to adjust the wrist angle of the orthosis, it should be modified to a neutral position. Some of the prefabricated orthoses have a compartment in which a metal or thermoplastic insert is placed, and the insert allows adjustments for wrist position. However, prefabricated orthoses that have their angles adjusted may become unstable, less rigid, and less comfortable than a custom-molded orthosis.[77]

Another consideration with the wrist immobilization orthotic provision is the amount of finger flexion allowed. Research suggests that finger flexion affects carpal tunnel pressure, especially when the fingers fully flex to form a fist.[4,13] The rationale is that the lumbrical muscles may sometimes enter the carpal tunnel with finger flexion.[20,67]

When orthoses are provided to clients with CTS, the clients should be instructed to avoid flexing their fingers "beyond 75% of a full fist."[4] Therefore therapists should check finger position with orthotic provision. Osterman and colleagues[54] advised therapists to fabricate a volar wrist orthosis with a metacarpal or MCP block to decrease finger flexion when CTS symptoms do not improve (Fig. 7.9). Recent research is finding positive results with this MCP-blocking wrist orthosis. Some studies[12,30] compared the wrist orthosis with MCP block to the traditional wrist orthosis. The study by Golriz et al.[30] (24 patients) found that after a wear period of 6 weeks both orthoses were equal in relationship to the impact on grip and pinch strength. However, the wrist orthosis with the MCP block showed more improvement with pain reduction and functional performance. The study by Bulut et al.[12] (54 patients) found significant improvement with resting pain, grip/pinch strength, and function when wearing the wrist orthosis with the MCP block. These studies suggest that therapists should consider research findings with respect to inclusion of the MCP block when fabricating a custom orthosis for CTS.

With wrist orthotic provision for a person who has CTS, the therapist considers home and occupational demands carefully, keeping in mind that the wrist contributes to the overall function of the hand.[63] If an orthosis is worn at work, durability of the orthosis and the ability to wash it may be salient. Some people may benefit from the fabrication of two orthoses (one for work and one for home), especially if their job demands are in an unclean environment. Many who use computers tolerate orthoses that support the wrist position in the plane of flexion and extension but allow 10 to 20 degrees of radial and ulnar deviation for effective typing. Fabricating a slightly wider metacarpal bar on a custom-made wrist orthosis allows for a small area of mobility on the radial and ulnar sides of the hand.[62] However, with this orthotic adaptation the client is instructed to be cautious when using a wrist orthosis with repetitive activity because it may cause proximal muscle pain or inflammation due to the altered biomechanics of the upper extremity. If increased pain or inflammation occurs, the therapist instructs the client to decrease orthotic use at the computer. Rather, the client should simulate the position of the wrists as if the client wearing the orthosis.[23] Finally, the client simulates work and home tasks while wearing the wrist immobilization orthosis, and the therapist checks for functional fit.[62]

Therapists consider orthotic-wearing schedules. Options of scheduling include nighttime wear only, wear during activities that irritate the condition, a combination of the latter two schedules, or constant wear. The AAOS and other researchers recommend nighttime wear at the minimum, and day wear during activities that aggravate the condition.[2] Individuals who sleep with the wrist flexed or extended may benefit from nighttime wear.[62] With nighttime wear, therapists caution clients to avoid pulling the straps too tight, which may inadvertently increase symptoms. In another study, subjects were found to benefit most from full-time wear of the orthosis, but adherence to the wearing schedule was an issue.[77] Length of time for orthotic wear may be prescribed by the person's physician. It is generally suggested that the orthosis be worn for 6 to 8 weeks with effectiveness of wear shown for up to 1 year.[43,52]

In addition to orthotic provision, researchers consider other interventions, such as neural gliding. A systematic review of 13 clinical trials meeting the inclusion criteria to evaluate the effectiveness of neural gliding exercises for CTS[8] found that limited evidence exists about the effectiveness of neural gliding. A conservative approach is recommended with the usage of wrist orthoses. Researchers suggest that neural gliding can be used as an adjunct intervention with a conservative approach to address pain and function.

Intervention combining lumbrical stretches along with wrist orthoses that have an MCP block may be an effective option for conservative management of CTS. Baker et al.[7] found that for mild to moderate CTS, a custom-fabricated wrist orthosis with an MCP block immobilizing the MCPs at 0 degrees combined with intensive lumbrical muscle stretches was more effective long term than the same MCP-blocking orthosis combined with general hand exercises or a traditional wrist cock-up orthosis combined with either lumbrical stretches or general stretches. A regimen of lumbrical stretches and provision of a wrist orthosis with an MCP block decreased the incidence of surgery.

Other effective intervention measures for CTS are the modification of activities (so that the person does not make excessive wrist and forearm motions, especially wrist flexion). It is also important to avoid sustained pinch or grip activities and to use good posture whenever possible with all ADLs. Because CTS is generically a disease of decreased blood supply to the soft tissues, an environment that is cold will additionally deprive nerves of blood. Thus staying warm is an important part of CTS care, and orthoses provide local warmth.[64] When conservative measures are ineffective, additional medical management includes corticosteroid injection or the possibility of surgery.

Wrist Orthotic Intervention Post Carpal Tunnel Surgery

Some therapists and physicians recommend[36] no wrist immobilization orthosis postoperatively to clients because of concerns about the impact of immobilization on joint stiffness and muscle shortening.[32] A recent Cochrane systematic review of rehabilitation after CTS surgical release of 22 trials and 1521 participants found either limited or low evidence for many postoperative interventions, including orthoses.[57]

Possible reasons for postoperative wrist orthotic provision may be to prevent extreme nighttime wrist postures (flexion and extension), to manage inflammation,[32] and to support the wrist during stressful activities. Other reasons include maintenance of gains from exercise,[47,65] prevention of tendon bowstringing, and facilitation of rest during the healing phase. Some therapists instruct clients to gradually wean from orthotic wear (when the orthosis is no longer meeting the person's therapeutic goals) to prevent stiffness and to allow the person to return to work and ADLs more quickly. Weaning is often done over the course of 1 week, gradually decreasing the hours of orthotic wear.[64]

A series of studies has been conducted to examine orthotic intervention for CTS. (Table 7.2 outlines some of the research evidence for CTS that can benefit from wrist orthoses.) Intervention for CTS is a relatively highly researched area. Therapists must stay current on the evidence that influences intervention approaches. Therapists should critically question how the research was performed and by whom as well as limitations.[45] Awareness of research also points to the fact that studies emphasize the importance of orthotic intervention with early intervention for mild to moderate CTS[53] because orthoses are less beneficial with ongoing parasthesias.[16]

Wrist Orthotic Intervention for Radial Nerve Injuries

Radial nerve injuries most commonly occur from fractures of the humeral shaft, fractures and dislocation of the elbow, or compressions of the nerve.[68] Other reasons for radial nerve injuries include lacerations, gunshot wounds, explosions, and amputations. The classic picture of a radial nerve injury is a wrist drop position whereby the wrist and MCP joints are unable to actively extend. If the wrist is involved, a physician may order a wrist orthosis to place the wrist in a more functional position. The exact wrist positioning is highly subjective, and it is up to the therapist and the client to decide on the amount of extension that maximizes function.

Commonly approximately 30 degrees of extension is considered a position of function for this condition because it facilitates optimum grip and pinch.[18] For nighttime wear a resting hand or hand immobilization orthosis (refer to Chapter 9) is fabricated to support the MCPs in extension and the thumb joints in extension. Although a wrist orthosis is one option for radial nerve injuries, there are many other options that therapists should critically consider. These include the location of the orthosis (volar versus dorsal), type of orthosis (e.g., wrist immobilization, tenodesis, or mobilization), and whether to fabricate one or two orthoses. More details about these other types of orthotic intervention options for a radial nerve injury are discussed in Chapter 14.

Wrist Orthotic Intervention for Tendinopathy, Tenosynovitis, and Tendinosis

Tendinopathy (deterioration of the tendon along with tiny microtears and collagen degeneration surrounding the tendon) typically refers to the disease of a tendon. Two terms have evolved to further describe tendon pathology. Tenosynovitis (inflammation of the tendon and its surrounding synovial sheath) clinically presents as pain, tenderness, weakness, and inflammation.[6] **Tendinosis** is defined as a noninflammatory "degeneration of the collagen tissue due to aging, microtrauma or vascular compromise."[5] Unlike tenosynovitis, which can often be successfully treated within several weeks, tendinosis can take several months to improve.

The term *tendinopathy* is used to refer to many tendon problems and can involve the muscles on the volar (flexor muscles) and dorsal (extensor muscles) surfaces of the forearm. A common site for tendinopathy is the lateral and medial elbow and rotator cuff tendons of the upper extremity.[37] Tendinopathy often leads to substitution patterns and muscle imbalance.[35] These conditions commonly occur because of cumulative and repetitive motions in work, home, and leisure activities. Having tendinopathy can result in an overuse cycle. The overuse cycle begins with friction, microscopic tears, pain, and limitations in motion, followed by resting the involved area, avoidance of use, and development of weakness. When activities resume, the cycle repeats itself.[35]

These conditions can benefit from conservative management, including wrist orthotic intervention. Resting the wrist in an orthosis helps to take tension off the muscle-tendon unit. Orthotic intervention for tendinopathy minimizes tendon excursion and thus decreases friction at the insertion of the muscles. Orthotic intervention can serve as a reminder to decrease engagement in painful activities. It is beneficial to ask clients to pay attention to those activities that are limited by an orthosis because they are often aggravating factors for tendinopathy. Thus clients should become more cognizant of aggravating activities and modify them so as not to enhance the condition.[64] Clients should also be cautioned not to tense their muscles and fight against the orthosis when wearing it or it may aggravate the tendinopathy. Rather, the muscles should be relaxed. Orthoses provided for tenosynovitis during acute flare-ups are worn as needed to avoid and reduce pain.

Text continued on p. 131

TABLE 7.2 Evidence-Based Practice About Wrist Orthotic Intervention

Author's Citation	Design	Number of Participants	Description	Results	Limitations
Carpal Tunnel Syndrome					
Baker, N. A., Moehlingm, K. K., Rubinstein, E. N., et al. (2012). The comparative effectiveness of combined lumbrical muscle splints and stretches on symptoms and function in carpal tunnel syndrome. *Archives of Physical Medicine and Rehabilitation, 93*(1), 1–10.	Randomized clinical trial	124 volunteer subjects with mild to moderate CTS	Subjects participated in a 4-week program of night orthotic intervention with either a prefabricated wrist cock-up or custom-fabricated lumbrical orthosis in neutral along with daily lumbrical stretches (either general or intensive). Subjects were randomly divided into four groups: 1. Lumbrical orthotic/lumbrical stretch group (intensive lumbrical intervention) 2. Lumbrical orthotic/general stretch group 3. General orthotic lumbrical stretch group 4. General orthotic/general stretch group	Subjects were evaluated with the CTQ and the DASH questionnaire. Researchers concluded that orthotic intervention along with the lumbrical stretches was more effective than orthotic intervention alone or stretches alone. The authors also concluded that it may take several months to resolve CTS symptoms and that function may show continual improvement after symptoms have halted. Subjects were followed up at 4, 12, and 24 weeks. At 24 weeks the group with the general orthosis along with lumbrical stretches demonstrated continual functional improvement. Surgery following these conservative interventions was only 25.5%.	Inclusion criteria did not specifically involve subjects with lumbrical tightness, nor did inclusion criteria require electrodiagnostic nerve conduction studies to confirm CTS. Subjects self-reported adherence to the study regimen. Subjects followed a prescribed regimen for only a 4-week time frame, which might have biased later results. There was no control group.
Bulut, G. T., Caglar, N. S., Aytekin, E., et al. (2015). Comparison of static wrist splint with static wrist and metacarpophalangeal splint in carpal tunnel syndrome. *Journal of Back and Musculoskeletal Rehabilitation, 28*(4), 761–767.	Randomized controlled trial	33 participants with diagnosis of CTS; 54 hands included in the study due to prevalence of CTS in both UE	One group of participants wore a neutral volar static wrist splint in 0–5 degrees of extension. The MCP joint, fingers, and elbow were allowed to move. In the other group, participants wore a neutral volar static wrist and MCP splint with wrist in 0–5 degrees of extension and MCP in 0–10 degrees of flexion. The fingers and elbow were allowed movement. Each participant was instructed to wear splint all night for duration of 4 weeks. Inclusion criteria included: a. Diagnosis of CTS according to subjective symptoms and physiological and electrophysiological examinations b. 18 years of age or older c. Ability to understand questionnaires	Participants were evaluated at baseline and at 4 weeks using electrophysiological tests, ViAS, grip and pinch strength, and CTS questionnaire. Researchers reported statistically significant improvements in ViAS, grip and pinch strength, and CTS questionnaire following 4-week nighttime wear of wrist MCP splint. When comparing the two groups, participants in the wrist MCP splint had significant improvements in pain, grip and pinch, and functional status portion of the CTS questionnaire when compared with the wrist splint group. However, there were no significant differences between these two groups on electrophysiological measures. Therefore researchers suggest a neutral wrist MCP splint is more effective than a neutral wrist splint in reducing pain and symptoms and improving function with individuals with CTS. When prescribing a splint to individuals with CTS, one should consider the position of the MCP joint.	The physician was blinded, but it is unclear if the clinician performing the outcome measures was blinded to the intervention. Study includes a smaller sample size, which creates difficulty with generalization. Researchers did not collect data on splint adherence. The study does not investigate long-term effects of the different splints.

Continued

TABLE 7.2   Evidence-Based Practice About Wrist Orthotic Intervention—cont'd

Author's Citation	Design	Number of Participants	Description	Results	Limitations
Goliz, B., Bani, M. A., Arazpour M., et al. (2016). Comparison of the efficacy of a neutral wrist splint and a wrist splint incorporating a lumbrical unit for the treatment of patients with carpal tunnel syndrome. *Prosthetics and Orthotics International, 40*(5), 617–623.	Quasiexperimental design	24 participants with mild or moderate CTS	Experimental group: Custom-molded wrist splint in neutral position with an extended trim line to allow for control of MCP (0–10 degrees of flexion). Control group: Custom-made neutral wrist splint. Participants in each group instructed to wear the splint at night and whenever possible during the day for duration of 6 weeks. Inclusion criteria included: a. Diagnosis of mild or moderate CTS b. Over 18 years of age c. Positive Tinel sign or Phalen maneuver d. Reported pain at night, numbness, and tingling in previous 12 months Researchers used a randomized allocation to assign participants to a group.	Researchers used the ViAS to evaluate pain, the DASH questionnaire to evaluate function, and grip and pinch (lateral) to evaluate strength. Each outcome measure was completed at baseline and at 6 weeks. Participants self-reported use of splint. Each group had a significant decrease in pain and an increase in pinch and grip strength and function. Participants using the wrist splint with MCP unit demonstrated significant decreases in pain and DASH score, suggesting better effectiveness than the neutral wrist splint in decreasing pain and improving function. There were no differences between the two group on pinch and grip strength.	This study explores only short-term effects of splint wear. In addition, the study had a relatively small sample size. It is unclear if the rater was blinded to the treatment intervention.
Hall, B., Lee, H. C., Fitzgerald, H., et al. (2013). Investigating the effectiveness of full-time wrist splinting and education in the treatment of carpal tunnel syndrome: A randomized controlled trial, *American Journal of Occupational Therapy, 67*(4), 448–459.	Randomized controlled trial	54 participants with CTS; 30 participants in treatment group; 24 participants in control group	Treatment group: Participants completed an 8-week conservative treatment program with full-time wear of wrist support splint with self-management education. The splint supported the wrist in a neutral position and allowed full finger and thumb movement. The two occupational therapists used clinical reasoning to select 1 of 4 types of wrist splints (3 prefabricated; 1 custom-made). For the educational component, participants attended 2 treatment sessions, 1 during first week and 1 additional session between weeks 2 and 4. Participants also received a follow-up phone call during week 7. Control group: Participants were assessed but did not receive intervention. Inclusion criteria included: a. Greater than 18 years of age b. Paresthesia in median nerve distribution at night or during day c. Clumsiness, grasp weakness, or sleep difficulties d. No medical intervention e. No conservative management in last 6 months f. No pregnancy Participants were randomly divided into groups via a blocking strategy.	Participants were evaluated with the Boston Questionnaire for the Assessment of Carpal Tunnel Symptom Severity, the ViAS, Jamar dynamometer, the Purdue Pegboard Test, the Semmes-Weinstein Monofilament (SWM), the Phalen test, and a satisfaction questionnaire. Participants averaged 89% compliance rate for nighttime wear and 81% compliance rate for daytime wear. The treatment group reported an improved understanding and confidence in ability to manage their condition. The treatment group also demonstrated greater improvements in severity of symptoms, functional status, perception of pain, and grip strength. Results indicated a positive correlation between symptom severity, functional status, and pain and desire for surgical intervention. The authors conclude that an 8-week, full-time wrist splint wear and a structured education program are key components for the treatment of CTS.	It is unclear how adherence rate of splint wear was assessed. This study was not blinded, and 2 occupational therapists delivered the experimental group interventions. Because of dropout, there is a different number of participants in the control and experimental groups. Bias could have affected results of report of deciding against surgery since participants were directly reporting this information to their treating occupational therapist.

Citation	Study Type	Description	Inclusion Criteria	Findings
Huisstede, B. M., van den Brink, J., Randsdorp, M. S., et al. (2018). Effectiveness of surgical and postsurgical interventions for carpal tunnel syndrome—a systematic review. *Archives of Physical Medicine and Rehabilitation.* 99(8):1660–1680.e21.	Literature review of randomized controlled trials	Review of effectiveness of surgical and postsurgical treatments of CTS. Participants varied per study. Sources of data included Cochrane library, PubMed, Embase, CINAHL, and PEDro.	Inclusion criteria included: a. Participants with CTS b. CTS not caused by acute trauma or systematic disease c. An intervention for CTS was evaluated d. Reported results on pain, function, or recovery. Two reviewers reviewed articles for inclusion, and 4 Cochrane reviews and 33 randomized controlled trials met this criteria. Topics included in the review were surgical treatment, such as timing of surgery and surgical techniques; nonsurgical treatments, such as splinting, steroid injection, medication, hand therapy, manual therapy, ultrasonography, nerve and tendon gliding exercises, and laser therapy; and postsurgical treatment.	There is moderate evidence that surgical intervention is more effective than splinting midterm and long-term. However, there is opposing evidence about the short-term effectiveness when comparing these interventions. There were no significant differences between a splint and soft bulky dressing following CTS release. European experts suggested splinting following surgery. However, need to continue studying postsurgical interventions for CTS. Researchers unable to statistically pool data due to heterogeneity of the included studies. Only 40% of the studies were considered to have high methodological quality. Only a few studies that incorporated a splinting intervention were included in this review. Therefore this review provides limited data about splinting with CTS.
Page, M. J., Massey-Westropp, N., O'Connor, D., et al. (2012). Splinting for carpal tunnel syndrome (review). *Cochrane Database Syst Rev.* 11;(7):CD010003.	Literature review of randomized and quasirandomized trials	Reviewed articles comparing the effectiveness of splinting versus no treatment, placebo, or another nonsurgical intervention for CTS. Sources of data included Cochrane Neuromuscular Disease Group Specialized Register, CENTRAL, NHS EED, DARE, MEDLINE, Embase, CINAHL, and AMED	Two reviewers selected articles for review based on specific inclusion criteria: a. Published and unpublished randomized or quasirandomized controlled trials b. Studies comparing splinting with no treatment or nonsurgical interventions or studies that compared two different types of splints c. All participants had a diagnosis of CTS19 studies with 1190 participants with CTS were included in the review.	In these 19 studies, treatment varied in duration, type, and routine of splint wear. The most common time frame for splint wear was between 2 and 4 weeks with nighttime wear as the most commonly prescribed schedule. Two of the studies in this review compared the use of a splint with no treatment, 5 studies investigated the effectiveness of different splint designs, 7 studies investigated the use of a wrist splint compared to another nonsurgical intervention, and 5 studies reviewed a wrist splint as a component with another nonsurgical intervention. Researchers reported there is limited evidence that a nighttime splint is more effective than wearing no splint in the short term. There is also insufficient evidence supporting the effectiveness or safety of a certain splint design and wearing schedule or of a wrist splint over other nonsurgical interventions. Only 3 of the studies measured long-term outcomes (greater than 3 months) of a wrist splint with CTS. Therefore more research is needed investigating the long-term effects of wrist splinting. The studies included in this review were heterogeneous, and the researchers were unable to pool data for comparison in meta-analysis. Only 1 study asked how much the participant actually wore splint. Only 3 studies looked at long-term "follow-up of the intervention. Only 2 studies reported a method of random sequence allocation (low risk of bias). Only 1 study reported patient blinding. Researchers suspected reporting bias in 10 studies.

Continued

TABLE 7.2   Evidence-Based Practice About Wrist Orthotic Intervention—cont'd

Author's Citation	Design	Number of Participants	Description	Results	Limitations
Peters, S., Page, M. J., Coppieters, M. W., et al. (2016). Rehabilitation following carpal tunnel release (review). *Cochrane Database Syst Rev*.17:2:CD004158.	Literature review of randomized controlled trials	Reviewed articles on effectiveness and safety of rehabilitation after CTS surgery when compared to other rehabilitation treatment, no treatment, or placebo treatment. Sources of data included: Cochrane Neuromuscular Specialised Register, the Cochrane Central Register of Controlled Trials, MEDLINE, Embase, CINAHL Plus, AMED, LILACS, PsycINFO, PEDro, the World Health Organization International Clinical Trials Registry Platform, the UK Clinical Research Network Study Portfolio, and ClinicalTrials.gov	Two reviewers selected articles for review based on specific inclusion criteria: a. All published and unpublished studies with randomized methods that compare postoperative rehabilitation with no treatment, placebo, or another rehabilitation intervention b. Study included participants with CTS who underwent CTS surgery c. All postoperative interventions 22 trials with 1521 participants with CTS were included in this review.	Two randomized controlled trials compared the effectiveness of immobilization versus a bulky dressing. Four randomized controlled trials compared the effectiveness of immobilization (with various types of wrist splints) versus mobilization. One randomized controlled trial compared a bulky dressing with a volar wrist splint orthosis in neutral position versus a light bandage. Overall, authors conclude there is limited and low-to very low-quality evidence that supports use of a variety of rehabilitation interventions after carpal tunnel release. One study found no statistically significant differences in hand function of participants with postoperative wrist orthosis versus bulky dressing with early mobilization. Another study found no statistically significant differences between wear of a wrist orthosis for 2 weeks versus a bulky dressing following carpal tunnel release surgery. No significant differences were found in the studies that compared immobilization with wrist splint versus early mobilization. In addition, one study reported adverse events in which 80% of participants reported discomfort with splint wear compared to 0 participants in the early mobilization group. (Orthosis data only pulled from article.)	The studies included in this review were heterogeneous, and the researchers were unable to pool data for comparison in meta-analysis. There are several low to very-low quality articles in this review. Two studies on immobilization with wrist splint reported incomplete data, while two additional studies comparing immobilization to early immobilization reported incomplete data. There was a lack of blinding in the study about wrist orthosis. Some studies examining wrist orthosis also lacked appropriate randomization. Only 4 of the 22 studies reported the primary outcome measure of interest.

Distal Radius Fracture (Colles Fracture)

Citation	Study Design	Sample	Methods	Results	Limitations
Grle, M., Milijko, M., Grle, I., et al. (2017). Early results of the conservative treatment of distal radius fractures—immobilization of the wrist in dorsal versus palmar flexion. *Medicinski Glasnik* 14(2), 236–243.	Prospective cohort study	122 patients with a distal radius fracture; however, only 100 participants completed the study; 50 participants per group	In the DF group, participants had wrist immobilized in approximately 20 degrees dorsal flexion and minimal ulnar deviation. In the PF group, participants had wrist immobilized in approximately 20 degrees of palmar flexion and minimal ulnar deviation. Each group wore the plaster splint for 4 weeks. Inclusion criteria included: a. Diagnosis of distal radius fracture b. Above 25 years of age Randomization is unclear.	Researchers used the following outcome measures at 4 weeks and 2 months after injury: radiological, clinical (ROM and grip strength), and functional parameters, wrist evaluation survey for wrist pain and function, and SF-12 questionnaire (quality of mental and physical health). Participants in the DF group had significantly greater ROM. Radiological examinations favored the DF group. However, both groups had positive radiological results. There was no difference on the wrist evaluation survey between the two groups. Participants in the DF group reported better physical component outcome on the SF-12 survey. Researchers conclude the forearm splint on the dorsal side that places wrist in dorsiflexion provides better early outcomes for radial fractures than wrist placed in palmar flexion.	There was a large dropout rate (22 participants). Blinding or randomization was not described. Researchers did not track data on adherence to splint wear and did not describe splint wear schedule. There was no control group.

Radial Nerve Injury

Citation	Study Design	Sample	Methods	Results	Limitations
Raquel, C.T., Miguel, G.M., Cristina, L.T. (2016). Effects on upper-limb function with dynamic and static orthosis use for radial nerve injury: A randomized trial. *Journal of Neurological Disorders, 4*(2), 2.	Randomized controlled trial	18 participants; 9 participants in static orthosis group and 9 participants in dynamic orthosis group	Researchers instructed participants to wear the splint during the day and to not remove the splint during daily activities. The splints were checked once per week. Participants in the static splint group wore a static volar orthosis that supported the wrist in 30 degrees of extension and thumb in opposition. Participants in the dynamic splint group wore a splint across the palmar arch that supported the wrist and the fingers and thumb had dynamic assistance with cuffs at the proximal phalanges. Inclusion criteria included: a. Adults with radial nerve lesion in dominant arm after humerus shaft fractures after surgical intervention b. 3 to 5 weeks after surgical interventions Participants randomized via software program.	The primary outcome measure was the DASH. Participants completed the DASH before splint fabrication and 1 month later. Participants in each group improved DASH scores between first and second assessment. However, participants in the static splint group demonstrated significantly better scores than participants in the dynamic splint group. Participants in the static splint group experienced further improvement in function.	Researchers had a small sample size and used only one outcome measure, creating difficulty with generalization. Researchers do not discuss blinding. It is also unclear if participants complied with splint wear.

Continued

TABLE 7.2 Evidence-Based Practice About Wrist Orthotic Intervention—cont'd

Author's Citation	Design	Number of Participants	Description	Results	Limitations
Rheumatoid Arthritis					
Ramsey, L., Winder, R.J., & McVeigh, J.G. (2014). The effectiveness of working wrist splints in adults with rheumatoid arthritis: A mixed methods systematic review. *Journal of Renabilitation Medicine, 46*(6), 481–492.	Mixed methods systematic review	Reviewed articles examining the effectiveness (function, strength, pain, and dexterity) of working wrist splints for individuals with RA. Reviewers searched 10 databases and followed the Preferred Reporting Items for Systematic Reviews and Meta-Analyses guidelines.	One researcher screened eligible studies and discussed and assessed with two additional researchers for consensus. Inclusion criteria included qualitative and quantitative studies published in English that explored effectiveness of working wrist splint with individuals with RA or studies that explored the experiences or perceptions of patients, therapists, or caregivers with a working wrist splint with RA. 23 studies with 1492 participants met inclusion criteria. Of these 23 studies, 9 randomized controlled trials were included.	Of these studies the most common outcomes assessed were hand function, grip and pinch strength, pain, and dexterity. Researchers conclude that there is strong quantitative evidence with support from qualitative evidence that working wrist splints are effective for reducing pain with individuals with RA. Moderate evidence exists that working wrist splints improved grip strength. However, there is concern that dexterity could be negatively affected, and there is insufficient evidence that working wrist splints are effective for improving function in RA. Article has a very nice chart of different types of prefabricated and custom-fabricated splints.	Studies were heterogeneous, and researchers were unable to complete meta-analysis. A wide variety of splints and of splint frequency and duration were included in systematic review; also a wide variety of outcome measures. Many studies lacked adequate blinding, randomization, and power.

AMED, Allied and Complementary Medicine Database; *CTQ,* Carpal Tunnel Symptom Severity and Function Questionnaire; *CTS,* carpal tunnel syndrome; *DARE,* Database of Abstracts of Reviews of Effects; *DASH,* Disabilities of the Arm, Shoulder, and Hand; *DF,* dorsal flexion; *MCP,* metacarpophalangeal; *NHS EED,* NHS Economic Evaluation Database; *PF,* palmar flexion; *RA,* rheumatoid arthritis; *ROM,* range of motion; *SF-12,* short form-12; *UE,* upper extremity; *VAS,* visual analog scale.
Contributed by Whitney Henderson.

Orthotic intervention to avoid pain is beneficial, but continuous orthotic usage prevents the nourishment of collagen that is associated with pain-free arcs of motion. Therefore, orthotic provision for these conditions should allow for removal for hygiene and pain-free range of motion (ROM) exercises followed by gradual weaning.[23]

Generally, when fabricating orthoses for flexor carpi radialis (FCR) or flexor carpi ulnaris (FCU) tendinopathy, it is recommended that the client's wrist be positioned at neutral or 10 degrees of flexion[23] to rest the tendons.[34] Therapists can fabricate a volar wrist orthosis for FCR and an ulnar gutter wrist orthosis for FCU. Wrist extensor tendinopathy, including extensor carpi radialis brevis (ECRB) or extensor carpi radialis longus (ECRL), benefits from a fabricated orthosis in 20 to 30 degrees of wrist extension because this normal resting position provides a balance between the flexors and extensors. For extensor carpi ulnaris (ECU) tendinopathy, therapists can fabricate an ulnar gutter wrist orthosis in 20 to 30 degrees of wrist extension.

Wrist Orthotic Intervention for Rheumatoid Arthritis

For clients with **rheumatoid arthritis (RA)**, general reasons for orthotic provision include pain control, edema reduction, and prevention of deformity.[27] Orthoses for RA provide mechanical joint support and enhance function. Sometimes they are used for postoperative positioning.[25] When an orthosis is prescribed for a person with RA, application of clinical reasoning helps to determine the objective(s) for provision as multiple purposes can exist for a single orthosis.[25]

Wrist immobilization orthoses for RA are typically fabricated in a functional position of 0 to 30 degrees of wrist extension, thus promoting synergistic wrist-extension and finger-flexion patterns. This position allows the greatest level of function in relationship to grip for ADLs.[46,56] Wearing a wrist orthosis may be used to control pain during activities.[38] Orthotic wear is especially helpful in protecting the wrist during demanding tasks.[72] For people with radiocarpal or midcarpal arthritis, a wrist orthosis fabricated out of thin ¹⁄₁₆-inch thermoplastic material is recommended.[38] For a total wrist arthrodesis a volar wrist orthosis is provided when the cast is removed (usually at approximately week 6 to 8 following surgery). Surgeons vary in their prescriptions for length of splint wear time based on tissue healing and patient needs.

Wrist orthotic intervention for a person with RA can be quite challenging because of the tendency for the carpal structures of the rheumatoid arthritic wrist to sublux volarly and ulnarly.[26] In addition, there can be related digital involvement to consider, such as MCP volar subluxation and/or ulnar drift. In the early stages of this ulnar drift, the wrist joint should be positioned as close to neutral with respect to radial and ulnar deviation as can be comfortably tolerated. However, some experts recommend positioning the wrist in slight ulnar deviation to promote more neutral MCP positioning.[23] With consistent access to the person, the therapist can progress the wrist into neutral on successive visits. This position helps eliminate the development of a zigzag deformity. The zigzag deformity develops when the carpal bones deviate ulnarly and the metacarpals deviate radially, which exacerbates the ulnar deviation of the MCP joints.[26] (See Fig. 7.10A for an illustration of the deformity and Fig. 7.10B for one orthotic suggestion.)

If only the MCP joints (not the interphalangeal (IP) joints) are involved, the therapist may consider fabricating a wrist orthosis in a neutral position that extends beyond the distal palmar crease and ends proximal to the proximal interphalangeal (PIP) crease to support the MCP joints.[58] Another recommendation for someone with a zigzag deformity is to fabricate an orthosis on the entire hand (see Chapter 9).

When fabricating a wrist orthosis for a person with RA, the therapist uses a thermoplastic material with a high degree of conformability and drapability to help prevent pressure areas. Alternatively, the long working time of highly rubber-based thermoplastic materials helps the therapist create a more cosmetic and well-fitting orthosis.[64] The therapist carefully monitors for the development of pressure areas over many of the small bones of the hand and wrist, as shown in Fig. 7.11.[26] Another consideration for orthosis fabrication for an individual who has RA is using an orthotic sock or stockinette underneath the orthosis or lining the orthosis with padding. If the individual has been on a steroid regimen for a long period of time, the skin is likely to be thinner and more fragile, which increases the potential for superficial burns during the orthotic intervention process.[19] Some people with RA may prefer a prefabricated orthosis that is easy to apply and is perceived to be more comfortable than a fabricated orthosis because it is made from softer material and has more flexibility. Further discussion later in this chapter addresses the functional implications of commercial or prefabricated wrist orthoses with RA.

Finally, a recently available systematic review of 23 qualifying studies (n = 1492) for wrist orthoses with RA provides insight about orthotic usage. Strong evidence exists that wrist orthoses provide pain reduction; moderate evidence exists for improved grip strength; and insufficient evidence exists on functional impact. Impaired dexterity associated with fine motor tasks was reported with wearing wrist orthoses. However, wrist orthoses assisted daily tasks that required strength, such as heavy lifting.[59] A Cochrane systematic review of occupational therapy for RA verified that in general orthoses for RA decrease pain.[75]

Wrist Orthotic Intervention for Fractures

A Colles fracture is a fracture of the distal radius usually occurring because of falling on an outstretched hand. Orthoses for Colles fractures are individualized, based on the person's skeletal and soft tissue status. The initial goal of rehabilitation after a fracture of the distal radius is to regain functional wrist extension.[41] To achieve this goal, fabricate the orthosis to position the wrist in slight extension. Wrist orthotic intervention post fracture provides protection, pain relief, and rest to the extremity.[49] Custom-fabricated orthoses are best because

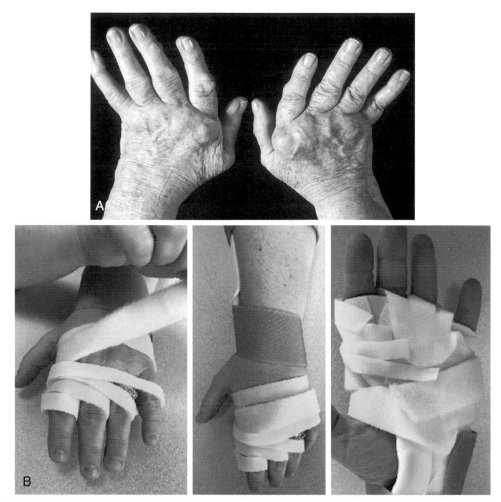

Fig. 7.10 A zigzag deformity with rheumatoid arthritis. B, An orthosis for a zigzag deformity that combines thermoplastic material and straps to help reposition the digits away from ulnar deviation into radial alignment and the wrist away from radial deviation into ulnar alignment. (A, Reprinted from the Clinical Slide Collection on the Rheumatic Diseases, copyright 1997. Used by permission of the American College of Rheumatology. From Cameron, M., & Monroe, L. [2007]. *Physical rehabilitation*, St. Louis: W.B. Saunders. B, Photos by Jeanine Beasley.)

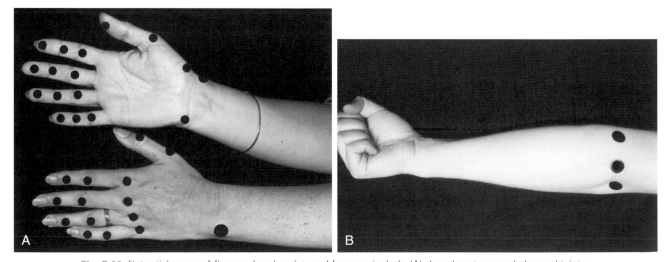

Fig. 7.11 Potential areas of fingers, hand, wrist, and forearm include (A) dorsal metacarpophalangeal joints, thumb web space, ulnar styloid, radial styloid, thumb carpometacarpal joint, center of palm (especially with flexion wrist contractures), and (B) proximal edge of orthosis. (From Fess, E. E., Gettle, K., Philips, C., et al. [2005]. *Hand and upper extremity splinting: Principles and methods* [3rd ed.]. St. Louis, MO: Mosby.)

prefabricated orthoses may not fit comfortably and may block ROM of the fingers and thumb.[40] Sometimes a serial static orthotic intervention approach may be necessary to regain PROM. (Refer to the discussion later in this chapter for more details about serial static orthotic intervention and also refer to Chapter 13.) With any open wound, therapists must follow wound precautions and physician preferences for management (see Chapter 5). If pins or hardware are present and an orthosis is ordered, the therapist fabricates an orthosis to avoid the area or creates a dome or bubble in the material to avoid contact with the open wound. Caution is taken to ensure that the orthosis stability and purpose is not compromised.

The therapist fabricates a well-designed custom dorsal or volar orthosis for Colles fractures. Moscony and Shank[49] recommend a volar wrist orthosis after the removal of a cast for approximately 1-2 weeks, whereas Laseter[40] recommends fabricating a dorsal wrist orthosis because it helps control edema and allows for functional motions of the finger joints. If the person needs more support, a circumferential wrist orthosis is considered.[41] Using a circumferential orthosis is highly supportive and very comfortable. The circumferential orthosis tends to limit forearm rotation more than a volar or dorsal wrist orthosis.[65] The client is weaned from any orthosis as soon as possible.[40,41] To encourage regaining function, Weinstock[79] recommends that the orthosis be part of therapeutic intervention until 30 to 45 degrees of active extension is obtained. If PROM of the wrist/forearm remains limited after approximately 6 to 8 weeks, it may be appropriate to discuss the possibility of mobilization orthotic provision with the physician (see Chapter 13).

Wrist orthoses are used with Colles fractures after surgery. External fixation, dorsal plating, and volar fixed-angle plating are examples of surgical fixation approaches. With surgically inserted dorsal plating, wrist orthoses are used to rest the wrist between exercises. Wrist orthoses may be indicated for rest and protection after volar fixed-angle plating insertion. The therapist collaborates with the referring physician on the orthotic-wearing schedule. For any of these surgical fixation procedures, static progressive wrist orthoses may be indicated to gradually improve wrist extension.[49]

Wrist Orthotic Intervention for Wrist Sprains

A grade I sprain results in a substance tear with minimal fiber disruption and no obvious tear of the ligament fibers. A mild grade II sprain results in tearing of the ligament fibers. Persons with grade I and II sprains may initially benefit from wearing a wrist immobilization orthosis. With grade I sprains the person will likely wear the orthosis for 3 weeks. For grade II sprains 6 weeks of wear may be indicated. This wrist orthosis helps rest the hand during the acute healing phase and removes stress from the healing ligament(s). The physician may allow removal during bathing, depending on severity.

Wrist Orthotic Intervention for Complex Regional Pain Syndrome Type I (Reflex Sympathetic Dystrophy)

Complex regional pain syndrome describes a complex grouping of symptoms impacting an extremity and characterized by extreme prolonged pain, diffuse edema, stiffness, trophic skin changes, and discoloration.[50] **Complex regional pain syndrome (CRPS) types I and II are terms coined by the World Health Organization (WHO) to distinguish between sympathetically mediated and non–sympathetically mediated pain.** CRPS type I is a sympathetically mediated pain[46] and refers to pain from an injury that lasts longer and hurts more than is anticipated. Type II refers to pain related to a nerve injury. Symptoms are similar for both types of pain.[50]

Orthotic intervention may be a part of the rehabilitation program for CPRS. However, the current approach for intervention is that orthoses are suggested only if it is painful for the person to perform functional movements. Typically, a volar wrist orthosis in functional extension as tolerated is provided.[23] The therapist applies clinical reasoning skills to determine which orthosis meets the various therapeutic goals. (Refer to the discussion on the use of resting hand orthoses with this condition in Chapter 9.) Other purposes for providing wrist immobilization orthoses in addition to pain relief are for muscle spasm relief, to promote circulation and tissue nutrition, and for regaining a functional resting wrist position.[61,76,78] Recovering a functional resting hand position is important for normal hand motions and for the prevention of deforming forces as a result of muscle imbalance. To increase wrist extension to a more functional position, the therapist may need to provide serial static wrist orthoses over time to achieve the goal of a functional resting wrist position.

WRIST JOINT CONTRACTURE: SERIAL ORTHOTIC INTERVENTION WITH A WRIST ORTHOSIS

When a wrist is not properly moving (such as after removal of a cast for a Colles fracture), the therapist may consider serial static wrist orthotic intervention.[60] With serial static orthotic intervention, the therapist intermittently remolds the orthosis to facilitate increases in wrist extension (Fig. 7.12). The orthosis is first applied with the wrist positioned at the maximal amount of extension that the current soft-tissue length allows and the person can tolerate. The person is instructed to wear the orthosis for long periods of time, with periodic removal for exercise and hygiene, until the wrist can move beyond that amount of extension.

The orthosis is readjusted to position the soft tissues at their maximum length.[21] Positioning living tissue at maximum length causes the tissue to remodel to a longer length.[63] This process is repeated until optimal wrist extension is regained. Thus serial static orthotic intervention is beneficial for PROM limitations because it provides long periods of low load stress at or near the end of the soft-tissue length.[63] Serial static wrist orthotic intervention is only one approach that can improve wrist PROM. Refer to Chapter 13 for other approaches, such as fabricating static progressive orthoses.

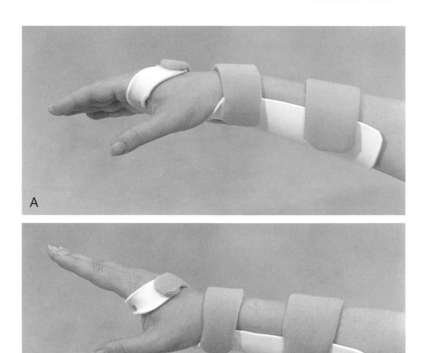

Fig. 7.12 A and B, Serial wrist orthotic intervention.

FABRICATION OF A WRIST IMMOBILIZATION ORTHOSIS

The initial step in the fabrication of a wrist immobilization orthosis (after evaluation of the person's hand) is the drawing of a pattern. Pattern making is important in customizing an orthosis because every person's hand is different in shape and size. Pattern making also saves time and minimizes waste of materials.

A common mistake of a novice therapist during fabrication of a wrist immobilization pattern is drawing the forearm trough narrower than the natural curve of the forearm muscle-bulk contour. This mistake can occur with anyone but especially with a person who has a large forearm. If the forearm trough is not one-half the circumference of the forearm, the orthosis will not provide adequate support. In addition, the therapist must follow the natural angle of the MCP heads with the pattern.

A volar wrist immobilization pattern presents another orthotic intervention option (Fig. 7.13A). It is sometimes called a *thumb-hole wrist orthosis*.[70] The therapist constructs the orthosis by punching a hole with a leather punch in the heated thermoplastic material and pushing the thumb through the hole. The therapist rolls the material away from the thumb and thenar eminence far enough that it does not interfere with functional thumb movement and yet allows adequate wrist support (see Fig. 7.13B). In one research study this thumb-hole wrist orthosis was found to be the most restrictive of wrist motion and slowest with dexterity

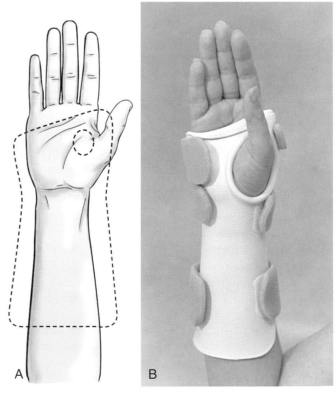

Fig. 7.13 A, A volar wrist immobilization pattern for a thumb-hole orthosis. B, A volar wrist immobilization thumb-hole orthosis.

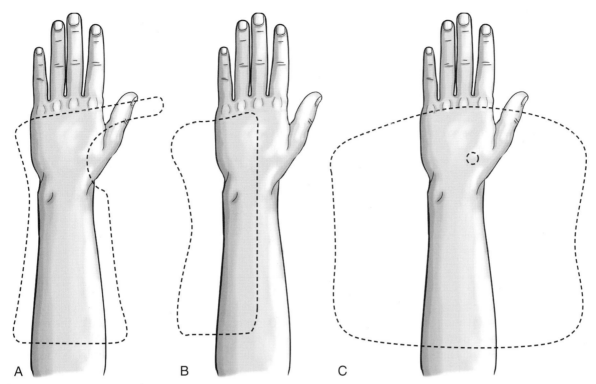

Fig. 7.14 A, A dorsal wrist immobilization pattern. B, An ulnar wrist immobilization pattern. C, A circumferential wrist immobilization pattern.

performance compared with volar and dorsal wrist orthoses with metacarpal bars.[70] Fig. 7.14A shows a pattern for a dorsal wrist immobilization orthosis. Fig. 7.14B is a pattern for an ulnar wrist immobilization orthosis. Fig. 7.14C depicts a pattern for a circumferential wrist immobilization orthosis.

Novice therapists may learn to fabricate orthosis patterns by following detailed written instructions and looking at pictures of patterns. As therapists gain experience, they can easily draw patterns without copying from pictures. (See Figs. 7.1–7.4 for pictures of completed orthosis products.) The following instruction is for construction of a volar wrist immobilization orthosis (Fig. 7.15 and Fig. 7.7) and is similar to instruction for a dorsal wrist immobilization orthosis (see Figs. 7.8 and 7.14A). Table 7.3 provides an overview of safety considerations for any wrist orthotic provision.

1. Position the person's hand palm down on a piece of paper. The wrist should be as neutral as possible with respect to radial and ulnar deviation. The fingers should be in a natural resting position (not flat) and slightly abducted. Draw an outline of the hand and forearm to the elbow.
2. While the person's hand is still on the paper, mark an A at the radial styloid and a B at the ulnar styloid. Mark the second and fifth metacarpal heads C and D, respectively. Mark the olecranon process of the elbow E. Remove the hand from the pattern. Mark two-thirds the length of the forearm on each side with an X. Place another X on each side of the pattern approximately 1 to 1½ inches outside and parallel to the two previous X markings for the approximate width of the orthosis, and label each F. These markings are to accommodate for the side of the forearm trough.

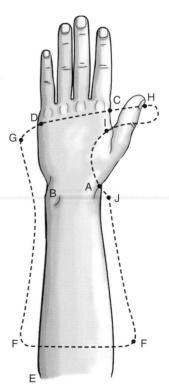

Fig. 7.15 A detailed pattern for a volar wrist immobilization orthosis.

3. Draw an angled line connecting the marks of the second and fifth metacarpal heads (C to D). Extend this line approximately 1 to 1½ inches from the ulnar side of the hand, and mark it G. On the radial side of the hand, extend the line straight out approximately 2 inches, and mark it H.

TABLE 7.3 **Patient Safety Considerations for Wrist Orthotic Intervention**

Orthotic Fabrication	Orthotic Wearing
• Avoid pressure points around the radial and ulnar styloids, the first web space, and the dorsal portion of the metacarpals. • Be aware of the temperature of the thermoplastic material when molding on the patient's wrist. Use a couple layers of cool damp paper towels or a stockinette as protection during the fabrication process. • Never apply the heat gun to the orthosis while the patient is wearing the orthosis. • Monitor wrist position while the thermoplastic material is cooling because sometimes patients reposition during the process. • For individuals with thin skin, consider lining the orthosis with padding or an orthotic liner to reduce pressure or skin irritation, or have the person wear a stockinette.	• Instruct patients to monitor skin for redness and report immediately to the therapist any irritation(s). • Educate patients on the importance of following the orthotic-wearing schedule. • Provide patients with information regarding safe storage and cleaning of the orthosis. • Instruct patients to never make their own adjustments to the orthosis and to inform the therapist of any discomfort.

---

4. On the ulnar side of the orthosis, extend the metacarpal line from G down the hand and forearm of the orthotic pattern, making sure the pattern follows the person's forearm muscle bulk. End this line at F.

5. Measure and place an I approximately ¾ inch below the mark for the head of the index finger (C). Extend a line parallel from I to the line between G and H. Curve this line to meet H. This area represents the extension of the metacarpal bar and usually measures approximately ¾ inch down from C to the outline on the other side of the metacarpal bar. Draw a curved line that simulates the thenar crease from I to A. Extend the line past A approximately 1 inch, and mark it J.

6. Draw a line from J down the radial side of the forearm, making sure the line follows the increasing size of the forearm. Curve out like drawing a "bell" to ensure that the orthosis design is adequate to fit the forearm. To ensure that the orthosis is two-thirds the length of the forearm, end the line at F.

7. For the bottom of the orthosis, draw a straight line connecting both F marks.

8. Make sure the pattern lines are rounded at H, G, J, and the two Fs to prevent any pressure or discomfort.

9. Cut out the pattern.

10. Position the person's upper extremity with the elbow resting on a pad (folded towel or foam wedge) on the table and the forearm in a neutral position—rather than in supination or pronation, which results in a poorly fitted orthosis. Make sure that the fingers are relaxed and the thumb is lightly touching the index finger. Place the wrist immobilization pattern on the person as shown in Fig. 7.16A. Check that the wrist has adequate support, with the pattern ending just proximal to the MCP joint. On the dorsal surface of the hand, check whether the hypothenar bar on the ulnar side of the hand ends just proximal to the fifth metacarpal head. The metacarpal bar on the radial side of the hand should point to the triquetrum or distal ulna bone after it wraps through the first web space. On the volar surface of the hand, check below the thumb carpometacarpal (CMC) joint to determine whether the pattern provides enough support at the wrist joint. Make sure the forearm trough is two-thirds the length and one-half the width of the forearm. Make necessary adjustments (i.e., additions or deletions) on the pattern.

11. Trace the pattern onto the sheet of thermoplastic material.

12. Heat the thermoplastic material.

13. Cut the pattern out of the thermoplastic material.

14. Measure the person's wrist using a goniometer to determine whether the wrist has been placed in the correct position. The therapist should instruct and practice with the person maintaining the correct position (see Fig. 7.16B).

15. Reheat the thermoplastic material.

16. Mold the form onto the person's hand. To fit the orthosis on the person, place the person's elbow in a resting position on a pad on the table with the forearm in a neutral position. Make sure the fingers are relaxed and the thumb is lightly touching the index finger (see Fig. 7.16C). The advantage of this approach is that the therapist can better monitor the wrist position visually during orthosis formation.

17. Make sure that the wrist remains correctly positioned as the thermoplastic material hardens. During the formation phase, roll the metacarpal bar just proximal to the distal palmar crease, and roll the thermoplastic material toward the thenar crease. Flare the distal end of the orthosis on a flat surface to prevent skin breakdown (see Fig. 7.16D).

18. Make necessary adjustments on the orthosis (see Fig. 7.16E–F).

19. Cut the Velcro into approximately ½-inch oval pieces for the metacarpal bar area and 1½-inch oval pieces for the forearm trough. Heat the adhesive with a heat gun to encourage adherence before putting them on the orthosis (see Fig. 7.16G). Using a solvent on the thermoplastic material, scratch the thermoplastic material to remove some of the nonstick coating to help with

adherence of the Velcro pieces For an adult, add two 2-inch straps on the forearm trough and one narrower strap on the dorsal surface of the hand, thus connecting the metacarpal bar on the radial side to the hypothenar bar on the ulnar side of the hand. A child's orthosis requires straps that are narrower than an adult's. The strap placed at the wrist is located exactly at the wrist joint and not proximal to it to ensure a good fit (see Fig. 7.16H).

Technical Tips for a Proper Fit

- Choose a thermoplastic material that has a high degree of conformability to allow a close fit and to prevent migration. Some therapists may prefer a rubber-based moderate drape thermoplastic material.
- Use caution when cutting a pattern out of thermoplastic material that stretches easily. Leave stretchable thermoplastic material flat on the table when cutting to prevent the material from stretching and the orthosis from losing

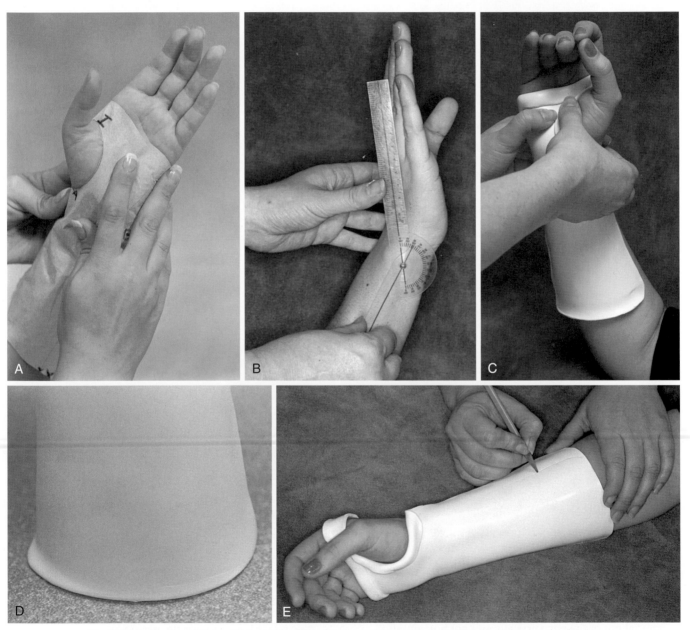

Fig. 7.16 A, Placing of the wrist immobilization pattern on the person. B, Before forming the orthosis, the therapist should measure the person's wrist with a goniometer to obtain the correct amount of extension. C, A position for molding the wrist immobilization orthosis. D, Flaring the distal end of the orthosis on a flat surface. E, Marking of the orthosis to make an adjustment. F, Cutting off excess thermoplastic material to make an adjustment. G, Heating of the Velcro tabs with a heat gun to help them adhere to the orthosis. H, The therapist should place two straps on the forearm trough with one at the wrist level, one approximately ⅔ down the trough, and one strap on the dorsal surface of the hand that connects the metacarpal bar to the hypothenar bar. (B from Reese, N. B., & Bandy, W. D. [2002]. Joint range of motion and muscle length testing. London: W.B. Saunders.)

(Continued)

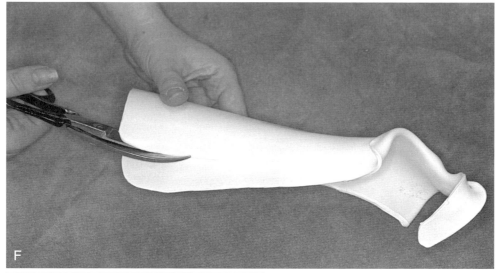

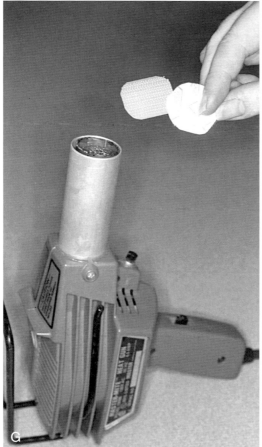

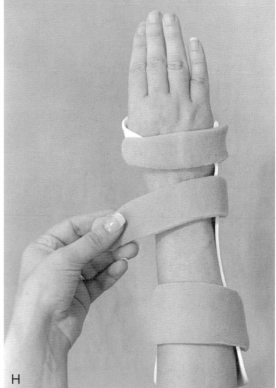

Fig. 7.16, cont'd

the original shape of the pattern and remember to take the material out of the pan vertically and not horizontally.

- When positioning the client, one option is to position the person's elbow joint on a towel with the elbow flexed 90 degrees and the forearm in neutral. Another option is to position the person's forearm resting on a rolled towel on a table in a supinated position, allowing the wrist to fall into extension. The first position allows for more careful observation of wrist position, but the orthotic material

may stretch. The second option provides a more comfortable relaxed position for the person.

- Mold the orthosis sequentially. For a volar wrist immobilization orthosis, form the hypothenar bar (Fig. 7.17A), wrap the metacarpal bar around the palm to the dorsal side of the hand (see Fig. 7.17B), roll down the metacarpal bar (see Fig. 7.17C), and then form the thenar area (see Fig. 7.17D). See the specific comments in this section for hints about each of these areas.

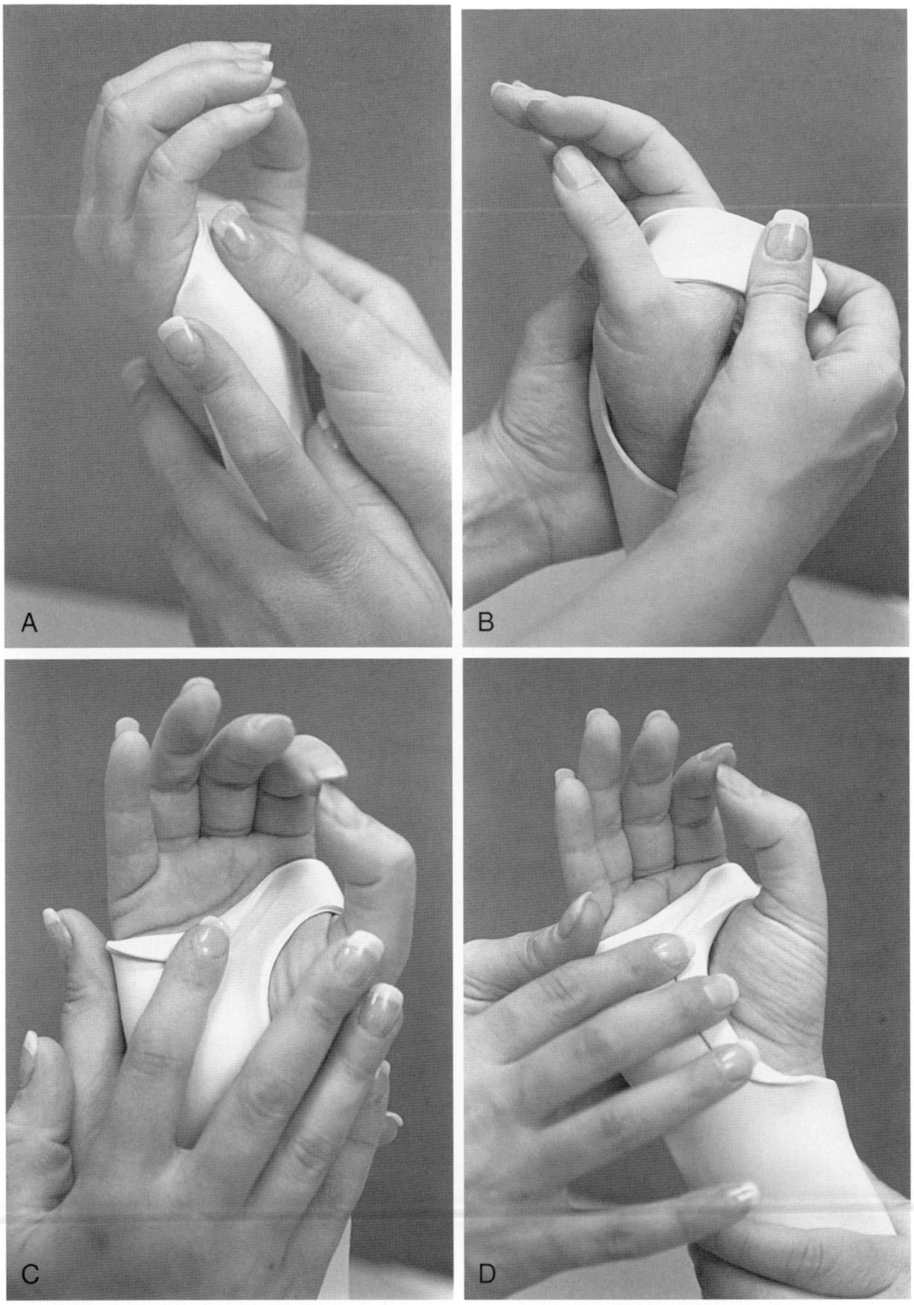

Fig. 7.17 A, The formation of the hypothenar bar. B, Wrapping the metacarpal bar around the palm. C, Rolling the metacarpal bar. D, Forming the thenar area.

- As the orthosis is being formed, be sure to follow the natural curves of the longitudinal, distal, and proximal arches. Having the person lightly touch the thumb to the index finger during molding helps conform the orthosis to the arches of the hand (see Fig. 7.16C). Mold the thermoplastic material to conform naturally to the center of the palm. Be careful not to flatten the transverse arch, which could cause metacarpal contractures. However, overemphasizing the transverse carpal arch can create a focal pressure point in the central palm that will be intolerable for the person.
- For a volar wrist immobilization orthosis, position the metacarpal bar on the volar surface just proximal to the distal

palmar crease. This position allows adequate wrist support and full MCP flexion. In addition, make sure the metacarpal bar follows the natural angle of the distal transverse arch (see Fig. 7.17C). On the dorsal surface, position the metacarpal bar just proximal to the natural angle of the MCP heads. A correctly conformed dorsal metacarpal bar helps to hold the wrist in the correct position. If the metacarpal bar does not conform and there is a gap, the wrist will be mobile. For comfort, some clients may prefer that the metacarpal bar is shorter and the strap longer on the dorsal surface due to the bony prominence of the metacarpals on the dorsum of the hand.
- Always determine whether the person has full finger flexion when wearing the orthosis by having him or her flex

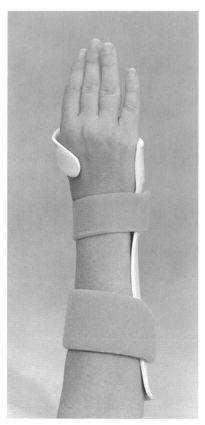

Fig. 7.18 The metacarpal bar and hypothenar bar help position and hold the wrist.

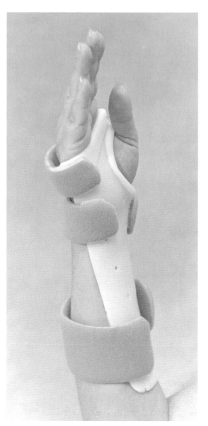

Fig. 7.19 This forearm trough was twisted.

the MCP joints. If any areas of the metacarpal bar are too high, the therapist makes adjustments.

- Make sure the hand and wrist are positioned correctly by taking into consideration the position of a normal resting hand. On volar and dorsal wrist immobilization orthoses, the metacarpal bar (which wraps around the radial side of the hand) and the hypothenar bar (on the ulnar side) help position and hold the wrist (Fig. 7.18). If adequate support is lacking on either side, the wrist may be in an incorrect position.
- A frequent fabrication mistake is to allow the wrist to deviate radially or ulnarly. This mistake can occur because of a lack of careful monitoring of the person's wrist position as the thermoplastic material is cooling. The therapist should closely monitor the wrist position in any orthosis that positions the wrist in neutral because it is easy for the wrist to move in slight flexion. A quick spot check before the thermoplastic material is completely cool can address this problem.
- If a mistake occurs with an orthotic material that easily stretches, be extremely careful with adjustments to avoid further compromising of wrist position. For thermoplastic material with memory, remold the entire orthosis rather than spot heating the wrist area because doing the latter tends to cause the material to buckle. Sometimes adjustments can be done by heating the entire orthosis made from material without memory.
- After the formation of the palmar and wrist part of the orthosis is complete, the therapist can begin to work on other areas of the orthosis, such as the forearm trough. A problem that

can easily be corrected just before the thermoplastic material is cooled is twisting of the forearm trough. If this problem is not corrected, the orthosis will end up with one edge of the forearm trough higher than the other (Fig. 7.19).

- After the thermoplastic material has cooled, determine whether the person can fully oppose the thumb to all fingers. The thenar eminence should not be restricted or flattened. Wrist support should be adequate to maintain the angle of the wrist. To check whether the thenar eminence area is rolled enough, have the person move the thumb in opposition to the little finger, and sustain the hold while evaluating the roll. Also observe that the thenar crease is visible to allow for full thumb mobility. Adjustments should be made to allow complete thumb excursion. Otherwise, a potential for a pressure sore to develop exists, especially in the area of the thumb web space (Fig. 7.20).
- Occasionally after the thermoplastic material is cooled, the therapist will note areas that are too tight in the forearm trough, which can potentially result in pressure sores. To easily correct this problem, the therapist pulls apart the sides of the forearm trough.

Troubleshooting Wrist Immobilization Orthoses

A careful practitioner must continuously think of precautions, such as checking for pressure areas. Precautions for making a wrist immobilization orthosis include the following:

- Be aware of and make adjustments for potential pressure points on the radial styloid, on the ulnar styloid, at the first web space, and over the dorsal aspects of the metacarpals.

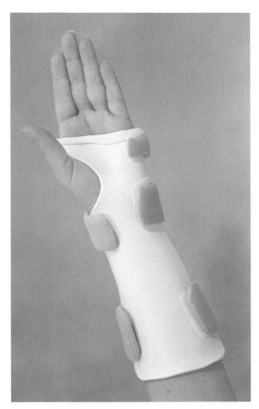

Fig. 7.20 This thenar web space was not rolled enough to allow full thumb excursion.

The thumb web space is a prime area for skin irritation because it is so tender. Some people cannot tolerate plastic in the first web space. The thermoplastic material must be cut back and replaced with soft strapping. Others can tolerate the plastic if it is rolled and extremely thin.[65] Instruct the person to monitor the skin for reddened areas and to communicate immediately about any irritation that occurs.

- Control edema before orthotic provision. For persons with sustained edema, avoid using constricting wrist orthoses. Instead, fabricate a wider forearm trough with wide strapping material.[18] Dorsal orthoses are better for edematous hands.[21,40] Carefully monitor persons who have the potential for edematous hands, and make necessary orthotic adjustments. As discussed earlier, a "continuous strap" made from flexible fabric is a good strapping option to help manage edema.
- For persons with little subcutaneous tissue and thin skin, carefully monitor the skin for pressure areas. Lining the orthosis with padding may help, but several adjustments may be necessary for a proper fit. Fabricating the orthosis over a thick orthotic liner, QuickCast liner, or a piece of stockinette can prevent skin irritation during orthotic fabrication.
- Make sure the orthosis provides adequate support for functional activities.

PREFABRICATED ORTHOSES

Prefabricated or commercially available wrist orthoses are commonly used in the treatment of CTS and RA.[26,72] A variety of prefabricated wrist orthoses are available, as shown in Fig. 7.21.

As discussed, conservative management of CTS includes positioning the wrist as close to neutral as possible to maximize the space in the carpal tunnel. The supportive metal or thermoplastic stay in most prefabricated wrist orthoses positions the wrist in extension. Therefore, an adjustment must be made to position the wrist in the desired neutral position. However, care must be taken when adjustments are made to ensure that the orthosis adequately fits and supports the hand.

Several options for prefabricated wrist orthoses are marketed for CTS. Options for the work environment include padding to reduce trauma from vibration, leather for added durability, and metal internal pieces that act to position the wrist. Prefabricated wrist immobilization orthoses are also effective for symptoms of CTS during pregnancy.[24]

Fabricating an orthosis for a person who has RA is most effective in the early stages and incorporates positioning, immobilization, and the assumed comfort of neutral warmth from a soft orthosis. The effects of RA can result in decreased joint stability, leading to decreased grip strength and the more obvious finger deformities.[26] When persons with RA wear wrist orthoses, they help decrease pain during ADLs.[70] Prefabricated wrist orthoses marketed for persons with RA are designed for easy application and to decrease ulnar deviation. Some orthoses include correction or protection for finger joints as well as for the wrist joint.

Therapists need to determine whether to fabricate a custom wrist orthosis or to use a commercial prefabricated wrist orthosis. There are many factors to consider with this decision, such as the impact of the prefabricated or custom orthosis on hand function, pain reduction, and degrees of immobilization that the orthosis provides.[22,55,73,74] Research helps therapists select the best orthosis for their clients. Collier and Thomas[22] studied the degree of immobilization of a custom volar wrist orthosis compared with three commercial prefabricated wrist orthoses. They found that the custom wrist orthosis allowed "significantly less palmar flexion and significantly more dorsiflexion" than the commercial orthoses. Thus, custom thermoplastic orthoses may block wrist motion better than prefabricated orthoses, which are more flexible.

Other studies considered the effect of commercial prefabricated orthoses on grip and dexterity,[17,70,73,74] work performance,[55] and proximal musculature.[14] Continued research needs to be done to analyze the efficacy of commercial orthoses, especially as newer ones are developed. Furthermore, as Stern and colleagues[72] found, no single type of wrist orthosis will be appropriate for all clients and that satisfaction with a prefabricated orthosis is often associated with therapeutic benefits, comfort, and utility. Therefore, it benefits therapists to stock a variety of prefabricated orthosis options in the clinic,[71] or therapists can provide information to clients so that they can procure the right orthosis for themselves. Box 7.1 provides some questions for therapists to contemplate when considering a prefabricated wrist orthosis or custom-made wrist orthosis. This information can also be used to educate clients to procure the right prefabricated orthosis for themselves.

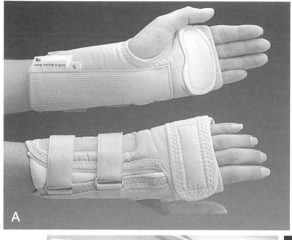
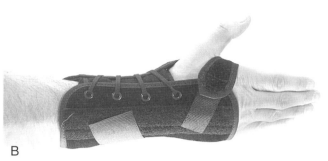
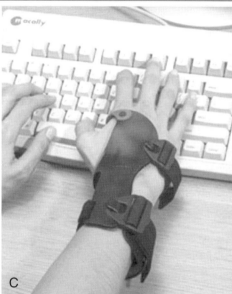
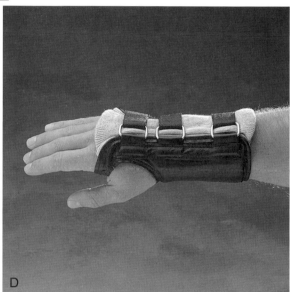

Fig. 7.21 A, This wrist orthosis has D-ring straps and immobilizes the MCPs (Rolyan® D-Ring Wrist Brace). B, This wrist orthosis has a unique strapping system with laces (Sammons Preston Rolyan® Laced Wrist Support). C, This lightweight orthosis can be used for carpal tunnel and other repetitive injuries (Sammons Preston Exolite Wrist Brace). D, The Rolyan® Workhard® D-Ring Wrist Brace is made of soft, pliable leather with ¼" padding for improved work durability. (Courtesy Performance Health, Warrenville, IL.)

BOX 7.1   Questions to Determine Use of Custom-Made Versus Prefabricated Wrist Orthosis

- Is time a factor? (Consider providing prefabricated orthoses; although with experience a custom orthosis can be made in a short time period.)
- Is cost a factor? (Consider costs with custom orthoses versus prefabricated orthoses.)
- Is fit a factor? (Consider whether the prefabricated orthosis is restricting too much motion, such as thumb opposition, or chafes the hand.[77] Or consider whether it is really doing what it is supposed to do, such as keeping the hand in neutral with carpal tunnel syndrome (CTS).[77]
- Is only wrist support required? (Consider either a custom or a prefabricated orthosis.)
- Is restriction of motion a factor? (Consider a custom orthosis.)
- Does the person need the orthosis only for pain relief, such as with arthritis? (Consider a prefabricated orthosis or a custom-made orthosis with padding.)

- Is the person involved in sports? (Consider a soft prefabricated orthosis to avert injury to other people.[10])
- Is wrist and hand edema a factor? (Consider fabricating a custom dorsal wrist orthosis, taking edema into consideration.)
- Is the weight of the orthosis a factor? (Consider custom fabricating an orthosis out of lighter thermoplastic material [1/16 inch] or a lightweight prefabricated orthosis.)
- What are the occupational demands of the person? (Consider a custom-fabricated orthosis if heavy labor is part of the person's life or a prefabricated orthosis if demands are minimal.[38] Consider the material out of which the prefabricated orthosis is fabricated. A prefabricated orthosis out of leather may provide adequate durability, support, protection, and comfort for job demands.)
- Has any research evidence on the orthoses being considered been accessed?

IMPACT ON OCCUPATIONS

For people with the diagnoses discussed in this chapter, supporting the wrist while allowing finger and thumb motions enables them to continue their life occupations. For example, a person with CTS wears a wrist orthosis to avoid extreme wrist positions when working and doing other occupations.

A person with arthritis obtains support and pain relief from wearing a wrist orthosis while doing functional activities. A person undergoing serial orthotic intervention after a Colles fracture to decrease stiffness will eventually be able to better perform meaningful occupations. Wrist orthoses can help many people maintain or eventually improve their functional abilities.

🔎 SELF-QUIZ 7.1ᵃ

For the following questions, circle either true (T) or false (F).

1. T F Wrist immobilization orthoses can be volar, dorsal, ulnar, or circumferential.
2. T F A wrist immobilization orthosis usually decreases wrist pain or inflammation, provides support, enhances digital function, and prevents wrist deformity.
3. T F All prefabricated orthoses are made to correctly fit someone who has carpal tunnel syndrome (CTS).
4. T F Some research suggests the value of early conservative intervention with orthotic intervention.
5. T F After removal of a cast for a Colles fracture, if motion is limited in the wrist, the therapist may consider serial orthotic intervention.
6. T F The therapist must follow standard intervention protocols exactly for any diagnosis that requires a wrist immobilization orthotic application.
7. T F With a wrist immobilization orthosis, the therapist usually positions the wrist in extreme extension, which promotes functional movement.
8. T F The hypothenar bar on a wrist immobilization orthosis helps to position the hand in a neutral resting position by preventing extreme ulnar deviation.
9. T F The therapist should position the volar wrist immobilization orthosis distal to the distal palmar crease.
10. T F If a mistake is made during fabrication of a volar wrist immobilization orthosis, in getting the correct wrist extension the therapist should spot heat the wrist area to make an adjustment.
11. T F People with CTS should be encouraged to perform strong finger flexion while wearing their orthoses to allow for finger mobility.

ᵃSee Appendix A for the answer key.

SUMMARY

As this chapter content reflects, appropriate wrist alignment is very important to maintaining a functional hand. A well-fitted orthosis can be a key element to assist with recovery from many conditions. Therefore, therapists should be aware of diagnostic indications, types, parts, and appropriate fabrication for wrist orthotic intervention. As always in clinical practice, the therapist needs to apply clinical reasoning, because each case is different. Finally, therapists should consider the person's occupations when providing a wrist orthosis.

REVIEW QUESTIONS

1. What are three main indications for use of a wrist immobilization orthosis?
2. When fabricating a wrist orthosis for a person with RA, what are some of the common deformities that can influence orthotic intervention?
3. When might a therapist consider serial orthotic intervention with a wrist immobilization orthosis?
4. What are the goals of wrist orthotic intervention with a Colles fracture?
5. What is the advantage of a volar wrist immobilization orthosis?
6. What is a disadvantage of a dorsal wrist immobilization orthosis?
7. What purpose does the hypothenar bar serve on a wrist immobilization orthosis?
8. What are two positions that the therapist can use for molding a static wrist orthosis, and what are the advantages of each?
9. Which precautions are unique to static wrist immobilization orthoses?
10. What are four questions that therapists could consider when deciding on a prefabricated wrist orthosis versus a custom-fabricated wrist orthosis?
11. What are some findings from the evidence that support wrist orthotic intervention for CTS?

REFERENCES

1. American Academy of Orthopaedic Surgeons: *Management of carpal tunnel syndrome evidence-based clinical practice guideline.* Retrieved from https://www.aaos.org/uploadedFiles/PreProduction/Quality/Guidelines_and_Reviews/guidelines/CTS%20CPG_2.29.16.pdf, 2016.

2. American Academy of Orthopaedic Surgeons: *Carpal tunnel syndrome.* Retrieved from http://orthoinfo.aaos.org/topic.cfm?topic=receivable5, 2016.

3. Bailey J, Cannon N, Colditz J, et al.: *Splint classification system,* Chicago, 1992, American Society of Hand Therapy.

4. Apfel E, Johnson M, Abrams R: Comparison of range-of-motion constraints provided by prefabricated splints used in the treatment of carpal tunnel syndrome: a pilot study, *J Hand Ther* 15(3):226–233, 2002.

5. Ashe MC, McCauley T, Khan KM: Tendinopathies in the upper extremity: a paradigm shift, *J Hand Ther* 17(3):329–334, 2004.

6. Biundo JJ: Tendinitis and tenosynovitis, *Merck Manual Professional Version.* Retrieved October, 19, 2017, from https://www.merckmanuals.com/professional/musculoskeletal-and-connective-tissue-disorders/bursa,-muscle,-and-tendon-disorders/tendinitis-and-tenosynovitis.

7. Baker NA, Moehlingm KK, Rubinstein EN, Wollstein R, Gustafsonk NP, Baratz M: The comparative effectiveness of combined lumbrical muscle splints and stretches on symptoms and function in carpal tunnel syndrome, *Arch Phys Med Rehabil* 93(1):1–10, 2012.

8. Ballestero-Pérez R, Plaza-Manzano G, Urraca-Gesto A, et al.: Effectiveness of nerve gliding exercises on carpal tunnel syndrome: a systematic review, *J Manipulative Physiol Ther* 40(1):50–59, 2017.

9. Braidotti F, Atzei A, Fairplay T: Dart-splint: an innovative orthosis that can be integrated into a scapho-lunate and palmar midcarpal instability re-education protocol, *J Hand Ther* 28(3):329–335, 2015.

10. Bell-Krotoski JA, Breger-Stanton DE: Biomechanics and evaluation of the hand. In Mackin EJ, Callahan AD, Skirven TM, et al.: *Rehabilitation of the hand and upper extremity,* ed 5, St. Louis, 2002, Mosby, pp 240–262.

11. Biese J: Therapist's evaluation and conservative management of rheumatoid arthritis in the hand and wrist. In Mackin EJ, Callahan AD, Skirven TM, et al.: *Rehabilitation of the hand and upper extremity,* ed 5, St. Louis, 2002, Mosby, pp 1569–1582.

12. Bulut GT, Caglar NS, Aytekin E, et al.: Comparison of static wrist splint with static wrist and metacarpophalangeal splint in carpal tunnel syndrome, *J Back Musculoskelet Rehabil* 28(4):761–767, 2015.

13. Brininger TL, Rogers JC, Holm MB, et al.: Efficacy of fabricated customized splint and tendon and nerve gliding exercises for the treatment of carpal tunnel syndrome: a randomized controlled trial, *Arch Phys Med Rehabil* 88(11):1429–1436, 2007.

14. Bulthaup S, Cipriani DJ, Thomas JJ: An electromyography study of wrist extension orthoses and upper-extremity function, *Am J Occup Ther* 53(5):434–444, 1999.

15. Burke D, Burke MM, Steward GW, et al.: Splinting for carpal tunnel syndrome: in search of the optimal angle, *Arch Phys Med Rehabil* 75(11):1241–1244, 1994.

16. Burke FD, Ellis J, McKenna H, et al.: Primary care management of carpal tunnel syndrome, *Postgrad Med J* 79(934):433–437, 2003.

17. Burtner PA, Anderson JB, Marcum ML, et al.: A comparison of static and dynamic wrist splints using electromyography in individuals with rheumatoid arthritis, *J Hand Ther* 16(4):320–325, 2003.

18. Cannon NC, et al.: *Diagnosis and treatment manual for physicians and therapists,* ed 4, Indianapolis, 2013, Hand Rehabilitation Center of Indiana.

19. Cannon NM: *Manual of hand splinting,* New York, 1985, Churchill Livingstone.

20. Cobb TK, An KN, Cooney WP: Effect of lumbrical muscle incursion within the carpal tunnel on carpal tunnel pressure: a cadaveric study, *J Hand Surg Am* 20(2):186–192, 1995.

21. Colditz JC: Therapist's management of the stiff hand. In Mackin EJ, Callahan AD, Skirven TM, et al.: *Rehabilitation of the hand and upper extremity,* ed 5, St. Louis, 2002, Mosby, pp 1021–1049.

22. Collier SE, Thomas JJ: Range of motion at the wrist: a comparison study of four wrist extension orthoses and the free hand, *Am J Occup Ther* 56(2):180–184, 2002.

23. Cooper C: *Personal communication,* January 2012.

24. Courts RB: Splinting for symptoms of carpal tunnel syndrome during pregnancy, *J Hand Ther* 8:31–34, 1995.

25. de Almeida PH, Pontes TB, Matheus JP, Muniz LF, da Mota LM: Occupational therapy in rheumatoid arthritis: what rheumatologists need to know? *Rev Bras Reumatol* 55(3):272–280, 2015.

26. Dell PC, Dell RB: Management of rheumatoid arthritis of the wrist, *J Hand Ther* 9(2):157–164, 1996.

27. Egan M, Brosseau L, Farmer M, et al.: Splints and orthosis for treating rheumatoid arthritis, *Cochrane Database of Systematic Reviews* (4):Art. No.: CD004018, 2001. https://doi.org/10.1002/14651858.CD004018.

28. Fess EE, Gettle KS, Philips CA, et al.: *Hand and upper extremity splinting principles and methods,* ed 3, St. Louis, 2005, Elsevier Mosby.

29. Gelberman RH, Hergenroeder PT, Hargens AR, et al.: The carpal tunnel syndrome: a study of carpal canal pressures,, *J Bone Joint Surg Am* 63(3):380–383, 1981.

30. Golriz B, Ahmadi Bani M, Arazpour M, et al.: Comparison of the efficacy of a neutral wrist splint and a wrist splint incorporating a lumbrical unit for the treatment of patients with carpal tunnel syndrome, *Prosthet Orthot Int* 40(5):617–623, 2016.

31. Hall B, Lee HC, Fitzgerald H, Byrne B, Barton A, Lee AH: Investigating the effectiveness of full-time wrist splinting and education in the treatment of carpal tunnel syndrome: a randomized controlled trial, *Am J Occup Ther* 67(4):448–459, 2013.

32. Hayes EP, Carney K, Mariatis Wolf J, et al.: Carpal tunnel syndrome. In Mackin EJ, Callahan AD, Skirven TM, et al.: *Rehabilitation of the hand and upper extremity,* ed 5, St. Louis, 2002, Mosby, pp 643–659.

33. Huisstede BM, Hoofvliet P, Randsdorp MS, et al.: Carpal tunnel syndrome. Part I: effectiveness of nonsurgical treatments—a systematic review, *Arch Phys Med Rehabil* 91(7):981–1004, 2010.

34. Idler RS: Helping the patient who has wrist or hand tenosynovitis. Part 2: managing trigger finger, de Quervain's disease, *J Musculoskelet Med* 14(2):62–65, 68, 74–75, 1997.

35. Kasch MC: Therapist's evaluation and treatment of upper extremity cumulative-trauma disorders. In Mackin EJ, Callahan AD, Skirven TM, et al.: *Rehabilitation of the hand and upper extremity,* ed 5, St. Louis, 2002, Mosby, pp 1005–1018.

36. Keith MW, Masear V, Chung KC, et al.: American Academy of Orthopaedic Surgeons clinical practice guideline on the treatment of carpal tunnel syndrome, *J Bone Joint Surg Am* 92:218–219, 2010.

37. Khan KM, Cook JL, Taunton JE, et al.: Overuse tendinosis, not tendonitis part 1: a new paradigm for a difficult clinical problem, *Phys Sportsmed* 28(5):38–48, 2000.

38. Kozin SH, Michlovitz SL: Traumatic arthritis and osteoarthritis of the wrist, *J Hand Ther* 13(2):124–135, 2000.

39. Kuo MH, Leong CP, Cheng YF, et al.: Static wrist position associated with least median nerve compression: sonographic evaluation, *Am J Phys Med Rehabil* 80(4):256–260, 2001.

40. Laseter GF: Therapist's management of distal radius fractures. In Mackin EJ, Callahan AD, Skirven TM, et al.: *Rehabilitation of the hand and upper extremity*, ed 5, St. Louis, 2002, Mosby, pp 1136–1155.

41. Laseter GF, Carter PR: Management of distal radius fractures, *J Hand Ther* 9(2):114–128, 1996.

42. LaStayo P: Ulnar wrist pain and impairment: a therapist's algorithmic approach to the triangular fibrocartilage complex. In Mackin EJ, Callahan AD, Skirven TM, et al.: *Rehabilitation of the hand and upper extremity*, ed 5, St. Louis, 2002, Mosby, pp 1156–1170.

43. LaBlanc KE, Cestia W: Carpal tunnel syndrome, *Am Fam Physician* 83(8):952–958, 2011.

44. Manente G, Torrieri F, Di Blasio F, Staniscia T, Romano F, Uncini A: An innovative hand brace for carpal tunnel syndrome: a randomized controlled trial, *Muscle Nerve* 8(8):1020–1025, 2001.

45. McClure P: Evidence-based practice: an example related to the use of splinting in a patient with carpal tunnel syndrome, *J Hand Ther* 16(3):256–263, 2003.

46. Melvin JL: *Rheumatic disease in the adult and child: occupational therapy and rehabilitation*, ed 3, Philadelphia, 1989, FA Davis.

47. Messer RS, Bankers RM: Evaluating and treating common upper extremity nerve compression and tendonitis syndromes... without becoming cumulatively traumatized, *Nurse Pract Forum* 6(3):152–166, 1995.

48. Moritomo H, Apergis E, Herzberg G, et al.: 2007 IFSSH committee report of wrist biomechanics committee: biomechanics of the so-called dart-throwing motion of the wrist, *J Hand Surg Am* 32(9):1447–1453, 2007.

49. Moscony AMB, Shank T: Wrist fractures. In Cooper C, editor: *Fundamentals of hand therapy: clinical reasoning and treatment guidelines for common diagnoses of the upper extremity*, ed 2, St. Louis, 2014, Elsevier.

50. National Institute of Neurological Disorders and Stroke: *Complex regional pain syndrome fact sheet*. Retrieved October 25, 2017 from https://www.ninds.nih.gov/Disorders/Patient-Caregiver-Education/Fact-Sheets/Complex-Regional-Pain-Syndrome-Fact-Sheet.

51. Nordenskiold U: Elastic wrist orthoses: reduction of pain and increase in grip force for women with rheumatoid arthritis, *Arthritis Care Res* 3(3):158–162, 1990.

52. Nuckols T, Harber P, Sandin K, et al.: Quality measures for the diagnosis and non-operative management of carpal tunnel syndrome in occupational settings, *J Occup Rehabil* 21(1):100–119, 2011.

53. Ono S, Chapham PJ, Chung KC: Optimal management of carpal tunnel syndrome, *Int J Gen Med* 3:235–261, 2010.

54. Osterman AL, Whitman M, Porta LD: Nonoperative carpal tunnel syndrome treatment, *Hand Clin* 18(2):279–289, 2002.

55. Pagnotta A, Baron M, Korner-Bitensky N: The effect of a static wrist orthosis on hand function in individuals with rheumatoid arthritis, *J Rheumatol* 25(5):879–885, 1998.

56. Palmer AK, Werner FW, Murphy D, et al.: Functional wrist motion: a biomechanical study, *J Hand Surg Am* 10(1):39–46, 1985.

57. Peters S, Page MJ, Coppieters MW, Ross M, Johnston V: Rehabilitation following carpal tunnel release, *Cochrane Database Syst Rev* (2): CD004158, 2016. https://doi.org/10.1002/14651858.CD004158.pub3.

58. Philips CA: Therapist's management of patients with rheumatoid arthritis. In Hunter JM, Mackin EJ, Callahan AD, editors: *Rehabilitation of the hand: surgery and therapy*, ed 4, St. Louis, 1995, Mosby, pp 1345–1350.

59. Ramsey L, Winder RJ, McVeigh JG: The effectiveness of working wrist splints in adults with rheumatoid arthritis: a mixed methods systematic review, *J Rehabil Med* 46(6):481–492, 2014.

60. Reiss B: Therapist's management of distal radial fractures. In Hunter JM, Mackin EJ, Callahan AD, editors: *Rehabilitation of the hand: surgery and therapy*, ed 4, St. Louis, 1995, Mosby, pp 337–351.

61. Saidoff DC, McDonough AL: *Critical pathways in therapeutic intervention: upper extremity*, St. Louis, 1997, Mosby.

62. Sailer SM: The role of splinting and rehabilitation in the treatment of carpal and cubital tunnel syndromes,, *Hand Clin* 12(2):223–241, 1996.

63. Schultz-Johnson K: Splinting the wrist: mobilization and protection, *J Hand Ther* 9(2):165–176, 1996.

64. Schultz-Johnson K: *Personal communication*, April 2006.

65. Schultz-Johnson K: *Personal communication*, April 1999.

66. Schwartz DA: An alternative fabrication method of the dart thrower's motion orthosis (also known as the dart orthosis), *J Hand Ther* 29(3):339–347, 2016.

67. Siegel DB, Kuzma G, Eakins D: Anatomic investigation the role of the lumbrical muscles in carpal tunnel syndrome, *J Hand Surg Am* 20(5):860–863, 1995.

68. Skirven T: Nerve injuries. In Stanley BG, Tribuzi SM, editors: *Concepts in hand rehabilitation*, Philadelphia, 1992, FA Davis, pp 323–352.

69. Stein CM, Svoren B, Davis P, et al.: A prospective analysis of patients with rheumatic diseases attending referral hospitals in Harare, Zimbabwe, *J Rheumatol* 18(12):1841–1844, 1991.

70. Stern EB: Grip strength and finger dexterity across five styles of commercial wrist orthoses, *Am J Occup Ther* 50(1):32–38, 1996.

71. Stern EB, Sines B, Teague TR: Commercial wrist extensor orthoses: hand function, comfort, and interference across five styles, *J Hand Ther* 7(4):237–244, 1994.

72. Stern EB, Ytterberg SR, Krug HE, et al.: Commercial wrist extensor orthoses: a descriptive study of use and preference in patients with rheumatoid arthritis, *Arthritis Care Res* 10(1):27–35, 1997.

73. Stern EB, Ytterberg SR, Krug HE, et al.: Finger dexterity and hand function: effect of three commercial wrist extensor orthoses on patients with rheumatoid arthritis, *Arthritis Care Res* 9(3):197–205, 1996.

74. Stern EB, Ytterberg SR, Krug HE, et al.: Immediate and short-term effects of three commercial wrist extensor orthoses on grip strength and function in patients with rheumatoid arthritis, *Arthritis Care Res* 9(1):42–50, 1996.

75. Steultjens EEMJ, Dekker JJ, Bouter LM, Schaardenburg DD, Kuyk MAMAH, Van den Ende ECHM: Occupational therapy for rheumatoid arthritis, *Cochrane Database Syst Rev* (1): Art.

No.: CD003114, 2004. https://doi.org/10.1002/14651858.CD003114.pub2.

76. Swan M: *A therapist's perspective on treating CRPS*. Retrieved from https://rsds.org/a-therapists-perspective-on-treating-crps/, 2007.

77. Walker WC, Metzler M, Cifu DX, et al.: Neutral wrist splinting in carpal tunnel syndrome: a comparison of night-only versus full-time wear instructions, *Arch Phys Med Rehabil* 81(4):424–429, 2000.

78. Walsh MT, Muntzer E: Therapist's management of complex regional pain syndrome (reflex sympathetic dystrophy). In Mackin EJ, Callahan AD, Skirven TM, et al.: *Rehabilitation of the hand and upper extremity*, ed 5, St. Louis, 2002, Mosby, pp 1707–1724.

79. Weinstock TB: Management of fractures of the distal radius: therapists commentary, *J Hand Ther* 12(2):99–102, 1999.

80. Weiss ND, Gordon L, Bloom T, et al.: Position of the wrist associated with the lowest carpal-tunnel pressure: implications for splint design, *J Bone Joint Surg Am* 77(11):1695–1699, 1995.

APPENDIX 7.1 CASE STUDIES

Case Study 7.1ᵃ

Read the following scenario and use your clinical reasoning skills to answer the questions based on information in this chapter.
Angela is a homemaker who began experiencing carpal tunnel syndrome (CTS) symptoms of numbness, grasp weakness, and paresthesias over the distribution of the median nerve. Angela went to her family physician, whose nurse provided her with a quick remedy. Not being familiar with the correct wrist positioning for CTS, the nurse placed a strip of thermoplastic material stretching down the dorsal aspect of Angela's forearm, wrist, and hand and wrapped it in gauze. After a while Angela began to complain about the thermoplastic strip feeling awkward during activities, such as using a knife to cut meat, because it was not supporting the wrist. Eventually Angela began to wake up in the middle of the night, noticing that her hand was again numb. Angela returned to her family physician. This time he referred her to a neurologist, who diagnosed her with CTS. The neurologist provided a cortisone shot and referred her to occupational therapy. The occupational therapist requested an order for a custom orthosis. At that point, Angela had doubts about wearing the orthosis. She asked for valid reasons for the custom orthosis versus a prefabricated orthosis. She stated in frustration, "Why don't I just go ahead and have surgery!"

1. Provide two reasons that the thermoplastic strip was not the best choice.

   _____

   _____

   _____

2. Describe the correct position for the custom orthosis that the therapist should fabricate for Angela.

   _____

   _____

3. What would be the suggested wearing schedule?

   _____

   _____

4. What precautions are important with orthotic wear?

   _____

   _____

   _____

5. How should the therapist address Angela's concerns about getting a custom orthosis and surgery? Include in the answer how you might present the research evidence to Angela.

   _____

   _____

   _____

6. Explain two advantages of using a custom-made orthosis compared to a prefabricated orthosis for CTS.

   _____

   _____

   _____

ᵃSee Appendix A for the answer key.

Case Study 7.2[a]

Read the following scenario and use your clinical reasoning skills to answer the questions based on information from this chapter.
Diane is a 52-year-old woman who was walking outside at dusk with a friend. She came up to an intersection without seeing the curb, and she fell with her right hand stretched out in front of her. She went to the emergency department, and a closed reduction approach with casting was used for her nondisplaced Colles fracture. After her cast was removed the physician ordered therapy for edema and pain control, range of motion (ROM), and fabrication of a wrist orthosis for the right upper extremity.

1. Diane comes to therapy with her right wrist in 15 degrees flexion. Her wrist can be passively extended to neutral. Describe the orthotic position for her right hand and the rationale for the position.

   _____

   _____

2. As Diane's ROM improves, how should the therapist revise the position of the orthosis?

   _____

   _____

3. At what point should the therapist discontinue wrist orthotic intervention?

   _____

   _____

---

[a]See Appendix A for the answer key.

APPENDIX 7.2 LABORATORY EXERCISES

Laboratory Exercise 7.1

1. Practice making a wrist immobilization orthotic pattern on another person. Use the detailed instructions provided to draw the pattern.
2. Using the outline for the left and right hand, draw a wrist immobilization pattern without the detailed instructions.

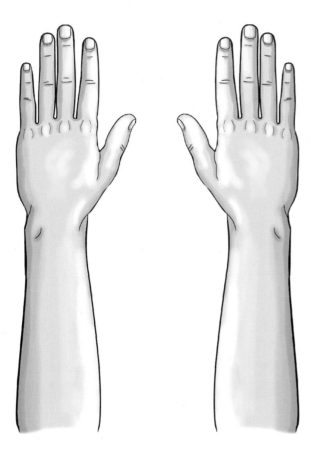

Laboratory Exercise 7.2[a]

Orthosis A

1. What problems can you identify regarding this orthosis?
2. What problems may arise from continual orthotic wear?

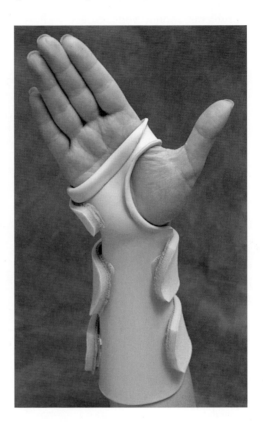

Orthosis B

You are supervising a student in clinical practice. You ask the student to practice making a wrist immobilization orthosis before actually fabricating an orthosis on a person. Orthosis B is a picture of the student's orthosis.

1. What problems should you address with the student regarding the orthosis?

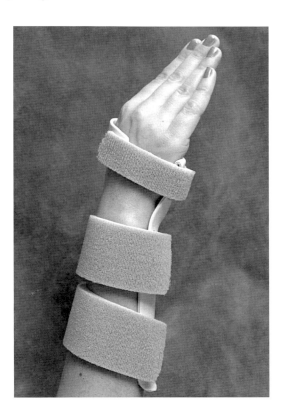

Orthosis C

Orthosis C was made for a 54-year-old woman working as a school bus driver. The person works full-time and has wrist extensor tendinopathy.

1. What problems can you identify regarding this orthosis?
2. What problems may arise from continual orthotic wear?

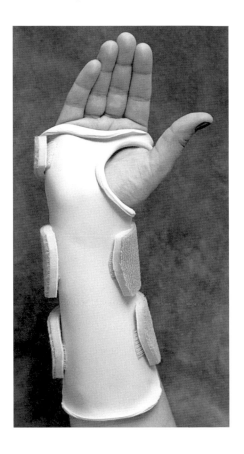

Laboratory Exercise 7.3

Practice fabricating a wrist immobilization orthosis on a partner. Before starting, determine the correct position for your partner's hand. Measure the angle of wrist extension with a goniometer to ensure a correct position. After fitting your orthosis and making all adjustments, use Form 7.1 as a self evaluation of the wrist immobilization orthosis, and use Grading Sheet 7.1 as a classroom grading sheet.

Laboratory Exercise 7.4ᵃ

The following picture is a volar-based wrist immobilization orthosis. Identify the parts of the orthosis that are marked.

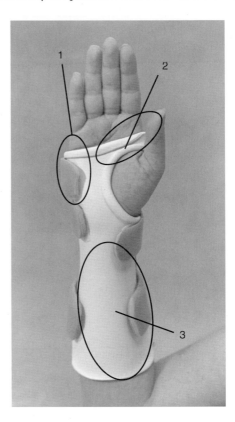

1. _____
2. _____
3. _____

ᵃSee Appendix A for the answer key.

APPENDIX 7.3 FORM AND GRADING SHEET

Form 7.1 Wrist Immobilization Orthosis

	Name: _____
Type of cone wrist and hand orthosis:	Date: _____
Volar platform ○ Dorsal platform ○	
Wrist position: _____	
After the person wears the orthosis for 30 minutes, answer the following questions. (Mark NA for nonapplicable situations.)	

Evaluation Areas				Comments
Design				
1. The wrist position is at the correct angle.	Yes ○	No ○	NA ○	
2. The wrist has adequate support.	Yes ○	No ○	NA ○	
3. The sides of the thenar and hypothenar eminences have support in the correct position.	Yes ○	No ○	NA ○	
4. The thenar and hypothenar eminences are not restricted or flattened.	Yes ○	No ○	NA ○	
5. The orthosis is two-thirds the length of the forearm.	Yes ○	No ○	NA ○	
6. The orthosis is one-half the width of the forearm.	Yes ○	No ○	NA ○	
Function				
1. The orthosis allows full thumb motions.	Yes ○	No ○	NA ○	
2. The orthosis allows full metacarpophalangeal (MCP) joint flexion of the fingers.	Yes ○	No ○	NA ○	
3. The orthosis provides wrist support that allows functional activities.	Yes ○	No ○	NA ○	

Straps				
1. The straps are secure and rounded.	Yes O	No O	NA O	
Comfort				
1. The orthosis edges are smooth with rounded corners.	Yes O	No O	NA O	
2. The proximal end is flared.	Yes O	No O	NA O	
3. The orthosis does not cause impingements or pressure sores.	Yes O	No O	NA O	
4. The orthosis does not irritate bony prominences.	Yes O	No O	NA O	
Cosmetic Appearance				
1. The orthosis is free of fingerprints, dirt, and pencil and pen marks.	Yes O	No O	NA O	
2. The thermoplastic material is not buckled.	Yes O	No O	NA O	
Therapeutic Regimen				
1. The person has been instructed in a wearing schedule.	Yes O	No O	NA O	
2. The person has been provided orthotic precautions.	Yes O	No O	NA O	
3. The person demonstrates understanding of the education.	Yes O	No O	NA O	
4. Client/caregiver knows how to clean the orthosis.	Yes O	No O	NA O	
5. The person is able to recognize signs of pressure and impingement.	Yes O	No O	NA O	

Discuss possible orthotic adjustments or changes that you should make based on the self-evaluation. (What would you do differently next time?)

_____

_____

_____

_____

Discuss possible areas to improve with clinical safety when fabricating the orthosis.

_____

_____

_____

_____

Grading Sheet 7.1 Wrist Immobilization Orthosis

	Name:
	Date:

Type of wrist immobilization orthosis:	
Volar ○	Dorsal ○

Wrist position: _____

Grade:

1 = Beyond improvement, not acceptable

2 = Requires maximal improvement

3 = Requires moderate improvement

4 = Requires minimal improvement

5 = Requires no improvement

Evaluation Areas						Comments
Design						
1. The wrist position is at the correct angle.	1	2	3	4	5	
2. The wrist has adequate support.	1	2	3	4	5	
3. The sides of the thenar and hypothenar eminences have support in the correct position.	1	2	3	4	5	
4. The orthosis is one-half the width of the forearm.	1	2	3	4	5	
5. The thenar and hypothenar eminences are not restricted or flattened.	1	2	3	4	5	
6. The orthosis is two-thirds the length of the forearm.	1	2	3	4	5	

Function						
1. The orthosis allows full thumb motion.	1	2	3	4	5	
2. The orthosis allows full metacarpophalangeal (MCP) joint flexion of the fingers.	1	2	3	4	5	
3. The orthosis provides wrist support that allows functional activities.	1	2	3	4	5	
Straps						
1. The straps are secure and rounded.	1	2	3	4	5	
Comfort						
1. The orthosis edges are smooth with rounded corners.	1	2	3	4	5	
2. The proximal end is flared.	1	2	3	4	5	
3. The orthosis does not cause impingements or pressure sores.	1	2	3	4	5	
4. The orthosis does not irritate bony prominences.	1	2	3	4	5	
Cosmetic Appearance						
1. The orthosis is free of fingerprints, dirt, and pencil and pen marks.	1	2	3	4	5	
2. The thermoplastic material is not buckled.	1	2	3	4	5	

Thumb Immobilization Orthoses

Helene L. Lohman

CHAPTER OBJECTIVES

1. Discuss important functional and anatomical considerations for orthotic intervention of the thumb.
2. Explain appropriate thumb and wrist positions for thumb immobilization orthoses.
3. Identify the three components of a thumb immobilization orthosis.
4. Describe the reasons for supporting the joints of the thumb.
5. Discuss the diagnostic indications for a thumb immobilization orthosis.
6. Discuss the process of pattern making and orthotic fabrication for a thumb immobilization orthosis.
7. Describe elements of a proper fit of a thumb immobilization orthosis.
8. Explain general and specific patient safety precautions for a thumb immobilization orthosis.
9. Use clinical reasoning to evaluate fit problems of a thumb immobilization orthosis.
10. Use clinical reasoning to evaluate a fabricated thumb immobilization orthosis.
11. Apply knowledge about thumb immobilization orthotic intervention to a case study.
12. Recognize the importance of evidence-based practice with thumb immobilization orthotic provision.
13. Describe the appropriate use of prefabricated thumb orthoses.

KEY TERMS

de Quervain tenosynovitis
hypertonicity
osteoarthritis (OA)

rheumatoid arthritis (RA)
scaphoid fracture

ulnar collateral ligament (UCL)
injury (skier's thumb or
gamekeeper's thumb)

On a winter vacation, Jill fell while snow skiing down a steep slope. She attempted to brace herself with an outstretched hand and an abducted thumb. Jill's thumb bent backward upon hitting the ground. After being helped down the slope, Jill was seen by a local orthopedic physician who diagnosed her with skier's thumb. The physician referred Jill to a local occupational therapy clinic where she was fitted for a hand-based thumb orthosis. The physician suggested that she follow up with additional physician monitoring and therapy once she returned to her home state.

Frequently prescribed for the thumb is a custom or prefabricated immobilization orthosis. The purpose of a thumb orthosis is to immobilize, protect, rest, and position one or all the thumb carpometacarpal (CMC), metacarpophalangeal (MCP), and interphalangeal (IP) joints while allowing the other digits to be free. A commonly recommended orthosis for the thumb is the thumb palmar abduction immobilization orthosis.[2] Other names for this orthosis are the *thumb spica orthosis,* the *short or long opponens orthosis,* the *CMC-MCP immobilization orthosis,*[71] or the *thumb gauntlet orthosis.*

Thumb immobilization orthoses can be divided into two broad categories: (1) forearm based and (2) hand based. Forearm-based thumb orthoses stabilize the wrist and the thumb. Stabilizing and supporting the thumb and wrist is beneficial for a painful wrist. Hand-based thumb orthoses provide stabilization for the thumb while allowing for wrist mobility. Forearm-based or hand-based thumb immobilization orthoses are often used to manage different conditions that affect the thumb's CMC, MCP, or IP joints.

Thumb conditions that may require a forearm-based orthosis include but are not limited to de Quervain tenosynovitis, rheumatoid arthritis (RA), **osteoarthritis (OA)**, scaphoid fracture, and hypertonicity. For example, for people who have de Quervain tenosynovitis, a forearm-based thumb orthosis provides rest, support, and protection of the tendons that course along the radial side of the wrist into the thumb joints. The therapist may also apply a forearm-based thumb immobilization orthosis postoperatively for control of motion in persons with RA after a joint arthrodesis or replacement. A thumb immobilization orthosis can position the thumb before surgery.[26]

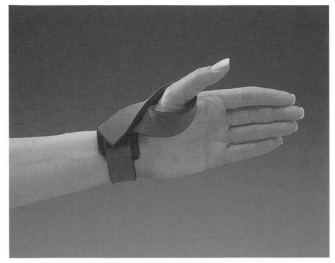

Fig. 8.1 Thumb orthosis for hypertonicity (Rolyan® Thump Loop). (Courtesy Performance Health, Warrenville, IL.)

Thumb conditions that may require a hand-based orthosis include but are not limited to traumatic thumb MCP joint injuries, such as sprains, MCP or IP joint dislocations, median nerve injury, and MCP ligament injuries, including the ulnar collateral ligament (UCL) (known as skier's/gamekeeper's thumb) and the radial collateral ligament (RCL). With the resulting muscle imbalance from a median nerve injury, the therapist may apply a hand-based thumb immobilization orthosis to keep the thumb web space adequately open. For **hypertonicity**, a thumb orthosis—sometimes called a *figure-eight thumb wrap* or *thumb loop orthosis* (Fig. 8.1)—facilitates hand use by decreasing the palm-in-thumb posture or palmar adduction that is often associated with this condition. Therefore, because the thumb orthosis is so commonly prescribed, it is important that therapists become familiar with its application and fabrication.

FUNCTIONAL AND ANATOMICAL CONSIDERATIONS FOR ORTHOTIC INTERVENTION OF THE THUMB

The thumb is essential for hand functions because of its overall importance to grip, pinch, and fine manipulation. The thumb's exceptional mobility results from the unique shape of its saddle joint (the CMC joint), the arrangement of its ligaments, and its intrinsic musculature.[6,15,65] The thumb provides stability for grip, pinch, and mobility because it opposes the fingers for fine manipulations.[68] Sensory input to the tip of the thumb is important for functional grasp and pinch.

A thorough understanding of the anatomy and functional movements of the thumb is necessary before the therapist attempts to fabricate a thumb orthosis. The most crucial aspect of the thumb immobilization orthotic design is the position of the CMC joint.[68] Positioning of the thumb in a thumb post (see Fig. 8.5) allows for palmar abduction and some opposition, which are critical motions for functional prehension. See Chapter 4 for a review of the anatomy and functional movements of the thumb.

FEATURES OF THE THUMB IMMOBILIZATION ORTHOSIS

The thumb immobilization orthosis prevents motion of one, two, or all of the thumb joints.[24] The orthosis has numerous design variations. Designs include volar (Fig. 8.2), dorsal (Fig. 8.3), or radial gutter (Fig. 8.4) depending on the person's condition and purpose of the orthosis. The orthosis may be hand based or wrist based, depending on the person's diagnosis, the anatomical structures involved, and the associated pain at the wrist. If the wrist is included, the wrist position varies according to the diagnosis. For example, with de Quervain tenosynovitis, the wrist is commonly positioned in 15 degrees of extension to take the pressure off the abductor pollicis longus and extensor pollicis brevis tendons.[10]

The orthotic components fabricated in the final product vary according to the thumb joints that are included. The orthotic design is based on the therapeutic goals for the person. The therapist must have a good understanding of the purpose and the fabrication process of the various orthotic components. Central to most thumb immobilization orthoses are three components: (1) the opponens bar, (2) the C bar, and (3) the thumb post (Fig. 8.5).[24] The opponens bar and C bar position the thumb, usually in some degree of palmar abduction. The thumb post, which is an extension of the C bar, immobilizes the MCP only or both the MCP and IP joints.

The position of the thumb in an orthosis varies from palmar abduction to radial abduction, depending on the person's diagnosis. With some conditions, such as arthritis, the therapist facilitates prehension by stabilizing the thumb CMC joint in palmar abduction and opposition. Certain diagnostic protocols, such as those for extensor pollicis longus (EPL) repairs, tendon transfers for thumb extension, and extensor tenolysis of the thumb, require the thumb to be in an extended and radial abducted position.[11] The thumb immobilization orthosis may do one of the following:

- Stabilize only the CMC joint
- Include the CMC and MCP joints
- Encompass all three joints (i.e., CMC, MCP, and IP)

The physician's order may specify which thumb joints to immobilize in the orthosis. In some situations, the therapist may be responsible for determining which joints the orthosis should stabilize. The therapist uses diagnostic protocols, strong knowledge of anatomy, and an assessment of the person's pain to make this decision. Certain diagnostic protocols (such as those for thumb replantations, tendon transfers, and tendon repairs) often require the inclusion of the IP joint in the orthosis.[61] Overall the therapist fabricates an orthosis that is the most supportive and least restrictive in movement.

DIAGNOSTIC INDICATIONS

Therapists fabricate thumb immobilization orthoses in general and specialized hand therapy practices. Specific

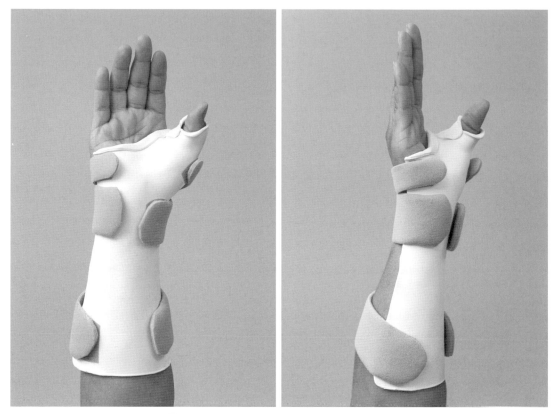

Fig. 8.2 A volar thumb immobilization orthosis.

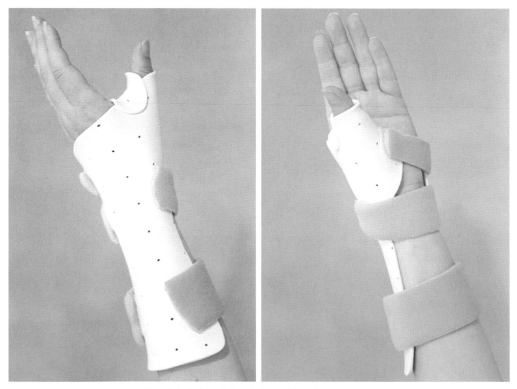

Fig. 8.3 A dorsal thumb immobilization orthosis.

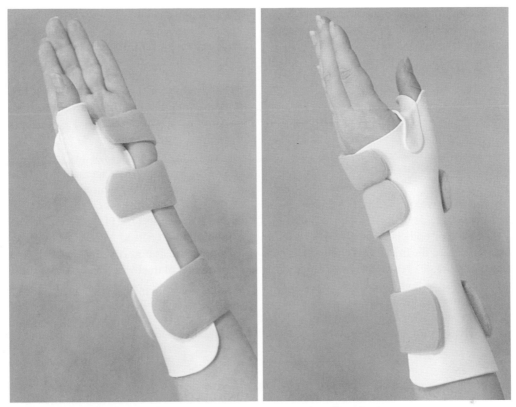

Fig. 8.4 A radial gutter thumb immobilization orthosis.

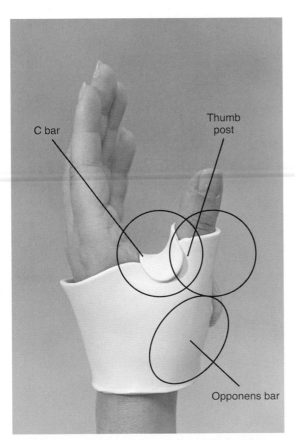

Fig. 8.5 The three components of a thumb immobilization orthosis. The opponens bar in conjunction with a C bar and a thumb post.

diagnostic conditions that require a thumb immobilization orthosis include, but are not limited to:

- Capsular tightness of the MCP and IP joints after trauma[a]
- Congenital adduction deformity of the thumb
- de Quervain tenosynovitis
- Distal radius fractures[a]
- EPL repairs[a]
- Extrinsic flexor or extensor muscle contracture[a]
- Flexor pollicis longus (FPL) repair[a]
- Hypertonicity
- Median nerve injuries
- MCP joint dislocations
- OA
- Posttraumatic adduction contracture[a]
- RA
- RCL or UCL strains
- Repair of MCP joint collateral ligaments[a]
- Scaphoid fractures[a]
- Stable fractures of the proximal phalanx of the first metacarpal[a]
- Tendon transfers[a]

Intervention for many of these conditions may require the expertise of experienced hand therapists. In clinical practice, therapists commonly treat persons who have de Quervain tenosynovitis, RA, OA, fractures, and ligament injuries. The

[a]Condition may require consultation with an experienced hand therapist.

orthoses for these conditions will be specifically discussed in this chapter. (Table 8.1 contains guidelines for these hand conditions.) The novice therapist should remember that physicians and experienced therapists may have their own guidelines for positioning and orthotic-wearing schedules. The therapist should also be aware that thumb palmar abduction may be uncomfortable for some persons. Therefore, the thumb may be positioned midway between radial and palmar abduction.

Orthotic Intervention for de Quervain Tenosynovitis

De Quervain tenosynovitis, which results from repetitive thumb motions and wrist ulnar deviation, is a form of tenosynovitis affecting the abductor pollicis longus (APL) and the extensor pollicis brevis (EPB) in the first dorsal compartment. People whose occupations involve repetitive wrist deviation and thumb motions (such as the home construction tasks of painting, scraping, wall papering, and hammering) are prone to this condition.[31] Any repetitive life activity that aggravates the wrist and thumb, such as typing on a computer, may lead

to this condition. De Quervain tenosynovitis is the most commonly diagnosed wrist tendonitis in athletes,[51] such as golfers.[39] People present with pain over the radial styloid, edema in the first dorsal compartment, and positive results from the Finkelstein test (Fig. 8.6). The Finkelstein test (also called the Eichhoff test) involves instructing the individual to clench the thumb in a fist and passively deviating the wrist in the ulnar direction,[4] with a positive test resulting in pain during the motion (see Fig. 8.6).

During the acute phase of de Quervain tenosynovitis, conservative therapeutic management involves immobilization of the thumb and wrist for symptom control[32] to rest the involved tendons.[32] This orthosis is classified by the American Society of Hand Therapists (ASHT) as a wrist extension, thumb CMC palmar abduction, and MCP flexion immobilization orthosis.[3] The orthosis may cover the volar or dorsal forearm or the radial aspect of the forearm and hand. The therapist positions the wrist in 15 degrees of extension, neutral wrist deviation, the thumb midway between palmar and radial abduction (40 to 45 degrees), and the thumb MCP joint in neutral.[10,20] Usually the IP joint is free for functional activities; however,

TABLE 8.1	Conditions That May Require a Thumb Immobilization Orthosis	
Hand Condition	**Type of Orthosis, Position**	**Wearing Schedule**
Soft Tissue Inflammation		
de Quervain tenosynovitis	During an acute flare-up the therapist provides a thumb immobilization orthosis (wrist extension, thumb CMC palmar abduction immobilization orthosis[3]). Orthosis can be long forearm-based or a radial gutter orthosis; the wrist is in 15 degrees of extension, the thumb CMC joint is palmarly abducted 40 to 45 degrees or midway between radial and palmar abduction, depending on person's tolerance, and the thumb MCP is positioned in neutral. Other positioning options are discussed in the chapter.	This person wears the orthosis during the night and as needed in the day to avoid pain and to rest the tendons. The orthosis is removed for pain-free occupations during the day to help remodel and nourish collagen formation.
Arthritis		
Rheumatoid arthritis: periods of pain and inflammation in the thumb joints	The therapist provides a forearm-based thumb immobilization orthosis (wrist extension, thumb CMC palmar abduction, and MCP flexion immobilization orthosis). The wrist is in 20 to 30 degrees of extension; the thumb CMC joint is either palmarly abducted 45 degrees or midway between radial and palmar abduction, depending on person's tolerance; and the MCP joint (if included) is in 5 degrees of flexion. Other specific orthoses for arthritic deformities are discussed in the chapter.	The person wears the orthosis continuously during periods of pain and inflammation with removal for exercise and hygiene. The therapist adjusts the wearing schedule according to the person's pain and inflammation levels.
Osteoarthritis		
CMC joint of the thumb	Orthotic approaches are individualized because there is no one recommended approach. Options include a hand-based thumb immobilization orthosis with the MCP joint immobilized or free, depending on the protocol. The thumb CMC joint is palmarly abducted to a position that the person can tolerate. Or, a hand-based orthosis that frees the thumb MCP joint for motion and stabilizes the first CMC joint in extension. A forearm-based orthosis can be provided for nighttime wear with scaphotrapezial joint involvement, or if the person requires more support.[16]	The person wears the orthosis continuously during an acute flare-up with removal for ROM and hygiene. Once pain has decreased, the orthosis can be selectively worn during activities to help position and stabilize the thumb.

TABLE 8.1 Conditions That May Require a Thumb Immobilization Orthosis—cont'd

Hand Condition	Type of Orthosis, Position	Wearing Schedule
Traumatic Injuries of the Thumb		
Skier's/Gamekeeper's thumb (UCL injury)	The therapist provides a hand-based thumb orthosis (MCP radial and ulnar deviation restriction orthosis).[3] The MCP joint is immobilized, the thumb CMC joint is palmarly abducted 40 degrees, and the MCP joint is in neutral. The thumb post for the hand-based orthosis can position the MCP joint in slight ulnar deviation to take the stress off the UCL. (It is important to position the thumb CMC joint in a position of comfort, which may not be exactly in the suggested degrees.)	• Grade I—The person wears the orthosis continuously for 3 to 4 weeks with removal for hygiene. • Grade II—The person wears the orthosis continuously for 4 to 5 weeks except for removal for hygiene. • Grade III—After immobilization in a cast the person is provided with the thumb immobilization orthosis and follows the same protocol described previously for grade I.
Golfer's thumb (RCL injury)	The therapist provides a hand-based thumb orthosis (MCP radial and ulnar deviation restriction orthosis).[3] The MCP joint is immobilized in palmar abduction, and the MCP joint is in neutral. Care is made to avoid ulnar stress at the MCP joint.	The wearing schedule is the same as for UCL injury, but follow physician preference.
Scaphoid fracture (stable and nondisplaced)	There are many variations of orthotics. One option is that the therapist provides a forearm volar or a dorsal/volar thumb immobilization orthosis (thumb CMC palmar abduction and MCP in 0 to 10 degrees flexion and the wrist in neutral).	The wearing schedule varies widely depending on the time after injury, the bone status, the physician preference, and the location of the fracture on the scaphoid. If the person has undergone a long course of casting and the physician is worried about bony union (this is often the case), initially the orthosis will be prescribed for continuous wear with removal for hygiene and to check the skin.
Hypertonicity	The therapist provides a thumb loop orthosis or a figure-eight thumb wrap orthosis, which can be customized out of thermoplastic or soft material. A prefabricated orthosis can also be used. With a prefabricated orthosis, a Neoprene strip is wrapped around the thumb web space and the hand to provide radial or palmar abduction while pulling the wrist into extension and radial deviation. Purchased thumb loops are available in sizes to fit premature infants to adults.	The wearing schedule varies according to the person's therapeutic needs. The orthosis should be removed and the skin should be carefully monitored at periodic intervals.

CMC, Carpometacarpal; *MCP*, metacarpophalangeal; *RCL*, radial collateral ligament; *ROM*, range of motion; *UCL*, ulnar collateral ligament.

the IP joint is included in the orthosis if the person is overusing the thumb or fights the orthosis, causing even more pain. Other recommendations exist for positioning. For example, Ilyas and colleagues[32] recommend conservative intervention by positioning the thumb in 30 degrees of abduction and 30 degrees of MCP flexion. Ultimately the position chosen for the thumb is the one that best relieves the person's symptoms.

Radial gutter or forearm-based thumb orthoses are worn during the night and as needed in the day during function to avoid pain and rest the tendons. The orthosis is removed for occupations that are pain-free during the day to help remodel and nourish collagen formation.[20] A prefabricated orthosis is recommended after the person's pain subsides[36,72] for work and sports activities,[2] or if the person does not want to wear a custom orthosis.[7] The study by Menendez and colleagues (N = 85) compared full-time wear of a thumb orthosis for de Quervain tenosynovitis to as-needed wear.[43] The investigators

found that there were no statistically significant differences in patient-reported outcomes with measures for disability, grip strength, pain, and treatment satisfaction between the group that wore the orthosis full time as compared to the group that wore the orthosis as needed. The investigators found that psychological factors such as depression and anxiety correlated with disability scores on the Disabilities of the Arm, Shoulder and Hand (DASH) questionnaire.

Most intervention for de Quervain tenosynovitis is done conservatively. However, if symptoms are not resolved, then surgery may be indicated. Postsurgical management of de Quervain tenosynovitis involves orthotic intervention, usually for 7 to 10 days.[51]

Research Evidence for de Quervain Tenosynovitis

Few studies have considered the efficacy of thumb orthotic intervention for de Quervain tenosynovitis, and results are

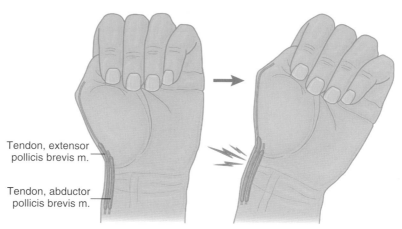

Fig. 8.6 The Finkelstein test is used to assess the presence of de Quervain tenosynovitis. (From Waldman SD. *Atlas of pain management injection techniques.* Philadelphia: Saunders; 2000.)

Tendon, extensor pollicis brevis m.

Tendon, abductor pollicis brevis m.

variable (Table 8.2). Most studies consider medical intervention approaches, such as nonsteroidal antiinflammatory drugs (NSAIDs) or corticosteroid injections, compared with conservative measures, such as orthoses. Two articles discuss systematic reviews of medical treatment options as compared to hand therapy. Cavaleri and colleagues[12] completed a systematic review with meta-analyses of six studies to compare corticosteroid injections with hand therapy. They considered orthoses and corticosteroid injections along with other approaches (e.g., acupuncture and general hand therapy). The investigators found that hand therapy and corticosteroid injections improved pain and function, but the combined intervention of orthoses and corticosteroid injections was most effective.

Richie and Briner[53] reviewed the literature to evaluate the evidence of treatment options for de Quervain tenosynovitis. They considered seven descriptive studies (N = 459 wrists) comparing effective treatments without control groups. They found the highest success rate for intervention of 83% for injection alone, followed by 61% for injection and orthotic intervention together, 14% for orthotic intervention alone, and 9% for rest or NSAIDs.[53] The authors concluded that the combination of injection and orthotic intervention resulted in a higher percentage of treatment failure (39%) compared with treatment failure of solely providing injections (17%). These authors did not discuss the limitations of the reviewed studies.

A recent quasi-experimental study completed by Nemati and colleagues[46] considered a new modified mobilization type of orthosis for de Quervain tenosynovitis. The investigators compared two types of orthotic intervention with two groups of subjects (N = 24). One group wore a modified forearm-based thumb orthosis that allowed for dynamic wrist flexion and extension with a hinge component—thus blocking wrist deviation. The other group wore a traditional static forearm-based orthosis. The investigators developed the modified dynamic orthosis to allow for wrist flexion and extension as muscles for those motions are not involved with wrist radial and ulnar deviation, which would aggravate de

Quervain tenosynovitis. After evaluation for pinch strength, pain, and function, the investigators found that both orthoses were equal. The investigators did, however, find that the study participants were more satisfied with the orthosis that allowed for wrist flexion and extension, as it was more comfortable (Fig. 8.7). More research needs to be completed to determine the efficacy of thumb orthotic intervention with de Quervain tenosynovitis. Therapists should review these studies as they can provide information about intervention efficacy.

Orthotic Intervention for Rheumatoid Arthritis

Rheumatoid arthritis (RA) is an autoimmune disease that often affects the joints symmetrically through recurring synovitis and tenosynovitis. The disease frequently presents in the thumb joints, particularly the MCP and CMC joints. Orthotic intervention for RA can reduce pain, slow deformity, and stabilize the thumb joints.[49] One perspective with orthotic intervention is to consider three stages of the disease. In each stage a different therapeutic goal is addressed even though the therapist may apply the same thumb immobilization orthosis.

The first stage involves an inflammatory process. The goal of orthotic intervention at this stage is to rest the joints and reduce inflammation. The person wears the thumb immobilization orthosis continuously during periods of inflammation and periodically thereafter for pain control as necessary. When the disease progresses in the second stage, the hand requires mechanical support because the joints are less stable and are painful with use. The person wears a thumb immobilization orthosis for support while engaging in daily activities and perhaps at night for pain relief. In the third stage, pain is usually not a factor, but the joints may be grossly deformed and unstable. In lieu of surgical stabilization a thumb immobilization orthosis may provide support to increase function during certain activities. At this stage, orthotic intervention is rarely helpful for the person at night, unless to help manage pain.[17] Another intervention approach is to provide the person who has arthritis with a rigid orthosis and a soft orthosis along with education for the benefits and activity uses of each type.[56]

TABLE 8.2 Evidence-Based Practice About Thumb Orthotic Intervention

Author's Citation	Design	Number of Participants	Description	Results	LIMITATIONS
Carpometacarpal Arthritis					
Aebischer, B., Elsig, S., & Taeymans, J. (2016). Effectiveness of physical and occupational therapy on pain, function and quality of life in patients with trapeziometacarpal osteoarthritis—a systematic review and meta-analysis. *Hand Therapy,* 21(1), 5–15.	Systematic review and meta-analysis	Researchers reviewed studies to determine the effectiveness of various occupational and physical therapy interventions with TMC OA. Sources of data included MEDLINE, CINAHL, OTseeker, Embase, PEDro, Cochrane Database of Systematic Reviews, CENTRAL	Two reviewers selected articles for review based on specific inclusion criteria: • RCT, quasi-randomized controlled trials, systematic reviews, case-control, observational, and pragmatic studies • Written in English, German, French, and Dutch • Studies that included adults with formal diagnosis of primary TMC OA • Interventions labeled as physical therapy, physiotherapy, or occupational therapy Twenty-two articles with 1179 total patients were included in this analysis.	Researchers were interested in the outcome measurements of pain, function, and quality of life. In this review, researchers compared 42 interventions. Participants in these studies experienced a reduction in pain with all but one intervention. Regardless of the type of splint, participants experienced positive pain results. Participants improved on functional outcome measures except for three studies that included the interventions of custom-made thermoplastic splint, joint protection, and custom-made thermoplastic long splint. Interventions that included exercises with and without splints had improved outcomes. In the meta-analysis, researchers found no differences between a prefabricated and a custom-made thermoplastic splint. None of the studies measured the outcome of quality of life. Overall, there is moderate to high-quality evidence for a positive effect of physical and occupational therapy interventions for pain with individuals with TMC OA. However, there is no statistical support for these interventions for improved function.	Each study included in this review had at least one high risk or unclear risk of bias. Eleven of the 27 research studies demonstrated a high risk in 2 or more of the 7 criteria. The studies included in this review demonstrated significant differences in design and outcome measures, making pooling of data difficult. Researchers reported that in some of the included studies, data were missing or contradictory to the studies' conclusions. Lastly, researchers used a subjective method to determine inclusion articles for the meta-analysis.

RCT, Randomized controlled trial; *TMC OA,* trapeziometacarpal osteoarthritis.
Contributed by Whitney Henderson.

Two common thumb deformities resulting from the arthritic process are boutonnière deformity (type I, MCP joint flexion and IP joint extension) and swan neck deformity (type 3, MCP extension or hyperextension and IP flexion).[15,45] Boutonnière deformity is believed to be the most common type of thumb deformity and is identified by MCP joint flexion and IP joint in hyperextension.[5] During the beginning stages of boutonnière deformity a circumferential Neoprene orthosis may be provided to support the MCP joint with the IP joint free to move.[15]

A swan neck deformity is identified by flexion of the IP joint and hyperextension of the MCP joint of the thumb. For early stages of swan neck deformity, a small custom-fitted dorsal thermoplastic orthosis over the MCP joint prevents MCP hyperextension.[15] Later dorsal and radial subluxation at the CMC joint causes CMC joint adduction, MCP hyperextension,

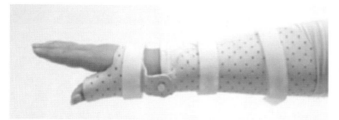

Fig. 8.7 This orthosis for de Quervain tenosynovitis allows for wrist flexion and extension, which increases client comfort, while still protecting the aggravated tendons. (From Nemati, Z., Javanshir, M, A., Saeedi, H., et al. [2017]. The effect of a new dynamic splint in pinch strength in de Quervain syndrome: a comparative study. *Disability and Rehabilitation: Assistive Technology, 12*[5], 457–461.)

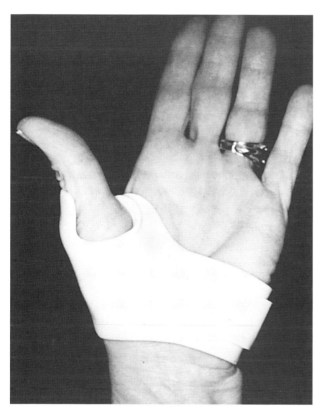

Fig. 8.8 This orthosis, which blocks metacarpophalangeal (MCP) hyperextension, is applied for advanced swan neck deformity. (From Colditz, J. C. [2002]. Anatomic considerations for splinting the thumb. In E. J. Mackin, A. D. Callahan, T. M. Skirven, et al. [Eds.], *Rehabilitation of the hand and upper extremity* [5th ed., pp. 1858–1874]. St. Louis: Mosby.)

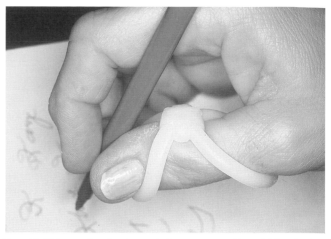

Fig. 8.9 This small orthosis can help a person with arthritis who has lateral instability of the thumb interphalangeal (IP) joint. (From Colditz, J. C. [2002]. Anatomic considerations for splinting the thumb. In E. J. Mackin, A. D. Callahan, T. M. Skirven, et al. [Eds.], *Rehabilitation of the hand and upper extremity* [5th ed., pp. 1858–1874]. St. Louis: Mosby.)

is classified by ASHT as a wrist extension, thumb CMC palmar abduction, and MCP extension immobilization orthosis.[3] Resting the hand in this position is extremely beneficial during periods of inflammation or if the thumb is unstable at the CMC joint.[38] Incorporating the wrist in a forearm-based thumb orthosis is appropriate when the client's wrist is painful or in the presence of wrist arthritic involvement.

When fabricating an orthosis on a person who has RA, be aware that the person may have fragile skin. Monitor all areas for potential skin breakdown, including the ulnar head, Lister tubercle, the radial styloid along the radial border, the CMC joint of the thumb, and the scaphoid and pisiform bones on the volar surface of the wrist.[21] Padding the orthosis for comfort to prevent skin irritation may be necessary.

The selected orthotic material should be easily adjustable to accommodate changes in swelling and repositioning as the disease progresses. Asking persons about their swelling patterns is important because orthoses fabricated during the day must allow enough room for nocturnal swelling. Thermoplastic material less than ⅛-inch thick is best for small hand orthoses. Orthoses fabricated from heavier thermoplastic material have the potential to irritate other joints.[41] Therapists should carefully evaluate all hand orthoses for potential stress on other joints and instruct persons to wear the orthoses at night, periodically during the day, and during stressful daily activities. However, therapists should always tailor any orthotic-wearing regimen to each person's therapeutic needs.

Orthoses for Carpomctacarpal Osteoarthritis

CMC joint arthritis can occur with OA or RA. CMC joint arthritis from OA is a common thumb condition, affecting 20% of men and women over age 40.[41,58,72] Pain from **OA** occurs at the base of the thumb or the saddle-shaped CMC joint—these joints facilitate thumb opposition. Pain at the CMC joint interferes with the person's ability to engage in normal functional activities because the CMC joint is the most critical joint of the thumb for function.[13,47] Precipitating

and IP flexion.[15] For this deformity Colditz[15] suggests fabricating a hand-based thumb immobilization orthosis that blocks MCP hyperextension (Fig. 8.8). With RA, laxity of the UCL at the IP and MCP joint can develop. Fig. 8.9 shows a functional orthosis, which can be used with RA or OA for lateral instability of the thumb IP joint. Prefabricated options are also available for both boutonnière and swan neck deformities.

One approach to orthotic intervention for a hand with arthritis is to immobilize the thumb in a forearm-based, thumb immobilization orthosis with the wrist in 20 to 30 degrees of extension, the CMC joint in 45 degrees of palmar abduction (if tolerated), and the MCP joint in neutral.[61] This orthosis factors include hypermobility, anatomical predisposition, repetitive grasping, pinching, use of vibratory tools, being postmenopausal, and having a family history of the condition.[41,49,58]

CMC arthritis occurs with the trapeziometacarpal joint (basal joint) and sometimes the scaphotrapezial joint. Both joints contribute to the mobility of the thumb.[49] Over time the dorsal aspect of the CMC joint is stressed by repetitive pinching and the strong muscle pull of the adductor pollicis and the short intrinsic thumb muscles. All together, these forces may cause the first CMC joint to sublux dorsally and radially. This subluxation typically results in the first metacarpal losing extension and becoming adducted. The MCP joint hyperextends to accommodate grasp.[17,41,56]

Orthoses are common interventions for conservative management of CMC arthritis to improve function[64] and are recommended by the American College of Rheumatology.[30] Orthoses help people with CMC arthritis manage pain, preserve their first web space, protect their joints, and provide stability for the intrinsic weakness of the capsular structures.[23] During the early stages of CMC arthritis, orthoses position the hand to prevent the thumb adduction deformity of the metacarpal head and the "dorsoradial subluxation of the metacarpal base on the trapezium."[49] Orthoses stabilize the thumb so that people can perform occupations.[49] Static orthoses are recommended for hypermobile or unstable joints, but not for fixed joints.[47]

Many orthotic options exist for people who have CMC OA. Orthotic options range from forearm orthoses (volar, radial gutter, or dorsal with the CMC and MCP joints included) to hand-based orthoses (with the CMC and MCP joints included, or only the CMC joint included). From a survey study of therapy practice with CMC arthritis, investigators found that therapists reported the most common application for CMC OA of hand-based orthoses followed by forearm orthoses.[48] Many custom-design options exist. One custom-fabricated orthotic option for CMC OA designed by Colditz[15] is a hand-based orthosis that allows for free motion of the thumb MCP joint and stabilizes the CMC joint to manage pain (Fig. 8.10). The wrist is not included in the orthotic design to allow for functional wrist motions (Fig. 8.11). Therapists should fabricate this hand-based orthosis solely for hands that have "a healthy MCP joint" because the MCP joint may sustain additional flexion pressure due to the controlled flexion position of the CMC joint.[42] Therapists must be attentive to wear on the MCP joint.[47] Colditz suggests an initial full-time wear of 2 to 3 weeks with removal for hygiene. Afterward the orthosis should be worn during painful functional activities.[16] Another option designed by Cantero-Tellez et al.[11a] offers support of the CMC and MCP thumb joints with a minimum amount of thermoplastic material on the dorsal surface. This design can be used for other diagnoses, such as thumb ligament injuries (Fig. 8.12). Melvin[41] suggests fabricating a dorsal hand-based thumb immobilization orthosis (thumb CMC palmar abduction immobilization orthosis [Fig. 8.13]),[2] with the primary therapeutic goal of restricting the mobility of the thumb

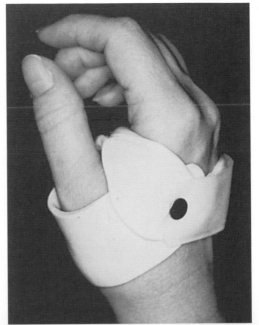

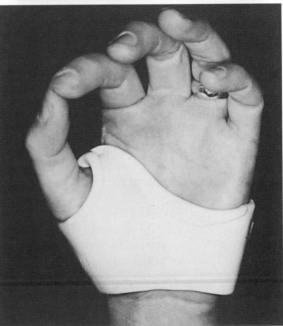

Fig. 8.10 An orthosis for rheumatoid arthritis (RA) or osteoarthritis that stabilizes only the carpometacarpal (CMC) joint. (From Colditz, J. C. [2002]. Anatomic considerations for splinting the thumb. In E. J. Mackin, A. D. Callahan, T. M. Skirven, et al. [Eds.], *Rehabilitation of the hand and upper extremity* [5th ed., pp. 1858–1874]. St. Louis: Mosby.)

joints to decrease pain and inflammation. The dorsal orthosis stabilizes the CMC and MCP joints in the maximal amount of palmar abduction that is comfortable for the person and allows for a functional pinch. Orthotic intervention of both joints in a thumb post stabilizes the CMC joint in abduction so that the base of the MCP is stabilized. With the orthosis on, the person should continue to perform complete functional tasks, such as writing, comfortably. This thumb immobilization orthosis may be fabricated from thin 1/16-inch or 3/32-inch) conforming thermoplastic material for a person with thin skin.

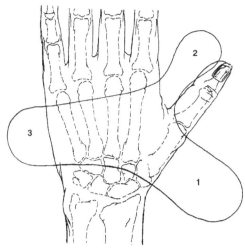

Fig. 8.11 A pattern for a thumb carpometacarpal (CMC) immobilization orthosis. (From Colditz, J. C. [2000]. The biomechanics of a thumb carpometacarpal immobilization splint: Design and fitting. *Journal of Hand Therapy, 13*[3], 228–235.)

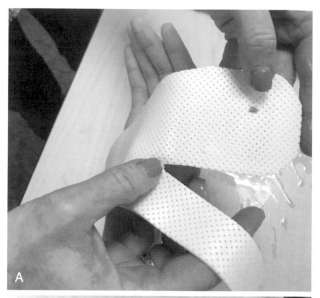

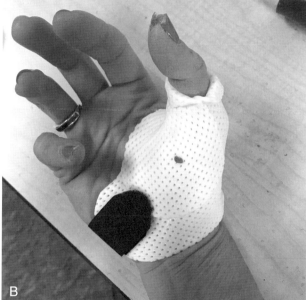

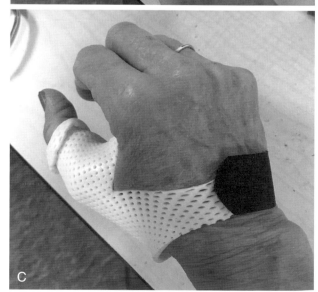

Fig. 8.12 This orthosis for carpometacarpal (CMC) arthritis supports the CMC and metacarpophalangeal (MCP) thumb joints with minimum thermoplastic material on the dorsal surface. (A-C Courtesy Debby Schwartz, OTD, OTR/L, CHT.)

Another consideration with any selected design for CMC arthritis is that the thumb is generally positioned in palmar abduction.[47] Based on cadaver research, people with a hypermobile MCP joint who are positioned with the thumb in 30 degrees of MCP flexion may experience reduced pressure on the palmar part of the trapeziometacarpal joint, an area prone to deterioration.[44] Poole and Pellegrini[50] recommend that the thumb be positioned in palmar abduction and 30 degrees MCP flexion. They postulate that the 30 degrees of flexion benefits the position of the trapeziometacarpal joint, allowing increased mobility for people in the earlier stages of the disease (stages I and II).

Because so many options exist for orthoses for CMC arthritis, therapists consider research evidence with design selection. Findings from systematic reviews of research evidence show that no one orthotic approach was better than another.[1,23] However, a finding from a scoping review of 14 publications was that, although the effectiveness of different orthoses still needs to be studied further, some evidence supports the use of a short hand-based design for pain reduction and improvement of function.[62] Furthermore, findings from another systematic review were that custom and prefabricated orthoses equally reduced pain. The investigators suggest that orthotic choice may depend on needs, such as a thermoplastic orthosis for harder work and a soft orthosis for activities of daily living (ADLs) and sleep.[1] Overall these reviews provide evidence that application of orthoses for CMC arthritis decreases pain and improves function.[23,33,35,62,63]

Prefabricated orthoses are also a consideration for CMC OA. However, some prefabricated orthoses should be used with caution, because positioning the thumb in abduction within the orthosis can increase MCP joint extension, which can worsen a possible deformity.[7] With a study of current therapy practice, the most frequently applied prefabricated orthoses for CMC OA were hand-based followed by forearm-based and thumb-based soft goods orthoses.[49] In a comparison study of a prefabricated thumb orthosis and a hybrid thumb

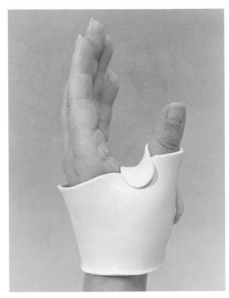

Fig. 8.13 A dorsal hand-based thumb immobilization orthosis (thumb carpometacarpal [CMC] palmar abduction immobilization orthosis).

orthosis made from thermoplastic and Neoprene material, the hybrid orthosis reduced pain to a statistically significant degree.[58] In another study considering custom as compared to prefabricated thumb orthoses, both types of orthoses were found to improve function and grip strength. The custom orthosis decreased pain more.[5] Hamann and colleagues[29] (N = 18 subjects with stage II and III CMC[22]) are the first researchers to consider the stabilization efficiency and function of prefabricated orthoses for CMC OA. Specifically, they studied four orthoses: BSN medical, Push Metagrip (PUSH) orthosis, Sporlastic orthosis (SPOR), and the Medi (MEDI) orthosis. The investigators found that the MEDI and the BSN orthoses provided the greatest amount of stabilization and motion restriction of the MCP joint. The PUSH provided the least amount of stabilization of the MCP joint. These findings may be based on the design of the orthoses studied as the MEDI and BSN included the MCP joint and the PUSH included solely the CMC joint. The SPOR, however, included both the CMC and MCP joints and had higher range of motion (ROM) and less stability in both joints. The PUSH orthosis stabilized only the CMC joint and allowed for the most functional movement that involved grasp/pinch. The MEDI orthosis stabilized the MCP and CMC joints and allowed for the least functional movements. Clients have different needs for stability and functionality. Applying results from such research can assist with clinical decision making. Grenier and colleagues completed a retrospective study (N = 48) of three orthoses considering functional pinch strength.[28] One of the three orthoses studied was the prefabricated Neoprene Comfort Cool orthosis. The other two thumb orthoses were the custom forearm radially based thumb spica orthosis immobilizing the CMC and MCP joints (similar to Fig. 8.4) and the Colditz design immobilizing the CMC joint (shown in Fig. 8.10). The research findings reported only the Colditz and Comfort Cool orthoses outcomes, as sample size was too small for the forearm thumb spica orthosis. The investigators found that wearing the custom Colditz design and the prefabricated Comfort Cool design resulted in an improvement in pinch strength with no statistical difference between the two orthoses. The investigators suggest that larger-scale research is needed to study the effectiveness of orthoses for CMC arthritis in relationship to their impact on function. However, therapists might consider findings from this study when choosing between fabricating a custom orthosis or providing a reasonably priced prefabricated orthosis.

Given the variety of orthotic options available, therapists must critically analyze which orthosis to provide (forearm based, hand based, dorsal or volar) and which thumb joints to immobilize (CMC or CMC and MCP). Critical thinking considerations include presence of pain, need for stability, work, and functional demands. Therapists consider findings from research of various designs. Ultimately orthotic provision must to be appropriate for the client's needs.[1,23,67] A client-centered approach may be most appropriate. Shankland and colleagues[57] (N = 60) studied application of a client-centered approach for intervention with people who presented with thumb CMC OA. Based on the provision of the Canadian Occupational Performance Measure (COPM), the investigators focused intervention on the participants' self-identified needs. The investigators found that a client-centered approach addressing pain with orthotic provision and other approaches along with meaningful activities resulted in improvement in all study measures (COPM, DASH questionnaire, total active range of motion [TAROM], lateral pinch strength, and the visual analog scale for pain). It is important to note that the study did not use a control group.

Finally, therapists might consider the type of orthosis for CMC OA provided based on nighttime or day wear. With a study protocol examining the impact of occupational therapy intervention with CMC OA, Kjeken and colleagues[34] selected the prefabricated Push Brace orthosis for daytime usage as it allows for good mobility and a custom-made thermoplastic hand-based orthosis to help support the thumb joints to avert subluxation and adduction for nighttime usage.

Orthoses for Carpometacarpal Joint Rheumatoid Arthritis

Some persons with RA who present with CMC joint involvement benefit from a hand-based thumb immobilization orthosis (thumb CMC palmar abduction immobilization orthosis),[2] as shown in Fig. 8.13.[16,41] If tolerated, position the thumb in enough palmar abduction for functional activities. With a hand-based thumb immobilization orthosis, if the IP joint is painful and inflamed, incorporate the IP joint into the orthosis. However, putting any material (especially plastic) over the thumb pad virtually eliminates thumb and hand function. The person wears this orthosis constantly for a minimum of 2 to 3 weeks with removal for hygiene and exercise. The wearing schedule is adjusted according to the person's pain and inflammation levels. Researchers found that for people who have RA and CMC arthritis an orthosis did not improve grip strength and that they required higher muscle loads with or without an orthosis to equalize the same muscle strength of healthy adults.[14] Therefore therapists need to consider carefully the purpose of a CMC orthosis when providing it to someone with RA.

On the other hand, some therapists stabilize the thumb CMC joint alone with a short hand-based orthosis that is properly molded and positioned (see Figs. 8.10 and 8.11). This orthosis works effectively on people who have CMC joint subluxation resulting in adduction of the first MCP joint and anyone with CMC arthritis who can tolerate wearing a rigid orthosis. This orthosis can also be used for CMC OA.[15,16]

Often when a physician refers a person who has RA for orthotic intervention, deformities have already developed. If the therapist attempts to place the person's joints in the ideal position of 40 to 45 degrees of palmar abduction, excessive stress on the joints may result. The therapist should always fabricate an orthosis for a hand affected by arthritis in a position of comfort.[16]

Orthoses for Ulnar Collateral Ligament Injury

A common thumb condition resulting in injury to the **ulnar collateral ligament (UCL)** at the MCP joint of the thumb is known as **skier's thumb** (acute injury) or **gamekeeper's thumb** (chronic injury).[20,29] *Gamekeeper's thumb* was the original name of the injury because gamekeepers stressed this joint when they killed birds by twisting their necks.[15]

The UCL helps stabilize the thumb by resisting radial stresses across the MCP joint.[69] The UCL can be injured if the thumb is forcibly abducted or hyperextended. This can occur when falling with an outstretched hand and abducted thumb, such as during skiing.[69] It can also occur during incidences in basketball, gymnastics, rugby, volleyball, hockey, and football.[24]

Treatment protocols depend on the extent of ligamental tear. There are protocols that involve immediate postoperative motion, and thus duration of casting and orthotic fabrication postoperatively varies widely. Injuries are classified by the physician as grade I, II, or III.[70] The following is one of many suggested orthotic intervention protocols for each grade of injury. This orthotic intervention protocol is accompanied by hand therapy.[70]

Grade I injuries, or those involving microscopic tears with no loss of ligament integrity, are positioned in a hand-based thumb immobilization orthosis with the CMC joint of the thumb in approximately 40 degrees of palmar abduction (or in the most comfortable amount of palmar abduction).[10] Some therapists position the thumb post for the hand-based orthosis so that the MCP joint is in slight ulnar deviation to take the stress off the UCL.[20] This orthosis is also called a *thumb MCP radial and ulnar deviation restriction orthosis.*[2] The purpose of this orthosis is to provide rest and protection during the healing phase. The person wears the orthosis continuously for 2 to 3 weeks with removal for hygiene purposes.

Grade II injuries involve a partial ligament tear, but the overall integrity of the ligament remains intact. The orthotic intervention protocol is the same as for grade I injuries, except that the thumb immobilization orthosis is worn for a longer time period (up to 4 or 5 weeks).

Grade III injuries involve a completely torn ligament and usually require surgery. A Stener lesion can occur in a high percentage of grade III UCL injuries when the end of the UCL is caught under the adductor policis muscle and is surgically repaired.[37] After the injury is casted, the cast is replaced by a thumb immobilization orthosis with the same protocol as described for grade I injuries. Typically, after surgery for a ruptured UCL (grade III) the person is immobilized in cast or a custom hand-based thumb orthosis. Rocchi and colleagues[55] developed and studied (N = 30) a modified hand-based orthosis that protects the UCL but allows for early controlled MCP joint flexion and extension motions. This orthosis has an open section on the palmar and dorsal sides of the MCP joint along with double thermoplastic reinforcement on the radial and ulnar sides of the MCP joint. The investigators divided the study participants into two groups with the control group wearing the standard hand-based thumb orthosis and the study group wearing the modified hand-based orthosis. Participants in the control group performed IP motions post surgery. Participants in the study group performed IP and MCP exercises post surgery frequently throughout the day. Although both groups demonstrated decreased pain post surgery, the group with the modified hand-based orthosis reported less pain on a visual analog scale at 2 and 6 months postoperatively. However, at 12 months postoperatively pain scores were equal between groups. Those participants wearing the modified orthosis had better functional scores, higher MCP ROM, fewer therapy sessions, and less lost time from work. Both the control group and the study group had equal MCP joint stability and pinch strength. The authors postulated that the application of the modified hand-based orthosis along with early controlled motions helps to restore function more quickly and therapists might explore its use in practice.

A unique "hybrid" orthosis was designed for athletes with a UCL injury who require orthotic intervention for protection during sports activities.[25] This orthotic design is a custom-made circumferential thermoplastic orthosis molded around the MCP joint and is held in place by a fabricated Neoprene wrap. The advantage of this orthotic design is that it provides MCP stability with the thermoplastic insert and allows for movement of other joints because of the Neoprene stretch. In addition, this orthosis helps control pain and allows for activities involving grip and pinch (Fig. 8.14). Therapists could either fabricate both parts of this orthosis or fabricate the circumferential orthosis and purchase a prefabricated Neoprene thumb wrap. For those who return to skiing soon after a UCL injury, researchers suggest fabricating a small thermoplastic orthosis held in place with tape inside a ski glove.[2] Finally, as with any therapeutic intervention, success is dependent on many factors (such as carefully following therapeutic protocols and good surgery techniques).

An RCL injury (or "golfer's thumb") is an injury that occurs less commonly than UCL injury[9] and requires a hand-based thumb immobilization orthosis. The orthosis is almost the same as for a UCL injury in a hand-based orthosis with a conforming thumb positioned in palmar abduction

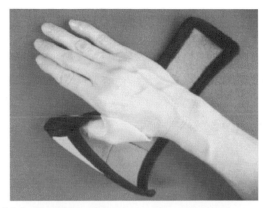

Fig. 8.14 A protective orthosis for an ulnar collateral ligament (UCL) injury that combines a custom-made circumferential thermoplastic orthosis molded around the metacarpophalangeal (MCP) joint, which is held in place by a fabricated Neoprene wrap. (From Ford, M., McKee, P., & Szilagyi, M. [2004]. A hybrid thermoplastic and Neoprene thumb metacarpophalangeal joint orthosis. *Journal of Hand Therapy, 17*[1], 64–68.)

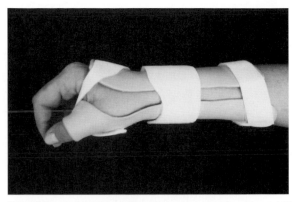

Fig. 8.15 This combination volar and dorsal orthosis adds stability to the healing scaphoid fracture. (From Fess, E. E., Gettle, K. S., Philips, C. A. , et al. [2005]. *Hand and upper extremity splinting: Principles and methods* [3rd ed.]. St. Louis: Elsevier Mosby.)

that protects the ligament. This orthosis is intended to protect the RCL from ulnar stress and alleviate pressure to the healing ligament.[60] The golfer who has injured a thumb and wants to return to the sport may find it difficult to play in a rigid orthosis. Rather than wearing a rigid orthosis during play, the person can be weaned from the orthosis in the same time as required for a UCL injury. The client learns how to wrap the thumb, which will be necessary for at least 1-year post injury,[56] or purchases a soft prefabricated orthosis.

Orthotic Interventions for Scaphoid Fractures

Fracture of the scaphoid bone is the second most common wrist fracture.[8] Similar to Colles fracture, **scaphoid fractures** usually occur because of a fall on an outstretched hand with the wrist dorsiflexed more than 90 degrees[27] and are a consequence of strong forces to the wrist.[19] Scaphoid fractures occur with impact sports, such as basketball, football, and soccer.[27,54,67] Clinically, persons who have a scaphoid fracture present with painful wrist movements and tenderness on palpation of the scaphoid in the anatomical snuffbox between the EPL and the EPB.[8]

Physicians cast the arm, and after the immobilization stage the hand may be positioned in an orthosis. There are many variations of orthotic options. One option is a volar forearm-based thumb immobilization orthosis[18] or a dorsal/volar forearm thumb immobilization orthosis. The thumb CMC joint is positioned in palmar abduction, the MCP joint is in 0 to 10 degrees flexion, and the wrist is in neutral.

Some clients (especially those in noncontact competitive sports) may benefit from a combination dorsal/volar thumb orthosis for added stability, protection, and pain and edema control (Fig. 8.15).[24] Therapists should educate clients that proximal scaphoid fractures take longer to heal, sometimes up to months, because of a poor vascular supply.[24,52] For people who play sports and have a healing scaphoid fracture, a soft commercial thumb immobilization orthosis may be used as a protective measure.[27]

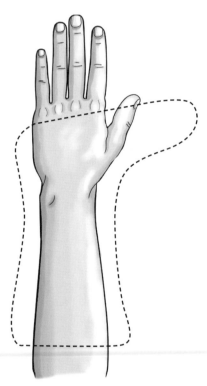

Fig. 8.16 A pattern option for either a volar or a dorsal thumb immobilization orthosis.

FABRICATION OF A THUMB IMMOBILIZATION ORTHOSIS

There are many approaches to fabrication of a thumb immobilization orthosis. Fig. 8.16 shows a pattern that can be used for either a volar or dorsal thumb immobilization orthosis. The radial design of the thumb immobilization orthosis[2] provides support on the radial side of the hand while stabilizing the thumb. This design allows some wrist flexion and extension but limits deviation.[41] The therapist usually places the thumb in a palmar abducted position so that the thumb pad can contact the index pad. The therapist leaves the IP joint free for functional movement but can adapt the orthotic pattern to include the IP joint if more support becomes necessary.

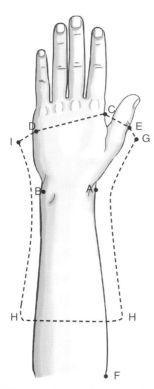

Fig. 8.17 A detailed pattern for a radial gutter thumb immobilization orthosis.

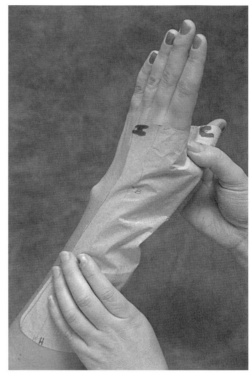

Fig. 8.18 To ensure proper fit, place the paper pattern on the person.

The thumb may be placed in a position of comfort (i.e., out of the functional plane) if the client does not tolerate the thumb placed in the functional position or when the physician does not want the thumb to incur any stress.

Fig. 8.17 shows a detailed radial gutter thumb immobilization pattern that excludes the IP joint. (See Fig. 8.4 for a photograph of the completed orthotic product.)

1. Position the forearm and hand palm down on a piece of paper. The fingers should be in a natural resting position and slightly abducted; the wrist should be neutral with respect to deviation. Draw an outline of the hand and forearm to the elbow. As you gain experience with pattern drawing, you will not need to draw the entire hand and forearm outline. The experienced therapist can estimate the placement of key points on the pattern.
2. While the person's hand is on the paper, mark an A at the radial styloid and a B at the ulnar styloid. Mark the second and fifth metacarpal heads C and D, respectively. Mark the IP joint of the thumb E, and mark the olecranon process of the elbow F. Then remove the person's hand from the paper pattern.
3. Place an X two-thirds the length of the forearm on each side. Place another X on each side of the pattern approximately 1 to 1½ inches outside and parallel to the two X markings for the appropriate width of the orthosis. Mark these two Xs H.
4. Draw an angled line connecting the second and fifth metacarpal heads (C to D). Extend this line approximately 1 to 1½ inches to the ulnar side of the hand, and mark it I.
5. Connect C to E. Extend this line approximately ½ to 1 inch. Mark the end of the line G.

6. Draw a line from G down the radial side of the forearm, making sure the line follows the increasing size of the forearm. To ensure that the orthosis is two-thirds the length of the forearm, end the line at H.
7. Begin a line from I, and extend it down the ulnar side of the forearm, making certain that the line follows the increasing size of the forearm. End the line at H.
8. For the proximal edge of the orthosis, draw a straight line that connects both H's.
9. Make sure the orthotic pattern lines are rounded at G, I, and the two H's to prevent any injury or discomfort.
10. Cut out the pattern.
11. Place the pattern on the person (Fig. 8.18). Make certain the orthosis' edges end midforearm on the volar and dorsal surfaces of the person's hand and forearm. Check that the orthosis is two-thirds the forearm length and one-half the forearm circumference. Check the thumb position, and make any necessary adjustments (e.g., additions, deletions) on the pattern.
12. Carefully trace with a pencil the thumb immobilization pattern on a sheet of thermoplastic material.
13. Heat the thermoplastic material.
14. Cut the pattern out of the thermoplastic material.
15. Reheat the material, mold the form onto the person's hand, and make necessary adjustments. Make sure the thumb is correctly positioned as the material hardens by having the person lightly touch the thumb tip to the pads of the index or middle fingers. Another approach is to provide light pressure over the plastic of the thumb MCP joint to align it in palmar abduction (Figs. 8.19 and 8.20).

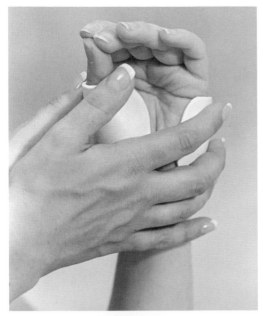

Fig. 8.19 Have the person lightly touch the thumb tip to the pads of the index and middle fingers to position the thumb in palmar abduction.

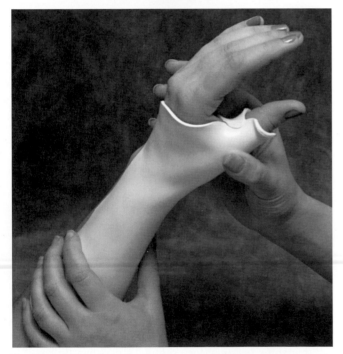

Fig. 8.20 Although the actual movement comes from the carpometacarpal (CMC) joint, provide light pressure on the thumb metacarpophalangeal (MCP) joint to position the thumb correctly in palmar abduction.

16. Add three 2-inch straps (one at the wrist joint, one toward the proximal end of the forearm trough, and one across the dorsal aspect of the hand) connecting the hypothenar bar to the metacarpal bar.

FABRICATION OF A DORSAL HAND-BASED THUMB IMMOBILIZATION ORTHOSIS

Hand-based thumb immobilization orthoses can be fabricated for people who have the following diagnoses: low

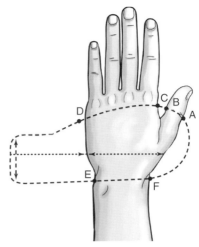

Fig. 8.21 A detailed pattern for a hand-based thumb immobilization orthosis.

median nerve injury, UCL or RCL injury of the MCP joint, CMC arthritis, and the potential for a first web space contracture. Each of these diagnoses may require placement of the thumb post in a different degree of abduction, based on protocols and comfort of the patient. With this orthosis the IP joint is usually left free for functional movement, unless extreme pain is present in the IP joint. However, if the IP joint is left free (especially during rigorous activity), it too can become vulnerable to stresses. This hand-based orthotic design is most appropriate for stabilizing the MCP joint because the position of the CMC is irrelevant. Finally, because this hand-based orthotic design incorporates the dorsal aspect of the palm, the therapist may need to add padding because the dorsal skin has a minimal subcutaneous layer and the boniness of the dorsal palm can cause skin breakdown.

Fig. 8.21 shows a detailed hand-based dorsal thumb immobilization pattern. (See Fig. 8.13 for a photograph of the completed orthotic product.)

1. Position the person's forearm and hand palm down on a piece of paper. Ensure that the client's thumb is radially abducted. The fingers should be in a natural resting position and slightly abducted. Draw an outline of the hand, including the wrist and a couple of inches of the forearm.

2. While the person's hand is on the paper, mark the IP joint of the thumb on both sides, and label it A (radial side of thumb) and B (ulnar side of the thumb), respectively. Then mark the second and fifth metacarpal heads C and D, respectively. Mark the wrist joint on the ulnar side of the hand E, and mark F on the radial side of the wrist. Remove the hand from the pattern.

3. Start in the web space. Draw an angled line connecting the marks of the second and fifth metacarpal heads (D to C). Then connect C to B and B to A. Curve the line around and angle it down to F. Connect F to E. Then extend the line out from E approximately equal to the length of the pattern on the hand. Go up vertically, curve the line around, and connect it to D. Make sure that all edges on this pattern are rounded.

4. Cut out the pattern, check fit, and make any adjustments. Make sure the pattern allows enough room for an adequately fitting thumb post.
5. Position the person's upper extremity with the elbow resting on the table and the forearm in a neutral position.
6. Trace the pattern onto a sheet of thermoplastic material.
7. Heat the thermoplastic material.
8. Cut the pattern out of the thermoplastic material.
9. Measure the CMC joint with a small goniometer to make sure it is in the correct position.
10. Reheat the thermoplastic material.
11. Mold the orthosis onto the person's hand. First form the thumb post around the thenar area. Make sure the thumb is correctly positioned as the material hardens. Allowances are made in the circumference of the thumb post to ensure that the client can move the thumb. This is particularly important when fabricating an orthosis from thermoplastic material that shrinks or has memory. Roll the volar part of the thumb post proximal to the thumb IP crease to allow adequate IP flexion. Then form the orthosis across the dorsal side of the hand from the thumb (radial side) to the ulnar side. Curving around the ulnar side, fit the thermoplastic material proximal to the distal palmar crease on the volar side of the hand. There will be just enough room between the thumb post and the end of the orthosis on the ulnar side to add a strap across the palm. Make sure the proximal end of the orthosis is flared to prevent skin breakdown.
12. After the thermoplastic material has hardened, check that the person can perform IP thumb flexion without impingement by the thumb post and that he or she can perform all wrist movements without interference by the proximal end of the orthosis. Adjust as necessary.
13. Add one strap across the palm.

Orthotic Intervention Pattern for Volar Forearm-Based Orthosis, Radial Gutter, and/or a Dorsal Hand-Based Thumb Immobilization Orthosis

This orthotic pattern is versatile because it can be used for the fabrication of three different thumb orthoses (i.e., volar-, radial- and dorsal-based) (Fig. 8.22). With a volar-based thumb immobilization orthosis for a proper fit, ensure that the pattern is fitted proximal to the distal palmar crease and follows the curves of the forearm. For a hand-based thumb immobilization orthosis, the dotted line on the pattern indicates the proximal end of the orthosis, which fits distal to the wrist joint. With this hand-based thumb immobilization orthosis, the section of the orthotic pattern that extends parallel to the ulnar side of the hand may need to be lengthened to fit around to the palmar (volar) side of the hand. For the radial gutter thumb immobilization orthosis, fit the pattern midforearm. Review the instructions earlier in the chapter for tips on general fabrication of radial gutter and dorsal hand-based thumb immobilization orthoses. For any of the three types of thumb orthoses, carefully check the pattern on the client before cutting out the thermoplastic material. The portion of the pattern that will cover the thenar eminence may need to be enlarged to fit the person's hand. In addition, to fit the thumb post pull the

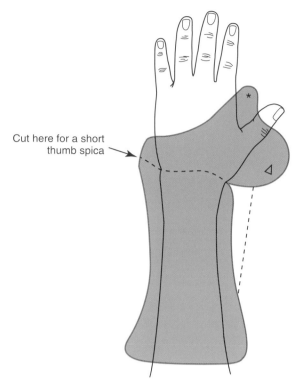

Cut here for a short thumb spica

Fig. 8.22 Pattern for a volar forearm-based orthosis, radial gutter orthosis, and/or a dorsal hand-based thumb immobilization orthosis. The dotted line on the radial side connecting the hand based piece to the forearm can help with fit on a forearm-based orthosis.

section that has a star drawn on it over the first web space and the section with a triangle on it around to the palmar (volar) aspect of the hand where it meets the "star" section.

Technical Tips for Proper Fit

1. Before molding the orthosis, place the person's elbow on a tabletop, positioned in 90 degrees of flexion and the forearm in a neutral position. Position the thumb and wrist according to diagnostic indications.
2. Monitor joint positions by measuring during and after orthotic fabrication. Place the thumb in a palmar abduction position as is comfortable for the person. The best way to position the thumb in palmar abduction for fabrication of an orthosis is to have the person lightly touch the thumb tip to the index or middle finger pad. Note that some persons (for example, a person who has RA) will find the thumb post more comfortable in a position between radial and palmar abduction.
3. Follow the natural curves of the longitudinal, distal, and proximal arches. Ensure the orthosis completely covers the thenar eminence. Be especially careful to check that the index finger has full flexion because of its close proximity to the opponens bar, C bar, and thumb post, and if necessary carefully roll the area just proximal to the proximal palmar crease.
4. With a volar forearm orthosis check that the distal end of the orthosis is positioned just proximal to the distal palmar crease and that it does not interfere with finger flexion. Also check that the forearm part of the orthosis is one-half the circumference of the forearm.

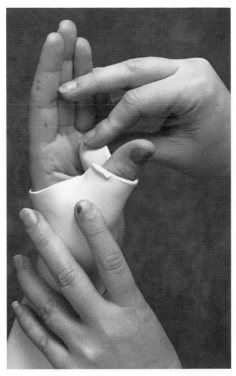

Fig. 8.23 Overlap the extra thermoplastic material into the thumb web space.

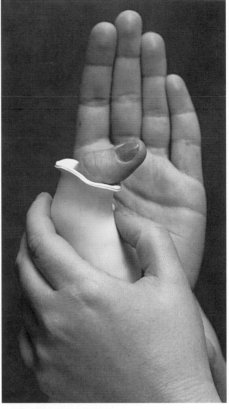

Fig. 8.24 Roll the distal end of the thumb post to allow full interphalangeal (IP) flexion.

5. For a radial gutter orthosis check that the forearm trough is correctly placed in midforearm (i.e., place a goniometer with the axis at midwrist, one arm extending between the third and fourth digits, and the other arm pointing toward the midforearm).

6. When molding the thumb post, overlap the thermoplastic material into the thumb web space (Fig. 8.23). Be certain the thumb IP joint remains in extension during molding to facilitate later orthotic application and removal. Be extremely careful in adjusting with a heat gun on the thumb post, or the result may be an inappropriate fit.

7. When applying thermoplastic material that shrinks during cooling and because the thumb is circumferential in shape, allowances must be made to ensure easy application and removal of the orthosis. The orthosis must provide enough support to the thumb in the thumb post. The thumb must not move excessively. There are several options to address the correct size of the thumb post. One is to have the person make very small thumb circles as the plastic cools, because this motion allows for some extra room.[56] Another option is to gently flare the thumb post with a narrow pencil[40] or popsicle stick. For people with larger thumb joints a paper towel can be placed in between where the pieces overlap to keep the thermoplastic material from adhering, so the orthosis is easier to take off.

8. Before the orthosis is completely cool, remove the orthosis from the thumb to ensure that the orthosis can be easily doffed and donned.

9. A thumb post can be fabricated with overlapping material that does not bond. This design method allows for adjustment to expand or contract the thumb post with Velcro straps that secure the post.[56]

10. For a thumb immobilization orthosis that allows IP mobility, make sure the distal end of the thumb post on the volar surface has been rolled to allow full IP flexion, yet remains high enough for full support (Fig. 8.24). When fabricating the thumb post, place the thermoplastic material slightly over the IP joint, and while stabilizing the thumb MCP joint have the person slowly flex the IP joint. Roll the distal end of the thumb post on the volar side to allow for full IP excursion. This technique results in a thumb post that is high enough for adequate support while not interfering with IP mobility.

11. Check that the distal end of the thumb post is just proximal to the IP joint and has not migrated lower. Make sure that the orthosis does not interfere with functional hand movements.

Patient Safety Tips and Precautions for Fabrication of Thumb Orthoses

The cautious therapist checks for areas of skin pressure over the distal ulna, the superficial branch of the radial nerve at the radial styloid, and the volar and dorsal surfaces of the thumb MCP joint. Specific precautions for the molding of the orthosis include the following:

- If the thumb post extends too far distally on the volar surface of the IP joint, the result is restriction of the IP joint flexion and a likely area for skin irritation.

- Because of its proximity to the opponens bar, C bar, and thumb post, the radial base of the first metacarpal and first web space has a potential for skin irritation.
- With a radial gutter orthosis, monitor the orthosis for a pressure area at the midline of the forearm on the volar and dorsal surfaces. Pull the sides of the forearm trough apart if it is too tight.
- Be careful to fabricate an orthosis that is supportive to the thumb's joints and is not too constrictive. Providing enough support allows the orthosis to meet therapeutic goals. Constriction results in decreased circulation and possible skin breakdown. Make allowances for edema when fabricating the thumb post.
- If using a thermoplastic material that has memory properties, be aware that the material shrinks when cooling Therefore the thumb post opening must remain large enough for comfortable application and removal of the orthosis. Refer to technical tips for suggestions on fabricating the thumb post.

IMPACT ON OCCUPATIONS

Having a workable thumb for grasp and pinch is paramount for functional activities. Research findings support the thumb's functional importance. Swigart and colleagues established that people with CMC arthritis had decreased involvement in crafts and changed their athletic involvement.[59a] With gamekeeper's thumb, lack of thenar strength and adequate pinch can impact daily functional activities, such as turning a key or opening a jar.[73]

Even with the stability provided by an orthosis, some people may find it more difficult to perform meaningful occupations. For example, Weiss and colleagues[66] found in their study (N = 25) that with some subjects the long thumb immobilization orthosis inhibited function and was more than necessary to meet therapeutic goals. Therefore, the goal of orthotic intervention is to improve function for meaningful activities. It is intended that with the benefits of orthotic wear and a therapeutic program the person will return to functional and meaningful activities.[73]

PREFABRICATED ORTHOSES

Deciding to provide a client with a prefabricated thumb orthosis requires careful reflection. Therapists critically consider the condition for which the orthosis is being provided, materials that the orthosis is made from, the design of the orthosis, and comfort factors. Therapists should remember that because prefabricated thumb orthoses are made for a mass population, the thumb positioning is often in some degree of radial abduction, which may or may not be the correct position for the patient. Furthermore, therapists should review the literature to determine whether a custom thumb orthosis is preferable over a prefabricated thumb orthosis to treat a condition.

Conditions

Prefabricated thumb orthoses are manufactured for a variety of conditions, including arthritis, thumb MCP collateral ligament injuries, de Quervain tenosynovitis, and hypertonicity. Orthotic types and positions for all these conditions have been discussed in this chapter (see Table 8.1).

Materials

Therapists should be aware of the characteristics of the wide variety of materials available for prefabricated thumb orthoses. Material firmness varies from soft to rigid. Soft materials are often used with thumb orthotic intervention because they can be easier to apply and provide a more comfortable fit for a client with a painful and edematous thumb IP joint than a rigid orthosis. Neoprene is a commonly used soft material for prefabricated orthoses. It has the advantage of providing hugging support with flexibility for function, but it has the disadvantage of retaining moisture next to the skin, increasing the possibility of skin breakdown. Another soft material used in prefabricated orthoses is leather. Leather orthoses absorb perspiration and are pliable; however, they often become odiferous and soiled. Some orthoses are lined with moisture-wicking material or are fabricated from perforated material to address this issue. Examples of prefabricated orthoses made from rigid materials are those fabricated out of thermoplastic, vinyl, or adjustable polypropylene materials.

An awareness of the orthosis' function, condition for which it is being used, and the client's occupational demands helps therapists critically determine the degree of material firmness to use. A prefabricated orthosis made from a rigid material might be very appropriate for a client engaged in sports or heavier work activities, or for any condition that requires a higher amount of support and protection. Finally, people who are allergic to latex require orthoses that are made from latex-free materials.

Design and Comfort

Like custom-fabricated thumb orthoses, prefabricated orthoses are either hand based or forearm based. The hand-based thumb immobilization designs provide support to the thumb joints through the circumferential thumb post component, thermoplastic material, or optional stays. The forearm-based immobilization designs derive some of their support from a longer lever arm. Prefabricated forearm-based orthoses contain many features that should be critically considered for client usage. Examples of these features are adjustable or additional straps and adjustable thumb stays to provide optimal support and fit. Some designs for both the forearm- and hand-based orthoses are hybrid designs. These orthoses usually have a softer outer layer with removable and adjustable inserts made from thermoplastic material to customize the fit.

Another consideration is the comfort of the prefabricated thumb orthosis. Factors to think about are adjustability, temperature, bulkiness, and padding of the possible orthotic selection. When adjusting the orthosis, therapists should account for the number and location of straps and types of strapping material to obtain an appropriate fit. For example, with a long thumb orthosis the therapist should consider whether the wrist straps provide adequate support. Considering temperature, the type of thermoplastic material that is used for the prefabricated orthosis is scrutinized as some materials are more breathable than others. Thumb orthoses made from Neoprene or other soft materials are usually more breathable than rigid thermoplastic materials. A prefabricated orthosis made from a breathable material might be a consideration for a person living or working in a hot environment. A person with arthritis might prefer a thumb orthosis that provides warmth. Padding may be an essential consideration with a person who has a tendency toward skin breakdown. Thumb immobilization orthoses may chafe the web space, so the therapist must monitor for fit and consider padding in that area. Some prefabricated thumb immobilization designs include added features, such as a gel pad for scar control or leather for added durability. Fig. 8.25 outlines prefabricated thumb orthotic options.

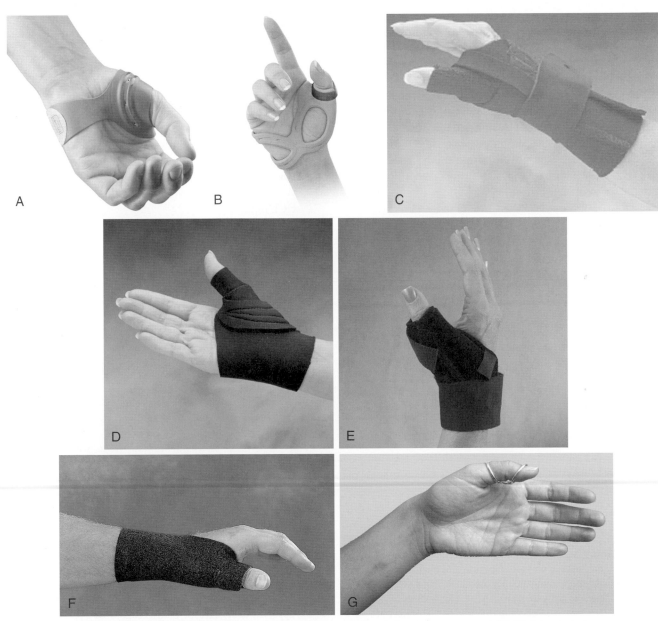

Fig. 8.25 A, This Push MetaGrip orthosis provides support of the carpometacarpal (CMC) joint to help with thumb osteoarthritis. It can be adjusted for fit and can be cleaned in a washing machine. (Courtesy of BraceLab.) B, The Actimove® Rhizo Forte provides support of the CMC and metacarpophalangeal (MCP) joints of the thumb. It can be adjusted for fit, and material is dirt and water repellent (©BSN medical, Inc.) C, This Comfort Cool® Wrist and Thumb CMC Restriction Orthosis is made from perforated Neoprene, which keeps the extremity cool. It has additional strapping at the wrist to allow for extra support. D, The Rolyan® Fabrifoam® Ultra CarpalGard™ offers semi-rigid support of the CMC joint while allowing for adjustable compression. (Courtesy Performance Health, Warrenville, IL.) E, The Sammons Preston Universal Thumb Orthosis has interchangeable flexible and rigid stays that provide the desired support of the thumb. (Courtesy Performance Health, Warrenville, IL.) F, The Rolyan® TakeOff® Thumb Support provides highly conformable, breathable, slip-resistant, and warm support. (Courtesy Performance Health, Warrenville, IL.)G, This SIRIS boutonnière helps position the IP joint. (Courtesy Silver Ring™ Splint Company.)

SUMMARY

Thumb orthotic intervention is commonly provided in clinical practice. Applying a critical analysis approach helps to determine the most optimal thumb orthotic intervention. It behooves therapists to be aware of the variety of orthoses (whether custom fabricated or prefabricated) to provide clients with orthoses that address specific conditions and occupational needs.

REVIEW QUESTIONS

1. What are the general reasons for provision of a thumb immobilization orthosis?
2. What are three common conditions that require thumb immobilization orthoses?
3. What are some clinical indications for including the thumb IP joint in a thumb immobilization orthosis?
4. What is an appropriate wearing schedule for a person with RA who wears a thumb immobilization orthosis?
5. What is the suggested position for a thumb orthosis for a person who has CMC joint arthritis? What joints are stabilized and why?
6. What does research evidence suggest about the application of orthoses for CMC joint arthritis in relationship to pain and functional outcomes?
7. Which type of thumb immobilization orthosis should a therapist fabricate for a person who has de Quervain tenosynovitis?
8. What does the research evidence for orthotic intervention of de Quervain tenosynovitis indicate?
9. Which type of thumb immobilization orthosis should be fabricated for an injury of the thumb UCL?
10. What is the orthotic-wearing schedule for each grade of a UCL injury?

❓ SELF-QUIZ 8.1ᵃ

For the following questions, circle either true (T) or false (F).
1. T F One purpose of a thumb immobilization orthosis is to protect the thumb.
2. T F Many studies have considered the efficacy of orthoses for de Quervain tenosynovitis.
3. T F A therapist should apply a thumb immobilization orthosis to a client only during the chronic phase of de Quervain tenosynovitis.
4. T F Fabricating either a long forearm thumb immobilization orthosis or a radial gutter thumb immobilization orthosis is best for a person who has de Quervain tenosynovitis.

5. T F Thermoplastic material more than 1/8-inch thick is best used for an orthosis for a person who has RA because this material adds more support.
6. T F If a person with RA has wrist pain, the therapist includes the wrist in the thumb immobilization orthosis.
7. T F Orthotic intervention for grade I ulnar collateral thumb injuries may require that the person wear the orthosis continuously for 2 to 3 weeks with removal only for hygiene.
8. T F The main purpose of orthotic intervention for an ulnar collateral thumb injury is to keep the web space open.
9. T F Fracture of the scaphoid bone requires orthotic intervention in a hand-based thumb immobilization orthosis.

ᵃSee Appendix A for the answer key.

REFERENCES

1. Aebischer B, Elsig S, Taeymans J: Effectiveness of physical and occupational therapy on pain, function and quality of life in patients with trapeziometacarpal osteoarthritis—A systematic review and meta-analysis, *Hand Ther* 21(1):5–15, 2016.
2. Alexy C, De Carlo M: Rehabilitation and use of protective devices in hand and wrist injuries, *Clin Sports Med* 17(3):635–655, 1998.
3. American Society of Hand Therapists: *Splint classification system*, Garner, NC, 1992, American Society of Hand Therapists.
4. Andréu J, Otón T, Silva-Fernández L, et al.: Hand pain other than carpal tunnel syndrome (CTS): the role of occupational factors, *Best Pract Res Clin Rheumatol* 25(1):31–42, 2011.
5. Bani MA, Arazpour M, Kashani RV, et al.: Comparison of custom-made and prefabricated neoprene splinting in patients with first carpometacarpal joint osteoarthritis, *Disabil Rehabil Assist Technol* 8(3), 2013. 323–237.
6. Belkin J, English C: Hand splinting: principles, practice, and decision making. In Pedretti LW, editor: *Occupational therapy: practice skills for physical dysfunction*, ed 4, St. Louis, 1996, Mosby, pp 319–343.
7. Biese J: Short splints: indications and techniques. In Mackin EJ, Callahan AD, Skirven TM, et al.: *Rehabilitation of the hand and upper extremity*, ed 5, St. Louis, 2002, Mosby, pp 1846–1857.
8. Cailliet R: *Hand pain and impairment*, Philadelphia, 1994, FA Davis.
9. Campbell PJ, Wilson RL: Management of joint injuries and intraarticular fractures. In Mackin EJ, Callahan AD, Skirven TM, et al.: *Rehabilitation of the hand and upper extremity*, ed 5, St. Louis, 2002, Mosby, pp 396–411.
10. Cannon NM: *Diagnosis and treatment manual for physicians and therapists*, ed 4, Indianapolis, 2001, The Hand Rehabilitation Center of Indiana.
11. Cannon NM: *Fundamentals of hand therapy: clinical reasoning and treatment guidelines for common diagnoses of the upper extremity*, Philadelphia, 2007, Elsevier.

11a. Cantero-Tellez R, Schwartz DA, Villafane JH, et al.: Short opponens orthosis: a whale of a design, *J Hand Ther* 30(1): 116–120, 2017.

12. Cavaleri R, Schabrun SM, Te, M, et al.: Hand therapy versus corticosteroid injections in the treatment of de Quervain's disease: a systematic review and meta-analysis, *J Hand Ther* 29:3–11, 2016.

13. Chaisson C, McAlindon TS: Osteoarthritis of the hand: clinical features and management, *J Musculoskelet Med* 14:66–68, 1997. 71–74, 77.

14. Chien-Hsiou L, Kai-Shun Y, Shih-Chen F: Optimal grasp distance and muscle loads for people with rheumatoid arthritis using carpometacarpal and metacarpophalangeal immobilization orthoses, *Am J Occup Ther* 71(1):1–9, 2017.

15. Colditz JC: Anatomic considerations for splinting the thumb. In Mackin EJ, Callahan AD, Skirven TM, et al.: *Rehabilitation of the hand and upper extremity*, ed 5, St. Louis, 2002, Mosby, pp 1858–1874.

16. Colditz JC: Arthritis. In Malick MH, Kasch MC, editors: *Manual on management of specific hand problems*, Pittsburgh, 1984, AREN Publications, pp 112–136.

17. Colditz JC: The biomechanics of a thumb carpometacarpal immobilization splint: design and fitting, *J Hand Ther* 13(3): 228–235, 2000.

18. Colditz JC: *Personal communication*, April 1995.

19. Cooney III WP: Scaphoid fractures: current treatments and techniques, *Instructional Course Lectures* 52:197–208, 2003.

20. Cooper C: *Personal communication*, June 2012.

21. Dell PC, Dell RB: Management of rheumatoid arthritis of the wrist, *J Hand Ther* 9(2):157–164, 1996.

22. Eaton RG, Littler W: Ligament reconstruction for the painful thumb carpometacarpal joint, *J Bone Joint Surg Am* 55:1655–1666, 1973.

23. Egan MY, Brousseau L: Splinting for osteoarthritis of the carpometacarpal joint: a review of the evidence, *Am J Occup Ther* 61:70–78, 2007.

24. Fess EE, Gettle KS, Philips CA, et al.: *Hand splinting principles and methods*, ed 3, St. Louis, 2005, Elsevier/Mosby.

25. Ford M, McKee P, Szilagyi M: A hybrid thermoplastic and neoprene thumb metacarpophalangeal joint orthosis, *J Hand Ther* 17(1):64–68, 2004.

26. Geisser RW: Splinting the rheumatoid arthritic hand. In Ziegler EM, editor: *Current concepts in orthosis*, Germantown, WI, 1984, Rolyan Medical Products, pp 29–49.

27. Geissler WB: Carpal fractures in athletes, *Clin Sports Med* 20(1):167–188, 2001.

28. Grenier ML, Mendonca R, Dallely P: The effectiveness of orthoses in the conservative management of thumb CMC joint osteoarthritis: an analysis of functional pinch strength, *J Hand Ther* 29(3):307–313, 2016.

29. Hamann N, Heidermann J, Heinrich K, et al.: Stabilization effectiveness and functionality of different thumb orthoses in female patients with first carpometacarpal joint osteoarthritis, *Clin Biomech* 29(10):1180–1176, 2014.

30. Hochberg MC, Altman RD, April KT, et al.: American college of Rehmatology 2012 recommendations for the use of non-pharmacolopgic and pharmacologic therapies in osteoarthris of the hand, hip and knee, *Arthritis Care Res* 4(64):465–474, 2012.

31. Idler RS: Helping the patient who has wrist or hand tenosynovitis. Part 2: managing trigger finger and de Quervain's disease, *J Musculoskelet Med* 14:62–65, 1997. 68, 74–75.

32. Ilyas AM, Ast M, Schaffer A, et al.: De Quervain tenosynovitis of the wrist, *J Am Acad Orthop Surg* 15(12):757–764, 2007.

33. Kjeken I, Smedslund G, Moe RH, et al.: Systematic review of design and effects of splints and exercise programs in hand osteoarthritis, *Arthritis Care Res* 63(6):834–848, 2011.

34. Kjeken I, Eide REM, Klokkeide A, et al.: Does occupational therapy reduce the need for surgery in carpometacarpal osteoarthritis? Protocol for a randomized controlled trial, *BMC Musculoskeletal Disorders* 17:1–15, 2016.

35. Kloppenburg M: Hand osteoarthritis-nonpharmacological and pharmacological treatments, *Nat Rev Rheumatol* 10(4), 2014. 242–241.

36. Lee MP, Nasser-Sharif S, Zelouf DS: Surgeon's and therapist's management of tendonopathies in the hand and wrist. In Mackin EJ, Callahan AD, Skirven TM, et al.: *Rehabilitation of the hand and upper extremity*, ed 5, St. Louis, 2002, Mosby, pp 931–953.

37. Mahajan M, Rhemrev SJ: Rupture of the ulnar collateral ligament of the thumb-a review, *Int J Emerg Med* 6–31, 2013.

38. Marx H: Rheumatoid arthritis. In Stanley BG, Tribuzi SM, editors: *Concepts in hand rehabilitation*, Philadelphia, 1992, FA Davis, pp 395–418.

39. McCarroll JR: Overuse injuries of the upper extremity in golf, *Clin Sports Med* 20(3):469–479, 2001.

40. McKee P, Morgan L: *Orthotics and rehabilitation: splinting the hand and body*, Philadelphia, 1998, FA Davis.

41. Melvin JL: *Rheumatic disease in the adult and child*, ed 3, Philadelphia, 1989, FA Davis.

42. Melvin JL: Therapist's management of osteoarthritis in the hand. In Mackin EJ, Callahan AD, Skirven TM, et al.: *Rehabilitation of the hand and upper extremity*, ed 5, St. Louis, Mosby, 2002, pp 1646–1663.

43. Menendez ME, Thornton E, Kent S, et al.: A prospective randomized clinical trial of prescription of full-time versus as-desired splint wear for de Quervain tendinopathy, *Int Orthop* 39(8):1563–1569, 2015.

44. Moulton MJ, Parentis MA, Kelly MJ, et al.: Influence of metacarpophalangeal joint position on basal joint-loading in the thumb, *J Bone Joint Surg Am* 83(5):709–716, 2001.

45. Nalebuff EA: Diagnosis, classification and management of rheumatoid thumb deformities, *Bull Hosp Joint Dis* 29(2):119–137, 1968.

46. Nemati Z, Javanshir MA, Saeedi H, et al.: The effect of a new dynamic splint in pinch strength in De Quervain syndrome: a comparative study, *Disabil Rehabil Assist Technol* 12(5):457–461, 2017.

47. Neumann DA, Bielefeld T: The carpometacarpal joint of the thumb: stability, deformity, and therapeutic intervention, *J Orthop Sports Phys Ther* 33(7):386–399, 2003.

48. O'Brien VH, McGaha JL: Current practice patterns in conservative thumb CMC joint care: survey results, *J Hand Therapy* 27(1):14–22, 2013.

49. Ouellette E: The rheumatoid hand: orthotics as preventive, *Semin Arthritis Rheum* 21(2):65–72, 1991.

50. Poole JU, Pellegrini VD Jr: Arthritis of the thumb basal joint complex, *J Hand Ther* 13(2):91–107, 2000.

51. Rettig AC: Wrist and hand overuse syndromes, *Clin Sports Med* 20(3):591–611, 2001.

52. Rettig ME, Dassa GL, Raskin KB, et al.: Wrist fractures in the athlete: distal radius and carpal fractures, *Clin Sports Med* 17(3):469–489, 1998.

53. Richie CA 3rd, Briner WW Jr.: Cortisosteroid infection for treatment of de Quervain's tenosynovities: a pooled quantitative literature evaluation, *J Am Board Fam Pract* 16(2):102–106, 2003.

54. Riester JN, Baker BE, Mosher JF, et al.: A review of scaphoid fracture healing in competitive athletes, *Am J Sports Med* 13(3):159–161, 1985.

55. Rocchi L, Merolli A, Morini G, et al.: A modified spica-splint in postoperative early motion management of skier's thumb lesion: a randomized clinical trial, *Eur J Phys Rehabil Med* 50: 49–47, 2014.

56. Schultz-Johnson K: *Personal communication*, June 2006.

57. Shankland B, Beaton D, Ahemed S, et al.: Effects of client-centered multimodual treatment on impairment, function, and satisfaction of people with thumb carpometacarpal osteoarthritis, *J Hand Ther* 30(3):307–313, 2017.

58. Sillem H, Backman CL, Miller WC, et al.: Comparison of two carpometacarpal stabilizing splints for individuals with osteoarthritis, *J Hand Ther* 24(3):216–226, 2011.

59. Skirven T, Osterman A, Fedorczyk J, et al.: *Rehabilitation of the hand and upper extremity*, ed 6, Philadelphia, 2011, Elsevier Mosby.

59a. Swigart CR, Eaton RG, Glickel SZ, et al.: Splinting in the treatment of arthritis of the first caropmetacarpal joint, *J Hand Surg Am* 24(1):86–91, 1999.

60. Tang P: Collateral ligament injuries of the thumb metacarpophalangeal joint, *J Am Acad Orthop Surg* 19(5):287–296, 2011.

61. Tenney CG, Lisak JM: *Atlas of hand splinting*, Boston/Toronto, 1986, Little, Brown & Co.

62. TQ de Almeida PH, MacDermid J, Pontes TB, et al.: Differences in orthotic design for thumb osteoarthritis and its impact on functional outcomes: a scoping review, *Prosthet Orthot Int* 41(4):323–335, 2017.

63. Valdes K, Marik T: A systematic review of conservative interventions for osteoarthritis of the hand, *J Hand Ther* 23(4):334–351, 2010.

64. Valdes K, Naughton N, Algar L: Linking ICF components to outcome measures for orthotic intervention for CMC OA: a systematic review, *J Hand Ther* 29(4):396–404, 2016.

65. Van Heest AE, Kallemeier P: Thumb carpal metacarpal arthritis, *J Am Acad Orthop Surg* 16(31):140–151, 2008.

66. Weiss S, LaStayo P, Mills A, et al.: Prospective analysis of splinting the first carpometacarpal joint: an objective, subjective and radiographic assessment, *J Hand Ther* 13(3):218–226, 2000.

67. Werner SL, Plancher KD: Biomechanics of wrist injuries in sports, *Clin Sports Med* 17(3):407–420, 1998.

68. Wilton JC: *Hand splinting: principles of design and fabrication*, London, 1997, WB Saunders.

69. Winzeler S, Rosenstein BD: Occupational injury and illness of the thumb, *AAOHN J* 44(10):487–492, 1996.

70. Wright HH, Rettig AC: Management of common sports injuries. In Hunter JM, Mackin EJ, Callahan AD, editors: *Rehabilitation of the hand*, ed4, St. Louis, 1995, Mosby, pp 1809–1838.

71. Yao J, Park M: Early treatment of degenerative arthritis of the thumb carpometacarpal joint, *Hand Clin* 24(3):251–261, 2008.

72. Zelouf DS, Posner MA: Hand and wrist disorders: how to manage pain and improve function, *Geriatrics* 50(3), 1995. 22–26, 29–31.

73. Zeman C, Hunter RE, Freeman JR, et al.: Acute skier's thumb repaired with a proximal phalanx suture anchor, *Am J Sports Med* 26(5):644–650, 1998.

APPENDIX 8.1 CASE STUDIES

Case Study 8.1[a]

Read the following scenario, and use your clinical reasoning skills to answer the questions based on information in this chapter.

Jack, a 10-year old boy, was skiing with his family on vacation. During one run on the bunny hill, he fell in a snow drift beside a tree with an outstretched right dominant hand and his thumb positioned in abduction. His thumb became painful and edematous. The physician diagnosed a partial tear of the ulnar collateral ligament (UCL; grade II) and casted the forearm, wrist, and thumb. After the cast is removed, a referral to therapy indicates the need for a thumb orthosis.

1. What type of orthosis should be selected? How should the thumb be positioned?

2. What is the purpose of the orthosis?

3. List three patient precautions to be aware of when creating this thumb immobilization orthosis.

4. What considerations should be made due to the patient's age?

5. What is the suggested wearing schedule?

6. Before the 4- to 5-week healing period is over, Jack's physician releases him to resume skiing. Jack is looking forward to skiing again. Jack's physician ordered the fabrication of an orthosis to wear while skiing. What type of orthosis might the therapist fabricate?

Case Study 8.2[a]

Read the following scenario, and use your clinical reasoning skills to answer the questions based on information in this chapter.

Margaret, a 58-year-old woman employed as a librarian, went to her physician complaining of thumb pain at the carpometacarpal (CMC) joint. She experiences pain while completing her activities of daily living (ADLs). This pain had occurred for less than 1 year. She was particularly concerned that the pain was being exacerbated by her job demands of manipulating, lifting, and carrying books. At home she was having difficulty with many of her ADLs and was concerned about not being able to knit or cross-stitch. Clinical examination revealed no additional pain or symptoms in the wrist, fingers, or other joints of the thumb. Margaret was diagnosed with osteoarthritis of the CMC joint. Her physician ordered therapy and fabrication of a thumb orthosis. The order was not specific and did not state which joints should be stabilized in the orthosis. No orthotic design was mentioned.

1. What type of orthosis might the therapist fabricate? Which thumb joints should be stabilized?

2. What is the purpose of the orthosis?

3. What is the suggested wearing schedule?

4. What factors must be considered when determining whether to provide a custom-made or a prefabricated orthosis?

5. Margaret discontinued therapy, and 3 years later her symptoms worsened due to continuing her hobby of needlework and her work and home demands. She presented with pain in her wrist and the thumb metacarpophalangeal (MCP) joint due to progression of the osteoarthritis. Describe an orthosis that the therapist might consider fabricating.

[a]See Appendix A for the answer key.

6. What position should the therapist place the thumb in the
   thumb post?

   _____

   _____

   _____

   _____

   _____

APPENDIX 8.2 LABORATORY EXERCISES

Laboratory Exercise 8.1[a]

These components are in various types of thumb immobilization orthoses. They are also part of other orthoses, such as the wrist cock-up and resting hand orthosis. Label the orthotic components shown in the following figure.

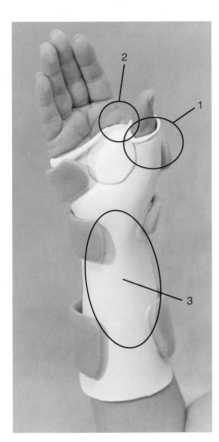

Laboratory Exercise 8.2

1. Practice making a pattern for a radial gutter thumb immobilization orthosis on another person. Use the detailed instructions on the previous pages to draw the pattern. Make necessary adjustments to the pattern after cutting it out.
2. Practice drawing a pattern for a radial gutter thumb immobilization orthosis on the following outlines of the hands without using detailed instructions. Label the landmarks.

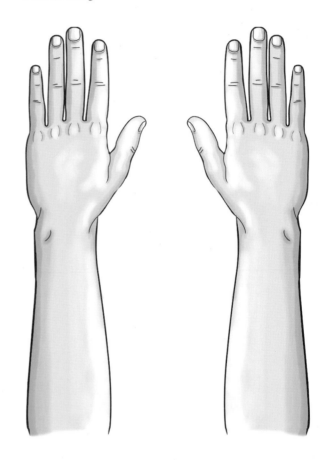

1. _____
   _____
2. _____
   _____
3. _____
   _____

Laboratory Exercise 8.3[a]

The following illustration shows a thumb immobilization orthosis for a 35-year-old woman working as an administrative assistant (secretary). She has a long history of rheumatoid arthritis (RA). Her physician ordered a thumb immobilization orthosis after she complained of thumb metacarpophalangeal (MCP) joint pain and inflammation. Keeping in mind the diagnostic protocols for thumb immobilization orthotic intervention, identify two problems with the illustrated orthosis.

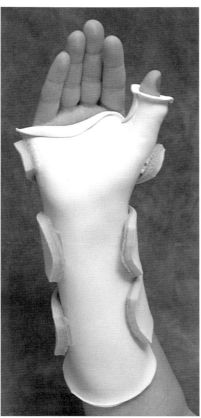

1. List two problems with this orthosis.

   a. _____
      _____

   b. _____
      _____

2. What problems might result from continual orthotic wear?

   _____
   _____
   _____
   _____
   _____

Laboratory Exercise 8.4

On a partner, practice fabricating a radial gutter or a volar forearm-based thumb immobilization orthosis that does not immobilize the thumb interphalangeal (IP) joint. Before starting, use a goniometer to ensure that the wrist is in 15 degrees of extension, the carpometacarpal (CMC) joint of the thumb is in 45 degrees of palmar abduction, and the MCP joint of the thumb is in 5 to 10 degrees of flexion. Check the finished product to ensure that full finger flexion and thumb IP flexion are possible after you fit the orthosis, and make all adjustments. Use Form 8.1 as a check-off sheet for a self-evaluation of the thumb immobilization orthosis. Use Grading Sheet 8.1 as a classroom grading sheet.

---

[a]See Appendix A for the answer key.

APPENDIX 8.3 FORM AND GRADING SHEET

Form 8.1 Thumb Immobilization Orthosis

	Name: _____
	Date: _____
Type of thumb immobilization orthosis:	
Volar ○ Dorsal ○ Radial gutter ○ Hand based ○	
Thumb joint position: _____	
After the person wears the orthosis for 30 minutes, answer the following questions. (Mark NA for nonapplicable situations.)	

Evaluation Areas				Comments
Design				
1. The wrist position is at the correct angle.	Yes ○	No ○	NA ○	
2. The thumb position is at the correct angle.	Yes ○	No ○	NA ○	
3. The thenar eminence is not restricted or flattened.	Yes ○	No ○	NA ○	
4. The thumb post provides adequate support and is not constrictive.	Yes ○	No ○	NA ○	
5. The orthosis is two-thirds the length of the forearm.	Yes ○	No ○	NA ○	
6. The orthosis is one-half the width of the forearm.	Yes ○	No ○	NA ○	
Function				
1. The orthosis allows full thumb interphalangeal (IP) flexion.	Yes ○	No ○	NA ○	
2. The orthosis allows full metacarpophalangeal (MCP) joint flexion of the fingers.	Yes ○	No ○	NA ○	
3. The orthosis provides wrist support that allows functional activities.	Yes ○	No ○	NA ○	
Straps				
1. The straps avoid bony prominences.	Yes ○	No ○	NA ○	
2. The straps are secure and rounded.	Yes ○	No ○	NA ○	

Comfort				
1. The edges are smooth with rounded corners.	Yes ○	No ○	NA ○	
2. The proximal end is flared.	Yes ○	No ○	NA ○	
3. The orthosis does not cause impingements or pressure sores.	Yes ○	No ○	NA ○	
Cosmetic Appearance				
1. The orthosis is free of fingerprints, dirt, and pencil and pen marks.	Yes ○	No ○	NA ○	
2. The orthosis is smooth and free of buckles.	Yes ○	No ○	NA ○	
Therapeutic Regimen				
1. The person has been instructed in a wearing schedule.	Yes ○	No ○	NA ○	
2. The person has been provided orthotic precautions.	Yes ○	No ○	NA ○	
3. The person demonstrates understanding of the education.	Yes ○	No ○	NA ○	
4. Client or caregiver knows how to clean the orthosis.	Yes ○	No ○	NA ○	

Discuss possible orthotic adjustments or changes that you should make based on the self-evaluation. What would you do differently next time?

_____

_____

_____

_____

Discuss possible areas to improve with clinical safety when fabricating the orthosis.

_____

_____

_____

_____

Grading Sheet 8.1 Thumb Immobilization Orthosis

	Name: _____
	Date: _____

Type of thumb immobilization orthosis:	
Volar O Dorsal O Radial gutter O Hand based O	
Thumb joint position: _____	
Grade: _____	
1 = Beyond improvement, not acceptable	
2 = Requires maximal improvement	
3 = Requires moderate improvement	
4 = Requires minimal improvement	
5 = Requires no improvement	

Evaluation Areas					
Design					
1. The wrist position is at the correct angle.	1	2	3	4	5
2. The thumb position is at the correct angle.	1	2	3	4	5
3. The thenar eminence is not restricted or flattened.	1	2	3	4	5
4. The thumb post provides adequate support and is not constrictive.	1	2	3	4	5
5. The orthosis is two-thirds the length of the forearm.	1	2	3	4	5
6. The orthosis is one-half the width of the forearm.	1	2	3	4	5
Function					
1. The orthosis allows full thumb motion.	1	2	3	4	5
2. The orthosis allows full metacarpophalangeal (MCP) joint flexion of the fingers.	1	2	3	4	5
3. The orthosis provides wrist support that allows functional activities.	1	2	3	4	5

Straps					
1. The straps avoid bony prominences.	1	2	3	4	5
1. The straps are secure and rounded.	1	2	3	4	5
Comfort					
1. The edges are smooth with rounded corners.	1	2	3	4	5
2. The proximal end is flared.	1	2	3	4	5
3. The orthosis does not cause impingements or pressure sores.	1	2	3	4	5
Cosmetic Appearance					
1. The orthosis is free of fingerprints, dirt, and pencil and pen marks.	1	2	3	4	5
2. The thermoplastic material is not buckled.	1	2	3	4	5

Comments:

_____

_____

_____

_____

_____

_____

Hand Immobilization Orthoses

Brenda M. Coppard

CHAPTER OBJECTIVES

1. List diagnoses that benefit from resting hand orthoses (hand immobilization orthoses).
2. Describe the functional or midjoint position of the wrist, thumb, and digits.
3. Describe the antideformity or intrinsic plus position of the wrist, thumb, and digits.
4. List the purposes of a resting hand orthosis (hand immobilization orthosis).
5. Identify the components of a resting hand orthosis (hand immobilization orthosis).
6. Explain the precautions to consider when fabricating a resting hand orthosis (hand immobilization orthosis).
7. Determine a resting hand (hand immobilization) orthotic-wearing schedule for different diagnostic indications.
8. Describe orthotic cleaning techniques that address infection control.
9. Apply knowledge about the application of the resting hand orthosis (hand immobilization orthosis) to a case study.
10. Use clinical judgment to evaluate a fabricated resting hand orthosis (hand immobilization orthosis).

KEY TERMS

antideformity position
complex regional pain syndrome (CRPS)

Dupuytren contracture
functional position

Ruth is a 53-year-old woman who has rheumatoid arthritis. Recently she experienced an exacerbation of her condition. She found it difficult to manage her job as a flight attendant, household, and activities of daily living due to pain and stiffness. Upon a referral to the therapy clinic, Ruth was asked if she had worn any orthoses in the past to rest her hands during periods of exacerbation.

Hand orthoses is a broad category of orthotic provision. This chapter overviews the most common types of hand immobilization orthoses for general practitioners. Commercial and customized hand immobilization orthoses are described. The purpose, component parts, and positions used for hand immobilization orthoses are described for common conditions such as rheumatoid arthritis (RA), hand burns, Dupuytren disease, and complex regional pain syndrome (CRPS).

Physicians commonly order resting hand orthoses, also known as *hand immobilization orthoses,*[1] *resting hand orthoses,* or *resting pan orthoses.* A resting hand orthosis is a static orthosis that immobilizes the fingers and wrist. The thumb may or may not be immobilized by the orthosis. Therapists fabricate custom resting hand orthoses or purchase them commercially. Some of the commercially available resting hand orthoses are prefabricated, preformed, and ready to wear. Table 9.1 outlines prefabricated orthoses for the wrist and hand. Others are available as precut resting hand orthotic kits that include the precut thermoplastic material and strapping mechanism. Each of these orthoses has advantages and disadvantages.

PREFORMED HAND ORTHOSES

Therapists order preformed commercial orthoses according to hand size (i.e., small, medium, large, and extra large) for the right or left hand. An advantage of premade orthoses is their quick application (usually only straps require adjusting). There is an advantage to ordering a preformed resting hand orthosis made from perforated material. The preformed orthosis has perforations only in the body of the orthosis. The edges are smooth because there are no perforations near the edges of the orthosis. However, if the perforated preformed or precut orthosis must be trimmed through the perforations, a rough edge may result. Perforations at the edges of orthoses are undesirable because of the discomfort they often create. Rough edges should be padded, smoothed, or flared.

TABLE 9.1   Examples of Wrist/Hand Orthoses

Therapeutic Objective	Description	
Resting hand orthoses immobilize the wrist, thumb, and metacarpophalangeal (MCP) joints to provide rest and reduce inflammation. The proximal interphalangeal (PIP) and distal interphalangeal (DIP) joints are free to move for functional tasks.	Similar to the resting hand orthotic design, orthoses can provide rest to the wrist, thumb, and MCP joints (Fig. 9.1). Padding and strapping systems can help control deviation of the wrist and MCPs. Orthoses are available in different sizes for the right and left hands.	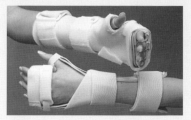 **Fig. 9.1** This orthosis is based on a resting hand design and is often used for individuals with rheumatoid arthritis (RA). (Rolyan Arthritis Mitt splint; courtesy Patterson Medical, Warrenville, Illinois.)
Designed to optimally position the hand in an intrinsic plus position after a burn injury.	Burn resting hand orthoses typically position the wrist in 20 to 30 degrees of extension, the MCP joints in 60 to 80 degrees of flexion, the PIP and DIP joints in full extension, and the thumb midway between radial and palmar abduction (Fig. 9.2).	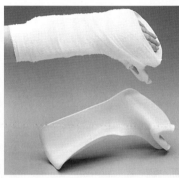 **Fig. 9.2** This resting hand orthosis positions the hand in an antideformity position for individuals with hand burns. (Rolyan Burn Splint; courtesy Patterson Medical, Warrenville, Illinois.)
Several orthoses are designed to manage spasticity.	Ball orthoses implement a reflex-inhibiting posture by positioning the wrist in neutral (or slight extension) and the fingers in extension and abduction. Cone orthoses combine a hand cone and a forearm trough, which maintains the wrist in neutral, inhibits the long finger flexors, and maintains the web space (Fig. 9.3). A resting hand orthosis positioning the hand in a functional position is advocated for spasticity (Fig. 9.4).	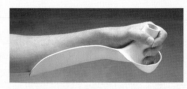 **Fig. 9.3** This cone orthosis is often used to help manage tone abnormalities. (Preformed Anti-Spasticity Hand Splint; courtesy North Coast Medical, Inc., Morgan Hill, California.) 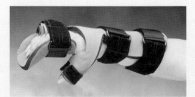 **Fig. 9.4** This resting hand orthosis is fabricated of soft materials and includes a dorsal forearm base design. (Progress Dorsal Anti-Spasticity Orthosis; courtesy North Coast Medical, Inc., Morgan Hill, California.)

A disadvantage of the commercial orthosis is a less-than-ideal fit for each person. With preformed orthoses the therapist has little control over joint position and the particular therapeutic angles, which may be different from the angles already incorporated into the orthotic design. The orthoses must be ordered for application on the right or left extremity, and the appropriate size needs to be factored. Unless there is accessible inventory on site, this often requires two sizes to be ordered to ensure appropriate fit, thus leading to additional cost and time delays.

PRECUT ORTHOTIC KITS

A resting hand orthotic kit typically contains strapping materials and precut thermoplastic material in the shape of a resting hand orthosis. Kits are available according to hand size (i.e., small, medium, large, and extra large). An advantage of using a kit is the time the therapist saves by the elimination of pattern making and cutting of thermoplastic material. Similar to premolded orthoses, precuts from perforated materials contain perforations in only the body of the orthosis. Precuts are interchangeable for right or left extremity application. The therapist has control over joint positioning. A disadvantage is that the pattern is not customized to the person. Therefore the precut orthosis may require many adjustments to obtain a proper fit.

CUSTOMIZED ORTHOSES

A therapist can customize a resting hand orthosis by making a pattern and fabricating the orthosis from thermoplastic material. The advantage is an exact fit for the person, which increases the orthosis' support and comfort. The therapist also has control over joint positioning. Furthermore, if a hand changes in shape (i.e., swelling, reduction), a therapist is skilled in modifying the existing orthosis without incurring additional cost for a replacement. A disadvantage is that customization may require more of the therapist's time to complete the orthosis and may be costlier. In addition, when a resting hand orthosis pattern is cut out of perforated thermoplastic material, it is difficult to obtain smooth edges because of the likelihood of needing to cut through the perforations (which causes a rough edge). Commercially available products, such as Rolyan Aquaplast Ultra Thin Edging Material, can be applied over the rough edges to create a smooth-edged reinforcement on orthoses fabricated from Aquaplast materials.[47]

Therapists must make informed decisions about whether they will fabricate or purchase an orthosis. Many products are advertised to save time and to be effective, but few studies compare orthotic materials when used by therapists with the same level of experience.[24] Lau[24] compared the fabrication of a resting hand orthosis with use of a precut orthosis; he compared the QuickCast (fiberglass material) with Ezeform thermoplastic material. The study employed second-year occupational therapy students as orthotic makers and first-year occupational therapy students as their clients.

The clients responded to a questionnaire addressing comfort, weight, and aesthetics. The orthotic makers also responded to a questionnaire asking about measuring fit, edges, strap application, aesthetics, safety, and ease of positioning. The analysis of timed trials revealed no significant difference in time required for fabricating the precut QuickCast and the Ezeform thermoplastic material. The thermoplastic material was rated safer than the fiberglass material. Because of the small sample, these results should be cautiously interpreted, and further studies are warranted.

PURPOSE OF THE RESTING HAND ORTHOSIS

The resting hand orthosis has three purposes: to immobilize, to position in functional alignment, and to retard further deformity.[28,59] When inflammation and pain are present in the hand, the joints and surrounding structures become swollen and result in improper hand alignment. Rest through immobilization reduces symptoms. The therapist may provide an orthosis for a person with arthritis who has early signs of ulnar drift by placing the hand in a comfortable neutral position with the joints in midposition. The resting hand orthosis may retard further deformity for some persons. Joints that are receptive to proper positioning may allow for optimal maintenance of range of motion (ROM).[59]

COMPONENTS OF THE RESTING HAND ORTHOSIS

The therapist must know the orthosis' components to make adjustments for a correct fit. Four main components constitute the resting hand orthosis: the forearm trough, the pan, the thumb trough, and the C bar (Fig. 9.5).[16]

Forearm troughs can be volar or dorsal based. The volar-based forearm trough at the proximal portion of the orthosis supports the weight of the forearm. Dorsally based forearm troughs are located on the dorsum of the forearm. The therapist applies biomechanical principles to make the trough approximately two-thirds the length of the forearm to distribute pressure of the hand and to allow elbow flexion when appropriate. The width is one-half the circumference of the forearm. The proximal end of the trough is flared or rolled to avoid a pressure area.

When a great amount of forearm support is desired, a volar-based forearm trough is the best design (Fig. 9.6). When the volar surface of the forearm must be avoided because of sutures, sores, rashes, or intravenous needles, a dorsally based forearm trough design is frequently used (Fig. 9.7). Dorsally based troughs are a beneficial design for applying a resting hand orthosis to a person with hypertonicity. The forearm trough is used as a lever to extend the wrist in addition to extending the fingers.

The pan of the orthosis supports the fingers and the palm. The therapist conforms the pan to the arches of the hand, thus helping to maintain such hand functions as grasping and cupping motions. The pan should be wide enough to house the width of the index, middle, ring, and little fingers when they are in a slightly abducted position. The sides of the pan should be curved so that they measure approximately ½ inch in height. The curved sides add strength to the pan and ensure that the

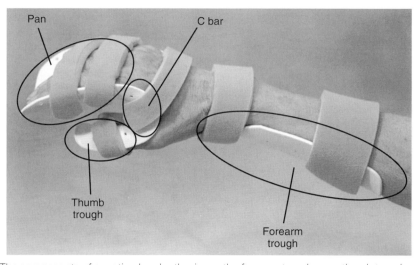

Fig. 9.5 The components of a resting hand orthosis are the forearm trough, pan, thumb trough, and C bar.

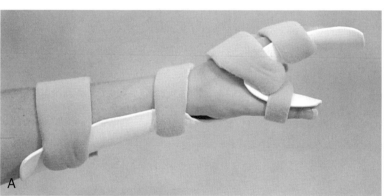

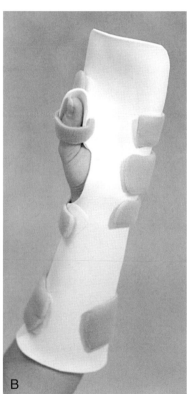

Fig. 9.6 Volar-based resting hand orthosis. A, Side view. B, Volar view.

fingers do not slide radially or ulnarly off the sides of the pan. However, if the pan's edges are too high, the positioning strap bridges over the fingers and fails to anchor them properly.

The thumb trough supports the thumb and should extend approximately ½ inch beyond the end of the thumb. This extension allows the entire thumb to rest in the trough. The width and depth of the thumb trough should be one-half the circumference of the thumb, which typically should be in a palmar abducted position. The therapist should attempt to position the carpometacarpal (CMC) joint in 40 to 45 degrees of palmar abduction[52] and extend the thumb's interphalangeal (IP) and metacarpal joints.

The C bar keeps the web space of the thumb positioned in palmar abduction. If the web space tightens, it inhibits cylindrical grasp and prevents the thumb from fully opposing the other digits. From the radial side of the orthosis, the thumb, the web space, and the digits should resemble a C (see Fig. 9.6).

RESTING HAND ORTHOSIS POSITIONS

Generally, two types of positioning are accomplished by a resting hand orthosis: a functional (midjoint) position and an antideformity (intrinsic plus) position. Diagnostic indication determines the general position used.

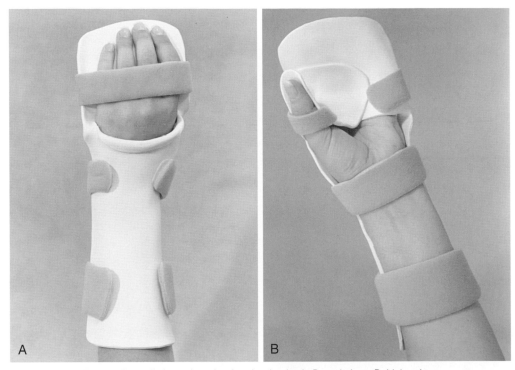

Fig. 9.7 Dorsally based resting hand orthosis. A, Dorsal view. B, Volar view.

Functional Position

To relieve stress on the wrist and hand joints, the resting hand orthosis positions the hand in a functional or midjoint position (Fig. 9.8). "The exact specifications of the functional position of the hand in a resting hand orthosis and the recommended joint positions vary."[24] One **functional position** that we suggest places the wrist in 20 to 30 degrees of extension, the thumb in 45 degrees of abduction (midway between palmar and radial abduction), the metacarpophalangeal (MCP) joints in 35 to 45 degrees of flexion, and all proximal interphalangeal (PIP) and distal interphalangeal (DIP) joints in slight flexion.

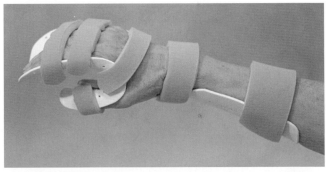

Fig. 9.8 A resting hand orthosis with the hand in a functional (midjoint) position.

Antideformity Position

The antideformity (also known as protected or safe) position is often used to place the hand in such a fashion as to maintain a tension/distraction of anatomical structures to avoid contracture and promote function. The **antideformity position** places the wrist in 15 to 20 degrees of extension, the thumb midway between radial and palmar abduction, the thumb IP joint in full extension, the MCPs at 50 to 80 degrees of flexion, and the PIPs and DIPs in full extension (Fig. 9.9).[55]

DIAGNOSTIC INDICATIONS

Several diagnostic categories may warrant the provision of a resting hand orthosis. Persons who require resting hand orthoses commonly have arthritis[2,12,37,39]; postoperative Dupuytren contracture release[13,41]; burn injuries to the hand[44], tendinitis, hemiplegic hand[40]; acquired brain injury[7]; hypertonic hand and wrist[33]; and tenosynovitis.[43] Table 9.2 lists evidence associated with hand orthoses related to a variety of diagnostic conditions.

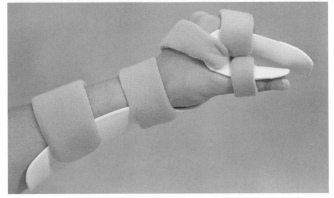

Fig. 9.9 A resting hand orthosis with the hand in an antideformity (intrinsic plus) position.

The resting hand orthosis maintains the hand in a functional or antideformity position, preserves a balance between extrinsic and intrinsic muscles, and provides localized rest to the tissues of the fingers, thumb, and wrist.[52] Although hand immobilization orthoses are commonly used, a paucity

TABLE 9.2   Evidence-Based Practice Related to Wrist Hand Orthoses

Author's Citation	Design	Number of Participants	Description	Results	Limitations
Arthritis					
Adams, J., Burridge, J., Mullee, M., et al. (2008). The clinical effectiveness of static resting splints in early rheumatoid arthritis: A randomized controlled trial. *Rheumatology, 47,* 1548–1553.	Prospective, randomized controlled trial	80	The purpose of this study was to determine the effectiveness of using static resting orthoses for patients with early stages of RA. All participants received occupational therapy treatment for their RA symptoms, including education in joint protection and hand and wrist exercises. The orthosis group was also provided with resting hand orthoses that positioned the hand in an intrinsic plus position to wear during periods of no activity.	No significant differences were noted in grip strength, MCP ulnar deviation, or pain level. One key area of difference was the patients' reported experience of morning stiffness. The orthosis group had a significantly lower number of patients reporting morning stiffness.	Limitations of this study include the fact that early stages of RA can cause difficulty with establishing effectiveness of an intervention, due to the likelihood that a condition was poorly controlled. Medication was considered in the results, but a second limitation is that it may have had a significant role in condition management between groups. The duration of the study may not have been long enough. Finally, there may be a better design for the orthoses used in the intervention.
Feinberg, J., & Brandt, K. D. (1981). Use of resting splints by patients with rheumatoid arthritis. *American Journal of Occupational Therapy, 35*(3), 173–178.	Retrospective study	50	50 patients with RA who had previously used an orthosis were identified for follow-up visits. The patients were identified as "compliant," meaning that they wore the orthosis 50% of the time or more, or "noncompliant," indicating they wore the orthosis less than 50% of the time. Factors that were addressed in this study included the effect of the orthosis on adherence to an orthosis-wearing schedule, as well as amounts of pain, morning stiffness, and ROM.	31 of 50 participants were deemed compliant, wearing their orthosis 50% or more of the time recommended by the therapist. Greatest compliance was found to be in patients between the ages of 40 and 70, as well as individuals who had been diagnosed with RA for 2 years or less. Overall most patients felt some benefit from wearing the orthoses, particularly during the initial phase of orthosis use. Long-term use of orthoses for pain management varied, depending on the patient's symptoms of RA.	Limitations of this study include the fact that orthoses were not of uniform design; they had been modified for the comfort of each patient. Additionally, there was a wide range of time from initial fitting of orthoses to the follow-up appointment (between 3 months and 34 months). A final limitation that may have affected results of this study was that there was a wide range of time since the patient had been diagnosed with RA.
Hand Burns					
Whitehead, C., & Serghiou, M. (2009). A 12-year comparison of common therapeutic interventions in the burn unit. *Journal of Burn Care & Research, 30*(2), 281–287.	Survey of 100 burn care facilities in the United States and Canada. Data collected included interventions (evaluation, positioning, orthoses, AROM, PROM, ambulation, and cross-training of therapists).	52 burn centers responded to survey	The survey to burn centers included responses from 61 occupational therapists and 75 physical therapists. Categories of the survey included: evaluation, positioning, orthoses, AROM, PROM, ambulation, and cross-training of therapists.	Regarding orthotic intervention, results show 95% of centers position patients with burns within 24 h of admission. Orthotic application is completed with 24 h of admission by 61% of centers. 73% reported they fabricate and apply orthoses in the operating room.	Respondents noted it was difficult to answer questions with a typical case scenario. No data were collected on the specific types or positions of orthoses.

Continued

Author's Citation	Design	Number of Participants	Description	Results	Limitations
Dupuytren Contracture					
Jerosch-Herold, C., Shepstone, L., Choinowski, A., J., et al. (2011). Night-time splinting after fasciectomy or dermo-fasciectomy for Dupuytren's contracture: A pragmatic, multi-centre, randomized controlled trial, *BMC Musculoskeletal Disorders, 12,* 136–144.	Prospective study	154	The purpose of this study was to evaluate the effectiveness of a night orthosis on function, finger extension, and patient satisfaction. Patients from five regional hospitals were randomized to receive hand therapy only or hand therapy plus using an orthosis at night.	This study found that there was no statistically significant difference in the recovery of patients who received the orthosis to use at nighttime and the patients who received hand therapy only.	Limitations of this study include the fact that the primary measure of outcome was based on patient report, and neither the patients nor the researchers assessing secondary outcomes were blinded.
Tone Reduction					
McPherson, J. J., Kreimeyer, D., Aalderks, M., et al. (1982). A comparison of dorsal and volar resting hand splints in the reduction of hypertonus. *American Journal of Occupational Therapy, 36(10),* 664–670.	Prospective study	10	The purpose of this study was to compare the effectiveness of dorsal- and volar-based resting hand orthoses on reducing abnormal muscle tone. All participants had hypertonus wrist flexors as sequelae of either a cerebrovascular accident, traumatic brain injury, or cerebral palsy.	This study found that both the dorsal- and volar-based resting hand orthoses were effective in reducing the amount of hypertonus. The group who wore the dorsal orthoses experienced a reduction of hypertonus equal to 7.25 lb of pull, and the volar-based orthoses resulted in a reduction of hypertonus equal to 7.0 lb of pull. This difference in reduction of hypertonus is not statistically significant.	Limitations of this study include the small sample size and the use of a measurement technique that does not "measure the hyper-reflexive status of the neuromuscular spindle" (p. 668).
Constraint-Induced Movement Therapy					
Uswatte, G., Taub, E., Morris, D., et al. (2006). Contribution of the shaping and restraint components of constraint-induced movement therapy to treatment outcome. *NeuroRehabilitation, 21(2),* 147–156.	Prospective study	17	The purpose of this study was to examine how various types of training (task-practice) and restraint (sling, half-glove, no restraint) affected outcomes of occupational therapy treatment. Participants were divided into four groups (sling and task practice, sling and shaping, half-glove and shaping, shaping only). Participants in the sling group had their less-affected arm placed in a resting hand orthosis/sling during the waking hours.	Results indicate that participants from all groups improved use of the more-impaired arm and experienced a reduction in time to complete bilateral tasks as a result of task training and restraint intervention. Immediately post treatment, no significant difference in assessment results was detected between the four groups. Two years following treatment, the sling and task participants demonstrated larger gains in assessment results as compared to the remaining groups.	After posttreatment assessment, different training intensity was given to the half-glove and shaping group than was given to the sling and shaping group. This may have altered the results of the 2-year follow-up assessment. A second limitation is that task-practice contains some important aspects of shaping. A third limitation is that the level of compliance with wearing the restraints was measured by self-report of the participants. Finally, the sample sizes of the groups in this study were small.

TABLE 9.2 Evidence-Based Practice Related to Wrist Hand Orthoses—cont'd

Author's Citation	Design	Number of Participants	Description	Results	Limitations
Acquired Brain Injury—Hypertonicity (Spasticity and Stiffness)					
Copley, J., Kuipers, K., Fleming, J., et al. (2013). Individualised resting hand splints for adults with acquired brain injury: A randomized, single blinded, single case design. *NeuroRehabilitation, 32.* 885–898.	Randomized, single-blinded, single-case design	10 Age range 18–80 y	5 patients in control group received no orthosis, and 5 patients in experimental group received an individualized resting hand orthosis. Measures included (1) PROM of wrist and fingers, (2) wrist and finger flexor muscles stiffness using the Modified Ashworth Scale of muscle spasticity, and (3) wrist and finger flexor muscle spasticity using the Modified Tardieu Scale of muscle spasticity.	Individualized resting hand orthoses provided to people with moderate hypertonicity and no contractures resulted positive effects for PROM, muscle stiffness, and spasticity.	Small sample size.

AROM, Active range of motion; *MCP,* metacarpophalangeal; *PROM,* passive range of motion; *RA,* rheumatoid arthritis; *ROM,* range of motion.

of literature exists on their efficacy. Thus it is a ripe area for future research. Therapists should consider the resting hand orthosis as a legitimate intervention for appropriate conditions despite the lack of evidence.

Rheumatoid Arthritis

Therapists often provide resting hand orthoses for people with RA during periods of acute inflammation and pain that require support and immobilization[3,34,59] for wear when their hands are not needed for activities.[25] The biomechanical rationale for orthotic intervention of acutely inflamed joints is to reduce pain by relieving stress and muscle spasms. However, it may not additionally prevent deformity.[3,14]

Typical joint placement in an orthosis for a person with RA is to position the wrist in 10 degrees of extension, the thumb in palmar abduction, the MCP joints in 35 to 45 degrees of flexion, and all the PIP and DIP joints in slight flexion.[35] For a person who has severe deformities or exacerbations from arthritis, the resting hand orthosis may also position the wrist at neutral or slight extension and 5 to 10 degrees of ulnar deviation.[17,29] The thumb may be positioned midway between radial and palmar abduction to increase comfort. These joint angles are ideal. Therapists use clinical judgment to determine what joint angles are positions of comfort for orthotic intervention.

Note that wrist extension varies from the typical 30 degrees of extension. When the wrist is in slight extension, the carpal tunnel is open—as opposed to being narrowed, with 30 degrees of extension.[35] Finger spacers may be used in the pan to provide comfort and to prevent finger slippage in the orthosis.[35] Finger spacers should not be used to passively correct ulnar deformity because of the risk for pressure areas.[35] In addition, once the orthosis is removed, there is no evidence that orthotic wear alters the deformity. However, it may prevent further deformity.

Acute Rheumatoid Arthritis

In persons who have acute RA the use of orthoses for purposes of rest during pain and inflammation is controversial.[12,34] Periods of rest (3 weeks or less) seem to be beneficial, but longer periods may cause loss of motion.[37] Persons with acute exacerbations wear orthoses full-time except for short periods of gentle ROM exercise and hygiene.[38] Biese[3] recommends that persons wear orthoses at night and part-time during the day. In addition, persons may find it beneficial to wear orthoses at night for several weeks after the acute inflammation subsides.[4]

Chronic Rheumatoid Arthritis

When the therapist provides an orthosis for a joint with chronic RA, the rationale is often based on biomechanical factors. "Theoretically, by realigning and redistributing the damaging internal and external forces acting on the joint, the orthosis may help to prevent deformity…or improve joint function and functional use of the extremity."[14] Therapists who provide orthoses to persons with chronic RA should be aware that prolonged use of a resting hand orthosis may also be harmful.[14] Studies on animals indicate that immobilization leads to decreased bone mass and strength, degeneration of cartilage, increase in joint capsule adhesions, weakness in tendon and ligament strength, and muscle atrophy.[14]

In addition to orthotic intervention, persons with RA benefit from a combination of management of inflammation, education in joint protection, muscle strengthening, ROM maintenance, and pain reduction.[14,27,38] Persons in late stages of RA who have skeletal collapse and deformity may benefit from the support of an orthosis during activities and at nighttime.[3,5] For example, a wrist or thumb orthosis might benefit the person during daytime activities and a resting hand orthosis for nighttime.

Compliance of persons with RA in wearing resting hand orthoses has been estimated at approximately 50%.[15] The degree to which a person's compliance with an orthotic-wearing schedule affects the disease outcome is unknown. However, research indicates that some persons with RA who wore their orthoses only at times of symptom exacerbation did not demonstrate negative outcomes in relation to ROM or deformities.[15]

Wearing schedules for resting hand orthoses vary depending on the diagnostic condition, orthotic purpose, and physician order (Table 9.3). Persons with RA often wear resting hand orthoses at night. A person who has RA may also wear a resting hand orthosis during the day for additional rest but should remove the orthosis at least once each day for hygiene and appropriate exercises. A person who has bilateral hand orthoses may choose to wear alternate orthoses each night.

Hand Burns

Burn care requires a team approach.[48] Occupational and physical therapists provide the orthotic and exercise interventions.[48] Despite the hands accounting for a small percentage of total body surface, they can have devastating effects on function.[55] Not all persons who sustain hand burns require an orthosis. Orthotic provision depends on burn depth degree as well as the person's tolerance for orthoses and overall therapy.[11] Initial evaluations are typically conducted in the first 48 to 72 hours after admission to a burn unit and/or hospital.[58] The timing of orthotic intervention for burns is important. Due to the contractile nature of scar tissue, the question to consider is if prophylactic orthotic intervention is necessary.[58] Literature suggests that the majority of therapists initiate orthotic intervention within the first 24 hours for burned hands and wrists.[58] Often the first orthotic intervention is provided within operating rooms.

Therapists do not position the person in the functional position after a hand burn. Instead, the therapist places the hand in the intrinsic plus or antideformity position[44] (see Fig. 9.9). The literature cites 43 orthoses to position the dorsally burned hand joints.[43] Despite the wide range of orthotic designs that exist for dorsal hand burns, it is common practice to use the antideformity position for acute hand burns.[43,58]

Positioning varies, depending on the surface of the hand that is burned. In general, the goal of providing an orthosis in the antideformity position is to prevent deformity by keeping structures whose length allows motion from shortening.

TABLE 9.3   Conditions That Require a Resting Hand Orthosis

Diagnosis	Suggested Wearing Schedule	Position
Rheumatoid Arthritis		
Acute exacerbation[a]	Fitted to maintain as close to a functional (midjoint) position as possible until exacerbation is over. Removed for hygiene and exercise purposes and worn during the day and at nighttime as necessary. Finger deformities must be taken into consideration if present.	• Wrist: Neutral or 20–30 degrees of extension depending on person's tolerance, 15–20 degrees of MCP flexion, all the PIP and DIP joints in slight flexion, and 5–10 degrees of ulnar deviation • Thumb: Position of comfort in between radial and palmar abduction
Hand Burns		
Dorsal or volar hand burns[a]	Generally, worn immediately after the burn injury. Continuously worn until healing begins and removed for dressing changes, hygiene, and exercises.	• Wrist: Volar or circumferential burn (15–30 degrees of extension), dorsal burn (0 degrees = neutral) • MCPs: Flexion of 50–80 degrees • PIP and DIP: Full extension • Thumb: Palmar abduction and extension
Acute phase	Initially, worn at all times except for therapy. Monitor fit for fluctuations in bandage bulk and edema. As ROM improves, decrease wearing time to allow for participation in activities.	Position as close to the previously indicated position as possible.
Skin graft phase	Worn after skin graft at all times for 5 days or with physician's order for removal.	Position as close to antideformity position as possible.
Rehabilitation phase	Orthosis worn during nighttime to maintain ROM. Wear should be limited during daytime to allow for participation in activities.	Position joints to oppose deforming forces.
Dupuytren disease contractures[a]	Worn after surgery and removed for hygiene and exercise. Worn at nighttime.	• Wrist: Neutral or slight extension • MCP, PIP, and DIPs: Full extension
Trauma		
Crush injuries of the hand	Fitted after the injury to reduce pain and edema and to prevent shortening of critical tissue and contracture formation. Worn at nighttime, and possibly worn as necessary during painful periods.	• Wrist: Extension of 0–30 degrees • MCPs: Extension of 60–80 degrees • PIP and DIPs: Full extension • Thumb: Palmar abduction and extension
Complex regional pain syndrome (CRPS)	Orthosis is worn at all times, initially with removal for therapy, hygiene, and ADLs (if possible). Person should be weaned from orthosis with pain reduction and improved motion.	Adjust to a position of comfort with the ideal position being (The orthosis should not cause more pain.): • Wrist: 20 degrees of extension, thumb in palmar abduction • MCPs: 70 degrees of flexion • PIPs: 0–10 degrees of extension
Acquired brain injury	2–4 h during the day; overnight wear if clients report wrist or finger tightness or malaligned posture while in bed. Consider discontinued use after 3 months.	Positioning should be individualized to place hypertonic muscles groups on low-load, prolonged stretch. Typically the wrist is 20 degrees extension. A more conservative position between 10 degrees of flexion and 20 degrees of wrist flexion may be used with signs of the wrist flexing out of the orthosis, fingers clawing into the orthosis, blanching of fingernails, hyperextension of the MCPs or IPs.

[a]Diagnosis may require additional types of orthotic intervention.
ADLs, Activities of daily living; *DIP,* distal interphalangeal; *MCP,* metacarpophalangeal; *PIP,* proximal interphalangeal; *ROM,* range of motion.

These structures are the collateral ligaments of the MCPs, the volar plates of the IPs, and the wrist capsule and ligaments. The dorsal skin of the hand maintains its length in the antideformity position. The thumb web space is also vulnerable to remodeling in a shortened form in the presence of inflammation and if tension of the structure is absent.

Experts in hand rehabilitation suggest the antideformity position for a palmar or circumferential burn places the wrist in 15 to 30 degrees of extension and 0 degrees (i.e., neutral) for a dorsal hand burn. For dorsal and volar burns the therapist should flex the MCPs into 50 to 80 degrees, fully extend the PIP joints and DIP joints, and place the thumb midway between radial and palmar abduction.[11,55] After a burn injury the thumb web space is at risk for developing an adduction contracture.[53] Therefore the position of choice for the thumb is midway between radial and palmar abduction, if tolerated.

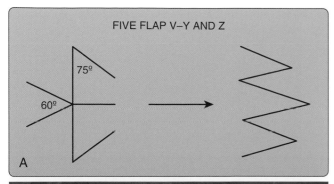

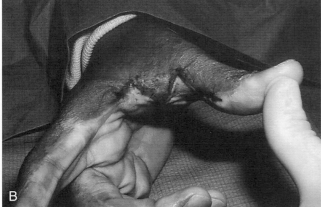

Fig. 9.10 A, B, Z-plasty to lengthen contracted web space. (From Simpson, R. L. [2011]. Management of burns of the upper extremity. In T. M. Skirven, A. L. Osterman, & J. M. Fedorczyk, et al. [Eds.], *Rehabilitation of the hand and upper extremity* [6th ed., p. 312]. St. Louis: Mosby.)

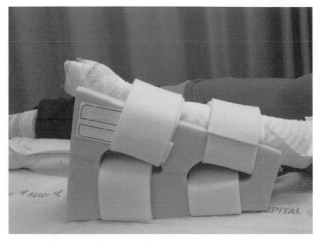

Fig. 9.11 Foam wedge to position for edema management. (From Tufaro, P. A., & Bondoc, S. L. [2011]. Therapist's management of the burned hand. In T. M. Skirven, A. L. Osterman, & J. M. Fedorczyk, et al. [Eds.], *Rehabilitation of the hand and upper extremity* [6th ed., p. 320]. St. Louis: Mosby.)

In cases in which the thumb index web space is contracted, a Z-plasty surgery may be performed[48] (Fig. 9.10). These joint angles are ideal. Some persons with burns may not initially tolerate these joint positions, and the hand should never be forced into the perfect intrinsic plus position.[11] When tolerable, the resting hand orthosis for the person who has hand burns can be adjusted more closely to the ideal position. As healing occurs, the orthosis is modified to maintain the palmar arches of the hand.[49] Stages of burn recovery should be considered with orthotic intervention. The phases of recovery are emergent, acute, skin grafting, and rehabilitation.

Emergent Phase

The emergent phase is the first 24 to 72 postburn hours.[55] From 8 to 12 hours after the burn, dorsal edema occurs and encourages wrist flexion, MCP joint hyperextension, and IP joint flexion.[10,55] Edema peaks up to 36 hours after the burn injury and begins to dissipate after 1 or 2 days. Usually the edema is resolved by 7 to 10 days after injury; however, destruction of the dorsal veins or lymphatic vessels may result in chronic edema.[55] Static orthosis intervention is initiated during the emergent phase to support the hand and maintain the length of vulnerable structures.[10] Positioning to counteract the forces of edema includes placing the wrist in 15 to 20 degrees of extension, the MCP joints in 70 to 90 degrees of flexion, and the PIP and DIP joints in full extension with the thumb positioned midway between palmar and radial

abduction and with the IP joint slightly flexed.[55] Positioning is important during the emergent phase.[55] Elevation of the extremity above the heart level can result in decreased arterial supply to the hand.[55] Additionally, excessive weight bearing on the olecranon of elbow should be avoided to prevent undue stress on the ulnar nerve. A foam wedge in which the forearm can rest assists in controlling edema to the hand (Fig. 9.11).

Children may sustain hand burns for many reasons, such as from a from fire, steam via vaporizers.[26] contact with a treadmill,[36] and glass-fronted fireplaces.[54] For children with dorsal hand burns, during the emergent phase the MCP joints may not need to be flexed as far as 60 to 70 degrees. For children under the age of 3 years, therapists may not need to provide an orthosis, unless it is determined that the wrist requires support.[9] Young children who have burned hands may not need orthoses because the bulky dressings applied to the burned hand may provide adequate support. If a child is age 3 years or older, orthotic intervention should be considered.

For any clients with hand burns a prefabricated resting hand orthosis in an antideformity position can be applied if a therapist cannot immediately construct a custom-made orthosis.[10] Prefabricated orthoses may be appropriate for superficial burns with edema for the first 3 to 5 days. For full-thickness burns with excessive edema, custom-made orthoses are necessary.[10,55] An orthosis applied in the first 72 hours after a burn may not fit the person 2 hours after application because of the significant edema that usually follows a burn injury.

The therapist closely monitors the person to make necessary adjustments to the orthosis. When fabricating a custom orthosis for a person with excessive edema, a therapist avoids forcing wrist and hand joints into the ideal position and risking ischemia from damaged capillaries.[10] With edema reduction, serial orthotic intervention may be necessary as digit, wrist, and hand ROM is gained toward the ideal position. Serial resting hand orthoses for persons with burns should conform to the person, rather than conforming persons to the orthoses.[10]

Persons with hand burns have bandages covering burn sites. "As layers of bandage around the hand increase, accommodation for the increased bandage thickness must be accounted for in the [orthotic] design, if it is to fit correctly."[42] To correct for bandage thickness the orthosis' bend corresponding to MCP flexion in the pan is formed more proximally.[42] Thus if commercially available orthoses are used initially, due to therapist time constraints, the forearm troughs will likely need to be pried open to increase their width to accommodate the hand's edema and bandage thickness.[55] For persons who are conscious, bandage changes and orthotic changes can be painful. Consider offering distractions to the person such as watching television or engaging with virtual reality and gaming devices.[55]

The initial orthotic provision for a person with hand burns is applied with gauze rather than straps. The gauze reduces the risk of compromising circulation. Soiled gauze is discarded during donning and doffing the orthosis. New gauze is applied for purposes of infection control. Orthoses on adults are removed for exercise, hygiene, and appropriate functional tasks. For children, orthoses are removed for exercise, hygiene, and play activities.[10]

Acute Phase

The acute phase begins after the emergent phase and lasts until wound closure.[10] Once edema begins to decrease, serial adjustments are made to the orthosis. Therefore it is advantageous to use thermoplastic material with memory properties. During the acute phase, therapists monitor the direction of deforming forces and adjust the existing orthosis or design an additional orthosis to "orient the collagen being deposited during the early stages of wound healing as well as maintain joint alignment."[9]

Healing wounds are also monitored, and the orthoses are evaluated for fit and for correct donning and doffing. As ROM is improved, the orthotic-wearing schedule is decreased during the day to provide time for activities that require hand use. If the person is unwilling or uncooperative in participating in self-care and supervised activities, the orthosis is worn continuously to prevent contractures. It is important for persons to wear orthoses at nighttime.

Skin Graft Phase

Before a skin graft, it is crucial to obtain full ROM. After the skin graft the site needs to be immobilized for 3 to 5 days postoperatively.[10,55] Usually an antideformity position resting hand orthosis is appropriate. The orthosis is often applied in the operating room or bedside to ensure immobilization of the graft.

Rehabilitation Phase

The rehabilitation phase occurs after wound closure or graft adherence until scar maturation.[10] The intervention goal for orthotic provision at this stage is to prevent contracture. Contractures from volar burns are wrist flexion, MP and IP flexion, and thumb adduction. Contractures from dorsal burns are wrist extension or flexion, MP and IP extension, and thumb adduction.[11] Throughout the person's rehabilitation after a burn, orthoses are donned over an extremity covered with a pressure garment. Orthoses may be used in conjunction with materials that manage scar formation, including silicone gel sheeting or elastomer/elastomer putty inserts. During

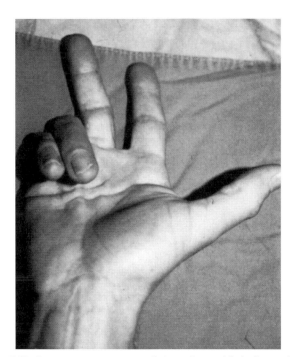

Fig. 9.12 Dupuytren contracture of the palm and little finger. Note the nodules and cord. (From Hurst L. [2011]. Dupuytren's disease: surgical management. In T. M. Skirven, A. L. Osterman, & J. M. Fedorczyk, et al. [Eds.], *Rehabilitation of the hand and upper extremity* [6th ed., p. 267]. St. Louis: Mosby.)

the rehabilitation phase, static (immobilization) and dynamic (mobilization) orthotic intervention may be needed. Plaster or synthetic material casting may also be considered.[9]

Persons commonly wear resting hand orthoses during the healing stages of burns. After wounds heal, persons may wear day orthoses with pressure garments or elastomer molds to increase ROM and to control scarring. In addition to daytime orthoses, it is important for the person to wear a resting hand orthosis at night to maintain maximum elongation of the healing skin and provide rest and functional alignment.

Dupuytren Disease

Dupuytren disease is a benign fibromatosis characterized by the formation of finger flexion contracture(s) with a thickened band of palmar and digital fascia.[19,30] Palpable nodules first develop in the distal palmar crease, usually in line with the finger(s). Slowly the condition matures into a longitudinal cord that is readily distinguishable from a tendon (Fig. 9.12).[19,30] In addition, pain and decreased ROM are the primary symptoms that often lead to impaired functional performance.[21] Dupuytren contractures are common and often severe in persons of Northern European origin. However, this disorder is present in most ethnic groups.[30] Epilepsy, diabetes mellitus, smoking, acquired immunodeficiency syndrome (AIDS), vascular disorders, and alcoholism are associated with Dupuytren contracture.[19,21,30,51] Persons with Dupuytren diathesis (a more aggressive form of the disease) often are male and have a family history of the disease, bilateral involvement, and lesions (e.g., plantar fibromatosis), with onset usually younger than 50 years.[18]

When a **Dupuytren contracture** is apparent, stretching or orthotic intervention that positions joints in extension does

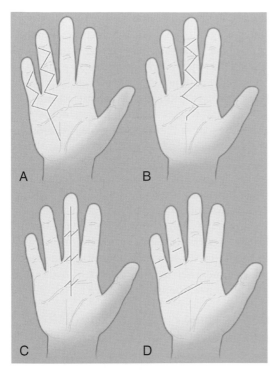

Fig. 9.13 Four basic skin incision patterns for Dupuytren fasciectomy. A, Zigzag. B, Littler-Brunner. C, Longitudinal. D, Transverse (open palm technique). (From Hurst L. [2011]. Dupuytren's disease: surgical management. In T. M. Skirven, A. L. Osterman, & J. M. Fedorczyk, et al. [Eds.], *Rehabilitation of the hand and upper extremity* [6th ed., p. 273]. St. Louis: Mosby.)

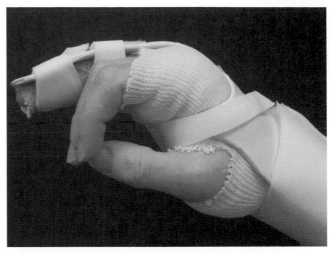

Fig. 9.14 Dorsal static protective orthosis for immediate wear post fasciectomy. The design allows for flexion, but not metacarpophalangeal (MCP) joint extension, in a controlled range preventing neurovascular and wound tension. The person exercises within the orthosis, strapping the interphalangeal (IP) joints to the dorsal hood between exercise sessions. (From Evans, R. B. [2011]. Therapeutic management of Dupuytren's contracture. In T. M. Skirven, A. L. Osterman, & J. M. Fedorczyk, et al. [Eds.], *Rehabilitation of the hand and upper extremity* [6th ed.]. St. Louis: Mosby.)

not delay the progression of the contracture.[19,30] However, recent studies indicate that injections of collagenase *Clostridium histolyticum* (CCH) are effective and safe interventions to reduce Dupuytren disease nodules.[8,45,46] Some research shows that an injection of CCH reduces the palmar nodule size and hardness.[8]

Surgery is performed to release severe Dupuytren contractures. Although surgery does not cure the disease, it is often indicated in the presence of painful nodules; uncomfortable induration (hardness); and MCP, PIP, or DIP joint contractures.[19,31] Surgical procedures to treat Dupuytren disease include fasciotomy, regional fasciectomy, and dermofasciectomy.[19,31,41] Fasciectomy options include open, closed, needle, and enzymatic.[19] Four incision patterns are used for Dupuytren fasciectomies (Fig. 9.13). The incision patterns include zigzag plasty, Littler-Bruner, Z-plasty, and transverse incisions. Most Dupuytren release surgeries are completed in an ambulatory or day surgery setting.[19]

Longitudinal follow-up studies report a recurrence after surgery is 100%.[32] Intermediate results of surgery may vary, depending on the affected joint.[30] For example, the MCP joint has a single fascial cord that is relatively easy to release. The PIP joint has four fascial cords that are difficult to release. In addition, the soft tissue around the PIP joint may contract and pull the joint into flexion, and components of the extensor mechanism may adhere to surrounding structures. The PIP joint of the little finger is the most difficult to correct. Flexion contractures at the DIP joint are uncommon but are difficult to correct for the same reasons as the PIP joint contracture. Contractures of the web spaces may be present, limiting the

motion of adjacent fingers. Web space contractures may also result in poor hygiene between the fingers.

Therapy and orthotic intervention begin 24 hours after surgery.[13] Postoperative orthotic intervention may include the fabrication of a dorsal static protective orthosis (Fig. 9.14).[13] The dorsal static protective orthosis positions the wrist at neutral, the MCP joints at 35 to 45 degrees of flexion, and the IP joints in relaxed extension.[13] Note that the digits receiving surgery release are the only digits included in the orthosis. The thumb is positioned in mild abduction if the first web space was a surgical site. Some therapists and physicians prefer a resting hand orthosis post Dupuytren release; the wrist is placed in a neutral or slightly flexed position. The MCP, PIP, and DIP joints are positioned in full extension. If the thumb is involved, it is incorporated into the orthosis. However, the uninvolved thumb usually does not need to be immobilized in the orthosis. Therefore the orthosis will not have a thumb trough component (Fig. 9.15). The thumb may be incorporated into the orthosis, particularly when the adjacent index finger has been released from a contracture. Note that the dorsal static protective orthosis is a no-tension approach to orthotic intervention. The protective orthosis is worn for 3 weeks. Daytime wear is discontinued. Then a volar hand-based extension orthosis (Fig. 9.16) with straps positioned over the MCP and PIP joints to maintain or improve extension is provided, and the person wears this orthosis during nighttime.[13]

Traditionally after a surgical release of a Dupuytren contracture, the person wears the initial orthosis continuously during both day and night with removal for hygiene and exercise. The orthosis is worn until the wounds completely heal. Orthoses are worn longer in the presence of a PIP contracture release. As the risk of losing ROM dissipates, the person may be weaned from orthotic use. Researchers reported that "no differences were observed in self-reported upper limb disability or active ROM between a group of patients who were all routinely

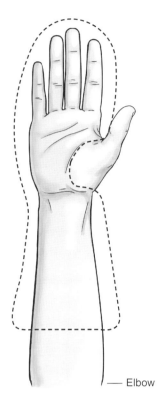

— Elbow

Fig. 9.15 A pattern for a resting hand orthosis after surgical release of Dupuytren contracture. Note that the thumb is not incorporated into the orthotic design.

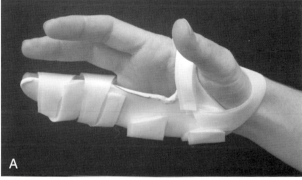

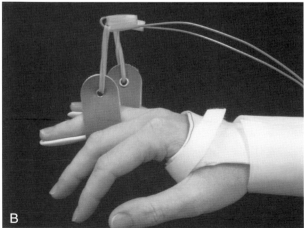

Fig. 9.16 A, Dynamic extension orthosis can be used during the day during weeks 2–4 for more difficult cases. B, A volar hand-based extension orthosis with straps over the metacarpophalangeal (MCP) and proximal interphalangeal (PIP) joints is used to maintain or improve extension. (From Evans, R. B. [2011]. Therapeutic management of Dupuytren's contracture. In T. M. Skirven, A. L. Osterman, & J. M. Fedorczyk, et al. [Eds.], *Rehabilitation of the hand and upper extremity* [6th ed.]. St. Louis: Mosby.)

splinted after surgery and a group of patients receiving hand therapy and only splinted if and when contractures occurred. Given the added expense of therapists' time, thermoplastic materials and the potential inconvenience to patients having to wear a device, the routine additional of night-time splinting for all patients after fasciectomy or dermofasciectomy is not recommended except where extension deficits occur"[20] (p. 136). Finally, orthoses other than a resting hand orthosis, such as volar or dorsal hand-based orthosis, for people with less extensive surgical procedures may be appropriate.[39]

Therapists working with persons who undergo a Dupuytren release must be aware of possible complications. Complications include excessive inflammation, wound infection, abnormal scar formation, joint contractures, stiffness, pain, and CRPS.[13,41] Occasionally in severe cases with complications, mobilization orthoses can be used when MCP and PIP joint extension are unsatisfactory and when multiple digit static orthoses are difficult for the person to don independently.[13]

Complex Regional Pain Syndrome (Reflex Sympathetic Dystrophy)

Complex regional pain syndrome (CRPS) is a term that describes posttraumatic pain that manifests by "inappropriate automatic activity and impaired extremity function."[22] Typical symptoms include the following[22]:

- Pain: Out of proportional intensity to the injury, often described as throbbing, burning, cutting, searing, and shooting
- Skin color changes: Blotchy, purple, pale, or red
- Skin temperature changes: Warmer or cooler compared with contralateral side
- Skin texture changes: Thin, shiny, and sometimes excessively sweaty
- Swelling and stiffness
- Decreased ability to move the affected body part

There are two types of CRPS. CRPS type I is usually triggered by tissue injury. The term applies to all persons with the symptoms listed previously but with no underlying peripheral nerve injury. CRPS type II is associated with the symptoms in the presence of a peripheral nerve injury.

The goal of rehabilitation for persons with CRPS is to eliminate one of the three etiological factors: pain, diathesis, and abnormal sympathetic reflex.[23,57] This is accomplished by minimizing ROM and strength losses, managing edema, and providing pain management so that the therapist can maximize function and provide activities of daily living (ADLs) and instrumental activities of daily living (IADLs) training for independence. The physician may be able to intervene with medications and nerve blocks.

As part of a comprehensive therapy regimen for CRPS, a resting hand orthosis may initially provide rest to the hand, reduce pain, and relieve muscle spasm.[23,57] Orthotic intervention during the presence of CRPS should be of a low force that does not exacerbate the pain or irritate the tissues.[56] Walsh and Muntzer[56] recommend that the resting hand orthosis position for the person be in 20 degrees of wrist extension, palmar abduction of the thumb, 70 degrees of MCP joint flexion, and 0 to 10 degrees of PIP joint extension. This is an ideal position, which persons with CRPS may not tolerate. Above all, therapists working with persons who have CRPS should avoid causing pain. Therefore the hand should be positioned in a position of comfort. Orthoses other than a resting hand orthosis may also be appropriate for this diagnostic population. (See Chapter 7 for a discussion of wrist orthotic intervention for CRPS.)

Resting hand orthoses provided to persons with CRPS are initially to be worn at all times with removal for therapy, hygiene, and (if possible) ADLs. As pain reduction and motion improvement occur, the amount of time that the person wears the orthosis is decreased.

Hand Crush Injury

To provide an orthosis for a crushed hand, position the wrist in 0 to 30 degrees of extension, the MCPs in 60 to 80 degrees of flexion, the PIPs and DIPs in full extension, and the thumb in palmar abduction and extension.[6] Placing a crushed hand into this position provides rest to the injured tissue and decreases pain, edema, and inflammation.[50]

Other Conditions

Resting hand orthoses are appropriate "for protecting tendons, joints, capsular and ligamentous structures."[25] These diagnoses usually require the expertise of experienced therapists and may warrant different orthoses for daytime wear and resting hand orthoses for nighttime use.

Therapists sometimes provide resting hand orthoses for persons who have increased tone or spasticity following a stroke or traumatic brain injury and who are at risk for developing contractures.[7,28] (See Chapter 15 for more information on orthotic intervention for a person who has an extremity with increased tone or spasticity.) Table 9.3 lists common hand conditions that may require a resting hand orthosis and includes information regarding suggested hand positioning and orthotic-wearing schedules. Beginning therapists should remember that these are general guidelines, and physicians and experienced therapists may have their own specific protocols for orthotic positioning and wearing.

FABRICATION OF A RESTING HAND ORTHOSIS

Beginning orthotic makers may learn to fabricate orthotic patterns by following detailed written instructions, by looking at pictures of orthotic patterns, or by looking at a ready-made sample. As beginners gain more experience, they will easily draw orthotic patterns without having to follow detailed instructions or pictures. Steps for fabricating a resting hand orthosis can be found in the following procedure. The therapist must also be sure to teach the wearer or caregiver to clean the orthosis when open wounds with exudate are present (Box 9.1).

PRECAUTIONS FOR A RESTING HAND ORTHOSIS

The therapist should take precautions when applying an orthosis to a person. If the diagnosis permits, the therapist should instruct the person to remove the orthosis for a ROM schedule to prevent stiffness and control edema.

BOX 9.1   Cleaning Techniques for Orthoses to Control Infection

During Orthotic Fabrication

1. After cutting a pattern from the thermoplastic material, re-immerse the plastic in hot water.
2. Remove and spray with quaternary ammonia cleaning solution.
3. Place the orthosis between two clean cloths to maintain heat and reduce the microorganism contamination from handling the material.
4. Use gloves when molding the orthosis to the person. Latex gloves are recommended. Vinyl gloves adhere to the plastic.

Donning an Orthosis in the Operating Room

Follow steps 1 through 4.

Clean the orthosis after the fit evaluation is completed, and place in a clean cloth during transportation.

Transport the orthosis only when the person receiving the orthosis is in the operating room.

Keep the orthosis in the clean cloth until it is needed in the operating room. The orthosis in the cloth should be kept off sterile surfaces in the operating room.

When the person leaves the operating room, all orthoses should be taken with him or her to the appropriate recovery room.

Data from Wright, M. P., Taddonio, T. E., Prasad, J. K., et al. The microbiology and cleaning of thermoplastic splints in burn care. *Journal of Burn Care & Rehabilitation, 10*(1), 79–83, 1989.

- The therapist monitors the person for pressure areas from the orthosis. With burns and other conditions resulting in open wounds, the therapist adjusts the orthosis frequently as bandage bulk changes.
- To prevent infection the therapist teaches the person or caregiver to clean the orthosis when open wounds with exudate are present. After removing the orthosis, the person or caregiver cleans it with warm soapy water, hydrogen peroxide, or rubbing alcohol and dries it with a clean cloth (see Box 9.1). Rubbing alcohol may be the most effective for removing skin cells, perspiration, dirt, and exudate.
- For a resting hand orthosis for a person in an intensive care unit (ICU), supplies and tools must be kept as sterile as possible. Careful planning about supply needs before going into the unit helps prevent repetitious trips. Enlist the help of a second person, aide, or therapist to assist with the orthotic process. The therapist working in a sterile environment follows the facility's protocol on universal precautions and body substance procedures. Prepackaged sterilized equipment can be used for orthotic provision. Alternatively, any equipment that can withstand the heat from an autoclave can be used.
- Depending on facility regulations, various actions may be taken to ensure optimal wear and care of an orthosis. The therapist considers the appropriate posting of the wearing schedule in the person's room. This precaution is especially helpful when others are involved in applying and removing the orthosis. A photograph of the person wearing the orthosis posted in the room or in the person's care plan in the chart may help with correct orthotic application. The therapist informs nursing staff members of the wearing schedule and care instruction.

- After providing an orthosis to a person in the ICU, the therapist follows up at least once after the orthosis' application regarding the fit and the person's tolerance of the orthosis. Orthoses on persons with burns require frequent adjustments. As the person recovers, the orthotic design may change several times.

- A person who has RA may benefit from an orthosis made from thinner thermoplastic (less than ⅛ inch). The thinner material reduces the weight over affected joints.[29]

PROCEDURE FOR FABRICATION OF A RESTING HAND ORTHOSIS

The first step in the fabrication of a resting hand orthosis is drawing a pattern similar to that shown in Fig. 9.17A.

1. Place the person's hand flat and palm down, with the fingers slightly abducted for a functional position or adducted for an intrinsic plus position. Trace the outline of the upper extremity from one side of the elbow to the other.

2. While the person's hand is on the piece of paper, mark the following areas: (1) the radial styloid A and the ulnar styloid B, (2) the CMC joint of the thumb C, (3) the apex of the thumb web space D, (4) the web space between the second and third digits E, and (5) the olecranon process of the elbow F.

3. Remove the person's hand from the piece of paper. Draw a line across, indicating two-thirds of the length of the forearm. Then label this line G. After doing this, extend line G approximately 1 to 1½ inches beyond each side of the outline of the arm. Then mark an H approximately 1 inch from the outline to the radial side of A. Mark an I approximately 1 inch from the outline to the ulnar side of B.

4. Draw a dotted vertical line from the web space of the second and third digits (E) proximally down the palm approximately 3 inches. Draw a dotted horizontal line from the bottom of the thumb web space (D) toward the ulnar side of the hand until the line intersects the dotted vertical line. Mark a J at the intersection of these two dotted lines. Mark an N approximately 1 inch from the outline to the radial side of D.

5. Draw a solid vertical line from J toward the wrist. Then curve this line so that it meets C on the pattern (see Fig. 9.17A). This part of the pattern is known as *the thumb trough*. After reaching C, curve the line upward until it reaches halfway between N and D.

6. Mark a K approximately 1 inch to the radial side of the index finger's PIP joint. Mark an L 1 inch from the top of the outline of the middle finger. Mark an M approximately 1 inch to the ulnar side of the little finger's PIP joint.

7. Draw the line that ends to the side of N through K, and extend the line upward and around the corner through L. From L, round the corner to connect the line with M, and then pass it through I. Continue drawing the line, and connect it with the end of G. Connect the radial end of G to pass through H. From H, extend the line toward C. Curve the line so that it connects to C (see Fig. 9.17A).

8. Cut out the pattern. Cut the solid lines of the thumb trough also. Do not cut the dotted lines.

9. Place the pattern on the person in the appropriate joint placement. Check the length of the pan, thumb trough, and forearm trough. Assess the fit of the C bar by forming the paper towel in the thumb web space. Make necessary adjustments (e.g., additions, deletions) on the pattern.

10. With a pencil, trace the pattern onto the sheet of thermoplastic material.

11. Heat the thermoplastic material.

12. Cut the pattern out of the thermoplastic material, and reheat it. Before placing the material on the person, think about the strategy that you will employ during the molding process.

13. Instruct the person to rest the elbow on the table. The arm should be vertical and the hand relaxed. Although some thermoplastic materials in the vertical position may stretch during the molding process, the vertical position allows the best control of the wrist position. Mold the plastic form onto the person's hand and make necessary adjustments. Cold water or vapocoolant spray can be used to hasten the cooling time. However, this is not appropriate for persons with open wounds, such as burns.

14. Add straps to the pan, the thumb trough, and the forearm trough (see Fig. 9.17B). One pan strap is located across the PIP joints; the other is just proximal to the MCP joints. The strap across the thumb lies proximal to the IP joint. The forearm has two straps: one courses across the wrist, and one is located across the proximal forearm trough. (See also Laboratory Exercise 9.1.)

Technical Tips for a Proper Fit

- For persons who have fleshier forearms, the pattern requires an allowance of more than 1 inch on each side. To be accurate, measure the circumference of the person's forearm at several locations and make the pattern corresponding to the location of the measurements one-half of these measurements.

- Check the pattern carefully to determine fit, particularly the length of the pan, thumb trough, and forearm trough and the conformity of the C bar. Moistening the paper towel pattern or a foil pattern allows detailed assessment of pattern fit.

- Select a thermoplastic material with strength or rigidity. Avoid materials with excessive stretch characteristics. The orthotic material must be strong enough to support the entire hand, wrist, and forearm. A thermoplastic material with memory can be reheated several times and is beneficial if the orthosis requires serial adjustments. To make an orthosis more lightweight, select a thermoplastic material that is perforated or is thinner than ⅛ inch, especially to manage conditions such as RA.

- Make sure the orthosis supports the wrist area well. If the thumb trough is cut beyond the radial styloid, the wrist support is compromised.

- Measure the person's joints with a goniometer when possible to ensure a correct therapeutic position before applying the thermoplastic material. Be cautious of positioning the wrist in too much ulnar or radial deviation.

- When applying the straps, be sure the hand and forearm securely fit into the orthosis. For maximal joint control, place straps across the PIPs, thumb IP, palm, wrist, and proximal forearm. Additional straps may be necessary, particularly for persons who have hypertonicity. Consider using gauze or elastic bandages to secure the orthosis when straps are not reasonable.

- Contour the orthotic pan to the hand to preserve the hand's arches. The pan should be wide enough to comfortably support the width of the index, middle, ring, and little fingers.

- Make sure the C bar conforms to the thumb web space (see Fig. 9.17C). The therapist may find it helpful to stretch the edge of the C bar and then conform it to the web space. Cut any extra material from the C bar as necessary.

- Verify that the thumb trough is long enough and wide enough. Stretch or trim the thumb trough as necessary.

- For fabrication of a dorsally based resting hand orthosis, the pattern remains the same—with the addition of a slit cut at the level of the MCP joints in the pan portion of the orthosis. The slit begins and ends about 1 inch from the ulnar and radial sides of the pan, as shown in Fig. 9.17D. When the orthosis is placed on the person, the hand inserts through the slit in such a way that the fingers rest on top of the pan portion and the forearm trough rests on the dorsal surface of the forearm. The edges of the slit require rolling or slight flaring away from the surface of the skin to prevent pressure areas. In addition, the thumb trough is a separate piece and must be attached to the pan and wrist portion of the orthosis. Thus material with bonding or self-adherence characteristics is important. (See also Laboratory Exercise 9.2.)

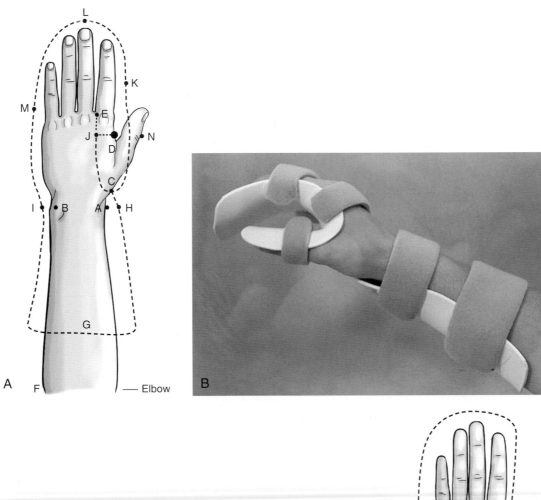

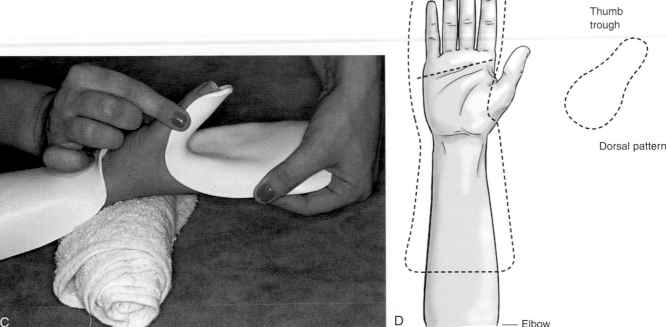

Fig. 9.17 Fabrication of a resting hand orthosis. A, Detailed pattern. B, Strap placement. C, C bar conformity to the thumb web space on a resting hand orthosis. D, Pattern for a dorsal-based resting hand orthosis.

REVIEW QUESTIONS

1. What are four common diagnostic conditions in which a therapist may provide a resting hand orthosis for intervention?

2. In what position should the therapist place the wrist, MCPs, and thumb for a functional resting hand orthosis?

3. For a person with RA who needs a resting hand orthosis, how should the joints be positioned?

4. When might a therapist use a dorsally based resting hand orthosis rather than a volar-based orthosis?

5. In what position should the therapist place the wrist, MCPs, and thumb for an antideformity resting hand orthosis?

6. What are the three purposes for using a resting hand orthosis?

7. What are the four main components of a resting hand orthosis?

8. Which equipment must be sterile to make a resting hand orthosis in a burn unit?

REFERENCES

1. American Society of Hand Therapists: *Splint classification system*, Garner, NC, 1992, American Society of Hand Therapists.

2. Beasley J: Therapist's examination and conservative management of arthritis of the upper extremity. In Skirven TM, Osterman AL, Fedorczyk JM, et al.: *Rehabilitation of the hand and upper extremity*, ed 6, Philadelphia, PA, 2011, Mosby.

3. Biese J: Therapist's evaluation and conservative management of rheumatoid arthritis in the hand and wrist. In Mackin EJ, Callahan AD, Skirven TM, et al.: *Rehabilitation of the hand: surgery and therapy*, ed 5, St. Louis, 2002, Mosby.

4. Boozer J: Splinting the arthritic hand, *J Hand Ther* 6(1):46, 1993.

5. Callinan NJ, Mathiowetz V: Soft versus hard resting hand splints in rheumatoid arthritis: pain relief, preference and compliance, *Am J Occup Ther* 50:347–353, 1996.

6. Colditz: *Personal communication*, 1995.

7. Copley J, Kuipers K, Fleming J, Rassafiani M: Individualised resting hand splints for adults with acquired brain injury: a randomized, single blinded, single case design, *NeuroRehabilitation* 32:885–898, 2013.

8. Costas B, Coleman S, Kaufman G, James R, Cohen B, Gaston RG: Efficacy and safety of collagenase clostridium histolyticum for Dupuytren disease nodules: a randomized controlled trial, BMC Musculoskelet Disord 18(1):374, 2017.

9. deLinde LG, Knothe B: Therapist's management of the burned hand. In Mackin EJ, Callahan AD, Skirven TM, et al.: *Rehabilitation of the hand: surgery and therapy*, ed 5, St. Louis, 2002, Mosby.

10. deLinde LG, Miles WK: Remodeling of scar tissue in the burned hand. In Hunter JM, Mackin EJ, Callahan AD, editors: *Rehabilitation of the hand: surgery and therapy*, ed 4, St. Louis, 1995, Mosby.

11. Deshaies L: Burns. In Cooper C, editor: *Fundamentals of hand therapy*, ed 2, St. Louis, 2014, Elsevier.

12. Egan M, Brosseau L, Farmer M, et al.: Splints/orthoses in the treatment of rheumatoid arthritis, *Cochrane Database Syst Rev* (1) CD004018, 2003.

13. Evans RB: Therapeutic management of Dupuytren's contracture. In Skirven TM, Osterman AL, Fedorczyk JM, et al.: *Rehabilitation of the hand and upper extremity*, ed 6, Philadelphia, PA, 2011, Mosby.

14. Falconer J: Hand splinting in rheumatoid arthritis, *J Hand Ther* 4(2):81–86, 1991.

15. Feinberg J: Effect of the arthritis health professional on compliance with use of resting hand splints by persons with rheumatoid arthritis, *J Hand Ther* 5(1):17–23, 1992.

16. Fess EE, Philips CA: *Hand splinting principles and methods*, ed 2, St. Louis, 1987, Mosby.

17. Geisser RW: Splinting the rheumatoid arthritic hand. In Ziegler EM, editor: *Current concepts in orthotics: a diagnosis-related approach to splinting*, Germantown, WI, 1984, Rolyan Medical Products.

18. Hindocha S, Stanley JK, Watson SJ, et al.: Dupuytren's diathesis revisited: evaluation of prognostic indicators for risk of disease recurrence, *J Hand Surg* 31(10):1626–1634, 2006.

19. Hurst L: Dupuytren's disease: surgical management. In Skirven TM, Osterman AL, Fedorczyk JM, et al.: *Rehabilitation of the hand and upper extremity*, ed 6, Philadelphia, PA, 2011, Mosby.

20. Jerosch-Herold C, Shepstone L, Chojnowski AJ, Larson D, Barrett E, Vaughn SP: Night-time splinting after fasciectomy or dermo-fasciectomy for Dupuytren's contracture: a pragmatic, multi-centre, randomized controlled trial, *BMC Musculoskelet Disord* 12:136, 2011.

21. Kaye R: Watching for and managing musculoskeletal problems in diabetes, *J Musculoskelet Med* 11(9):25–37, 1994.

22. Koman LA, Li Z, Smith BP, et al.: Complex regional pain syndrome: types I and II. In Mackin EJ, Callahan AD, Skirven TM, et al.: *Rehabilitation of the hand: surgery and therapy*, ed 5, St. Louis, 2011, Mosby.

23. Lankford LL: Reflex sympathetic dystrophy. In Hunter JM, Mackin EJ, Callahan AD, editors: *Rehabilitation of the hand: surgery and therapy*, ed 4, St. Louis, 1995, Mosby.

24. Lau C: Comparison study of QuickCast versus a traditional thermoplastic in the fabrication of a resting hand splint, *J Hand Ther* 11:45–48, 1998.

25. Leonard J: Joint protection for inflammatory disorders. In Hunter JM, Schneider LH, Mackin EJ, et al.: *Rehabilitation of the hand: surgery and therapy*, ed 3, St. Louis, 1990, Mosby.

26. Lonie S, Baker P, Teixeira R: Steam vaporizers: a danger for paediatric burns, *Burns* 421850–1853, 2016.

27. Lucas B: Supporting the older person with wrist and hand problems, *Nurs Resident Care* 15(2):88–91, 2013.

28. Malick MH: *Manual on static hand splinting*, Pittsburgh, 1972, Hamarville Rehabilitation Center.

29. Marx H: Rheumatoid arthritis. In Stanley BG, Tribuzi SM, editors: *Concepts in hand rehabilitation*, Philadelphia, 1992, FA Davis.

30. McFarlane RM: The current status of Dupuytren's disease, *J Hand Ther* 8(3):181–184, 1995.

31. McFarlane RM, MacDermid JC: Dupuytren's disease. In Mackin EJ, Callahan AD, Skirven TM, et al.: *Rehabilitation of the hand: surgery and therapy*, ed 5, St. Louis, 2002, Mosby.

32. McGrouther D: Dupuytren's contracture. In Green D, Hotchkiss R, Pederson W, et al.: *Green's operative hand surgery*, ed 5, Edinburgh, 2005, Churchill-Livingstone, pp 159–185.

33. McPherson JJ, Kreimeyer D, Aalderks M, et al.: A comparison of dorsal and volar resting hand splints in the reduction of hypertonus, *Am J Occup Ther* 36(10):664–670, 1982.

34. Melvin JL: *Rheumatic disease: occupational therapy and rehabilitation*, ed 2, Philadelphia, 1982, FA Davis.

35. Melvin JL: *Rheumatic disease in the adult and child: occupational therapy and rehabilitation*, Philadelphia, 1989, FA Davis.

36. Noffsinger DL, Johnson SR, Wheeler K, Shi J, Xiang H, Groner JI: Exercise treadmills: a cause of significant hand burns in young children, *J Burn Care Res* 38(4):215–219, 2016.

37. Ouellette EA: The rheumatoid hand: orthotics as preventative, *Semin Arthritis Rheum* 21:65–71, 1991.

38. Philips CA: Therapist's management of persons with rheumatoid arthritis. In Hunter JM, Mackin EJ, Callahan AD, editors: *Rehabilitation of the hand: surgery and therapy*, ed 4, St. Louis, 1995, Mosby.

39. Pitbladdo K, Taggart L: The neurological hand. In Cooper C, editor: *Fundamentals of hand therapy*, ed 2, St. Louis, 2014, Elsevier.

40. Pizzi A, Carlucci G, Falsini C, et al.: Application of a volar static splint in poststroke spasticity of the upper limb, *Arch Phys Med Rehabil* 86:1855–1859, 2005.

41. Prosser R, Conolly WB: Complications following surgical treatment for Dupuytren's contracture, *J Hand Ther* 9(4):344–348, 1996.

42. Richard R, Schall S, Staley M, et al.: Hand burn splint fabrication: correction for bandage thickness, *J Burn Care Rehabil* 15(4):369–371, 1994.

43. Richard R, Staley M, Daugherty MB, et al.: The wide variety of designs for dorsal hand burn splints, *J Burn Care Rehabil* 15(3):275–280, 1994.

44. Salisbury RE, Reeves SU, Wright P: Acute care and rehabilitation of the burned hand. In Hunter JM, Schneider LH, Mackin EJ, et al.: *Rehabilitation of the hand: surgery and therapy*, ed 3, St. Louis, 1990, Mosby, pp 831–840.

45. Sanjuan-Cervero R, Carrera-Hueso FJ, Oliver-Mengual S, Ramon-Barrios MA, Peimer CA, Fikri-Behbrahim N: Skin laceration in collagenase *Clostridium histolyticum* treatment for Dupuytren's contracture, *Orthop Nurs* 37(2):144–153, 2018.

46. Simón-Pérez C, Alía-Ortega J, García-Medrano B, et al.: Factors influencing recurrence and progression of Dupuytren's disease treated by collagenase *Clostridium histolyticum*, *Int Orthop* 42:859–866, 2018.

47. Sammons Preston Rolyan: *Hand rehab catalog*, Bolingbrook, IL, 2005, Sammons Preston Rolyan.

48. Simpson RL: Management of burns of the upper extremity. In Skirven TM, Osterman AL, Fedorczyk J, et al.: *Rehabilitation of the hand and upper extremity*, ed 6, Philadelphia, PA, 2011, Mosby.

49. Skirven TM, Osterman AL, Fedorczyk JM, et al.: *Rehabilitation of the hand and upper extremity*, ed 6, Philadelphia, PA, 2011, Mosby.

50. Stanley BG, Tribuzi SM: *Concepts in hand rehabilitation*, Philadelphia, 1992, FA Davis.

51. Swedler WI, Baak S, Lazarevic MB, et al.: Rheumatic changes in diabetes: shoulder, arm, and hand, *J Musculoskelet Med* 12(8):45–52, 1995.

52. Tenney CG, Lisak JM: *Atlas of hand splinting*, Boston, 1986, Little, Brown & Co.

53. Torres-Gray D, Johnson J, Mlakar J: Rehabilitation of the burned hand: questionnaire results, *J Burn Care Rehabil* 17(2):161–168, 1996.

54. Toor J, Crain J, Kelly C, Verchere C, Fish J: Pediatric burns from glass-fronted fireplaces in Canada: a growing issue over the past 20 years, *J Burn Care Res* 37(5):c483–c488, 2016.

55. Tufaro PA, Bondoc SL: Therapist's management of the burned hand. In Skirven TM, Osterman AL, Fedorczyk J, et al.: *Rehabilitation of the hand and upper extremity*, ed 6, Philadelphia, PA, 2011, Mosby.

56. Walsh MT, Muntzer E: Therapist's management of complex regional pain syndrome (reflex sympathetic dystrophy). In Mackin EJ, Callahan AD, Skirven TM, et al.: *Rehabilitation of the hand: surgery and therapy*, ed 5, St. Louis, 2002, Mosby.

57. Walsh MT: Therapist's management of complex regional pain syndrome. In Skirven TM, Osterman AL, Fedorczyk J, et al.: *Rehabilitation of the hand and upper extremity*, ed 6, Philadelphia, PA, 2011, Mosby.

58. Whitehead C, Serghiou M: A 12-year comparison of common therapeutic interventions in the burn unit, *J Burn Care Res* 30(2):281–287, 2009.

59. Ziegler EM: *Current concepts in orthotics: a diagnostic-related approach to splinting*, Germantown, WI, 1984, Rolyan Medical Products.

APPENDIX 9.1 CASE STUDIES

Case Study 9.1[a]

Read the following scenario, and use your clinical reasoning skills to answer the questions based on information in this chapter.

Juan, a 39-year-old man with bilateral dorsal hand burns, has just been admitted to the intensive care unit (ICU). Juan has second- and third-degree burns resulting from a torch exploding in his hands. He is receiving intravenous pain medication and is not alert. Approximately 14 hours have passed since his admission, and you just received orders to fabricate bilateral hand orthoses.

1. Which type of orthosis is appropriate for dorsal hand burns?
   a. Bilateral resting hand orthoses with the hand in a functional (midjoint) position
   b. Bilateral resting hand orthoses with the hand in an antideformity (intrinsic plus) position
   c. Bilateral wrist cock-up orthoses
2. What is the appropriate wrist position?
   a. Neutral
   b. 15 to 30 degrees of flexion
   c. 15 to 30 degrees of extension
3. What is the appropriate metacarpophalangeal (MCP) position?
   a. 50 to 80 degrees of extension
   b. 50 to 80 degrees of flexion
   c. Full extension
4. What is the appropriate thumb position?
   a. Radial abduction
   b. Palmar abduction
   c. Midway between palmar and radial abduction
5. Which of the following statements is false regarding the orthosis process for the previous scenario?
   a. The supplies should be sterile.
   b. An extremely stretchable material is necessary to fabricate the orthoses over the bandages.
   c. The therapist should give an orthotic-wearing schedule to the ICU nurse for inclusion in the treatment plan.

Case Study 9.2[a]

Read the following scenario, and use your clinical reasoning to answer the questions based on information from this chapter and previous chapters.

Ken is a 45-year-old right-hand–dominant man with diabetes mellitus and Dupuytren disease. He underwent an elective surgical procedure to release proximal interphalangeal flexion contractures in his right ring and little fingers. The physician used a Z-plasty open palm technique. Ken returns from the surgical suite, and you receive an order to "evaluate, treat, and provide orthosis." Ken is an accountant who is married with a 16-year-old son.

1. What diagnosis in Ken's past medical history is associated with Dupuytren disease?
2. What orthotic designs are appropriate for Ken's condition?
3. What therapeutic position will be used in the orthotic design?
4. What wearing schedule will you give Ken?
5. You notice that Ken's bandage bulk is considerable. How will you design the orthosis to accommodate for bandage thickness? What type of thermoplastic material properties will you choose?
6. How frequently will Ken require therapy?
7. What support systems may Ken require for rehabilitation from this surgery?

APPENDIX 9.2 LABORATORY EXERCISES

Laboratory Exercise 9.1 Making a Hand Orthosis Pattern

1. Practice making a resting hand orthosis pattern on another person. Use the detailed instructions provided to draw the pattern. Cut out the pattern, and make necessary adjustments.
2. Use the outline of the following hands to draw the resting hand orthosis pattern without using the detailed instructions.

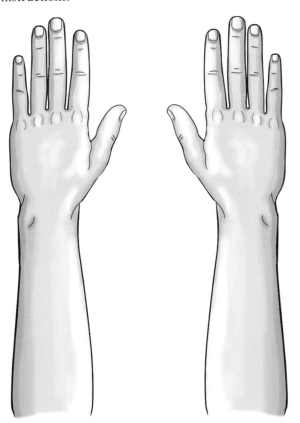

Laboratory Exercise 9.2 Identifying Problems With Orthoses[a]

There are three persons who sustained burns on their hands. Their wounds have healed, and they must wear orthoses at night to prevent contractures. The therapist fabricated the following orthoses. Look at each picture and identify the problem with each.

1. What is the problem with this orthosis?[a]

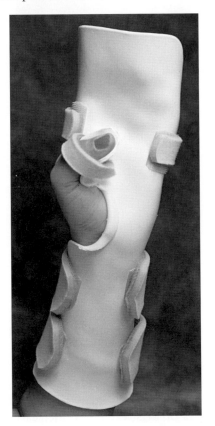

2. What is the problem with this orthosis?

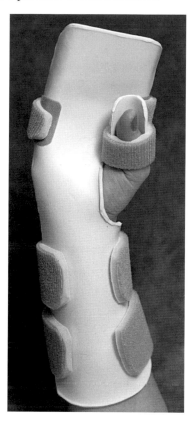

3. What is the problem with this orthosis?

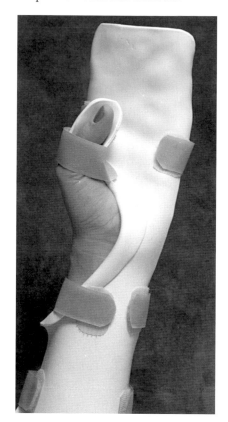

Laboratory Exercise 9.3 Fabricating a Hand Orthosis

Practice fabricating a resting hand orthosis on a partner. Before starting, determine the position in which you should place your partner's hand. Use a goniometer to measure the angles of wrist extension, metacarpophalangeal (MCP) flexion, and thumb palmar abduction to ensure a correct position. After fitting the orthosis and making all adjustments, use Form 9.1 as a self-evaluation check-off sheet. Use Grading Sheet 9.1 as a classroom grading sheet. (Grading Sheet 9.1 may also be used as a self-evaluation sheet.)

APPENDIX 9.3 FORM AND GRADING SHEET

Form 9.1 Resting Hand Orthosis

	Name: _____	
	Date: _____	

Position of resting hand orthosis:		
Functional position (midjoint) ○	Antideformity position (intrinsic plus) ○	
Answer the following questions after the person wears the orthosis for 30 minutes. (Mark NA for nonapplicable situations.)		

Evaluation Areas				Comments
Design				
1. The wrist position is at the correct angle.	Yes ○	No ○	NA ○	
2. The metacarpophalangeals (MCPs) are at the correct angle.	Yes ○	No ○	NA ○	
3. The thumb is in the correct position.	Yes ○	No ○	NA ○	
4. The wrist has adequate support.	Yes ○	No ○	NA ○	
5. The pan is wide enough for all the fingers.	Yes ○	No ○	NA ○	
6. The length of the pan and thumb trough is adequate.	Yes ○	No ○	NA ○	
7. The orthosis is two-thirds the length of the forearm.	Yes ○	No ○	NA ○	
8. The orthosis is half the width of the forearm.	Yes ○	No ○	NA ○	
9. Arches of the hand are supported and maintained.	Yes ○	No ○	NA ○	
Function				
1. The orthosis completely immobilizes the wrist, fingers, and thumb.	Yes ○	No ○	NA ○	
2. The orthosis is easy to apply and remove.	Yes ○	No ○	NA ○	
Straps				
1. The straps are rounded.	Yes ○	No ○	NA ○	
2. Straps are placed to adequately secure the hand/arm to the orthosis.	Yes ○	No ○	NA ○	

Comfort				
1. The edges are smooth with rounded corners.	Yes ○	No ○	NA ○	
2. The proximal end is flared.	Yes ○	No ○	NA ○	
3. The orthosis does not cause impingements or pressure areas.	Yes ○	No ○	NA ○	
Cosmetic Appearance				
1. The orthosis is free of fingerprints, dirt, and pencil or pen marks.	Yes ○	No ○	NA ○	
2. The orthosis is smooth and free of buckles.	Yes ○	No ○	NA ○	
Therapeutic Regimen				
1. The person has been instructed in a wearing schedule.	Yes ○	No ○	NA ○	
2. The person has been provided with orthosis precautions.	Yes ○	No ○	NA ○	
3. The person demonstrates understanding of the education.	Yes ○	No ○	NA ○	
4. Client/caregiver knows how to clean the orthosis.	Yes ○	No ○	NA ○	

Discuss adjustments or changes you would make based on the self-evaluation.
_____
_____
_____

Discuss possible areas to improve with clinical safety when fabricating the orthosis.
_____
_____
_____

Grading Sheet 9.1 Resting Hand Orthosis

	Name:
	Date:

Position of resting hand orthosis:		
Functional position (midjoint) ○	Antideformity position (intrinsic plus) ○	

Grade: _____

1 = Beyond improvement not acceptable

2 = Requires maximal improvement

3 = Requires moderate improvement

4 = Requires minimal improvement

5 = Requires no improvement

Evaluation Areas						Comments
Design						
1. The wrist position is at the correct angle.	1	2	3	4	5	
2. The metacarpophalangeals (MCPs) are at the correct angle.	1	2	3	4	5	
3. The thumb is in the correct position.	1	2	3	4	5	
4. The wrist has adequate support.	1	2	3	4	5	
5. The pan is wide enough for all the fingers.	1	2	3	4	5	
6. The length of the pan and thumb trough is adequate.	1	2	3	4	5	
7. The orthosis is two-thirds the length of the forearm.	1	2	3	4	5	
8. The orthosis is half the width of the forearm.	1	2	3	4	5	
9. Arches of the hand are supported and maintained.	1	2	3	4	5	
Function						
1. The orthosis completely immobilizes the wrist, fingers, and thumb.	1	2	3	4	5	
2. The orthosis is easy to apply and remove.	1	2	3	4	5	

Straps						
1. The straps are rounded.	1	2	3	4	5	
2. Straps are placed to adequately secure the hand/arm to the orthosis.	1	2	3	4	5	
Comfort						
1. The edges are smooth with rounded corners.	1	2	3	4	5	
2. The proximal end is flared.	1	2	3	4	5	
3. The orthosis does not cause impingements or pressure areas.	1	2	3	4	5	
Cosmetic Appearance						
1. The orthosis is free of fingerprints, dirt, and pencil or pen marks.	1	2	3	4	5	
2. The orthosis is smooth and free of buckles.	1	2	3	4	5	

Elbow and Forearm Immobilization Orthoses

Salvador Bondoc
John Jackson

CHAPTER OBJECTIVES

1. Define anatomical and biomechanical considerations for orthotic intervention of the elbow and forearm.
2. Discuss clinical/diagnostic indications for elbow and forearm immobilization orthoses.
3. Identify the components of elbow immobilization orthoses.
4. Describe the fabrication process for an anterior and posterior elbow orthosis.
5. Review the precautions for elbow and forearm immobilization orthoses.
6. Use clinical reasoning to evaluate a problematic elbow or forearm immobilization orthosis.
7. Use clinical reasoning to evaluate a fabricated elbow or forearm immobilization orthosis.
8. Apply knowledge about the application of elbow or forearm immobilization orthoses to a case study.

KEY TERMS

anterior elbow immobilization orthosis
anterior transposition
concomitant injury
cubital tunnel syndrome
distal humerus
elbow instability
Essex-Lopresti fracture

medial and lateral epicondyles
Monteggia fracture
olecranon process
open reduction internal fixation (ORIF)
posterior elbow immobilization orthosis
radial head

subcutaneous
submuscular
"terrible triad" injury
tendinosis
tennis elbow
valgus
varus

Devon was playing basketball in a recreation league and fell on his outstretched hand. When he went to the emergency department, he was diagnosed with a dislocation of the ulnohumeral joint. The physician explained to Devon that the ulnohumeral joint played an important role in stabilizing the elbow. He subsequently was immobilized in a cast. After the cast was removed, Devon had difficulty reaching due to pain and stiffness at the elbow. This difficulty limited his ability to do many of his daily living activities, work, and play basketball. Devon's provider referred him for occupational therapy. During his first therapy session the occupational therapist explained that stiffness of the elbow was a common complication after an elbow cast removal. Both the therapist and Devon collaborated on priority goals to help Devon regain his motion, alleviate his pain, and most importantly resume his usual daily life activities and return to work and playing basketball again.

ANATOMICAL AND BIOMECHANICAL CONSIDERATIONS

The mechanical analog of the elbow joint is a simple hinge. Yet the sagittal plane motion of flexion and extension is produced by two articulations with different arthrokinematic properties: the humeroulnar and the humeroradial joints. The humeroulnar articulation consists of the trochlear notch of the proximal ulna and the trochlea of the distal humerus. The humeroradial articulation is formed by the fovea of the proximal radius and the capitellum of the distal humerus. These joint structures share a singular capsule along with the proximal radioulnar joint (PRUJ) and are highly congruent.[16] Although the PRUJ is anatomically linked to the humeroradial and humeroulnar articulations, the motion produced is functionally distinct. The PRUJ along with the distal radioulnar joint at the wrist forms a singular longitudinal axis that affords pronation and supination of the forearm.[15] With the high congruence of the joint surfaces, any fracture or dislocation affecting the joint surfaces could lead to loss of available range of motion in either or both extension-flexion and supination-pronation. Furthermore, given the single-capsule configuration of the elbow joint complex, prolonged immobilization could further accentuate the loss or restriction in the range of motion in all three elbow joints.

During range-of-motion assessment, normal elbow flexion produces a soft end feel with the contact of the soft tissues and the volar surfaces of the forearm and arm.

Meanwhile, elbow extension produces a hard end feel as the olecranon process of the ulna comes into contact with the olecranon fossa of the distal humerus. The forearm tends to deviate laterally when the forearm is supinated during elbow extension. The **valgus** angulation of the elbow, also known as *the carrying angle,* is 10 to 15 degrees from the longitudinal axis of the humerus and is attributed to the distal expansion of the medial aspect of the trochlea.[16,22] This valgus angle must be considered when applying immobilization or mobilization orthoses to the elbow in extension. In the absence of trauma or underlying pathology, an elbow in excessive valgus position (typically observed with prolonged weight bearing in elbow extension and forearm supination) may lead to a disruption or laxity of the medial collateral ligament.

Throughout the ranges of elbow flexion and extension, the medial and lateral collateral ligament complexes also contribute to the stability of the elbow joint. Elements of the medial collateral ligament complex produce valgus (medial) restraint from maximum extension to 120 degrees of flexion.[24] Meanwhile, the lateral (ulnar) collateral ligament complex remains taut throughout the range of motion and is further accentuated when the elbow undergoes **varus** stress.[20] Given the contribution of the collateral ligament complex to elbow stability, injury to either or both ligaments could also alter elbow alignment and range of motion.

The volar surface of the elbow is filled with soft tissue and features a transverse crease that, depending on a person's muscle mass and elbow joint complex laxity, may lie on a flat or concave surface when the elbow is in full extension. This volar area is bordered by the biceps brachii superiorly, the bellies of the brachioradialis, the common hand extensors laterally, and the common hand flexors medially. The landscape of the dorsal elbow surface is bony. When the elbow is in 90 degrees of flexion, the center points of the **olecranon process** and the **medial and lateral epicondyles** form a triangular configuration. These bony prominences are potential sources of irritation and must be protected during orthotic fabrication and fitting.

CLINICAL INDICATIONS AND COMMON DIAGNOSES

Immobilization orthoses for the elbow and the forearm are commonly constructed to protect and support healing structures following a traumatic injury to the bones, muscles, ligaments, and related soft tissues. These conditions are managed either conservatively or surgically. Conservative management may involve manipulation or closed reduction before immobilization and is often indicated for simple fractures. Surgical interventions vary based on the client's presentation and goals, surgeon's choice, and available resources. The more common surgical fixation procedures involve open reduction with internal fixation using plates and screws and/or wiring. Other surgical procedures used for the elbow include hinged

external fixation, arthroplasty (joint replacement), and nerve transposition. In cases of external fixations an additional elbow immobilization orthosis may be unnecessary.

An elbow immobilization orthosis may be indicated to manage pain and support unstable structures (e.g., arthritis), restrict motion and provide rest (e.g., ulnar nerve entrapment), or to prevent loss of or to improve motion (e.g., elbow stiffness and contractures) through progressive application. Elbow orthoses for the purpose of immobilization may be commercially prefabricated or custom made. The appropriate choice of orthosis depends on the clinical indication and the preferences of the surgeon, therapist, and client. Table 10.1 provides a summary and comparison of conditions for which an elbow immobilization orthosis is indicated.

Elbow Fractures and Dislocation

Traumatic fractures of the elbow may occur to the distal humerus, proximal ulna, proximal radius, or any combination. The incidence of elbow fractures is almost evenly distributed to the aforementioned structures with distal humerus and proximal radius being more common.[14] Fractures are often complicated by **concomitant injury** to surrounding soft tissues, blood vessels, or nerves. More complex forms of elbow fractures involve the articular surfaces and may include joint dislocations. However, joint dislocations may occur from disruptions in soft tissue support without fractures. Complex elbow injuries, if not properly treated, have a poor prognosis with recurrent instability, stiffness, and pain.[12]

Distal Humerus Fractures

Fractures to the **distal humerus** constitute approximately a third of all elbow fractures.[14] Intra-articular fractures may occur to one or both condyles because they articulate with the ulna or radius and result from compression forces across the elbow. Extra-articular fractures are typically supracondylar (above the condyles) or transcondylar (across the condyles above the articular surfaces) in nature. These fractures generally result from a fall on an outstretched hand.[10] Conservatively treated simple, nondisplaced fractures or postsurgical elbow fixation of more complex, unstable fractures are immobilized in a long arm cast or posterior elbow orthosis. A posterior elbow orthosis (Fig. 10.1) is designed to position the elbow at 90 degrees flexion and forearm in neutral. The duration of orthotic use may depend on the speed of bone and soft tissue healing. In many cases there is an overlap between immobilization orthoses for healing and mobilization orthoses to prevent or manage soft tissue tightness. Therapists must collaborate with the client's physician to ensure timeliness of intervention.

Proximal Radius Fractures

Proximal radius fractures are the most common of all elbow fractures.[24] In one estimate,[14] at least a third of all elbow fractures occur in the **radial head** and neck. These elbow fractures occur by axial loading on a pronated forearm with the elbow in more than 20 degrees of flexion. The severity of the fracture and the client's contexts determine intervention. Simple or

TABLE 10.1   Conditions That Require an Elbow Immobilization Orthosis

Condition	Suggested Wearing Schedule	Type of Orthosis and Position
Elbow fractures	After removal of postoperative dressing, the therapist fabricates an elbow immobilization orthosis. The orthosis is worn at all times and removed for exercises and hygiene, if permitted.	Distal humerus fracture: posterior elbow orthosis to position the elbow in 90 degrees of flexion and forearm in neutral. Proximal radius fracture: posterior elbow orthosis to position the elbow in 90 degrees of flexion and forearm in neutral for rest and protection. Proximal ulnar fracture: elbow is braced or dorsally positioned in 30–45 degrees of flexion to minimize the passive tension on the triceps.
Elbow arthroplasty	After removal of postoperative dressing, the therapist fabricates an elbow immobilization orthosis or fits the client for a brace. The orthosis is worn at all times and removed for protected range-of-motion exercises until the joint is stable.	Posterior elbow orthosis or a commercial (Bledsoe-type brace or Mayo elbow brace) in 90 degrees of flexion.
Elbow instability	After removal of postoperative dressing, a posterior elbow immobilization orthosis in 120 degrees of flexion is provided. The client is not permitted to remove the orthosis unsupervised.	Posterior elbow orthosis 100–120 degrees of flexion or brace locked in 110–120 degrees. If it is a posterolateral rotatory instability, position the forearm in pronation; otherwise, maintain the forearm in neutral. In any case, extend the custom orthosis to support the wrist for comfort.
Biceps/triceps repair		Biceps tear: conservative management is often indicated for partial tears using an elbow brace or posterior immobilization orthosis. This orthosis places the elbow in 90 degrees flexion with the forearm in neutral to supination. Postoperative bracing or orthotic provision is indicated for full tears with the forearm in supination. The supinated position is necessary to minimize the mechanical impingement of the distal biceps. The posterior placement is necessary to allow the elbow to rest and minimize biceps activity. Triceps repair: conservative management is often indicated for partial tears using an elbow brace or immobilization orthosis. This orthosis places the elbow in 90 degrees flexion with the forearm in neutral. Postoperative bracing or orthotic provision is indicated for full tears with the forearm in neutral. The supinated position is necessary to minimize the mechanical impingement of the distal biceps.
Cubital tunnel syndrome	Nighttime wear	Conservative: anterior elbow extension orthosis with elbow positioned in −30 degrees extension; or a posterior elbow orthosis with elbow positioned in −30 degrees extension and padding at the olecranon and to the medial epicondyle to create a space (noncontact) between the orthosis and the cubital tunnel area. Postoperative: posterior long arm orthosis with elbow positioned in 70–90 degrees flexion and forearm neutral for subcutaneous transposition and forearm in slight pronation with submuscular transposition.
Tennis elbow	Daytime wear	Combination of counterforce brace and wrist immobilization orthosis with the wrist in 20–30 degrees of extension.

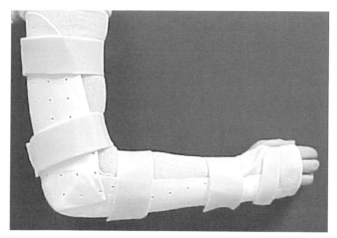

Fig. 10.1 Posterior elbow orthosis with elbow in 90 degrees flexion.

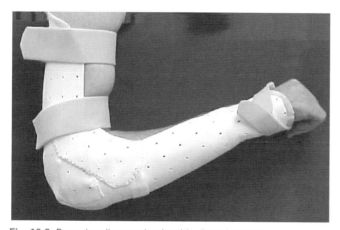

Fig. 10.2 Posterior elbow orthosis with elbow in 120 degrees flexion.

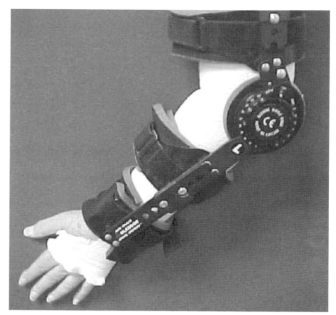

Fig. 10.3 Bledsoe brace. (Courtesy Bledsoe Brace Systems, Grand Prairie, Texas.)

minimally displaced radial head fractures with no evidence of mechanical block are often treated with gentle active mobilization early in the recovery period using a **posterior elbow immobilization orthosis** (see Fig. 10.1). This orthosis positions the elbow in 90 degrees of flexion and forearm in neutral for rest and protection. Displaced radial fractures may be treated surgically depending on the presence of mechanical block and the number of fracture segments.[17] Surgeons may elect to use an **open reduction internal fixation (ORIF)** technique or radial head replacement. In either case, clients need to be immobilized with a cast or commercially available brace immediately following the surgery. Immobilization orthotic provision may continue following cast removal, depending on the client's condition (e.g., rate of healing, joint stability, presence of concomitant collateral ligament injury) and the surgeon's preference. For clients with ORIFs the objective is to maintain the stability of the radial fixation by immobilizing the elbow in greater than 90 degrees flexion with the forearm in neutral or pronated position (Fig. 10.2). As the client improves, the elbow angle may be adjusted toward extension. For clients with radial head arthroplasties, the choice of immobilization is largely dependent on the integrity of the supportive ligaments and capsule. Some surgeons may opt for commercially available adjustable hinged braces, such as the

Bledsoe brace (Fig. 10.3), or a therapist may fabricate a custom hinged elbow device that may be adjusted or locked in the direction of both flexion and extension.

Proximal Ulnar Fractures

Most proximal ulnar fractures occur either at the olecranon or the coronoid process. Olecranon fractures typically result from a direct impact or from a hyperextension force.[3] Olecranon fractures are often amenable to ORIF using a plate and screws or tension wiring.[6] Many olecranon fractures involve the triceps either by rupture or avulsion. Following acute management surgically or conservatively (closed reduction), the elbow is braced or dorsally positioned in 30 to 45 degrees flexion to minimize the passive tension on the triceps. Fractures of the coronoid process are more complex and associated with significant instability.[13] (This topic is described later.) Approaches to management are varied[2] and include a more conservative cast immobilization or progressive hinged external fixation for several weeks. In such cases the purpose of rehabilitative orthotic provision shifts toward mobilization after cast removal due to stiffness.

Forearm Fractures

Many complex elbow fractures affecting the proximal radius and ulna result in disruption of the proximal and/or distal radioulnar joint(s). Radial head fractures associated with disruption of the interosseous membrane and dislocation of the distal radioulnar joint are also termed **Essex-Lopresti fractures.** Proximal ulnar fractures along with the dislocation of the radial head at the PRUJ are also known as **Monteggia fractures.** The objective of managing these fractures is to restore the joint articulation and kinematics for elbow and forearm mobility. The initial aim of management is to stabilize the forearm by restricting rotation. Restriction may be accomplished through bracing, orthoses, or casting that extends

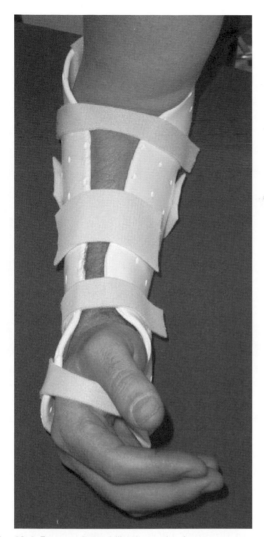

Fig. 10.4 Forearm immobilization orthosis, sugar tong type.

throughout the upper limb proximal to the elbow and distal to the wrist. Examples of the orthoses used to immobilize the forearm and wrist and restrict the elbow include a sugar tong orthosis (Fig. 10.4) and a Muenster orthosis. Both examples enable some degree of elbow motion typically within the functional range of 30 to 130 degrees of sagittal motion.

Elbow Dislocations

Dislocations of the elbow are common and may occur with or without fractures. Dislocations without fractures are considered simple, whereas dislocations with fractures (typically of avulsion type) are considered complex. Nearly all elbow dislocations, simple and complex, occur in posterior or posterolateral directions,[5] resulting in joint instability. A common pattern of complex **elbow instability** results from a dislocation of the ulnohumeral joint and injury to the varus and valgus stabilizers of the elbow and the radial head.[11] This injury occurs due to a forceful fall on an outstretched hand. If a coronoid avulsion fracture is involved, the condition is termed a **"terrible triad" injury.**

To prevent instability, simple dislocations are managed in one or more of the following options: (1) cast immobilization,

(2) surgical repair of ruptured collateral ligaments, or (3) early mobilization following a reduction or repair procedure. Clients who undergo an early mobilization program with or without ligament repair require supportive orthotic provision during periods of rest. Wolff and Hotchkiss[23] described a conservative approach to managing a postreduction elbow dislocation to prevent lateral instability using active mobilization within limits of pain and orthotic provision. The immobilization orthosis places the elbow in 100 to 120 degrees of elbow flexion with the forearm in neutral to a fully pronated position. An alternative is a commercially available hinged brace that stabilizes the elbow while at rest and may be adjusted during exercise.

Biceps Rupture

Distal biceps tendon rupture is uncommon and occurs more frequently to the long head branch within the shoulder. Such injury occurs more often in middle-aged men. The typical mechanism of injury is eccentric loading of the biceps while the elbow is in a flexed position.[18] Conservative management is often indicated for partial tears, using an elbow brace or immobilization orthosis. This orthosis places the elbow in 90 degrees flexion with the forearm in neutral to supination. Postoperative bracing or orthotic provision is indicated for full tears with the forearm in supination. The supinated position is necessary to minimize the mechanical impingement of the distal biceps. Seiler and colleagues[21] observed that 85% of the PRUJ space is occupied by the biceps tendon when the forearm is pronated. They theorized that repetitive pronation contributes to the pathophysiology of the distal biceps rupture through mechanical shearing and hypovascularization. Whether the client's elbow is conservatively or surgically managed, the orthosis or brace is progressively adjusted into extension as gentle exercises are introduced and upgraded over a typical course of tendon healing of 4 to 8 weeks.

Triceps Repair

Conservative management for a triceps repair is often indicated for partial tears using an elbow brace or immobilization orthosis. This orthosis places the elbow in 90 degrees flexion with the forearm in neutral. Postoperative bracing or orthotic provision is indicated for full tears with the forearm in neutral. The supinated position is necessary to minimize the mechanical impingement of the distal biceps.

Cubital Tunnel Syndrome

Cubital tunnel syndrome is the second most common site of nerve compression in the upper extremity.[1,19] Anatomically, the ulnar nerve is susceptible to injury at the elbow secondary to its superficial location situated between the medial epicondyle of the humerus and the olecranon. Injury to the nerve may occur as a result of trauma or prolonged or sustained motion that compresses the nerve over time.[7] Ulnar nerve entrapment following a trauma may arise immediately or gradually due to tethering of the nerve as it courses through a region that may be occupied by edema or adherent scar. Symptoms include pain and paresthesias (numbness, tingling) in the fourth and fifth digits of the hand. In advanced

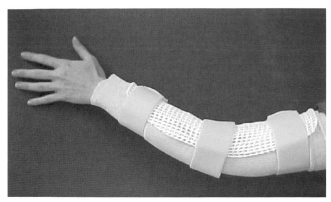

Fig. 10.5 Anterior elbow orthosis with elbow in −30 degrees of extension.

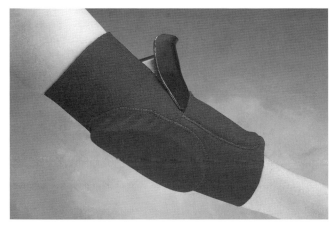

Fig. 10.6 Pil-O-Splint. (Courtesy North Coast Medical, Gilroy, California.)

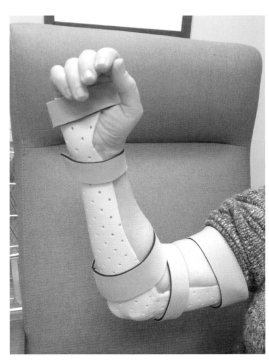

Fig. 10.7 Comfort Cool ulnar protector. (Courtesy North Coast Medical, Gilroy, California.)

Surgical Decompression of High Ulnar Nerve Injury

If conservative management of cubital tunnel syndrome is not successful or if compression of the ulnar nerve is too severe, causing distal muscle wasting and intolerable sensory discomfort on the part of the client, then surgery may be indicated. This surgical procedure includes **anterior transposition** of the ulnar nerve. Two main methods to accomplish this procedure include subcutaneous and submuscular transposition.[25] The **subcutaneous** method includes moving the ulnar nerve anteriorly medial to the median nerve and below subcutaneous fascia in the forearm. A posterior long arm orthosis with the elbow in 70 to 90 degrees flexion and the forearm in neutral is indicated. The **submuscular** method includes moving the ulnar nerve anteriorly and placed in a muscular bed, most commonly the flexor-pronator muscle origin. A posterior long arm orthosis with the elbow in 70 to 90 degrees flexion and the forearm in slight pronation is commonly used.

Elbow Stiffness

Stiffness is a common consequence of trauma to the elbow joint complex whether managed conservatively or surgically. Elbow stiffness may be a common consequence for clients with osteoarthritis. Elbow stiffness may be classified as intrinsic or extrinsic.[4] Intrinsic elbow stiffness may have intra-articular pathology, such as partial arthrodesis or loss of cartilaginous lining (i.e., osteoarthritis), or may be due to a loss of articular congruency from a less than accurate reduction and fixation after a fracture or dislocation. End range-of-motion assessment of intrinsic stiffness often yields a "bone-on-bone" end feel. On the other hand, extrinsic elbow stiffness is a result of

stages, weakness and atrophy of the hypothenar muscles and thumb adductor may be seen (see Chapter 14).

Conservative management focuses on avoiding postures and positions that aggravate the symptoms. Clients are instructed to avoid repetitive or sustained elbow flexion. A nighttime anterior elbow extension orthosis is fabricated with the elbow positioned in 30 to 45 degrees of flexion (Fig. 10.5). If the exposed cubital tunnel region remains irritated, a posterior elbow orthosis with a "belly gutter" to the posteromedial aspect of the elbow may be an option. There are commercially available soft orthotic devices, such as the Pil-O-Splint (North Coast Medical, Gilroy, CA) (Fig. 10.6) and the Comfort Cool ulnar protector (North Coast Medical) (Fig. 10.7), that offer additional alternatives if a thermoplastic orthotic device is not tolerated by the client. In one cadaver study by Apfel and Sigafoos,[26] three types of orthoses braces were all successful in preventing less than 90 degrees of elbow flexion. These are the Pil-O-Splint, Hely and Weber cubital brace, and a folded towel splint. In addition to the use of an effective orthosis design, the management of cubital tunnel syndrome should incorporate behavior modification on the part of the client, such as minimizing excessive elbow flexion and weight bearing on a flexed elbow to reduce pressure or traction on the ulnar nerve. Rigid night orthotic wear and activity modification have been found to be a successful treatment for cubital tunnel syndrome.[28]

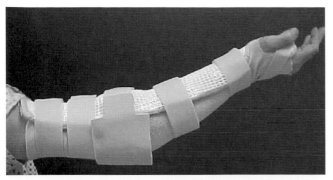

Fig. 10.8 A serial static elbow extension orthosis.

contractures to the surrounding capsular, ligamentous, and adjacent soft tissue structures, including skin, muscle, and tendon. Often the elbow is held in midflexion post injury. As the body undergoes the phases of healing (i.e., inflammatory response to repair and remodeling), tenacious edema, scarring, pain, and immobilization all contribute to the elbow's propensity to develop contractures of the soft tissues. To address this problem, early intervention is indicated through the controlled active motion and orthotic provision or bracing that provides low-load and prolonged stretch.[8]

There are two general approaches to orthotic provision that incorporate low-load and prolonged stretch to address elbow stiffness: (1) static progressive or serial static orthoses (Fig. 10.8) and (2) dynamic orthoses. The mechanism behind static progressive or serial static orthoses is stress relaxation (i.e., when the tissue is stretched, the load needed to maintain the stretched state decreases and becomes better tolerated). The mechanism behind dynamic orthotic provision is creep, in which load is constantly applied to cause a change in the viscoelastic properties of tissues.[4] In a systematic review by Veltman and colleagues,[27] static progressive orthotic wear resulted in an average change of 36 degrees among 160 patients, and dynamic orthosis resulted in an average change of 37 degrees among 72 patients. Rehabilitative management using orthoses for elbow stiffness is effective, but it is also time extensive and requires consistent client follow-through with the orthotic-wearing schedule and home program of range-of-motion and stretching exercises to be successful. Although both orthotic approaches are well supported by evidence, therapists should be attuned to the client's preferences and ability to follow up to better achieve wearing tolerance and adherence.

When there is substantial fibrosis and maturation of scars, extrinsic contractures may be resistant to orthotic provision or bracing and may require open or arthroscopic release. Intrinsic contractures may respond only to rehabilitative management when anatomically possible. To achieve full range of motion of the elbow, tissue release and joint arthroplasty may be necessary.[4]

Tennis Elbow

Tennis elbow, or lateral epicondylosis, is not only very prevalent with tennis players (and athletes that compete in racquet sports) but also with everyday people who perform repetitive wrist and gripping hand movements.[29] It involves overuse of

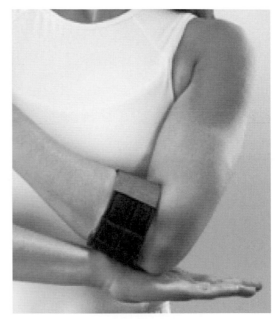

Fig. 10.9 Counterforce brace. (From Rizzone, K., Gregory, A (2013). Using casts, splints and braces in the emergency department. *Clinical Pediatric Emergency, 14*(4), 340-348.)

the forearm extensor muscles causing strain or microtears to the common extensor muscles, especially the extensor carpi radialis brevis.[29] As a result, clients report tenderness and pain at the lateral epicondyle and/or at the common extensor tendon area, especially when grasping objects. Clients may also experience decreased grip strength and posterolateral pain with resisted supination. If not diagnosed early and treated appropriately with immobilization and activity modification, the microtears may not sufficiently heal or could worsen, leading to chronic scarring of the muscle tendon or **tendinosis.**

There are two common orthotic approaches for the acute treatment of lateral epicondylitis: a wrist immobilization (cock-up) orthosis with the wrist at 20 to 30 degrees extension (see Chapter 7) and a counterforce brace (Fig. 10.9), both of which are readily available commercially at supermarkets or pharmacies. Studies comparing both orthoses yield conflicting results. One such study concluded that the use of a counterforce brace or sleeve was more effective at reducing pain with grip compared with a wrist orthosis.[29] Another study involving 42 participants showed that the wrist immobilization was better for pain relief compared with the forearm counterforce brace.[31] Both studies[29,31] did not examine long-term effects. This is critical because lateral epicondylitis is known to be a recurrent condition.

One study reported a novel orthotic design that incorporated both counterforce bracing and wrist immobilization, with restriction of forearm supination by way of a spiral forearm-wrist design, and made a positive impact on the symptoms of tennis elbow.[30] In this study the new spiral orthosis was worn for a total of 4 weeks.[30] Although this study had a small sample, subjects did show significant increase in grip strength, functional use of the hand, and decrease in pain.

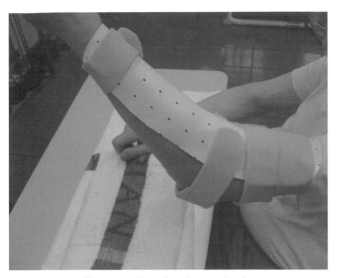

Fig. 10.10 Posterior elbow orthosis.

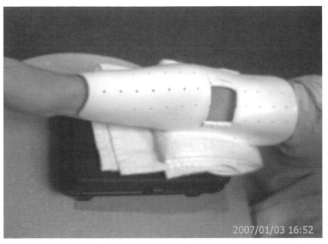

Fig. 10.11 Anterior elbow immobilization orthosis.

FEATURES OF ELBOW AND FOREARM ORTHOSES

Posterior Elbow Orthosis

A posterior elbow orthosis (Fig. 10.10) is a common orthotic choice for many acute posttraumatic and postsurgical elbow conditions, especially when positioning the elbow at 70 to 120 degrees flexion. The orthosis is easy to wear and offers rest and protection to painful and healing structures. Because of the prominent bony prominences located at the posterior elbow, measures to avoid pressure or provide pressure relief should be built into the orthotic design. Edema, a common consequence of elbow injury and surgery, must also be accommodated into the orthotic design and managed through compression sleeves. Sleeves will keep the skin, which is covered by the orthosis, dry.

Anterior Elbow Orthosis

An anterior elbow orthosis is indicated in situations where there is a posterior wound that cannot tolerate posterior pressure or contact. If positioning the elbow at less than 70 degrees of flexion, then an anterior orthosis may be considered. An anterior elbow orthosis is also used to prevent or correct elbow flexion contractures. Following a contracture release of a stiff elbow, an anterior elbow orthosis is used as a serial static orthosis to slowly gain extension of the elbow over time by remolding the orthosis in increased extension at weekly intervals. In addition, the anterior design is effective in blocking elbow flexion, such as with ulnar nerve compression neuropathies.

For extension contractures of 35 to 30 degrees, an anterior elbow extension orthosis is fabricated for use when the client is at rest (Fig. 10.11). As the position of comfort tends to be in flexion, it is recommended to gradually increase the wearing schedule to allow the client to get used to keeping the elbow in extension. During the fabrication process the orthosis may be molded to create a small space near the cubital fossa. During application the client may apply additional stretch to the elbow by attempting to

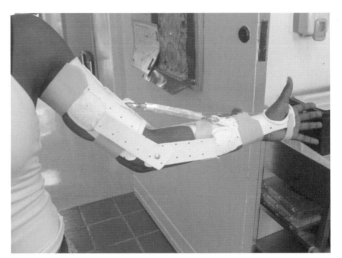

Fig. 10.12 Anterior elbow immobilization orthosis with a cubital window.

fully approximate the cubital fossa against the orthosis. If needed, a design modification of creating a cubital window may provide the client a visual guide (Fig. 10.12). As the client's elbow extension increases, the anterior elbow orthosis may be remolded to further provide static stretch until the goal is attained.

Static Progressive Elbow Extension

For flexion contractures of greater than 35 degrees, a static progressive elbow orthosis is either fabricated or provided. An effective design for a static progressive elbow extension orthosis is a custom turnbuckle orthosis (Fig. 10.13).[9] This orthosis features a long radial gutter distally, an anterior arm trough proximally, a pair of hinges, and a turnbuckle. The expandable adjustment of the turnbuckle rods affords incremental stretch. It should be noted that fabrication of this static progressive orthosis requires experience, expertise, and time. Simpler alternatives to the turnbuckle orthosis are commercially available, including the Mayo elbow universal brace (Fig. 10.14) and the JAS elbow orthosis (Fig. 10.15). Both braces are adjustable to the desired range and degree of stretch.

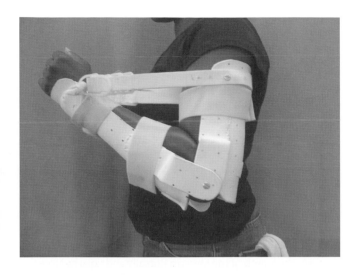

Fig. 10.13 Static progressive elbow orthosis with a turnbuckle.

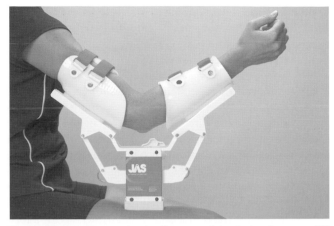

Fig. 10.15 JAS elbow orthosis. (Courtesy Joint Active Systems, Effingham, Illinois.)

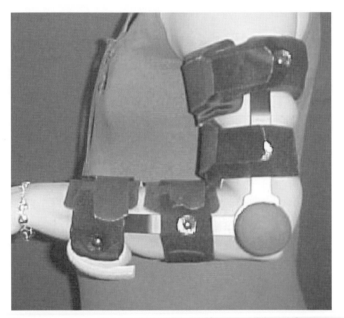

Fig. 10.14 Mayo elbow universal brace. (Courtesy Aircast, Summit, New Jersey.)

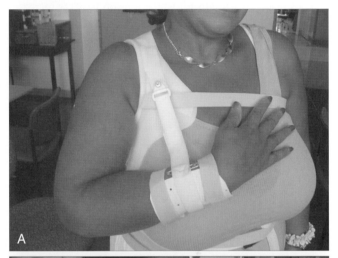

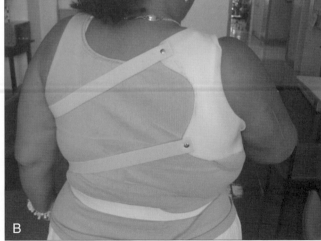

Fig. 10.16 Custom, static progressive elbow flexion orthosis, front (A) and back (B).

Static Progressive Elbow Flexion

For flexion contracture that prevents a client from achieving greater than 90 degrees of flexion, a custom static progressive elbow flexion orthosis is indicated (Fig. 10.16). This orthosis is referred to as the *"come-along" orthosis.* This orthosis features an ulnar gutter distally, a dorsal arm trough proximally, a pair of hinges, and strapping with an embedded series of D-rings. The straps with D-rings may be progressively advanced to provide the requisite flexion stretch. The therapist must assess the onset of ulnar nerve symptoms (e.g., report of numbness and tingling along the ulnar side of the hand and medial forearm) with prolonged elbow flexion. If such symptoms occur, the therapist examines and addresses the potential cause, including scar adhesions and edema that may restrict ulnar nerve gliding. An alternative to the use of D-straps is bungee cords (Fig. 10.17). However, with bungee cords the therapeutic mechanism changes from static

progressive stress relaxation to dynamic orthotic provision creep (see Chapter 13).

For flexion contracture that prevents a client with minimal elbow flexion motion (<90 degrees), a "holster-and-cuff" design is recommended (Fig. 10.18). The main biomechanical difference between this orthosis and the static progressive "come-along" orthosis is the length of the proximal moment arm. In a class I lever where the axis or fulcrum is in the middle of the effort and weight, the mechanical advantage favors the effort with a longer moment arm (Fig. 10.19). Again, the fabrication of these static progressive flexion orthoses requires experience, expertise, and time.

When the limitations are multidirectional, it may be necessary to fabricate multiple static orthoses for each limitation. The therapist must exercise a depth of reasoning in prioritizing which movement direction should be emphasized. Key considerations include the client's goals, severity of deficit, and response to active interventions, such as exercises, manual therapy, and therapeutic activities. It must be noted that for true physiological change to occur in the contractured tissues, the client must adhere to the wear regimen. Initially, clients are instructed to wear the orthosis for 2-hour intervals for a total of 6 to 8 hours daily. At first only short intervals are tolerated. The goal is to develop a tolerance for longer intervals. Clients may also be instructed to adjust the tension to allow increased motion as tolerated. When more than one orthosis is required, the client may alternate the orthoses during the day or wear one during the day and the other at night for sleeping. The orthotic regimen is highly individualized and tailored to meet the specific needs and limitations of each client. Off-the-shelf prefabricated static progressive flexion/extension orthoses are currently available and are effective in many cases. The shape of the client's arm, the degree of joint stiffness, and the firmness of joint end feel impact the fit and effectiveness of commercial orthoses.

Forearm Restriction

Restriction of forearm rotation is needed due to shaft fractures of the forearm or fracture-dislocation of the elbow or wrist. An orthosis that is nearly circumferentially positioned to the distal humerus and extending distally to include the wrist provides immobilization to the forearm. Two common designs are a sugar tong (see Fig. 10.4) and the Muenster-type orthosis. Both orthoses cover the length of the forearm dorsally and volarly. Note that with these orthoses the wrist is positioned in neutral or near neutral and restricted from sagittal plane movement. The elbow is partially restricted in the sagittal plane.

FABRICATION OF A POSTERIOR ELBOW IMMOBILIZATION ORTHOSIS

The initial step in the fabrication of an elbow immobilization orthosis is the drawing of a pattern. Elbow orthotic patterns differ from hand patterns in that measurements of the client's arm, elbow, forearm, wrist, and hand are taken and recorded. A pattern is drawn based on the recorded measurements. Tools and materials required to fabricate the orthosis include:
- Perforated $\frac{1}{8}$- to $\frac{3}{16}$-inch thermoplastic material with moderate elasticity, conformability, and bonding
- $\frac{1}{8}$-inch polycushion padding
- 1- to 2-inch strap
- 2- or 3-inch stockinette
- Tape measure
- Marker
- Scissors

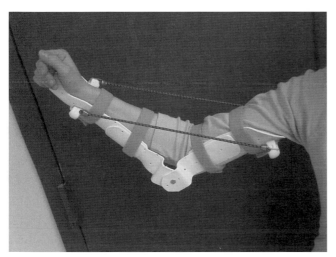

Fig. 10.17 Progressive elbow flexion orthosis using bungee cords.

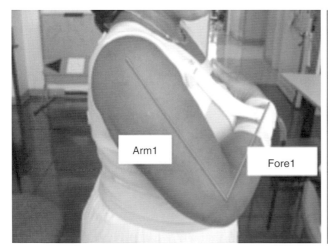

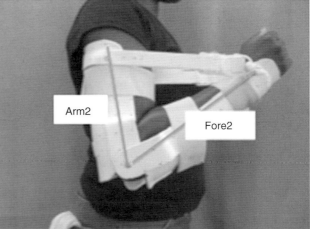

Mechanical Advantate (MA)
MA = Arm 1/Fore1
MA > 1, where Arm1 > Fore1

Mechanical Advantate (MA)
MA = Arm 2/Fore2
MA > 1, where Arm2 > Fore2

Fig. 10.18 Holster and cuff design orthosis.

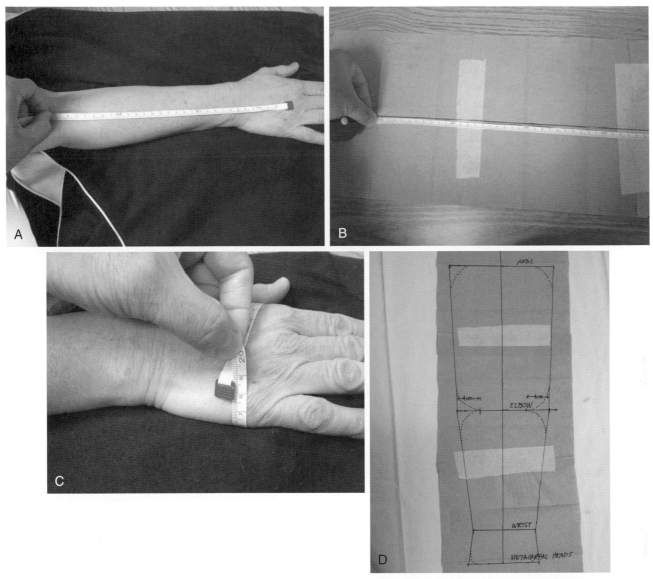

Fig. 10.19 Static progressive "come-along" orthosis. A, Measurement from distal palmar crease (DPC) to 2 cm distal to axillary fold. B, Drawing line along noted anatomical points. C, Drawing a perpendicular line at DPC. D, Measurements taken at anatomical landmarks.

PROCEDURE FOR FABRICATION OF A POSTERIOR ELBOW IMMOBILIZATION ORTHOSIS

The following steps describe the fabrication process for a posterior elbow immobilization orthosis in 90 degrees of flexion. The angle of the orthosis is determined by the structures to be protected.

1. Create a pattern by taking the following steps:
   a. Using a tape measure, measure the length of the upper extremity from the distal palmar crease (DPC), along the ulna and up to approximately 2 cm distal to the axillary fold (see Fig. 10.19A). Take note of the points corresponding to the DPC, ulnar styloid, olecranon process, and proximal arm.
   b. Draw a straight line on the paper using the length determined earlier (see Fig. 10.19B). Mark the anatomical points stated earlier along the straight line.
   c. Measure two-thirds of the circumference of the hand at the palmar crease (see Fig. 10.19C). Draw a perpendicular line at the DPC point by the straight line referenced in step 1b This straight line should bisect the perpendicular line.

   d. Repeat step 1c on the remaining measurement points: around the wrist by the ulnar styloid, around the elbow by the olecranon, and around the arm above the biceps (see Fig. 10.19D).
   e. Cut slits along the olecranon line approximately one-third of the width on both sides.
2. Cut the paper pattern from the paper and measure it on the client in the correct orthotic position. Make sure that the pattern covers the correct length from the DPC to the proximal arm. Ensure the correct girth at the anatomical points identified in step 1a. Once the pattern is deemed satisfactory, trace it on the thermoplastic material and cut the material (Fig. 10.20). If the material is too rigid to be cut, the material may be lightly heated to the point that it may be cut using a pair of scissors. Repetitive heating of the material may cause a loss of rigidity or durability.

Continued

PROCEDURE FOR FABRICATION OF A POSTERIOR ELBOW IMMOBILIZATION ORTHOSIS—cont'd

3. Position the client for orthotic provision. The ideal position is the client in supine with the shoulder and elbow in 90 degrees of flexion (Fig. 10.21). This position takes advantage of gravity to produce an easier and more precise drape of the thermoplastic material. Alternatively, the client may be lying prone with the shoulder abducted in 90 degrees and the forearm dangling over the edge of the plinth/bed.
4. Using disks cut out from polycushion, pad the following bony prominences: olecranon, lateral and medial epicondyles, and the ulnar head at the wrist (Fig. 10.22).
5. Cover the padding with a layer of stockinette to prevent it from adhering to the thermoplastic material. If the client has fragile or sensitive skin (e.g., allergic reaction to adhesives), an additional stockinette may be applied before sticking the polycushion pads on the bony prominences.
6. The material is heated according to the manufacturer's suggested duration. The material is removed and patted dry.
7. Carefully drape the material over the arm in the proper position described in step 3. Allow the material to rest on the client's limb before smoothing (Fig. 10.23).
8. The overlap between the arm and forearm troughs is pinched and smoothed first (Fig. 10.24). Then proceed with ensuring proper drape on the rest of the limb segments. A common error is for the client to extend the elbow slightly during the molding process, causing loss of the flexion angle. Using the noninjured hand, the client supports the limb by the wrist.
9. Once the material has cooled, the padding and stockinette are removed.
10. The elbow seams are smoothed, the edges flared, and the spaces for pressure relief over the bony prominences are further deepened by gently pushing the material (Fig. 10.25).
11. An alternative padding using the same thickness may be reinserted to the interior of the orthosis.
12. The fit is checked, and adjustments are made as needed.
13. Apply the following straps: proximal upper arm; distal upper arm, proximal to the elbow; proximal forearm; wrist and metacarpals (Fig. 10.26).
14. Reapply the orthosis, and recheck the fit (Fig. 10.27). If the elbow needs further reinforcement, a small thermoplastic strip may be cut, heated, and applied along corner edges of the elbow.
15. Educate the client in proper donning/doffing, skin checks and precautions, wearing schedule, and care of the orthosis.

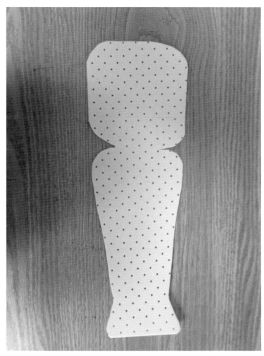

Fig. 10.20 Trace pattern and cut out.

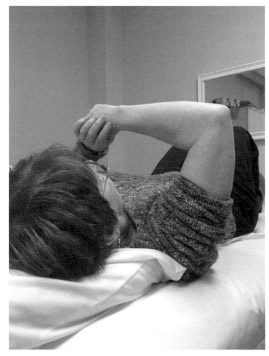

Fig. 10.21 Supine position of client for orthotic provision.

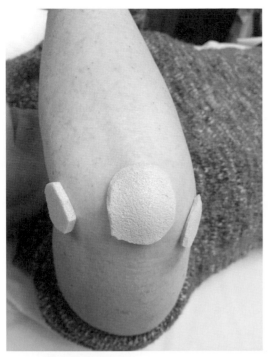

Fig. 10.22 Padding bony prominences.

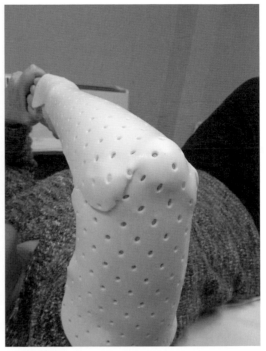

Fig. 10.24 Overlapping the arm and forearm troughs.

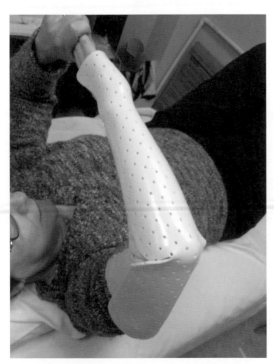

Fig. 10.23 Draping material over the arm.

TECHNICAL TIPS FOR A PROPER FIT

- Select a thermoplastic material that is rigid enough to support the elbow yet conforms well to the arm and joint.
- Align the thermoplastic material along the arm. Make sure to properly position the material before molding.

- An elastic wrap may be used to hold the material in place and free up the therapist's hands to support the arm in the correct position. Ensure that the pressure is even throughout the troughs. When using materials that are highly moldable, a wrap may leave unsightly imprints throughout the orthosis.
- Determine that the client has full range of motion of the shoulder and the hand when wearing the orthosis by having the client move in all planes.
- Ensure that the elbow, forearm, and/or wrist joints are in the correct angle during the molding process by checking the joint angles with a goniometer before the material cools.
- Make sure that the orthosis extends as proximal to the axilla as possible, particularly on the lateral side. This position provides adequate support and leverage to properly immobilize the elbow. Make sure the medial side of the proximal portion clears the axilla to prevent irritation.
- If a mistake occurs, it is better to remold the entire orthosis rather than spot heat/fix one area.
- If the material is not rigid enough, reinforce the orthosis with a material that has low memory. Make sure that when adding reinforcements like struts or exoskeletons, the orthosis is actually worn by the client.
- If the client is not adhering to the wear schedule, there is a tendency for the orthosis to curl inward (reducing circumferential opening).
- Use wide straps to properly secure the arm and the forearm in the orthosis. Consider using a figure-eight strap for clients with larger limb girth.

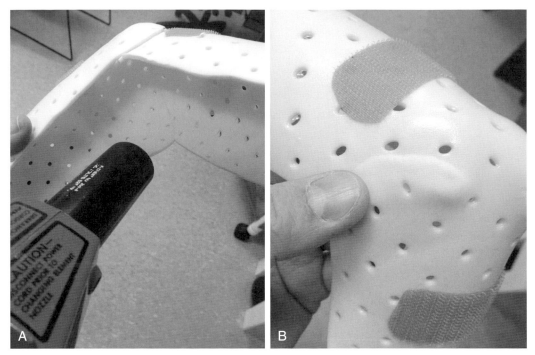

Fig. 10.25 Seams are smoothed (A), and ends are flared (B).

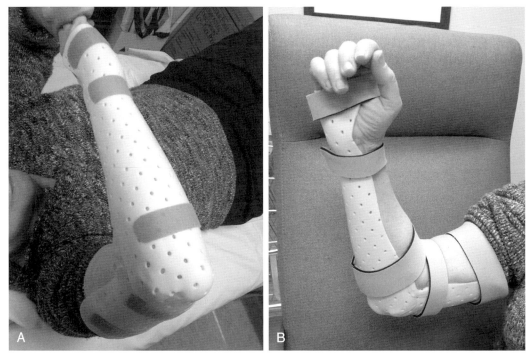

Fig. 10.26 A and B, Strap application.

PRECAUTIONS FOR ELBOW IMMOBILIZATION ORTHOSES

- Pad all bony prominences.
- Smooth or flare all edges. For a client with sensitive skin, add moleskin or thin padding as needed. Linings must be monitored for organic grime, dirt, and stains.
- Edema in the elbow is common after injury or surgery. Make sure the client is scheduled for a follow-up visit

within several days to modify and adjust the orthosis to accommodate for changes in edema.
- When applying an orthosis over an incision site that is not yet fully closed, make sure to cover the site with nonstick dressing. This protective dressing prevents moisture from transferring to the site from the orthosis.
- Open, draining, or infected wounds should not be covered by orthoses in order to allow for aeration and avoid pressure. Alternative orthoses should be explored.

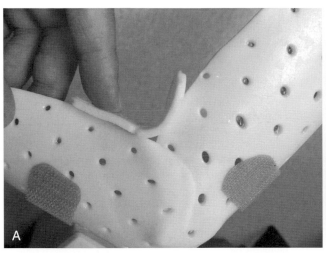
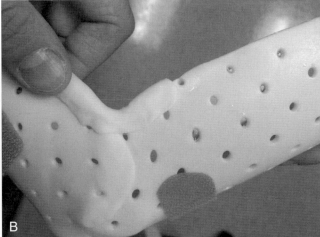

Fig. 10.27 Rechecking fit for needed reinforcement. A, Applying reinforcement. B, Adhering reinforcement to orthosis.

SELF-QUIZ 10.1[a]

For the following questions, circle either true (T) or false (F).

1. T F Elbow immobilization orthoses can be posterior or anterior.
2. T F It is better that the wrist be left free in forearm immobilization orthoses to allow for more functional motion.
3. T F Thinner and highly perforated material is preferable for postsurgical elbow orthoses to provide comfort and cooling.
4. T F Following a proximal radius fracture, the elbow can be immobilized in either a brace or posterior elbow orthosis.
5. T F Posterior elbow orthoses are preferred for increasing extension.
6. T F The angle of elbow immobilization is dictated by the client's comfort.
7. T F Olecranon fractures are positioned in 90 degrees of flexion.
8. T F An anterior elbow orthosis is appropriate for preventing or correcting elbow flexion contractures and for blocking elbow flexion.
9. T F The best orthosis for an extension contracture of the elbow of greater than 30 degrees is a serial static elbow extension orthosis.
10. T F Generally, biceps tendon repairs are immobilized with the elbow in complete extension.
11. T F Postoperative treatment of cubital tunnel includes positioning the elbow in 30 to 45 degrees of flexion.

[a]See Appendix A for the answer key.

REVIEW QUESTIONS

1. What are the main indications for elbow immobilization orthoses?
2. What are the precautions for elbow orthotic provision?
3. When might a therapist consider serial orthotic provision with an elbow immobilization orthosis?
4. What are the purposes of immobilization orthotic provision of the elbow?
5. What are the advantages and disadvantages of a custom orthosis over a commercial orthosis for the elbow?
6. What are the indications for anterior elbow orthotic provision?
7. What are the optimal positions for molding a posterior elbow orthosis?

REFERENCES

1. Blackmore S: Therapist's management of ulnar nerve compression at the elbow. In Mackin EJ, Callahan AD, Skirven TM, et al.: *Rehabilitation of the hand and upper extremity*, ed 5, St. Louis, 2000, Mosby.
2. Budoff JE: Coronoid fractures, *J Hand Surg Am* 37(11):2418–2423, 2012.
3. Cabanela MF, Morrey BF: Fractures of the olecranon. In Morrey BF, editor: *The elbow and its disorders*, ed 3, Philadelphia, 2000, Saunders, pp 365–379.
4. Charalambos CP, Morrey BF: Posttraumatic elbow stiffness, *J Bone Joint Surg* 94A:1428–1437.
5. de Haan J, den Hartog D, Tuinebreijer WE, et al.: Functional treatment versus plaster for simple elbow dislocations, *BMC Musc Dis* 11:263–270, 2010.

6. Edwards SG, Cohen MS, Lattanza LL, et al.: Surgeon perceptions and outcomes regarding proximal ulna fixation: a multicenter experience, *J Should Elb Surg* 12:1637–1643, 2012.

7. Fess E, Gettle K, Philips C, et al.: Splinting for work, sports and the performing arts. In Fess E, Gettle K, Philips C, et al.: *Hand and upper extremity splinting: principles and methods*, ed 3, St. Louis, 2005, Mosby, pp 470–471.

8. Flowers KR, LaStayo P: Effect of total end range time on improving passive range of motion, *J Hand Ther* 7(3):150–157, 1994.

9. Gelinas JJ, Faber KJ, Patterson SD, et al.: The effectiveness for turnbuckle splinting for elbow contractures, *J Bone Joint Surg Br* 82(1):74–78, 2000.

10. Hoisington SA, Murthy VL: Forearm fractures. In Hoppenfeld S, Murthy VL, editors: *Treatment and rehabilitation of fractures*, Philadelphia, 2000, Lippincott Williams and Williams, pp 169–190.

11. Hotchkiss R: Fractures and dislocations of the elbow. In Green DP, editor: *Rockwood and Green's fractures in adults*, ed 4, Philadelphia, 1996, Lippincott-Raven.

12. Liu HH, Wu K, Chang CH: Treatment of complex elbow injuries with a postoperative custom-made progressive stretching static elbow splint, *J Orthop Trauma* 20(6):400–404, 2006.

13. McKee RC, McKee MD: Complex fractures of the proximal ulna: the critical importance of the coronoid fragment, *Inst Course Lect* 61:227–233, 2012.

14. Morrey BF: Anatomy of the elbow joint. In Morrey BF, editor: *The elbow and its disorders*, ed 3, Philadelphia, 2000, Saunders, pp 13–42.

15. Neumann DA: The elbow and forearm complex. In Kisner C, Colby LA: *Therapeutic exercise foundations and techniques*, ed 6, Philadelphia, FA Davis.

16. Oatis CA: *Kinesiology: the mechanics and pathomechanics of human movement*, Philadelphia, 2004, Lippincott Williams and Williams.

17. Pike JM, Athwal GS, Faber KJ, et al.: Radial head fractures—an update, *J Hand Surg Am* 34(3):557–565, 2009.

18. Quach T, Jazayeri R, Sherman OH, et al.: Distal biceps tendon injuries—current treatment options, *Bull NYU Hosp Jt Dis* 68(2):103–111, 2010.

19. Rayan G: Ulnar nerve compression, *Hand Clinics* 8:325, 1992.

20. Ruch DS, Papadonikolakis A: Elbow instability and arthroscopy. In Trumble TE, Budoff JE, Cornwall R, editors: *Hand, elbow and shoulder: core knowledge in orthopedics*, St. Louis, 2004, Mosby, pp 510–521.

21. Seiler 3rd JG, Parker LM, Chamberland PD, et al.: The distal biceps tendon: two potential mechanisms involved in its rupture: arterial supply and mechanical impingement, *J Shoulder Elbow Surg* 4(3):149–156, 1995.

22. Smith LK, Weiss EL, Lehmkuhl LD: *Brunnstrom's clinical kinesiology*, ed 5, Philadelphia, 1996, FA Davis.

23. Wolff AL, Hotchkiss RN: Lateral elbow instability: nonoperative, operative, and postoperative management, *J Hand Ther* 19(2):238–243, 2006.

24. Yoon A, Athwal GS, Faber KJ, et al.: Radial head fractures, *J Hand Surg Am* 37(12):2626–2634, 2012.

25. Moscony A: Peripheral nerve problems. In Cooper C, editor: *Fundamentals of hand therapy*, ed 2, St. Louis, 2014, Elsevier Mosby, pp 299–300.

26. Apfel E, Sigafoos GT: Comparison of range-of-motion constraints provided by splints used in the treatment of cubital tunnel syndrome—a pilot study, *J Hand Ther* 19(4):384–392, 2006.

27. Veltman ES, Doornberg JN, Eygendaal D, van den Bekerom MPJ: Static progressive versus dynamic splinting for posttraumatic elbow stiffness: a systematic review of 232 patients, *Arch Orthop Trauma Surg* 135:613–617, 2015.

28. Shah CM, Calfee RP, Gelberman RH, Goldfarb CA: Outcomes of rigid night splinting and activity modification in the treatment of cubital tunnel syndrome, *J Hand Surg* 38A:1125–1130, 2013.

29. Jafarian FS, Demneh ES, Tyson SF: The immediate effect of orthotic management on grip strength of patients with lateral epicondylosis, *J Orthop Sports Phys Therapy* 39(6):484–490, 2009.

30. Najafi M, Arazpour M, Aminian G, Curran S, Madani SP, Hutchins SW: Effect of a new hand-forearm splint on grip strength, pain, and function in patients with tennis elbow, *Prosthet Orthot Int* 40(3):363–368, 2016.

31. Garg R, Adamson GJ, Dawson PA, Shankwiler JA, Pink MM: A prospective randomized study comparing a forearm strap brace versus a wrist splint for the treatment of lateral epicondylitis, *Hand (New York)* 19(4):508–512, 2010.

APPENDIX 10.1 CASE STUDIES

Case Study 10.1[a]

Read the following scenario, and use your clinical reasoning skills to answer the questions based on information in this chapter.

Laura is a 47-year-old attorney who slipped on the ice and fractured and dislocated her left elbow. She was first treated at the local emergency department, where the elbow was casted. One week later, she underwent open reduction internal fixation (ORIF) to the radial head, which repaired the ruptured lateral ligament of the elbow. Two days post surgery she is referred for therapy (before discharge from the hospital) for a posterior elbow orthosis in 110 to 120 degrees of flexion. Laura lives alone and has two active dogs for pets.

1. Describe the appropriate orthosis for Laura. List all of the joints to include in this orthosis.
2. How should the client be positioned for fabrication of this orthosis?
3. Which bony prominences require extra protection in the orthosis? How is this accomplished?
4. What wearing schedule should be provided to Laura?

Case Study 10.2

Read the following scenario, and use your clinical reasoning skills to answer the questions based on information from this chapter.

Marissa is a 42-year-old office clerk who is referred for therapy with a diagnosis of ulnar neuropathy of the left hand. She reports waking up in the middle of the night with tingling sensation to the ulnar side of the forearm and hand lasting for 10 to 15 minutes. There is no atrophy of the intrinsic hand muscles of the left hand. There is a significant difference in strength of grip and pinch between the two hands. Further examination reveals a positive Tinel sign to the ulnar nerve at the cubital tunnel region and positive symptoms of tingling following 30 seconds of sustained elbow flexion.

Frank is a 55-year-old factory worker who underwent an ulnar nerve anterior submuscular transposition surgery 10 days ago. The patient has just had his sutures removed, and the surgeon has referred Frank to occupational therapy services for evaluation and treatment and fabrication of an elbow orthosis.

Bob is a 37-year old taxicab driver who sustained a terrible triad injury of the right elbow from a non–work-related car accident. He underwent open reduction internal fixation (ORIF) of the distal humerus, coronoid process, and proximal radius. A hinged external fixator was applied for 11 to 12 weeks. He was referred to therapy to improve his range of motion and facilitate return to work. He came to therapy 2 weeks after external fixator removal without an orthosis or brace. His elbow range of motion is currently 50/120. Bob performs his self-care activities independently. His main concern is being able to drive his taxi again.

1. What orthosis or brace is most appropriate for each client?
2. What wearing schedule and instructions should be provided to each client?

APPENDIX 10.2 LABORATORY EXERCISES

Laboratory Exercise 10.1 Making an Elbow Shell Pattern

1. Practice making a posterior elbow shell pattern on another person. Use the detailed instructions provided to take measurements and draw the pattern.
2. Cut out the pattern, and check for proper fit.

Laboratory Exercise 10.2 Fabricating an Elbow Orthosis

Practice fabricating an elbow immobilization orthosis on a partner. Before starting, determine the correct position for the partner's elbow. Measure the angle of elbow flexion/extension with a goniometer to ensure correct position. After fitting the orthosis and making adjustments, use Form 10.1 as a self-evaluation of the elbow immobilization orthosis, and use Grading Sheet 10.1 as a classroom grading sheet.

[a] See Appendix A for the answer key.

APPENDIX 10.3 FORM AND GRADING SHEET

Form 10.1 Elbow Immobilization Orthosis

	Name: _____
	Date: _____
Type of elbow immobilization orthosis:	
Posterior	Anterior
Elbow position: _____	
After the person wears the orthosis for 30 minutes, answer the following questions. (Mark NA for nonapplicable situations.)	

Evaluation Areas				Comments
Design				
1. The elbow position is at the correct angle.	Yes	No	NA	
2. The elbow has adequate medial and lateral support (two-thirds the circumference of the elbow).	Yes	No	NA	
3. The orthosis supplies sufficient proximal/lateral support (1 inch proximal to axillary crease).	Yes	No	NA	
4. The orthosis is two-thirds the circumference of the upper arm.	Yes	No	NA	
5. Distally the orthosis extends to the distal palmar crease (DPC).	Yes	No	NA	
6. The orthosis is two-thirds the circumference of the forearm.	Yes	No	NA	
Function				
1. The orthosis allows full thumb and digit motion.	Yes	No	NA	
2. The orthosis allows full shoulder motion.	Yes	No	NA	
3. The orthosis provides adequate elbow support to properly secure the elbow in the orthosis and prevent elbow motion.	Yes	No	NA	
Straps				
1. The straps are secure.	Yes	No	NA	
2. The straps are adequate in length.	Yes	No	NA	
Comfort				
1. The orthosis' edges are smooth with rounded corners.	Yes	No	NA	
2. The proximal and distal ends are flared.	Yes	No	NA	
3. The orthosis does not cause impingements or pressure sores.	Yes	No	NA	
4. The orthosis does not irritate bony prominences.	Yes	No	NA	
Cosmetic Appearance				
1. The orthosis is free of fingerprints, dirt, and pencil and pen marks.	Yes	No	NA	
2. The orthotic material is not buckled.	Yes	No	NA	
Therapeutic Regimen				
1. The person was instructed in a wearing schedule.	Yes	No	NA	
2. The person was provided orthotic precautions.	Yes	No	NA	
3. The person demonstrates understanding of the education.	Yes	No	NA	
4. Client/caregiver knows how to clean the orthosis.	Yes	No	NA	

Discuss possible orthosis adjustments or changes you should make based on the self-evaluation. (What would you do differently next time?)

Discuss possible areas to improve clinical safety when fabricating the orthosis.

Grading Sheet 10.1 Elbow Immobilization Orthosis

	Name: _____
	Date: _____

Type of elbow immobilization orthosis:		
Posterior	Anterior	

Elbow position: _____

Grade:

1 = Beyond improvement, not acceptable

2 = Requires maximal improvement

3 = Requires moderate improvement

4 = Requires minimal improvement

5 = Requires no improvement

Evaluation Areas						Comments
Design						
1. The elbow position is at the correct angle.	1	2	3	4	5	
2. The elbow has adequate medial and lateral support (two-thirds the circumference of the elbow).	1	2	3	4	5	
3. The orthosis supplies sufficient proximal/lateral support (1 inch proximal to axillary crease).	1	2	3	4	5	
4. The orthosis is two-thirds the circumference of the upper arm.	1	2	3	4	5	
5. Distally the orthosis extends to the distal palmar crease (DPC).	1	2	3	4	5	
6. The orthosis is two-thirds the circumference of the forearm.	1	2	3	4	5	
Function						
1. The orthosis allows full thumb and digit motion.	1	2	3	4	5	
2. The orthosis allows full shoulder motion.	1	2	3	4	5	
3. The orthosis provides adequate elbow support to properly secure the elbow in the orthosis and prevents elbow motion.	1	2	3	4	5	
Straps						
1. The straps are secure.	1	2	3	4	5	
2. The straps are adequate in length.	1	2	3	4	5	
Comfort						
1. The orthosis' edges are smooth with rounded corners.	1	2	3	4	5	
2. The proximal end is flared.	1	2	3	4	5	
3. The orthosis does not cause impingements or pressure sores.	1	2	3	4	5	
4. The orthosis does not irritate bony prominences.	1	2	3	4	5	
Cosmetic Appearance						
1. The orthosis is free of fingerprints, dirt, and pencil and pen marks.	1	2	3	4	5	
2. The orthotic material is not buckled.	1	2	3	4	5	

Orthoses for the Shoulder

William P. Finley

CHAPTER OBJECTIVES

1. Review general shoulder anatomy and biomechanical considerations for immobilization.
2. Identify shoulder immobilization orthoses, slings, and braces.
3. Discuss common shoulder diagnoses that require immobilization.
4. Review precautions for shoulder immobilization.
5. Apply biomechanical consideration for orthotic, sling, and brace application.
6. Demonstrate clinical judgment in the provision of shoulder immobilization devices.
7. Apply knowledge of shoulder immobilization devices to a case study.
8. Fabricate a proximal humerus cap orthosis.

KEY TERMS

acromion
AMBRI
appendicular skeleton
axial skeleton
Bankart lesion
Bankart repair

clavicular facet
coracohumeral ligament
figure-eight orthosis
glenoid fossa
open reduction internal fixation
  (ORIF)

osteoporotic fracture
subluxation
superior labrum tear from anterior
  to posterior (SLAP)
transverse humeral ligament
TUBS

Mr. Smith was walking with his wife on a busy city street when he fell onto the side of his arm. He was immediately rushed to the emergency department and was diagnosed with a humeral fracture, and surgery was recommended. Mr. Smith had recently retired and was experiencing various other medical conditions that did not make him a strong surgical candidate. As such, he decided to proceed with nonoperative management. Mr. Smith was placed in a sling and sent to occupational therapy for a proximal humerus cap orthosis and light passive range-of-motion exercises.

ANATOMICAL AND BIOMECHANICAL CONSIDERATIONS

The shoulder complex is unlike any other structure in the human body. The shoulder is composed of four joints, which perform coordinated intricate movement patterns within a large range of motion (ROM) and with significant strength. The bony anatomy of the shoulder consists of the sternum, clavicle, scapula, and humerus. The four joints of the shoulder are the: sternoclavicular joint, acromioclavicular (AC) joint, scapulothoracic joint, and the glenohumeral joint (Fig. 11.1).[19]

The sternoclavicular joint is technically the link between the **axial skeleton** and **appendicular skeleton** and is composed of the medial end of the clavicle, the **clavicular facet** of the sternum, and the superior border of the cartilage of the first rib. The movements of this small joint are elevation and depression, protraction and retraction, and axial rotation. An articular disk and a dense amount of tissue stabilize this joint, which makes direct injuries or dislocations rare, but a lack of motion can result in a loss of end-range motions for shoulder flexion and abduction.[16]

The articulation between the lateral end of the clavicle and the **acromion** of the scapula forms the AC joint. The small movements of this joint are upward and downward rotation, horizontal plane rotation, and sagittal plane rotation. This small joint is highly predisposed to osteoarthritis and is at high risk of dislocation in the athletic population.[12]

The scapulothoracic joint is not considered a true joint as it is formed between the anterior surface of the scapula and the posterior-lateral wall of the thorax. Although it is technically not the link between the axial and appendicular skeleton, it is the foundation of force transmission and motion between the larger core muscles and the upper extremity. The scapulothoracic joint relies on the surrounding musculature for stabilization. The kinematics consist of elevation

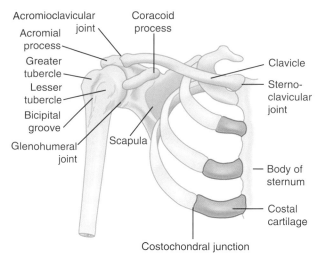

Fig. 11.1 Anatomy of the shoulder complex. (From Phelps, K., & Hassed, C. (2011). *General practice: The integrative approach.* Sydney: Churchill Livingstone/Elsevier.)

and depression, protraction and retraction, and upward and downward rotation.[19] Due to the large amount of muscular involvement, scapula dyskinesis plays a major role in many shoulder injuries and pain pathologies.[11]

The final joint of the shoulder complex, the glenohumeral joint is formed by the head of the humerus and the concavity of the **glenoid fossa.** The basic anatomical motions of this dynamic joint include abduction and adduction, flexion and extension, and internal and external rotation. There are considerable accessory motions that occur at this joint such as roll, spin, and slide. Due to the mobility of this joint, tissue stabilization is of utmost importance. The glenohumeral joint is stabilized by the capsular ligaments, **coracohumeral ligament, transverse humeral ligament,** glenoid labrum, and the surrounding musculature.[19] Due to demands placed on this mobile joint, it is predisposed to dislocations, and the surrounding tissues are vulnerable to various traumatic and nontraumatic injuries.[29]

Immobilization of the shoulder is more problematic than other parts of the body due to the possibility of adhesive capsulitis (frozen shoulder syndrome) and scapular dyskinesis (alteration of the static and/or dynamic positioning of the scapula), which significantly interferes with the rehabilitation process.[20,21] When immobilizing the shoulder, proper fit, positioning, wear time, and client education are necessary components. Incorrect or prolonged immobilization has long-term deleterious effects.[12] Therefore, when immobilizing the shoulder, the therapist considers numerous variables to minimally impact the client's rehabilitation.

COMMON DIAGNOSES

There are several diagnoses that often require shoulder orthotic intervention (Table 11.1). Diagnoses include proximal humeral fractures, shoulder **subluxation** and instability syndrome, rotator cuff (RTC) repairs, **superior labrum anterior to posterior (SLAP)** and Bankart repairs, AC dislocations, clavicle fractures, and axilla contractures.

Proximal Humerus Fractures

Proximal humeral fractures are a common orthopedic injury, typically affecting the older adult population, and can have a significant impact on all functional activities. The proximal humeral fracture is universally referred to as an **osteoporotic fracture** and can lead to extreme pain and high levels of deformity. Incidences vary from 105 to 342 per 100,000 persons per year.[2] Proximal humeral fractures vary in severity and are graded as one-part, two-part, three-part, or four-part. Generally one- and two-part proximal humeral fractures are managed conservatively. Three- and four-part proximal humeral fractures are managed surgically.[2] Current evidence on immobilization and rehabilitation for one- and two-part fractures is very positive with 77% to 88% of patients having good to excellent results based on ROM).[10] In contrast, researchers report a significant decrease in quality of life when comparing nonsurgical to surgical management of three-part proximal humerus fractures.[23] Four-part proximal humerus fractures will have fracture lines along the humeral head, greater tuberosity, lesser tuberosity, and humeral shaft; three out of four parts will be displaced with respect to the fourth; and surgery is almost always indicated.[5]

The severity of fracture plays a crucial role in determining the need for surgical intervention, orthotic provision, and/or immobilization time frame. Because a humeral fracture is a common injury in the older adult, one must consider prior level of function and comorbidities to develop an intervention. Regardless of intervention the elder population requires some form of immobilization of the shoulder complex. The recommended immobilization time frame can range from 1 to 7 weeks, depending on severity of fracture.[5] The most common immobilization for humeral fractures is a traditional sling with the arm placed in adduction and internal rotation and/or a proximal humerus cap orthosis (Figs. 11.2 and 11.3)

Shoulder Subluxation and Instability Syndrome

Shoulder instability syndrome is another common orthopedic condition that may or may not warrant immobilization. Many people with mild to moderate instability syndrome function without pain or disability. Instability syndrome becomes problematic when it leads to subluxation(s). There are two main types of classification for shoulder instability/subluxation: **TUBS** (**T**raumatic etiology, **U**nidirectional instability, **B**ankart lesion, whereby **S**urgery is required) and **AMBRI** (**A**traumatic, **M**ultidirectional instability, **B**ilateral, **R**ehabilitation, **I**nferior capsule shift), whereby rehabilitation is the treatment of choice.[3]

A TUBS injury is likely to be traumatic in nature and often leads to a Bankart repair requiring immobilization of up to 6 weeks. These clients are positioned in varying degrees of abduction and varying degrees of rotation. Recent studies recommend a neutral to externally rotated position, compared with the more traditional internally rotated position.[33]

Clients with an AMBRI classification usually have a small or flat glenoid fossa, capsular tissue migration, weak RTC muscles, malpositioning of the humeral head, and/or neuromuscular and proprioceptive deficits. Multiple factors such as

TABLE 11.1 Evidenced-Based Practice About Shoulder Immobilization Orthoses

Author Citation	Design	Number of Participants	Description	Results	Limitations
Axillary Burn Injuries					
Jang, K. U., Choi, J. S., Mun, J. H., et al. (2015). Multi-axis shoulder abduction splint in acute burn rehabilitation: A randomized controlled pilot trial. *Clinical Rehabilitation, 29*(5), 439–446. https://doi.org/10.1177/0269215514547653	RCT	24 patients from an inpatient burn center who had sustained shoulder burns within the previous 30 days were randomized into two groups.	*Splint group:* Patients wore a multiaxis shoulder abduction splint, which positioned the shoulder as close as possible to a 90-degree abduction angle at all times, unless receiving hygiene care or undergoing medical procedures. *Nonsplint group:* Patients did not receive a splint. Both groups received comparable medical treatment and exercises (active/passive mobilization and stretching for 30 min 2×/day). Shoulder ROM was measured at baseline and each week over a 4-week period.	The splint group achieved significant improvements in shoulder abduction angle compared with the nonsplint group. There were no differences in shoulder flexion or external rotation angles between groups.	Limitations of this study include its small sample size, and ROM was the only study outcome. Functional outcomes remain unknown. Long-term impacts of this splint were not explored.
Kolmus, A. M., Holland, A. E., Byrne, M. J., et al. (2012). The effects of splinting on shoulder function in adult burns. *Burns, 38*(2012), 638–644. https://doi.org/10.1016/j.burns.2012.01.010	RCT	52 adult patients with axillary burns were randomized into a splint group or a control group.	*Splint group:* Patients wore a shoulder splint, which positioned the shoulder in 90 degrees abduction at all times for 6 weeks, except during hygiene, dressing changes, and exercise participation. For an additional 6 weeks, participants wore the splint overnight only. Individuals also participated in a daily exercise program that involved stretching, strengthening, and functional upper extremity training. *Control group:* Patients performed the daily exercise program for 12 weeks. *Outcome measures:* shoulder abduction and flexion, QOL (Burn Specific Health Scale-Brief), UE function (UEFI and Grocery Shelving Task), and adherence (questionnaires).	There were no statistically significant differences between groups for ROM, QOL, or function at any point in time. There were no clinically important differences among groups on any outcome measure at week 12. Splint adherence was generally poor, with only 16% adherent at week 12. There were not any differences between groups in terms of exercise adherence at weeks 1, 3, or 12; however, the splint group had a tendency to adhere to the exercises more at week 6 in comparison to the control group. Ultimately, the addition of the shoulder splint to an exercise program did not improve clinical outcomes in participants.	This was the first RCT exploring the impacts of a shoulder splint in conjunction with a daily exercise program in individuals with axillary burns. Due to poor splint adherence, it is difficult to generate strong conclusions regarding the splint's effect.

Continued

TABLE 11.1 Evidenced-Based Practice About Shoulder Immobilization Orthoses—cont'd

Author Citation	Design	Number of Participants	Description	Results	Limitations
Clavicle Fractures					
Tamaoki, M. J., Matsunaga, F. T., Ferreira da Costa, A. R., et al. (2017). Treatment of displaced midshaft clavicle fractures: Figure-of-eight harness versus anterior plate osteosynthesis. *Journal of Bone and Joint Surgery, 99*(14), 1159–1165.	RCT	117 adults with displaced midshaft clavicle fractures who were randomized into a nonsurgical group or a surgical group.	*Nonsurgical group:* Participants wore a figure-eight harness and were educated about skin care, brace management, and using the affected limb as much as able. *Surgical group:* Participants underwent open reduction and anterior plate osteosynthesis. Following surgery, they remained immobilized via sling for 7–10 days before AROM was initiated. Both groups underwent the same rehabilitation program, which included elbow/wrist/hand AROM starting the first day, PROM after the seventh day, followed by shoulder AROM as tolerated. *Outcome measures:* UE function at 6 months (DASH), pain, time to return to work or previous activities, patient satisfaction with cosmetic results, radiographic findings, and presence of complications.	There were no differences in UE function, pain, or mean time to return to work or activities between groups. There were no restrictions in shoulder ROM at the final assessment in either group. Mean amount of bone shortening secondary to malunion was greater in the nonsurgical group than that in the surgical group ($P < .001$). All fractures within the surgical group healed, whereas 7 individuals on the nonsurgical group developed fracture nonunion ($P = .004$). 7 patients in the surgical group experienced paresthesia, as compared to 1 patient in the nonsurgical group ($P = .036$). No statistically significant differences regarding dissatisfaction with cosmetic results or shoulder droop were detected across groups. More individuals in the nonsurgical group reported shoulder malpositioning, shortening, and bone prominence ($P = .020$, $P < .001$, $P < .001$).	Only one functional outcome was assessed within this study. It is also possible that results may change with longer follow-up, particularly in cases where shortening and malunion were noted. Authors note that cost-effective analysis and stratification or block randomization for fracture types was not performed within this trial.
Woltz, S., Stegeman, S. A., Krijnen, P., et al. (2017). Plate fixation compared with nonoperative treatment for displaced midshaft clavicular fractures: A multicenter randomized controlled trial. *Journal of Bone and Joint Surgery, 99-A*(2), 106–112.	RCT	160 patients with displaced midshaft clavicle fractures were randomized into a nonoperatively treated group or an operatively treated group	*Nonoperative treatment group:* For the first 2 weeks, individuals wore a sling and were instructed to perform pendulums, followed by AROM up to the horizontal plane. At 6 weeks, patients were permitted to engage in full ROM and strengthening exercises. *Operative treatment group:* Individuals underwent surgical intervention within 3 weeks of injury and followed the same postoperative mobilization protocol as those in the nonoperative treatment group. *Outcomes of interest:* nonunion, adverse events and secondary operations, pain, arm function, satisfaction with cosmetic appearance, and general health status.	Arm function, as measured by Constant scores and DASH scores, were similar across both treatment groups at 1 year. Regarding general health status, SF-36 physical component scores were somewhat lower in the nonoperative group at 6 weeks ($P = .03$). At 6 weeks, pain scores were also higher in the nonoperatively treated group ($P = .04$). 5% of those in the operatively treated group and 18% of those in the nonoperative group claimed dissatisfaction with cosmetic results. At 1 year, 2.4% of patients in the operatively treated group and 23.1% patients in the nonoperative treatment group developed nonunion ($P < .0001$). Secondary operation rates due to adverse events did not differ significantly between groups (15.7% in the nonoperative treatment group; 10.7% in the operative group). 19.2% of patients in the operative group experienced persistent numbness of the skin surrounding the surgical site 1 year following surgery.	Authors note that there was an imbalance between both groups (n = 86 within the operative group; n = 74 within the nonoperative treatment group). Several patients were lost to follow-up, which could contribute to bias and reduce the power associated with the data gathered from functional outcomes. Surgical treatment protocols differed across hospitals. The radiographic images were also read by treating surgeons, which could

Author Citation	Design	Number of Participants	Description	Results	Limitations
Shoulder Subluxation/Dislocation					
Nadler, M., & Pauls, M. M. H. (2017). Shoulder orthoses for the prevention and reduction of hemiplegic shoulder pain and subluxation: Systematic review. *Clinical Rehabilitation, 31*(4), 444–453. https://doi.org/10.1177/0269215516648753	Systematic review	8 studies consisting of 186 participants in total (1 RCT, 1 quasi-RCT, 1 before/after controlled study, 5 observational studies) *Inclusion criteria:* English language and studies composed of adults with stroke that assessed impact of shoulder orthoses on vertical subluxation and shoulder pain	Authors investigated whether orthoses prevent or reduce vertical subluxation and hemiplegic shoulder pain, whether differing types of orthoses are equally effective, whether there were any adverse effects associated with wearing shoulder orthoses, and whether they were well tolerated. A descriptive synthesis was performed using data gathered from studies that met inclusion criteria. *Outcomes of interest:* immediate repositioning of the humeral head, reduced subluxation after prolonged wear, decreased pain, reduced ROM, onset/increase of spasticity, increased hand edema, patient satisfaction, and tolerance to the orthosis.	None of the studies investigated whether shoulder orthoses can *prevent* subluxation from developing. Findings from three studies provided minimal evidence to support that shoulder orthoses can improve or reverse subluxation following prolonged wear. Orthoses that only provided support at the proximal UE were least effective, whereas orthoses providing whole arm support or proximal and distal support were more effective in minimizing subluxation. Three studies suggested modest improvements in pain measures for the majority of patients who wore a shoulder orthosis. Two studies provided evidence to suggest good patient tolerance and moderately high compliance levels to wearing a shoulder orthosis. Results from three studies did not show any increase in shoulder contracture following orthotic wear. One trial found that there were not any increases in spasticity following the use of a shoulder orthosis for hemiplegia, and another trial noted significant improvements in edema.	A descriptive synthesis was necessary, since the data was heterogeneous and ineligible for meta-analysis. There was only one RCT included within this review. Authors claim there could have been some subjectivity and bias with recruitment, intervention, and assessment methods in the included observational studies. Future studies should incorporate large sample sizes with blinded assessors and randomization for recruitment and allocation of participants. More studies exploring the effects of early application of shoulder orthoses, duration of wear, and long-term implications are warranted.

Continued

TABLE 11.1 Evidenced-Based Practice About Shoulder Immobilization Orthoses—cont'd

Author Citation	Design	Number of Participants	Description	Results	Limitations
Humeral Fractures					
Matsunaga, F. T., Tamaoki, M. J., Matsumoto, M. H., et al. (2017). Minimally invasive osteosynthesis with a bridge plate versus a functional brace for humeral shaft fractures. *Journal of Bone and Joint Surgery, 99-A(7)*, 583–592.	RCT	110 patients randomized into the surgery group (bridge plate) or the nonoperative group (functional brace)	*Nonoperative treatment group:* Participants first underwent a closed reduction and immobilization via coaptation U-splint from the axilla to the elbow. A functional brace was applied after 2 weeks, which permitted shoulder and elbow ROM, and worn until fracture consolidation was confirmed. *Surgical group:* The upper limb was immobilized via coaptation splint until ready to undergo anterior-access bridge plate osteosynthesis. Following surgery, these individuals wore a sling until their first evaluation. Both groups received similar rehabilitation programs involving A/PROM of the elbow and pendulums as tolerated early on. IR and ER were allowed 6 weeks postintervention. *Outcomes Measures:* DASH scores, scores on the SF-36 life quality questionnaire, complications of treatment, Constant-Murley scores for the shoulder, pain, and radiographic results.	Those in the surgical group achieved significantly higher DASH scores at 6 months (*P* = .046). Statistically significant differences were not seen in any domains of the SF-36, Constant-Murley scores, or VAS pain scores. Severe complications were noted in 10 patients within the nonoperative treatment group (23%), as compared to 0 within the surgical group. 15% of those in the nonoperative group experienced nonunion. 7 patients within the surgical group also experienced complications that did not require additional intervention, and 5 patients in the nonoperative group developed contact dermatitis from the brace. Those who wore the functional brace also demonstrated significantly greater final angular displacement on anteroposterior radiographs (10.5 degrees) when compared with those who underwent surgery (2.0 degrees).	16 patients were lost to follow-up. Nonunions could have contributed to lower scores on some of the outcomes used. For example, individuals with nonunion could have achieved lower DASH scores because they were still recovering from a corrective surgery. Authors also noted decreased external validity, as the study took place in one center.

AROM, Active range of motion; *DASH,* Disabilities of the Arm, Shoulder, and Hand; *ER,* external rotation; *IR,* internal rotation; *QOL,* quality of life; *RCT,* randomized controlled trial; *ROM,* range of motion; *SF-36,* Short Form-36; *UE,* upper extremity; *UEFI,* Upper Extremity Functional Index; *VAS,* visual analog scale.

Contributed by Andrea Coppola.

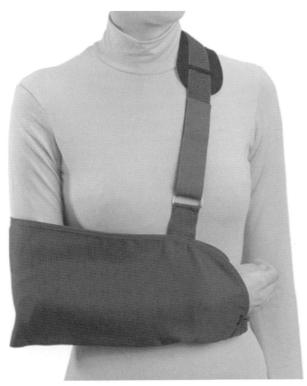

Fig. 11.2 Traditional shoulder sling (adduction and internal rotation). (Courtesy of DJO, LLC.)

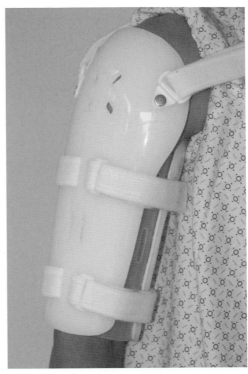

Fig. 11.3 Sarmiento proximal humeral cap orthosis with cross-body strap. (Courtesy of Brian Laney, OT, CHT.)

mechanism of injury and number of previous subluxations affect the decision for the position and length of immobilization. Although recent studies contradict the traditional adducted and internally rotated sling position, the internally rotated position is the most frequently used position to stabilize the shoulder (see Fig. 11.2). Generally for a first dislocation incident the client is immobilized for a slightly longer period, but usually not greater than 4 weeks. When dislocations are recurrent for a client, a much shorter time spent in the traditional adducted internally rotated sling position is recommended. These clients may be in a sling for less than 1 week; this is recommended to avoid further anterior capsule laxity and posterior capsule tightness.

Rotator Cuff Repairs

RTC pathology represents up to 70% of shoulder pain disorders, and there are approximately 250,000 repairs performed annually, making it one of the most common orthopedic procedures.[15,24] In the nonathletic population, RTC repair is generally recommended for those with medium, large, and massive/full-thickness RTC tears. There is a surgical option for partial-thickness or small RTC tears, but it is usually reserved for the young, overhead athlete.[1,11]

Immobilization following RTC repair is necessary for 2 to 6 weeks with varying levels of activity and rehabilitation in the acute phase. Immobilization of the shoulder is multifactorial, but for RTC repairs the major concern is the amount of tension being placed on the surgically repaired tendon(s). Increased tension on the repaired RTC is associated with a higher rate of repair failure.[7] Through cadaveric studies,

researchers report the optimal posture of the shoulder following RTC repair is elevation of 21 to 45 degrees and external rotation of 18 to 23 degrees.[17] Although there is limited evidence to support an abducted and externally rotated position when using pain and function as outcomes, this evidence supports the notion of changing the traditional sling design.[7] Thus immobilization positions have significant variation.[18]

Multiple studies compared various shoulder immobilization positions following RTC repair.[4,7,17] Due to increased tension on the superior and posterior RTC, the traditional internally rotated and adducted position is not recommended for RTC repair. Currently there is no agreement upon optimal position to immobilize the shoulder following RTC repair. This is most likely due to significant anatomical variations among clients. It is recommended to immobilize clients with RTC repairs in slight abduction and in a neutral to a slightly externally rotated position (Fig. 11.4).[4,7,17]

Superior Labrum Tear From Anterior to Posterior and Bankart Repairs

SLAP and Bankart lesions are not as prevalent as RTC disorders. However, they account for 6% to 12% of those who seek medical treatment for shoulder pain. They are more common in young males who are overhead athletes, military personnel, and/or extreme athletes.[22,25] SLAP and Bankart tears are generally managed surgically, especially when the biceps tendon is involved. A nonsurgical option for small, partial, or type I tears exists, but type II, III, and IV need to be managed surgically as the labrum will not heal on its own when separated from the glenoid.[30]

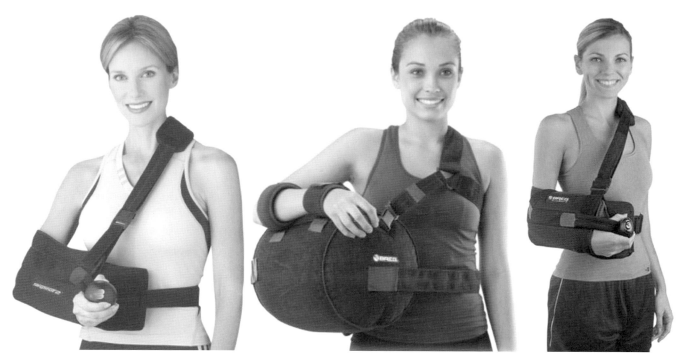

Fig. 11.4 Breg braces, demonstrating various degrees of shoulder abduction and external rotation. (Courtesy of Breg, Inc.)

SLAP and Bankart repairs are required with extensive damage to the labrum. Due to the poor vascularity of the glenoid labrum, surgical intervention is usually indicated. These injuries are often the result of multiple dislocations occurring over a long period of time or one traumatic injury. Such injuries are commonly related to sports, falls, and more traumatic events (e.g., motor vehicle or bicycle accidents).[32]

Immobilization following labrum repairs is recommended for 4 to 6 weeks with progressive rehabilitation. Positioning following SLAP and Bankart repair varies. There is no universally accepted position after these procedures.[28,35] As with RTC repairs, a shift was made from the traditional adducted and internally rotated sling to a position of abduction and external rotation (see Fig. 11.4). Although some studies support the abducted and externally rotated position, it is not universally accepted.[31]

Acromioclavicular Dislocations and Clavicle Fractures

Injuries to the AC joint and clavicle are a common problem in the young athlete. Clavicular fractures account for 2.6% to 4% of all fractures.[14,21,27] The AC joint is susceptible to dislocation during falls, particularly with the arm in an adducted position. There is also risk of injury to the AC joint and clavicle when falling on an outstretched hand. The AC joint is often impacted by motor vehicle or bicycle accidents and sports injuries. These injuries are managed surgically or nonsurgically depending on the type of dislocation or grouping of fractures.

Immobilization for an AC dislocation ranges from 4 to 8 weeks and includes various devices. The most commonly used device is some type of figure-eight shoulder immobilizer (Fig. 11.5). A figure-eight immobilizer is necessary following

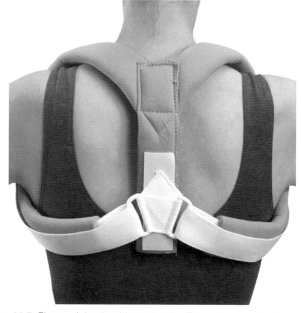

Fig. 11.5 Figure-eight shoulder orthosis. (From Rizzone, K., Gregory, A (2013). Using casts, splints and braces in the emergency department. *Clinical Pediatric Emergency*, 14(4), 340-348.)

an AC or clavicular injury due to the superior migration of the proximal clavicle. The figure-eight places the clavicle and/or AC joint in proper anatomical alignment to allow tissue healing. The figure-eight device may be used in combination with a traditional shoulder sling and/or a control strap (Fig. 11.6). The distal control strap provides additional inferior pressure and is commonly used with a more severe AC joint dislocation.[13]

Nonsurgical treatment is generally preferred when treating AC and clavicular injuries, but there is a lack of consistency in

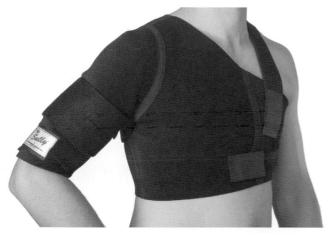

Fig. 11.6 Acromioclavicular (AC) separation strap. (Courtesy of DJO, LLC.)

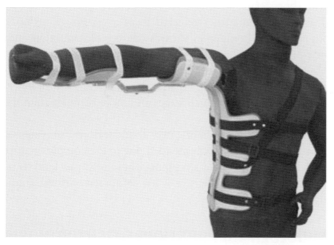

Fig. 11.7 Example of an airplane orthosis. (From Alok Su Rahul Ranjan et al: Peripheral Nerve Injuries. In *Textbook of orthopedics*, ed 1, 2018, Elsevier.)

immobilization techniques and protocols. Research indicates that 94% of US surgeons preferred a simple sling, whereas 88% of German surgeons preferred the figure-eight straps.[6,26] Systematic reviews investigating these immobilization techniques are inconclusive, particularly for middle third clavicular fractures.[14] Regardless of the exact immobilization technique, proper anatomical alignment is the key to tissue healing and preventing further deformity.

Axilla Contractures

Axillary contractures are extremely challenging and problematic in the rehabilitation of upper extremity burns. Axillary contractures are classified by the severity and tissue involvement. Regardless of the classification, some type of orthotic provision is required to prevent future contracture development and to increase functional shoulder motion, particularly for abduction.[8,19]

The airplane orthosis is most often used for the prevention of axilla contractures. Airplane orthoses are available commercially as prefabricated orthoses, or they can be fabricated

by the clinician. The purposes of the airplane orthosis are to increase the abduction angle of the glenohumeral joint, increase tissue elasticity, and prevent further contracture.[9] Construction and application vary significantly, depending on the client's goals. Clients generally need some form of an airplane orthosis for 3 to 6 months following a contracture to the axilla (Fig. 11.7). Custom airplane orthoses are challenging to fabricate. Fabrication requires multiple materials/supplies. The process requires the time of at least two clinicians. Therefore a prefabricated airplane orthosis is generally recommended.

Due to the size of the airplane orthosis, adherence to the wearing schedule tends to be a major concern. Clients report discomfort and decreased function, particularly while navigating the community.[9] Poor adherence is detrimental to the recovery process, resulting in further contracture development and the need for additional surgical procedures. Many attempts to increase comfort of the airplane orthosis have been made to improve adherence to the wearing schedule.[9,34] Changes include lightweight prefabricated devices and variations that allow for functional adjustments based on occupational needs. The airplane orthosis is challenging for the client to put on/take off and to comply with usage, particularly during community reintegration. The clinician must (1) educate the client about the importance of adherence and (2) must consider all activities of daily living when designing the airplane orthosis.

SHOULDER ORTHOSES

Proximal Humerus Cap Orthoses

A proximal humerus cap orthosis is indicated for fractures to the proximal humeral shaft and/or post **open reduction internal fixation (ORIF)** of a proximal to mid-humeral fracture. The purpose of the proximal humeral cap orthosis is to provide circumferential compression while allowing gravity to assist with bone alignment. The orthosis also protects the fracture or injury site while the client engages in occupations and/or navigates the community. This orthosis allows full ROM of the elbow, forearm, and wrist; therefore the client is instructed in distal upper extremity therapeutic exercises for motion. By allowing distal ROM, the proximal humeral cap orthosis increases functional use and decreases edema in the distal upper extremity.

The proximal humerus cap orthosis continues to evolve as orthotic material and prefabricated devices become stronger, lighter, and more comfortable. Multiple vendors offer prefabricated proximal humerus cap orthoses that require the clinician to measure the upper extremity at various locations to determine the appropriate size. If fabricating a custom proximal humerus cap orthosis, provide a compression sleeve or garment to increase circumferential support. The clinician determines whether a cross-chest strap is appropriate (Fig. 11.8; see Fig. 11.3).

AIRPLANE ORTHOSES

The airplane orthosis is often used in burn rehabilitation to prevent axilla contractures. The client is positioned in abduction (see Fig. 11.7). The airplane orthosis is generally a dynamic or static progressive design, and the clinician

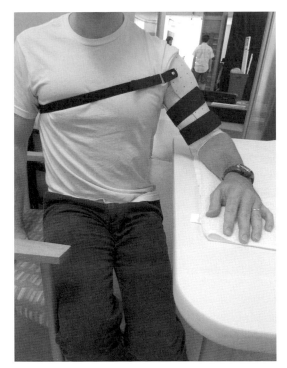

Fig. 11.8 Humeral cap orthosis with cross-body strap.

continues to increase the abduction angle as the client progresses throughout rehabilitation.

Custom airplane orthoses are complex and time/labor intensive to fabricate. Due to advancements in prefabrication design, measuring and purchasing a prefabricated orthosis is recommended for most clients. Multiple companies (e.g., Breg, Ability, Rehabmart) sell airplane orthoses with various designs and features. The clinician may need to make slight modifications to these products to increase comfort.

ADDUCTION AND INTERNAL ROTATION SLING

The adduction and internal rotation sling, or standard upper extremity sling, is the most often used shoulder immobilization device (see Fig. 11.2). Slings place the client in shoulder adduction and internal rotation with the forearm across the abdomen. Slings are commercially available in multiple variations and sizing options. Slings are indicated for postoperative clients and with nonoperative management of subluxations, fractures, muscular tears, and impingements.[12] Most clients are discharged from the emergency department or a medical office with a standard over-the-shoulder sling. Some designs offer additional support straps, such as a cross-chest strap.

Purchasing prefabricated adduction and internal rotation slings is recommended due to economic cost and ease of use. The clinician is responsible for adjusting and fitting the sling properly to the client. Fitting includes an appreciation of bilateral scapula and shoulder positioning. The elbow should rest and be supported in the sling, while providing

a slight compression to the glenohumeral joint. Excessive compression often leads to upper trapezius overactivation, impingement, and/or scapula dyskinesis.[29] Appreciation of the contralateral side is recommended as contralateral compensation often leads to additional shoulder and postural problems.[13,29] When the client is viewed within the sling, shoulders should align without significant elevation and the scapulae should be flush against the thorax with the inferior angles in alignment and equal distance to the spine.

ABDUCTION AND/OR EXTERNAL ROTATION SLING

The abduction and/or external rotation sling has been increasing in popularity in recent years (see Fig. 11.4). Several studies defend the use of the abducted and/or externally rotated position to improve glenohumeral positioning and healing, with short-term and long-term functional improvements.[4,7,35] This brace (sometimes referred to as a *gunslinger orthosis*) supports the shoulder in various degrees of abduction and/or external rotation. The abduction and/or external rotation brace is indicated postoperatively with various shoulder surgeries, particularly labral repairs. The abduction and/or external rotation brace is much larger and more complex than the traditional arm sling.

A commercial, prefabricated abduction and/or external rotation orthosis is recommended due to the complex nature of design, support, and strapping. These orthoses tend to be significantly more expensive when compared with the traditional sling.

SHOULDER SUPPORT FIGURE-EIGHT ORTHOSIS

The figure-eight orthosis, often referred to as the *figure-eight brace or strap,* is indicated following a proximal or midclavicular fracture (see Fig. 11.5). In the event of a distal clavicular fracture and/or AC joint dislocation, the figure-eight orthosis is used with the addition of a stability control strap to provide additional support to the distal clavicle and AC joint (see Fig. 11.6). The figure-eight orthosis supports the healing clavicle and/or AC joint in proper anatomical alignment and prevents superior migration of the proximal clavicle. The brace is used in nonoperative and postoperative management of clavicular and AC joint injuries.

The figure-eight orthosis is another device in which a commercially prefabricated brace is recommended. Various companies (e.g., BraceAbility, Ossur, Orthotic Shop) sell the figure-eight orthosis at relatively low prices. Some braces are available in one size fits all, whereas others require the clinician to measure the client for a proper size. In general, every brace fits snugly, and the straps are large and padded. When using the additional control strap, the client is educated about proper tension as this strap is often more elastic and results in an increased compressive force. The control strap should provide enough compression to stabilize the distal clavicle and/or AC joint, but shoulder alignment should remain equal to the contralateral side.

PROCEDURE FOR FABRICATION OF A PROXIMAL HUMERUS CAP ORTHOSIS

1. Place the client in a compression sleeve (elastic tubular bandage) with elbow supported on table in slight assisted abduction.
2. Design a pattern by taking the following measurements (Fig. 11.9):
   a. Part 1
   1. Use a tape measure to measure the distance from the posterior AC joint to the superior lateral epicondyle. Subtract approximately 2 inches when designing the pattern.
   2. Draw a vertical line on the paper using the length determined in the previous measurement.
   3. Measure the distance from the anterior to the posterior axilla. Subtract approximately 2 inches when designing the pattern.
   4. Draw a line across the paper using the width determined in the previous measurement. This will form the superior aspect of the orthosis.
   5. Measure the circumference of the superior biceps. Divide by 2 when designing the pattern.
   6. Draw a line across the paper inferior to the previous line. This will be in the middle of the orthosis.
   7. Measure the circumference of the inferior biceps. Divide by 2 when designing the pattern.
   8. Draw a line across the paper inferior to the previous line. This will be located toward the inferior border of the orthosis.
   b. Part 2
   1. Measure the distance from the axilla to the medial epicondyle. Subtract approximately 2 to 4 inches when designing the pattern.
   2. Draw a vertical line using the length determined in the previous measurement.
   3. Measure the circumference of the superior biceps. Divide by 2 when designing the pattern.
   4. Draw a horizontal line using the measurement determined in the previous measurement. This will be the superior aspect of the orthosis.
   5. Measure the circumference of the inferior biceps. Divide by 2 when designing the pattern.
   6. Draw a horizontal line using the measurement determined in the previous measurement. This will be the inferior aspect of the orthosis.
3. Round off the edges, and create a slight dome superiorly.
4. Cut the pattern from the paper (Fig. 11.10).
5. Place the paper pattern on the client to approximate size/fit.
6. Transfer the design from the paper to lightweight ⅛-inch perforated thermoplastic material (Fig. 11.11).
7. Heat the thermoplastic material for part 1. Ensure that the material is safe for contact. Mold to the client using the drapability of the material. Allow the material to cool, and then remove from the client.
8. Heat the thermoplastic material for part 2. Ensure that the material is safe for contact, and mold to the client using the drapability of the material (Fig. 11.12).
9. Place part 1 and part 2 on the client (give a very small stretch to the material before application). Approximate strap locations at anterior and poster deltoid, superior biceps and triceps, and inferior biceps and triceps (Fig. 11.13; see Fig. 11.12).
10. Rivet the posterior strap in place and anterior turnbuckle for the cross-body strap.
    a. Create a turnbuckle by folding approximately 4 inches of strapping material around a 1-inch plastic buckle (Fig. 11.14).
    b. Using a riveter (Fig. 11.15), punch holes on the overlapping strap and through the splinting material (Fig. 11.16).
    c. Remove the small circular material that the riveter punched out of the strap and the splint material.
    d. Place the flat end of the rivet on the inside of the splint, and push the other end through the straps and splinting material.
    e. Use flat pliers to push the metal rivets together (Figs. 11.17 and 11.18).
11. Pad the metal surfaces of the rivets on the inside of the orthosis (Figs. 11.19 and 11.20).
12. Place hook on the corresponding surface of part 2 (see Fig. 11.8).
13. Adjust to the client. Ensure that the orthosis is snug with 1 inch of space between part 1 and part 2.
14. Ensure full ROM at the elbow and that no irritation to the axilla or the thorax is present.
15. Add padding to the inferior boarders if showing signs of irritation.
16. Ask the client to practice putting on and taking off the orthosis, while maintaining shoulder motion precautions.

Technical Tips for Proper Fit
- Use a compression garment.
- Give the material a slight stretch before applying it to the client. This will allow the material to slightly recoil and then contour to the client.
- Pad the metal surfaces of the rivets on the inside of the orthosis.
- Pad the inferior border of part 1 and part 2 if the client shows signs of irritation.
- Prepare all material in advance of the client session. Have the turnbuckles cut and ready to be riveted. Have the rivets set up, and have the moleskins cut (Fig. 11.21). Have all the strapping material and turnbuckles prepared (if not already completed).
- Use a table to place your client's elbow in slight abduction and elbow/forearm resting on the table while fabricating the orthosis. This will support the humeral head in a slightly abducted position during orthotic fabrication (see Fig. 11.12).

Precautions for the Shoulder Cap Orthosis
- Assess for signs of irritation on the shoulder and the thorax from orthosis contact.
- If using an additional body strap, assess for irritation on the contralateral side.
- Ensure that the client has full elbow ROM without making contact with the orthosis, particularly for end-range elbow flexion.
- Ensure that the client is aware of precautions and can follow precautions while putting on/taking off the orthosis.
- Ensure that there is at least 1 inch of space between part 1 and part 2 on both sides of the orthosis. This will allow the client to tighten or loosen the orthosis to account for fluctuations in edema without needing to create a second orthosis.
- Review tightening and loosening of the orthosis with the client to ensure compliance.

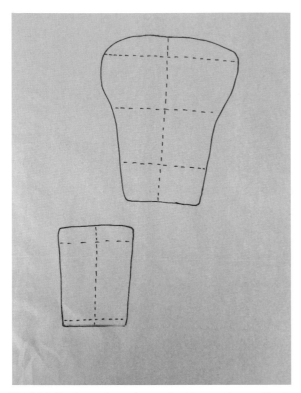

Fig. 11.9 Design patterns for proximal humeral cap orthosis.

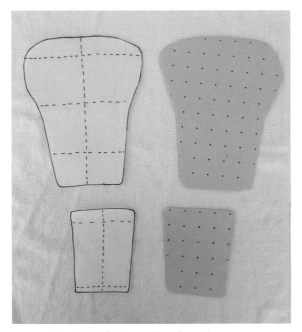

Fig. 11.10 Cut the pattern from the paper.

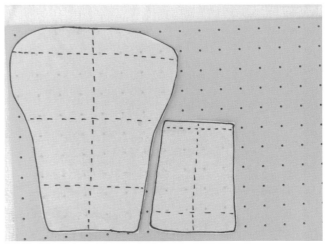

Fig. 11.11 Tracing patterns onto thermoplastic material.

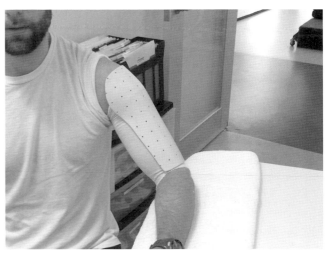

Fig. 11.12 Mold to the client using the drapability of the material (proximal humeral orthosis part 2).

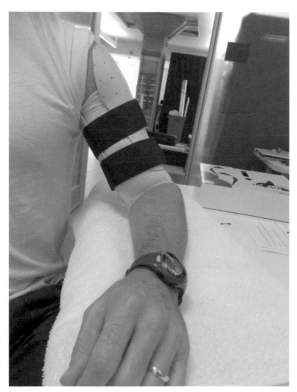

Fig. 11.13 Proximal humeral cap orthosis part 1 and part 2 with strapping.

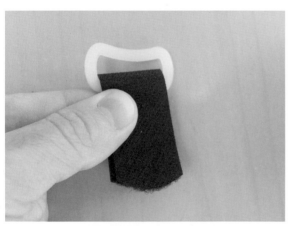

Fig. 11.14 Turnbuckle.

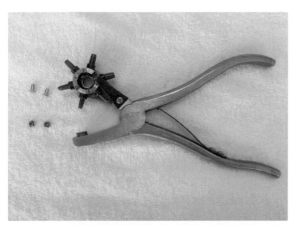

Fig. 11.15 Riveter and rivets.

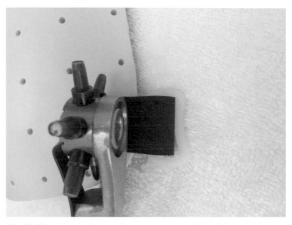

Fig. 11.16 Riveting holes to line up turnbuckle with hole in splinting material.

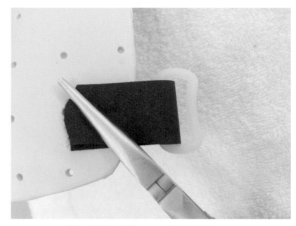

Fig. 11.17 Pliers pushing in rivets.

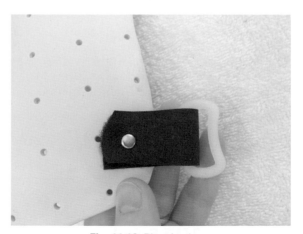

Fig. 11.18 Rivet in place.

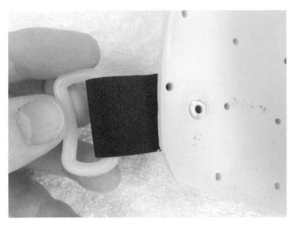

Fig. 11.19 Interior surface of rivet (side contacting client before padding).

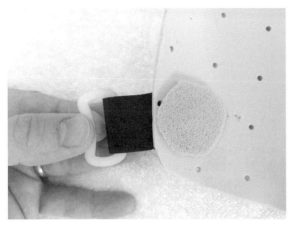

Fig. 11.20 Interior surface of rivet with padding over all metal.

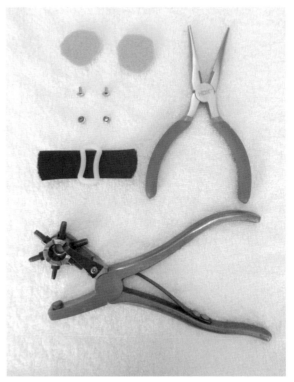

Fig. 11.21 Riveter and set-up equipment.

🔲 SELF-QUIZ 11.1ᵃ

For the following questions, circle either true (T) or false (F).
1. T F The shoulder complex is composed of five joints.
2. T F The scapulothoracic joint is not considered a true joint.
3. T F Type I, II, III, and IV proximal humeral fractures will require surgical intervention.
4. T F Following a shoulder subluxation, clients should be immobilized for 4 weeks or less
5. T F The preferred immobilization position following a labral repair is internal rotation and adduction.
6. T F Clinicians must be aware of frozen shoulder syndrome and scapular dyskinesis when immobilizing the shoulder.

7. T F Compliance issues are highly prevalent with the airplane orthosis due to its large size and decreased function while in use.
8. T F The figure-eight orthosis should have thin ridged straps.
9. T F Use of an internal rotation/adduction sling should compress the humeral head, resulting in shoulder hiking.
10. T F AC joint separations will require an additional support strap when managed nonoperatively.

ᵃSee Appendix A for the answer key.

REVIEW QUESTIONS

1. What are the four joints that constitute the shoulder complex?
2. What are the main indicators for shoulder immobilization orthoses?
3. What are two possible deleterious effects of prolonged or incorrect shoulder immobilization?
4. What are the advantages of providing a prefabricated orthosis for shoulder immobilization?

5. What are the advantages of a custom orthosis for shoulder immobilization?
6. What diagnoses require a humeral cap orthosis?
7. What shoulder position should a client be in following a SLAP repair?
8. Approximately how long is a client immobilized following a first incident of shoulder dislocation?

REFERENCES

1. Belangero PS, Ejnisman B: *Arce: a review of rotator cuff classifications in current use. Shoulder concepts 2013: consensus and concerns*, 2013, pp 5–13.
2. Burkart KJ, Dietz SO, Bastian L, et al.: The treatment of proximal humeral fracture in adults, *Dtsch Arzebl Int* 110:591–597, 2013.
3. Cavanaugh JT, Rodeo SA: Nonoperative rehabilitation for shoulder instability, *Tech Shoulder Elbow Surg* 15(1):18 24, 2014.
4. Conti M, Garofalo R, Castagna A: Does a brace influence clinical outcomes after arthroscopic rotator cuff repair?, *Musculoskelet Surg* 3136(99), 2015. RTC 3.
5. Handoll H, Brealey S, Rangan A, et al.: The ProFHER (PROximal Fracture of the Humerus: Evaluation by Randomisation) trial – a pragmatic multicentre randomised controlled trial evaluating the clinical effectiveness and cost-effectiveness of surgical compared with non-surgical treatment for proximal fracture of the humerus in adults, *Health Technol Assess* 19(24):1–280, 2015.
6. Heuer HJ, Boykin RE, Petit CJ, et al.: Decision-making in the treatment of diaphyseal clavicle fractures: is there agreement among surgeons? Results of a survey on surgeons' treatment preferences, *J Shoulder Elbow Surg* 23(2), 2014.
7. Hollman F, Wolterbeek N, Zijl JA, et al.: Abduction brace versus antirotation sling after arthroscopic cuff repair: the effects on pain and function, *Arthroscopy*(17)749–806, 2017. - RTC.
8. Ibrahim-Walash AM, Kishk TF, Ghareeb FM: Treatment of postburn axillary contracture, *Menoutia Med J*(27)278–283, 2014.
9. Jang KU, Choi JS, Hyeon J, et al.: Multi-axis shoulder abduction splint in acute burn rehabilitation: a randomized controlled pilot trial, *Clin Res* 29(5):439–446, 2015.
10. Jordan RW, Modi CS: A review of management options for proximal humeral fractures, *Open Orthop J* 8(1):148–156, 2014.
11. Kibler WB, Ludewig PM, Mcclure PW, et al.: Clinical implications of scapular dyskinesis in shoulder injury: the 2013 consensus statement from the 'scapular summit', *Br J Sports Med* 47(14):877–885, 2013.
12. Kibler WB, Mcmullen J, Uhl T: Shoulder rehabilitation strategies, guidelines, and practice, *Oper Tech Sports Med* 20(1):103–112, 2012.
13. Lenza M, Belloti JC, Andriolo RB, et al.: Conservative interventions for treating middle third clavicle fractures in adolescents and adults, *Cochrane Database Syst Rev*, 2014.
14. Lenza M, Presente-Tanihuch LF: Ferretti, M: Figure-of-eight bandage versus arm sling for treating middle-third clavicle fractures in adults: study protocol for a randomized controlled trial, *BioMed Central* 22(17), 2016.
15. Mather RC, Koenig L, Acevedo D, et al.: The societal and economic value of rotator cuff repair, *J Bone Joint Surg Am* (95):1993–2000, 2013.
16. Martetschlager F, Warth RJ, Millett PJ: Instability and degenerative arthritis of the sternoclavicular joint, *Am J Sports Med* 42(4):999–1008, 2013.
17. McElvany MD, McGoldrick E, Gee AO, et al.: Rotator cuff repair: published evidence on factors associated with repair integrity and clinical outcome, *Am J Sports Med* 43(2):491–500, 2014.
18. Nassiri M, Egan C, Mullet H: Compliance with sling-wearing after rotator cuff repair and anterior shoulder stabilization, *Shoulder Elbow* 3(3):188–192, 2011.
19. Neumann DA: *Shoulder complex in neumann DA: kinesiology of the musculoskeletal system foundations for physical rehabilitation*, 2002, pp 91–132. St. Louis.
20. Neviaser A, Stupay K: Management of adhesive capsulitis, *ORR Orthope Res Rev* 83, 2015.
21. Nordqvist A, Petersson C. The incidence of fractures of the clavicle. *Clin Orthop Relat Res* (300):127–132, 1994. Cited by: Lenza M, Taniguchi LF, Ferretti M. Figure-of-eight bandage versus arm sling for treating middle-third clavicle fractures in adults: study protocol for a randomised controlled trial. Trials. 2016;17(1):229.
22. Noreski MA, Cohen SB: Epidemiology of shoulder injuries in overhead athletes, *Sports Injur Shoulder Elbow*23–34, 2015.
23. Olerud P, Ahrengart L, Ponzer S, et al.: Internal fixation versus nonoperative treatment of displaced 3-part proximal humeral fractures in elderly patients: a randomized controlled trial, *J Shoulder Elbow Surg* 20(5):747–755, 2011.
24. Oliva F, Osti L, Padulo J, Maffulli N: Epidemiology of the rotator cuff tears: a new incidence related to thyroid disease, *Muscles Ligaments Tendons J* 3(3):309–314, 2014.
25. Omid R: A SLAP tear epidemic? *J Bone Joint Surg Am Orthop Highlight Shoulder Elbow* 2(12), 2012.
26. Pieske O, Dang M, Zaspel J, Beyer B, Löffler T, Piltz, S: Midshaft clavicle fractures–classification and therapy. Results of a survey at German trauma departments, *Der Unfallchirurg* 111(6):387–394, 2008. https://doi.org/10.1007/s00113-008-1430-z. Cited by: Heuer, H. D., Boykin, R. E., Petit, C. J., Hardt, J., & Millett, P. J. (2014). Decision-making in the treatment of diaphyseal clavicle fractures: is there agreement among surgeons? Results of a survey on surgeons' treatment preferences. *J Shoulder Elbow Surg* 23(2): e23–e33. https://doi.org/10.1016/j.jse.2013.04.016.
27. Postacchini F, Gumina S, De Santis P, Albo F. Epidemiology of clavicle fractures. *J Shoulder Elbow Surg* 11(5):452–456, 2002 Sep 1. Cited by: Lenza M, Taniguchi LF, Ferretti M. Figure-of-eight bandage versus arm sling for treating middle-third clavicle fractures in adults: study protocol for a randomised controlled trial. *Trials*. 2016;17(1):229.
28. Rossy W, Sanchez G, Sanchez A, et al.: Superior labral anterior-posterior (SLAP) tears in the military: a clinical review of incidence, diagnosis, and treatment compared with the civilian population, *Orthop Surg* 8(6):503–508, 2016. – SLAP 1.
29. Severini G, Ricciardi A, Cacchio A: Principles of shoulder rehabilitation, *Shoulder Arthroscopy*73–82, 2013.
30. Shin S, Rao N, Seo MJ: Is SLAP repair necessary? Clinical outcomes of symptomatic SLAP lesion in non-athletic patients with conservative treatment, *J Shoulder Elbow Surg* 24(4), 2015.
31. Smith BI, Bliven KC, Morway GR, et al.: Management of primary anterior shoulder dislocations using immobilization, *J Athl Train* 50(5):550–552, 2015.
32. Sugaya H: Multidirectional instability and loose shoulder in athletes, *Sports Injur Shoulder Elbow*237–250, 2015.
33. Wilk KE, Macrina LC, Reinold MM: Nonoperative rehabilitation for traumatic and atraumatic glenohumeral instability, *In Shoulder Instability: A Comprehensive Approach* 108–112, 2012.
34. Williams T, Berenz T: Postburn upper extremity occupational therapy, *Hand Clin* 22(2):293–304, 2017.
35. Yin B, Levy D, Meadows M, et al.: How does external rotation bracing influence motion and functional scores after arthroscopic shoulder stabilization? *Clin Orthop Rel Res* 2389–2396, 2013.

APPENDIX 11.1 CASE STUDY

Case Study 11.1[a]

Read the following scenario, and use your clinical reasoning skills to answer the questions based on information in this chapter.

Lauren is a 27-year-old woman who works at a marketing firm. She has also been a dancer her whole life and currently competes in small weekend dancing competitions. One week ago she felt her right shoulder dislocate while practicing with her partner. As this has happened to her at least five times in the past 10 years, she performed a self-manual reduction and followed up with her doctor later in the week. Her doctor is concerned that she has damaged her labrum. Lauren would like to attempt occupational therapy (OT) and then consider surgery later in the year.

She arrives at OT without an orthosis and reports fear of re-dislocation with dance moves requiring any overhead or behind-back motion. Besides the fear of a re-dislocation, she has mild discomfort. She can complete all activities of daily living (ADLs) and instrumental IADLs (IADLs) and work with modified independence. She has not returned to dancing, but that is her goal for therapy.

1. What orthosis would be the most appropriate for Lauren?
2. What is the orthosis-wearing schedule for Lauren?
3. What are some of the concerns with this type of immobilization orthosis?
4. What should Lauren be educated about regarding this orthosis?

APPENDIX 11.2 LABORATORY EXERCISE

Laboratory Exercise 11.1 Fabricating a Custom Proximal Humerus Cap Orthosis

Practice fabricating a proximal humerus cap orthosis. Follow the outlined guidelines that address positioning, materials required, and measurements. After fabrication:

- ensure comfort,
- check for ability to put on/take off independently,
- evaluate elbow range of motion,
- evaluate client's ability to perform pendulum exercises, and
- use Form 11.1 to perform a self-evaluation. Use Grading Sheet 11.1 as a classroom grading sheet.

---

[a] See Appendix A for the answer key.

APPENDIX 11.3 FORM AND GRADING SHEET

Form 11.1

	Name: _____
	Date: _____

Proximal Humerus Cap Orthosis

After the client wears the orthosis for 30 minutes, answer the following questions.
(Mark NA for nonapplicable situations.)

Evaluation Areas				Comments
Design				
1. The shoulder is positioned correctly.	Yes	No	NA	
2. The proximal arm has approximately two-thirds coverage.	Yes	No	NA	
3. The orthosis provides compression.	Yes	No	NA	
4. The orthosis is proximal to the epicondyles.	Yes	No	NA	
5. The acromioclavicular joint is not being irritated.	Yes	No	NA	
Function				
1. The orthosis allows for pendulum exercises.	Yes	No	NA	
2. The orthosis allows full elbow range of motion.	Yes	No	NA	
3. The orthosis provides support and compression.	Yes	No	NA	
4. The client can put on/take off independently	Yes	No	NA	
Straps				
1. The straps are secure.	Yes	No	NA	
2. The straps do not irritate the thorax.	Yes	No	NA	
Comfort				
1. The edges are smooth without causing irritation.	Yes	No	NA	
2. There are no pressure sores.	Yes	No	NA	
3. The thorax is not irritated by the medial border.	Yes	No	NA	
4. All bony prominences are cleared.	Yes	No	NA	
Cosmetic Appearance				
1. All marks have been removed.	Yes	No	NA	
2. There are no fingermarks or indentations.	Yes	No	NA	
Therapeutic Regimen				
1. The client is aware of the wearing schedule.	Yes	No	NA	
2. The client is educated on precautions.	Yes	No	NA	
3. The client verbalizes understanding.	Yes	No	NA	
4. The client demonstrates ability to put on/take off properly.	Yes	No	NA	
5. The client is aware of how to clean and maintain the orthosis.	Yes	No	NA	

Discuss possible orthotic adjustments or changes that you should make based on the self-evaluation.
(What would you do differently next time?)

Discuss possible areas to improve clinical safety when fabricating the orthosis.

Grading Sheet 11.1

	Name: _____
	Date: _____

Proximal Humerus Cap Orthosis
Grade:
1 = Beyond improvement, not acceptable
2 = Requires maximal improvement
3 = Requires moderate improvement
4 = Requires minimal improvement
5 = Requires no improvement

Evaluation Areas						Comments
Design						
1. The shoulder is positioned correctly.	1	2	3	4	5	
2. The proximal arm has approximately two-thirds coverage.	1	2	3	4	5	
3. The orthosis provides compression.	1	2	3	4	5	
4. The orthosis is proximal to the epicondyles.	1	2	3	4	5	
5. The acromioclavicular joint is not being irritated.	1	2	3	4	5	
Function						
1. The orthosis allows for pendulum exercises.	1	2	3	4	5	
2. The orthosis allows full elbow range of motion.	1	2	3	4	5	
3. The orthosis provides support and compression.	1	2	3	4	5	
4. The client can put on/take off independently	1	2	3	4	5	
Straps						
1. The straps are secure.	1	2	3	4	5	
2. The straps are not irritating the thorax.	1	2	3	4	5	
Comfort						
1. The edges are smooth without causing irritation.	1	2	3	4	5	
2. There are no pressure sores.	1	2	3	4	5	
3. The thorax is not irritated by the medial border.	1	2	3	4	5	
4. All bony prominences are cleared.	1	2	3	4	5	
Cosmetic Appearance						
1. All marks have been removed.	1	2	3	4	5	
2. There are no fingermarks or indentations.	1	2	3	4	5	
Therapeutic Regimen						
1. The client is aware of the wearing schedule.	1	2	3	4	5	
2. The client is educated on precautions.	1	2	3	4	5	
3. The client verbalizes understanding.	1	2	3	4	5	
4. The client demonstrates ability to put on/take off properly.	1	2	3	4	5	
5. The client is aware of how to clean and maintain the orthosis.	1	2	3	4	5	

Orthotics for the Fingers

Kristin Valdes

CHAPTER OBJECTIVES

1. Explain the functional and anatomical considerations of orthotics for the fingers.
2. Identify diagnostic indications for using finger orthoses.
3. Describe a mallet finger.
4. Describe a boutonnière deformity.
5. Describe a swan neck deformity.
6. Name three structures that provide support to the stability of the proximal interphalangeal (PIP) joint.
7. Explain the purpose of buddy straps.
8. Apply clinical reasoning to evaluate finger orthoses in terms of materials used, strapping type and placement, and fit.
9. Discuss the process of making a mallet orthosis, a gutter orthosis, and a PIP hyperextension block orthosis, a three-point PIP extension orthosis, a trigger finger orthosis, and a distal interphalangeal stabilization orthosis.

KEY TERMS

boutonnière deformity
buddy straps
central slip
collateral ligaments
extensor lag
finger sprain

flexion contracture
fusiform swelling
lateral bands
mallet finger
oblique retinacular ligament (ORL)
osteoarthritis

swan neck deformity
terminal extensor tendon
transverse retinacular ligament
trigger finger
volar plate (VP)

Marge is a 74-year-old right-hand–dominant woman who retired from her job. She likes to crochet and knit. She has pain and swelling of her index and small finger distal interphalangeal (DIP) joints. Her physician diagnosed her with osteoarthritis of the fingers and sent her to occupational therapy for evaluation and treatment. At her initial evaluation she reports night DIP joint pain interferes with her sleep. She reports she does not understand why her physician sent her to therapy, and she thinks she just needs to "live with the pain." She was grateful to learn that there is evidence to support that DIP orthoses relieve pain at the DIP joints, and she is anxious to see if they will help.

Depending on the diagnosis, finger problems may require orthotics that cross the hand and wrist, or they may be treated with orthotics that are smaller. This chapter describes the smaller orthoses that are finger-based, crossing the proximal interphalangeal (PIP) and/or distal interphalangeal (DIP) joint, leaving the metacarpophalangeal (MCP) joint free.

FUNCTIONAL AND ANATOMICAL CONSIDERATIONS OF ORTHOTICS FOR THE FINGERS

The PIP and DIP joints are hinge joints. These joints have **collateral ligaments** on each side that provide joint stability and restraint against deviation forces. The radial collateral ligament protects against ulnar deviation forces, and the ulnar collateral ligament protects against radial deviation forces. On the palmar (or volar) surface is the **volar plate (VP)**, which is a fibrocartilaginous structure that prevents hyperextension. As the extensor mechanism of the digits crosses over the PIP joint, it branches into three bands: the **central slip** and two **lateral bands.** The central slip attaches to the middle phalanx, and the lateral bands attach to the distal phalanx. The central slip crosses the PIP joint dorsally and is part of the PIP joint dorsal capsule. It is implicated in boutonnière deformities. The lateral bands, which are contributions from the intrinsic muscles, and the **transverse retinacular ligament** are additional structures that contribute to the delicate balance of the extensor mechanism at the PIP joint. They are implicated in boutonnière deformities and swan neck deformities. The **terminal extensor tendon** attaches to the distal phalanx and is implicated in **mallet finger** injuries.

For all finger injuries and postsurgical interventions, it is always important to prioritize edema control to prevent fibrosis of the edema and adherence between anatomical structures. Treatment for edema can often be incorporated into the orthotics process. Examples of this would be the use of self-adherent compressive wrap under the orthosis, application of a finger compression sleeve, or using self-adherent compressive wrap to secure the orthosis on the finger. For diagnoses that require orthotic application 24 hours a day but permit washing of the digit, it may be appropriate to fabricate one orthosis for shower use and another one for the rest of the day. In general, thinner low-temperature thermoplastic (LTT) (¹⁄₁₆ inch or thinner) is typically used on digits because it is less bulky yet strong enough to support or protect these relatively small body parts. On a stronger person or a person with larger hands, ³⁄₃₂-inch material may be better to use than a ¹⁄₁₆-inch thickness. Choosing perforated versus nonperforated thermoplastic material is partly a matter of personal choice, but therapists should use caution with perforated materials because the edges may be rougher, and there can be the possibility of increased skin problems or irregular pressure, particularly if there is edema. Another material available for use is Orficast Thermoplastic Tape. It is a unique textile-like thermoformable taping material. It offers extreme comfort for clients and is very easy to use. This knitted hybrid fabric is ideal for all applications of finger and/or thumb orthoses.

Because finger orthoses are so small, there is an increased possibility of their being pulled off during sleep or during activity. It may be necessary to tape them in place in addition to using Velcro straps. The therapist or patient must be careful not to apply the tape circumferentially so as not to cause a tourniquet effect. An alternative solution is to use a long Velcro strap to anchor the orthosis around the hand or wrist.

DIAGNOSTIC INDICATIONS

Commonly seen diagnoses that require finger orthoses are mallet fingers, boutonnière deformities, swan neck deformities, **trigger finger**, painful **osteoarthritis** (OA) of DIP joints, PIP flexion contractures, and finger sprains. These diagnoses are discussed separately in terms of orthotic indications with consideration of wearing schedule and fabrication tips. Prefabricated orthotic options will also be addressed.

Mallet Finger

A mallet finger presents as a digit with a droop of the DIP joint (Fig. 12.1). This posture often occurs because of axial loading with the DIP extended or else by a flexion force to the fingertip. The terminal tendon is either torn or avulsed with a piece of bone, causing a droop of the DIP joint. A laceration of the finger can also disrupt the terminal tendon.

With a mallet injury, the DIP joint can usually be passively extended to neutral, but the client is not able to actively extend it. This is called a DIP **extensor lag.** If the DIP joint

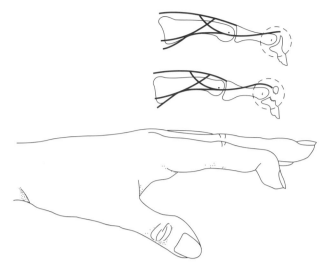

Fig. 12.1 Mallet finger deformity. (From American Society for Surgery of the Hand. [1983]. *The hand: Examination and diagnosis* [2nd ed.]. Edinburgh, Scotland: Churchill Livingstone.)

cannot be passively extended fully, this is called a DIP **flexion contracture.** It is unlikely for the DIP joint to develop a flexion contracture early on, but this can be seen in more long-standing cases.

Orthoses for Mallet Finger

The goal of orthotics for mallet finger is to prevent DIP flexion. Some physicians prefer the DIP joint to be supported in slight hyperextension to prevent extensor lag, whereas others prefer a neutral DIP position. The therapist should clarify the requested position of the DIP joint with the physician. If hyperextension is desired, care must be taken not to excessively hyperextend the joint, because this may compromise blood flow to the area. Either way, it is important that the orthosis does not impede PIP flexion unless there are specific associated issues, such as a secondary swan neck deformity, that would justify limiting the PIP joint's mobility. The PIP joint may also need to be included in the orthosis if the involved digit is very short and the length of the required device is not practical to maintain the required contact with the digit.

The DIP joint should be supported 24/7 for approximately 6 to 8 weeks[12] to allow the terminal tendon to heal. The joint should not be left unsupported or be allowed to flex for even a moment during this 6-week interval. It can be challenging to achieve this continuous DIP support because there is also the need for skin care. Sometimes providing two orthoses will improve adherence because the patient can remove the wet orthosis used in the shower and replace it with a dry orthosis that has already been "set up" for application. Practice application of the device with the client so there is a thorough understanding of techniques used to support the DIP joint while performing skin hygiene and when applying and removing the orthosis. The therapist may also consider casting the mallet finger. Tocco et al.[10] used QuickCast to immobilize 30 mallet fingers for 6 weeks if the injury was less than 21 days old and 8 weeks for chronic injuries. Tocco et al.[10] found

TABLE 12.1	Evidence-Based Practice About Silver Ring Orthoses				
Author's Citation	Design	Number of Participants	Description	Results	Limitations
Saito, K. & Kihara, H. (2016). A randomized control trial of the effect of 2-step orthosis treatment for a mallet finger of tendinous origin. *Journal of Hand Therapy, 29,* 433–439.	Randomized controlled trial	54 subjects	Subjects were randomized into either a two-step or figure-eight–type orthosis group. The two-step immobilization group underwent initial immobilization using an orthosis with the PIP joint in flexion and the DIP joint in slight hyperextension for 3 weeks. After 3 weeks the two-step group wore just a conventional device that immobilized only the DIP joint in slight hyperextension	The residual extensor lag of the two-step group was a mean difference of 8.9 degrees better than the control group. This result was statistically significant.	Study included only new cases of tendinous mallet finger, so the effect on bony mallet fingers is unknown. Small sample size.

DIP, Distal interphalangeal; *PIP,* proximal interphalangeal.

that full-time immobilization of type I mallet fingers using QuickCast was more effective than the traditional approach of instructing the patient in home-based splint removal for skin hygiene. Please refer to Chapter 19 for more information regarding casting.

After approximately 6 to 8 weeks of continual support and with medical clearance, the client is weaned off the orthosis. The orthosis is usually still worn at night for several weeks. At this time it is important to watch for the development of a DIP extensor lag; if this is noticed, resume use of the orthosis and consult the physician. Table 12.1 presents a study on the efficacy of using two-step orthosis treatment for mallet finger.

Boutonnière Deformity

A **boutonnière deformity** is a finger that postures with PIP flexion and DIP hyperextension (Fig. 12.2). A boutonnière deformity can result from axial loading, tendon laceration, burns, or arthritis. The central slip is disrupted, which leads to the imbalance of the extensor mechanism as the lateral bands displace volarly. If not treated in a timely manner, the PIP joint extensor lag may become a flexion contracture. In addition, the DIP joint may lose flexion motion due to tightness of the **oblique retinacular ligament (ORL),** also called the *ligament of Landsmeer.*

Orthotics for Boutonnière Deformity

The goal of orthotics for boutonnière deformity is to maintain PIP joint extension while keeping the MCP and DIP joints free for approximately 6 to 8 weeks. If there is a PIP flexion contracture, a prefabricated dynamic three-point extension orthosis might be used, or a static orthosis can be adjusted serially with the goal of achieving full passive PIP extension. There are various types of orthoses for boutonnière deformity, including simple volar gutter orthoses or DeRoyal LMB Dynamic Wire-Foam Spring Extension Assist. Fig. 12.3 demonstrates some common options of orthotics for the PIP joint in extension while keeping the DIP joint free. In some cases, including the DIP joint in the orthosis

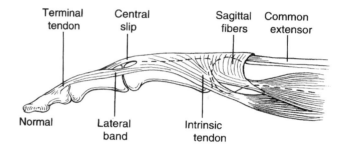
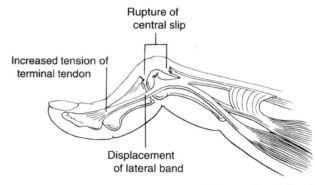

Fig. 12.2 Normal anatomy and anatomy of boutonnière deformity. (From Burke, S. L., Higgins, J., McClinton, M. A., et al. [2006]. *Hand and upper extremity rehabilitation: A practical guide* [3rd ed.]. St. Louis, MO: Churchill Livingstone.)

may be preferable because this will increase the mechanical advantage. It is usually acceptable to do this if the ORL is not tight.

Serial casting is also an option with this diagnosis (Fig. 12.4). This technique when using plaster cast material requires training and practice before being used on clients. Orficast Thermoplastic Tape is easier to apply because the material is heated in water and simply wrapped around the digit (Fig. 12.5). After 6 to 8 weeks of support and with medical clearance, the client is weaned off the orthosis. At this time, it is important to watch for loss of PIP extension. If this is noted, adjust orthotic usage accordingly.

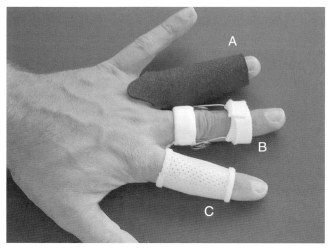

Fig. 12.3 Extension orthoses. A, Tube. B, Capener. C, Custom. (From Burke, S. L., Higgins, J., McClinton, M. A., et al. [2006]. *Hand and upper extremity rehabilitation: A practical guide* [3rd ed.]. St. Louis, MO: Churchill Livingstone.)

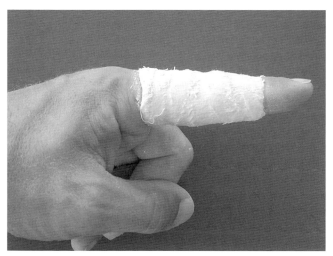

Fig. 12.4 Serial cast. (From Burke, S. L., Higgins, J., McClinton, M. A., et al. [2006]. *Hand and upper extremity rehabilitation: A practical guide* [3rd ed.]. St. Louis, MO: Churchill Livingstone.)

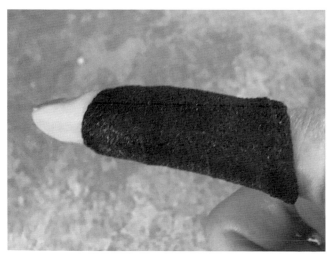

Fig. 12.5 Serial orthosis fabricated from Orficast. (Courtesy Kristin Valdes.)

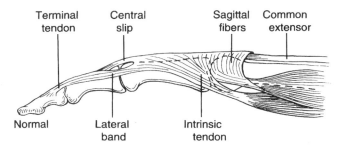

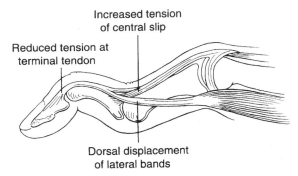

Fig. 12.6 Normal finger anatomy and anatomy of swan neck deformity. (From Burke, S. L., Higgins, J., McClinton, M. A., et al. [2006]. *Hand and upper extremity rehabilitation: A practical guide* [3rd ed.] St. Louis, MO: Churchill Livingstone.)

Swan Neck Deformity

A **swan neck deformity** is seen when the finger postures with PIP hyperextension and DIP flexion (Fig. 12.6). The swan neck deformity at the PIP and DIP is the opposite of the boutonnière deformity. It may be possible to correct the PIP and DIP joints passively, or they may be fixed in their deformity positions. There are multiple possible causes of this deformity that may occur at the level of the MCP, the PIP, or the DIP joints. As with a boutonnière deformity, the result is an imbalance of the extensor mechanism, but with a swan neck deformity the lateral bands displace dorsally. In addition to other traumatic causes, it is not uncommon for people with rheumatoid arthritis to demonstrate swan neck deformities.

Orthoses for Swan Neck Deformity

The goal of orthoses for swan neck deformity is to prevent PIP hyperextension and to promote DIP extension while not restricting PIP flexion. Three-point and silver ring orthoses are shown in (Fig. 12.7). These orthoses prevent PIP hyperextension but allow PIP flexion. They can be either custom formed or prefabricated.

Trigger Finger

Flexor tendons normally glide easily through the sheath and under pulleys. When a tendon becomes inflamed and swollen, its ability to slide freely is limited, and the finger can lock when attempting to extend the finger after making a fist. Bending the finger or thumb can make it snap or pop. Rheumatoid arthritis, gout, and diabetes also can contribute to the presence of trigger

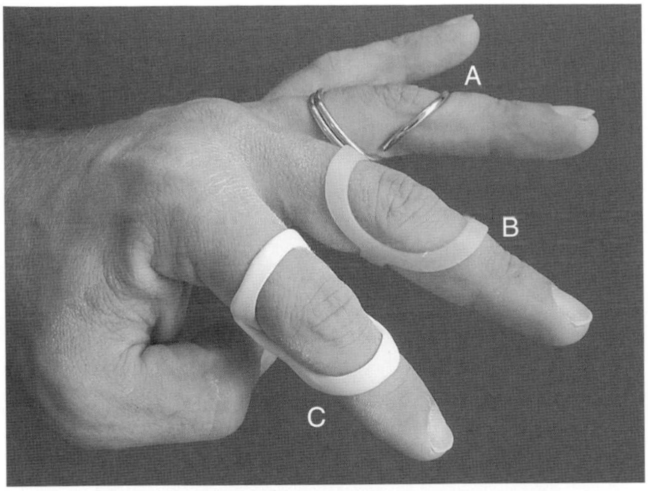

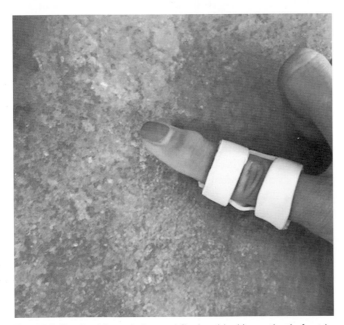

Fig. 12.7 Proximal interphalangeal hyperextension block (swan neck) orthoses. A, Custom-ordered silver ring orthosis. B, Prefabricated polypropylene Oval-8 orthosis. C, Custom low-temperature thermoplastic orthosis. (From Burke, S. L., Higgins, J., McClinton, M. A., et al. [2006]. *Hand and upper extremity rehabilitation: A practical guide* [3rd ed.]. St. Louis, MO: Churchill Livingstone.)

Fig. 12.8 Proximal interphalangeal flexion–blocking orthosis for trigger finger. (Courtesy Kristin Valdes.)

finger. The lifetime risk of developing trigger finger is between 2% and 3% but increases to up to 10% in diabetics.[9]

Finger Orthosis for Trigger Finger

Valdes[11] reported successfully managing trigger finger using a finger-based orthotic device (Fig. 12.8). The decision to use a single-digit orthosis was based on the understanding that blocking PIP flexion would restrict flexor tendon movement through the affected A1 pulley while leaving the palm unrestricted. A thumb-based orthosis can immobilize the interphalangeal (IP) joint but keep the thumb tip as free as possible for improved prehension and tactile discrimination. The orthoses are custom fabricated using thermoplastic material.

Osteoarthritis of Distal Interphalangeal Joint

OA can be a common occurrence at the DIP joints, resulting in deformity and pain. Deformity, either radial or ulnar deviation at the joint, or loss of full extension (extension lag) is common. Functional deficits and reduced quality of life are well documented in those with DIP joint disease, particularly when associated with other hand joint involvement.[7] Aesthetic concerns from hand OA also cause considerable distress, and their presence correlates with reduced health-related quality of life.[5]

Orthoses for Osteoarthritis of Distal Interphalangeal Joint

Two studies[6,13] examined the use of wearing a customized gutter DIP orthosis and the effect on pain. The studies demonstrated that wearing a customized DIP orthosis significantly reduces pain. The device can also be fabricated from the Orficast tape and can be slipped on and off easily by the patient. The Ikeda et al.[6] study demonstrated a large effect size of 2.59 for the reduction of pain after wearing the DIP orthosis. Watt et al.[13] found that short-term nighttime DIP joint splinting is a safe, simple treatment modality that reduces DIP joint pain and improves extension of the digit and does not appear to give rise to noncompliance, increased stiffness, or joint restriction.

Proximal Interphalangeal Flexion Contracture

The PIP joint is the structure producing the largest range of motion in the hand,[8] accounting for 85% of the grasping capabilities of the fingers. PIP joint contractures are common finger injuries seen by therapists following joint dislocation, subluxation, synovitis, ligament damage, soft tissue injury, or prolonged edema of the hand.

Orthoses for Proximal Interphalangeal Flexion Contracture

The reason for orthotic intervention varies but may include increasing function, preventing deformity, correcting deformity, protecting healing structures, restricting motion, and allowing for tissue growth and remodeling. The LMB spring wire (DeRoyal Industries), Reverse Knuckle Bender (Bunnell), Joint Jack (Joint Jack Company), Capener splint (LifeTec Inc.), and the Dynasplint (Dynasplint Systems, Inc.) are prefabricated mobilizing orthotics that aid in PIP extension. Custom low-profile orthoses and serial casting are also options available to therapists. Recent studies[2–4] that provided a wearing schedule of a minimum of 6 hours of a Capener device for 8 to 17 weeks obtained the greatest improvements in extension deficits of the PIP joint. The mean extension gain was 21 degrees. The force of the orthosis should be low enough that the client senses the tension but feels no pain. Clients should be instructed to remove the device intermittently for finger range of motion (ROM) exercises to prevent tissue injury. Clients should be instructed to watch for swelling, cyanosis, or tingling, which may indicate that too much force is being applied.

Finger Proximal Interphalangeal Sprains

Clients may ignore **finger sprains,** but they can be very painful and functionally debilitating with potential for chronic swelling and stiffness and a surprisingly long recovery time.

Grade	Description	Treatment
Mild grade I sprain	No instability with AROM or PROM; macroscopic continuity with microscopic tears. The ligament is intact, but individual fibers are damaged.	Immobilize the joint in full extension if comfortable and available; otherwise immobilize in a small amount of flexion. When pain has subsided, begin AROM, and protect with buddy taping or buddy strapping.
Grade II sprain	Abnormal laxity with stress; the collateral ligament is disrupted. AROM is stable, but passive testing reveals instability.	Immobilize the joint in full extension for 2 to 4 weeks. The physician may recommend early ROM, but avoid any lateral stress.
Grade III sprain	Complete tear of the collateral ligament along with injury to the dorsal capsule or the VP. The finger has usually dislocated with injury.	Early surgical intervention is often recommended.

AROM, Active range of motion; *PROM,* passive range of motion; *ROM,* range of motion; *VP,* volar plate.

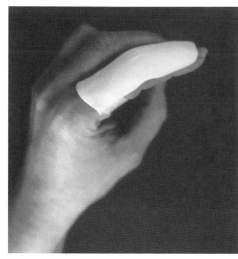

Fig. 12.9 Dorsal gutter orthosis blocking approximately 20 to 30 degrees of proximal interphalangeal extension. (From Fess, E. E., Gettle, K., Philips, C., et al. [2005]. *Hand and upper extremity splinting: Principles and methods* [3rd ed.]. St. Louis, MO: Mosby.)

Uninjured digits are at risk of losing motion and function, which further complicates the picture. Prompt treatment can favorably affect the client's outcome and expedite return to occupations impacted by the injury.

PIP sprains are graded in terms of severity, from grade I to III. Table 12.2 describes these grades and identifies proper treatment. PIP joint dislocations are also described in terms of the direction of joint dislocation (e.g., dorsal, lateral, or volar). PIP joint sprains are associated with **fusiform swelling,** which is fullness at the PIP that tapers proximally and distally. Edema control is critical with this diagnosis.

Orthoses for Finger Proximal Interphalangeal Sprains

The goal of orthoses for finger PIP sprains is to support the PIP joint and promote healing and stability. Orthotic options for the injured PIP joint with extension limitations are similar to those used for boutonnière deformities. If there is a PIP flexion contracture, then a dynamic or serial static PIP extension orthosis is used, or serial casting may be considered. If there has been a VP injury, then a dorsal gutter is fabricated to block approximately 20 to 30 degrees of PIP extension while allowing PIP flexion (Fig. 12.9).

Buddy straps (Fig. 12.10) are used to promote motion and support the injured digit. There are many different styles to choose from. An offset buddy strap may be needed, especially for small finger injuries due to the length discrepancy between the small and ring fingers.

The physician will indicate what arc of motion is safe, according to the injury and joint stability. It is important not

to apply lateral stress to the injured tissues. For example, if the index finger has an injury to the radial collateral ligament, avoid ulnar stress on it. Lateral pinch would also be problematic in this instance. Sometimes it is necessary to custom fabricate a PIP gutter that corrects lateral position as well. Fig. 12.11 shows a digital orthosis that provides lateral support. A silver ring orthosis can also be used to prevent lateral stress to the joint without interfering with joint mobility.

PIP finger sprains are at risk for stiffness and are prone to developing flexion contractures. For this reason, a night PIP extension orthosis is often appropriate to use. But this type of injury may also present problems achieving PIP/DIP flexion as well. In this instance, orthoses can be provided along with exercises to gain flexion passive range of motion (PROM). Examples of flexion orthoses are shown in Fig. 12.12. The force applied by the device should be low enough that the client senses the tension but feels no pain, and tissue tolerances should be monitored carefully.

PRECAUTIONS FOR FINGER ORTHOTICS

- Monitor skin for signs of maceration and/or pressure on both the finger affected and adjacent fingers that contact with the orthosis.
- Check orthotic edges and straps for signs of tightness.
- Provide written instructions, and practice with clients so that they are following guidelines of orthotics care and use correctly.
- If the orthosis is circumferential, circulation should be assessed with pressure to the digit to assess capillary refill.

OCCUPATION-BASED ORTHOTICS

Some finger orthoses may help with hand function by decreasing pain and providing stability. However, many finger orthoses can certainly interfere with daily hand use.

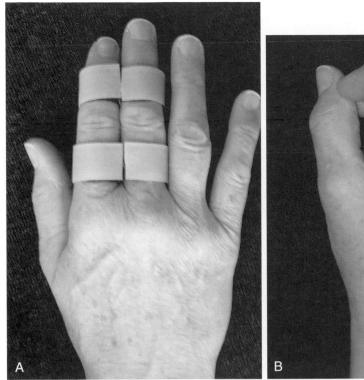

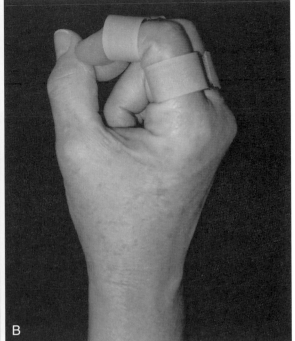

Fig. 12.10 A and B, Examples of buddy straps for proximal interphalangeal collateral ligament injuries. (From Burke, S. L., Higgins, J., McClinton, M. A., et al. [2006]. *Hand and upper extremity rehabilitation: A practical guide* [3rd ed.]. St. Louis, MO: Churchill Livingstone.)

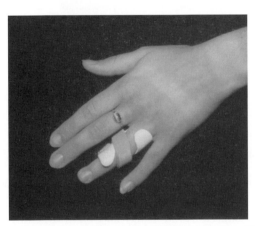

Fig. 12.11 Proximal interphalangeal extension orthosis with lateral support. (From Fess, E. E., Gettle, K., Philips, C., et al. [2005]. *Hand and upper extremity splinting: Principles and methods* [3rd ed.]. St. Louis, MO: Mosby.)

Understandably, clients may be tempted to remove their orthoses to participate in activities they enjoy. To help prevent this from happening, therapists should incorporate an occupation-based approach.

Examples of Occupation-Based Finger Orthoses

An elderly retired man enjoyed woodworking but was unable to use his woodworking tools comfortably due to arthritis-related pain and instability of the index finger PIP joint. He expressed interest in a PIP joint protective orthosis to help him use his tools. To determine the best position of the PIP joint orthosis, he brought his tools to therapy and demonstrated the finger position he needed. An orthosis was made that provided support during this task.

A client with a mallet injury came to the clinic with maceration under the orthosis. He stated that he was wearing his orthosis in the shower and keeping the wet orthosis on his finger all day. In addition to reviewing skin care guidelines and practicing safe protected donning and doffing of the orthosis, an additional orthosis was made to use while showering. This allowed him to apply a dry orthosis after his shower. With this solution, he could avoid further skin maceration.

FABRICATION OF A DORSAL-VOLAR MALLET ORTHOSIS

The dorsal-volar mallet orthosis is indicated for a mallet injury. Fig. 12.13A represents a detailed pattern that can be

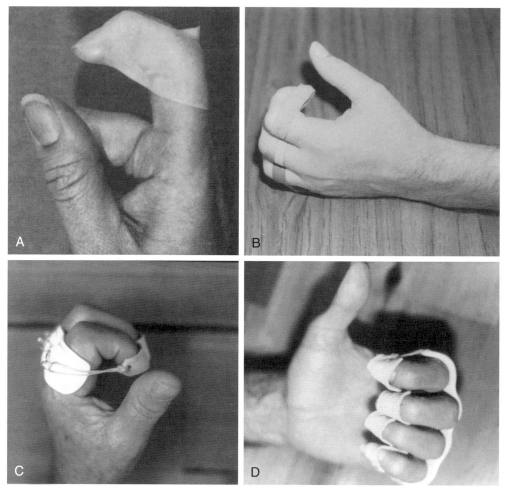

Fig. 12.12 A to D, Examples of proximal interphalangeal/distal interphalangeal flexion orthoses. (From Fess, E. E., Gettle, K., Philips, C., et al. [2005]. *Hand and upper extremity splinting: Principles and methods* [3rd ed.]. St. Louis, MO: Mosby.)

used for any finger. Fig. 12.13B shows a completed orthosis. This orthosis has some adjustability for fluctuations in edema, which can be advantageous. Nonperforated ³⁄₃₂-inch material works well for this orthosis. An alternative orthotic design is a DIP gutter orthosis. Fig. 12.13C represents a detailed pattern for this alternative orthosis.

1. Mark the length of the finger from the PIP joint to the tip.
2. Mark the width of the finger.
3. Cut out the pattern, and round the four edges.
4. Trace the pattern on a sheet of thermoplastic material.
5. Warm the material slightly to make it easier to cut the pattern out of the thermoplastic material.
6. Heat the thermoplastic material.
7. Apply the material to the client's finger, clearing the volar PIP crease. Be gentle with the amount of hand pressure over the dorsal DIP because this is usually quite tender.
8. Maintain the DIP in extension or slight hyperextension, depending on the physician's order.
9. Allow the material to cool completely before removing the orthosis.
10. Ensure proper fit of the orthosis. The orthosis should stay in place securely with a thin ½-inch Velcro strap.

11. Trim the edges as needed.
12. Smooth all edges completely.

Technical Tips for Proper Fit of Mallet Orthoses

1. Finger orthoses may seem easy to make because they are small. However, it may take extra time to fabricate them precisely. Do not be surprised if you wind up needing extra time to make and fine-tune these small orthoses.
2. Ordinary Velcro loop straps may feel bulky on small finger orthoses. Thinner strap material that is ½-inch wide and less bulky can be very effective for finger orthoses.
3. If an orthosis slips, consider using paper tape to apply the device to the finger and self-adherent elastic wrap, rather than Velcro strapping.

Safety Tips for Mallet Orthoses

1. Device must be removed by the patient and finger washed to prevent skin maceration.
2. If the patient has a pin to repair a bony mallet finger, protect the pin with a cap of material to prevent jarring of the pin.

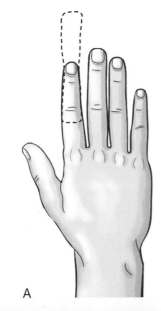

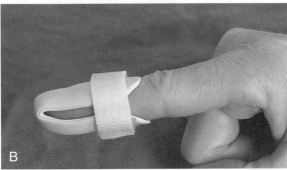

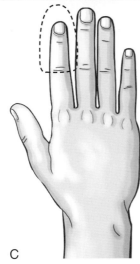

Fig. 12.13 A, Dorsal-volar mallet orthosis pattern. B, Completed dorsal-volar mallet orthosis. C, Distal interphalangeal gutter orthosis pattern.

PREFABRICATED MALLET ORTHOSES

If there has been surgery and the client has a percutaneous pin, the orthosis must accommodate the pin. The DIP orthosis can be a volar gutter orthosis, a dorsal-volar orthosis, or a stack orthosis. A prefabricated AlumaFoam orthosis is sometimes used, but there may be inconveniences and skin issues associated with the

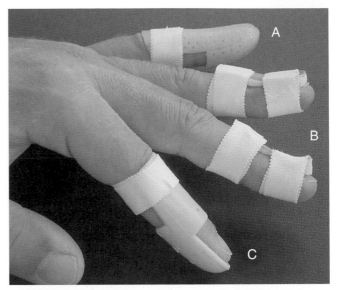

Fig. 12.14 Mallet orthoses. A, Custom thermoplastic. B, Aluma-Foam. C, Stack. (From Burke, S. L., Higgins, J., McClinton, M. A., et al. [2006]. *Hand and upper extremity rehabilitation: A practical guide* [3rd ed.]. St. Louis, MO: Churchill Livingstone.)

adhesive tape that is used to secure it. Prefabricated or custom fabricated stack orthoses need to be monitored for clearance at the dorsal distal edge, because this is an area prone to tenderness and edema related to the injury (Fig. 12.14).

Mallet Finger Impact on Occupation

Mallet injuries can result in awkward hand use and can also limit the freedom of flexion of uninvolved digits. It is important to teach clients to maintain active PIP motion of the involved digit and to use compensatory skills, such as relying on uninjured fingertips for sensory input.

FABRICATION OF A PROXIMAL INTERPHALANGEAL GUTTER ORTHOSIS

A PIP gutter orthosis is indicated for a PIP sprain injury. Fig. 12.15A represents a detailed pattern that can be used for any finger. Fig. 12.15B shows a completed orthosis. Nonperforated $^{3}/_{32}$-inch material works well for this orthosis.

1. Mark the length of the finger from the web space to the DIP joint.
2. Mark the width of the finger, adding approximately ¼ to ½ inch on each side, depending on the size of the digit.
3. Cut out the pattern, and round the four edges.
4. Trace the pattern on a sheet of thermoplastic material.
5. Warm the material slightly to make it easier to cut the pattern out of the thermoplastic material.
6. Heat the thermoplastic material.
7. Position the client's hand with the palm up to allow the material to drape.
8. Apply the material to the client's finger, clearing the MCP and DIP creases and positioning the PIP joint in the desired position. (This is typically the available passive extension.) Be gentle with the amount of hand pressure used over the PIP joint and over the sides of the joint.

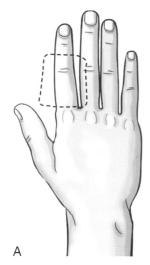

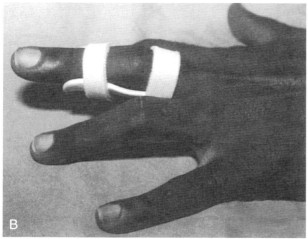

Fig. 12.15 A, Proximal interphalangeal gutter orthosis pattern for fabrication. B, Completed orthosis. (From Clark, G. L. [1998]. *Hand rehabilitation: A practical guide* [2nd ed.]. New York, NY: Churchill Livingstone.)

9. Roll the edges of the orthosis as needed for comfort and clearance of MCP and DIP joint motions.
10. Allow the material to cool completely before removing the orthosis.
11. Ensure proper fit of the orthosis.
12. Trim the edges as needed.
13. Smooth all edges completely.

Technical Tips for Proper Fit of a Proximal Interphalangeal Gutter Orthosis

1. Straps must fit closely enough to provide a secure fit. Consider using one long Velcro strap that wraps around the digit two to three times for better fit.
2. Modify the height of finger orthotic edges so that straps can have contact with the skin. If the edges are too high, the straps will not be effective.
3. If the goal is to achieve full PIP extension, consider placing a strap directly over the PIP joint, but be careful to closely monitor skin tolerance.

Safety Tip for Proximal Interphalangeal Orthosis

1. Straps should not be too tight because this can cause edema.

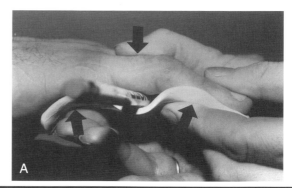

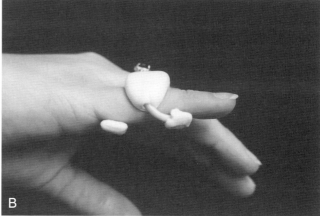

Fig. 12.16 A, Prefabricated proximal interphalangeal (PIP) extension orthosis that crosses the distal interphalangeal (DIP). B, Prefabricated PIP extension orthosis with DIP free. (From Fess, E. E., Gettle, K., Philips, C., et al. [2005]. *Hand and upper extremity splinting: Principles and methods* [3rd ed.]. St. Louis, MO: Mosby.)

Prefabricated Proximal Interphalangeal Orthoses

Fig. 12.16 shows examples of prefabricated PIP extension orthoses. Remember that prefabricated orthoses do not always fit well or accommodate edema. Also, there can be problems with distribution of pressure, skin tolerance, and excessive joint forces.

Impact of Proximal Interphalangeal Injuries on Occupations

PIP joint injuries can limit the flexibility and function of the entire hand. Reaching into the pocket or grasping a tool may be impeded. Pain can interfere with the comfort of doing a simple but socially significant task such as a handshake. Rings may no longer fit over the injured joint. Early appropriate therapy can help restore these functions to clients.

FABRICATION OF A PROXIMAL INTERPHALANGEAL HYPEREXTENSION BLOCK (SWAN NECK ORTHOSIS)

The PIP hyperextension block orthosis is indicated for a finger with a flexible swan neck deformity. Fig. 12.17A represents a detailed pattern that can be used for any finger. Fig. 12.17B shows a completed orthosis. An alternate orthotic design involves wrapping a thin strip or tube of thermoplastic material in a spiral fashion (see Fig. 12.17C).

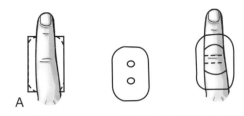

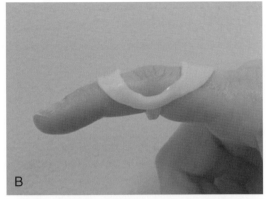

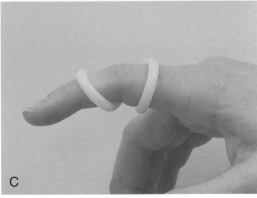

Fig. 12.17 A, Proximal interphalangeal (PIP) hyperextension block orthosis pattern. B, Completed PIP hyperextension block orthosis. C, Spiral design PIP hyperextension block orthosis.

A properly fitting orthosis effectively blocks the PIP in slight flexion when the finger is actively extended and allows unrestricted active PIP flexion. A thin (1/16 inch) nonperforated thermoplastic material (such as Orfit or Aquaplast) works well for this orthosis. It is especially important to minimize bulk if multiple fingers need orthoses on the same hand. The orthoses must not get caught on each other.

1. Mark the length of the finger from the web space to the DIP joint.
2. Mark the width of the finger, adding approximately 1/4 inch on each side.
3. Cut out the pattern, and round the four edges.
4. Trace the pattern on a sheet of thermoplastic material.
5. Cut the pattern out of the thermoplastic material. Cutting thin material does not require heating of the plastic first.
6. Mark location for holes, leaving an approximately 1/4- to 1/2-inch bar of material in the center of the orthosis.
7. Punch holes.
8. Apply a light amount of lotion to the finger to enable the material to slide over the finger easily.
9. Heat the thermoplastic material.

10. Slightly stretch the holes so that they are just large enough to slide the finger through. Be careful not to overstretch because the orthosis will be too loose.
11. Slide the material over the finger, weaving the finger up through the proximal hole and down through the distal hole.
12. Center the volar thermoplastic bar directly under the PIP joint, and the dorsal distal and proximal ends of the orthosis over the middle and proximal phalanges.
13. As the orthosis is formed on the finger, keep the PIP in slight flexion (approximately 20 to 25 degrees).
14. Roll the edges of the volar thermoplastic bar as needed to allow unrestricted PIP flexion.
15. Fold the lateral sides of the orthosis volarly and contour the material to the finger.
16. Allow the material to cool completely before removing the orthosis.
17. Ensure proper fit of the orthosis. The orthosis should be loose enough to slide over the PIP joint yet snug enough to not migrate or twist on the finger. The orthosis should allow full PIP flexion and effectively prevent the PIP from going into hyperextension.
18. Trim the edges as needed.
19. Smooth all edges completely.

Technical Tips for Proper Fit of the Hyperextension Block (Swan Neck Orthosis)

1. A common mistake is to allow the PIP joint to go into extension while fabricating the orthosis. Closely monitor the PIP position to make sure that it remains in slight flexion during the fabrication process.
2. If the PIP joint is enlarged or swollen, it may be very difficult to slide the orthosis off the finger once it is made. This can be avoided by gently sliding the orthosis back and forth over the PIP joint a few times before the thermoplastic material is fully cooled.
3. Because this orthosis is meant to enable function, make sure to minimize orthotic bulk by flattening the volar PIP bar and lateral edges as much as possible so that the edges do not impede the grasping of objects.

Safety Tip for Hyperextension Block Orthosis

1. Ensure that the device is not too tight because this will cause excessive edema and make the device difficult to remove.

Swan neck orthoses are commercially available, and they offer some advantages over custom-fabricated thermoplastic orthoses. They are more durable, less bulky, and often more cosmetically pleasing to clients. Therapists use ring sizers to determine the size needed for each finger. Custom-ordered ring orthoses made of silver or gold (Fig. 12.18) are attractive, unobtrusive, and flexible enough to be adjusted for fluctuations in joint swelling; however, they are costlier. Prefabricated orthoses made of polypropylene (Fig. 12.19) are a less expensive alternative that offer durability and a streamlined fit. Their fit can be slightly modified by a therapist using a heat gun, but they cannot be adjusted by clients in response to variations in joint swelling.

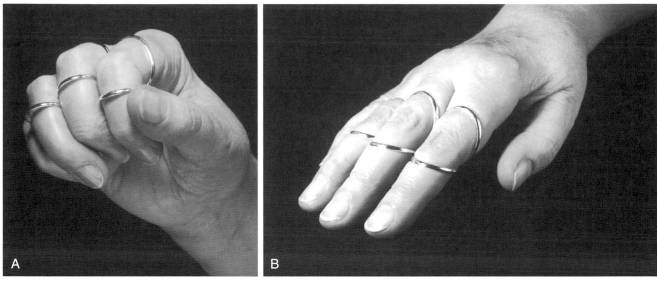

Fig. 12.18 A and B, Custom-ordered proximal interphalangeal hyperextension block orthoses. (From Skirven, T. M., Callahan, A. D., Osterman, A. L., et al. [2002]. *Hunter, Mackin & Callahan's rehabilitation of the hand and upper extremity* [5th ed.]. St. Louis, MO: Mosby.)

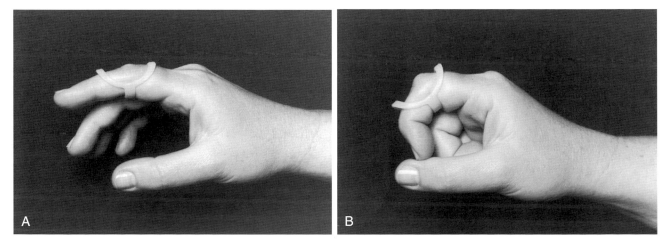

Fig. 12.19 A and B, Prefabricated proximal interphalangeal hyperextension block orthoses. (From Skirven, T. M., Callahan, A. D., Osterman, A. L., et al. [2002]. *Hunter, Mackin & Callahan's rehabilitation of the hand and upper extremity* [5th ed.]. St. Louis, MO: Mosby.)

IMPACT OF SWAN NECK DEFORMITIES ON OCCUPATIONS

Swan neck deformities often cause difficulty with hand closure. PIP tendons and ligaments can catch during motion, and the long finger flexors have less mechanical advantage to initiate flexion when the PIP starts from a hyperextended position. A PIP hyperextension block should improve the client's hand function by allowing the PIP to flex more quickly and easily, enabling the ability to grasp objects.

FABRICATION OF A THREE-POINT PROXIMAL INTERPHALANGEAL EXTENSION LOW-PROFILE ORTHOSIS

Boccolari and Tocco[1] provided directions for an orthosis that is suitable for PIP joint flexion contractures of a single digit and can be modified to accommodate contractures as severe as 70 degrees from full extension. The device provides equal pressure distribution and is low profile.

Materials

1. 5 × 5 cm thin elastic thermoplastic material for the proximal plate (e.g., 1.6-mm Aquaplast or 2.0-mm Orfit Classic), ends slightly distal to the palmar distal crease
2. 3 × 3 cm T-shaped piece of similar thermoplastic material for the distal cuff
3. 40-cm long 1.6-mm copper-coated steel welding rod
4. Round-tipped pliers or 90-degree wire bender
5. Wire cutter
6. 1 × 2 cm adhesive hook Velcro
7. 1 × 15 cm nonadhesive loop Velcro

Fabrication Procedure[1]*

1. "Position the pliers or wire bender at the half point of the copper wire and bend the wire to 90 degrees (Fig. 12.20A).
2. Measure the width of the frame by placing the edge of the bent wire on one side of the PIP crease (see Fig. 12.20B), leaving a space of 0.5 cm between it and the finger (see Fig. 12.20C). Do not use the DIP crease to measure, to avoid underestimating the width of the frame and later be faced with difficulties in assembling the distal cuff onto the frame.
3. Bend the wire at a 90-degree angle to obtain a reverse U-shape.
4. At 0.5 cm from these bending points (bilaterally), tilt the U-shaped portion 90 degrees anteriorly on a sagittal plane (see Fig. 12.20D). This will avoid hyperextending the PIP joint beyond the neutral position after achieving full passive PIP joint extension—the longitudinal portion of the frame will lie midway on either side of the finger once the joint has recovered full extension.
5. Place the U-shaped portion just proximal to the DIP crease to measure the *length* of the frame before applying another bilateral 90-degree anterior tilt to the frame (similar to step 4). The frame must be tilted just distal to the web space of the finger (see Fig. 12.20E–F) http://www.jhandtherapy.org/cms/attachment/2001330725/2005179457/gr7.jpg
6. Bend the wire 90 degrees in the opposite direction 0.5 cm from the previous bending points on each side to redirect the proximal rods toward the wrist (see Fig. 12.20G).
7. Curve the two proximal endings toward each other to end the frame just proximal to the distal palmer crease (or proximal crease when splinting the index finger (see Fig. 12.20H).
8. Wrap the 5 × 5 cm square piece of thermoplastic material around the proximal portion of the frame and cut the excess material around the frame (see Fig. 12.20I).
9. Place the reverse T-shaped thermoplastic piece over the DIP crease (see Fig. 12.20J). Before it hardens, lay the distal portion of the frame over the T-shaped piece just proximal to the DIP crease. Flip the distal portion of the T-shaped piece over the resting rod (see Fig. 12.20K). The cuff is not fixed to the copper wire, rather it is molded around it. This technique allows the distal cuff to rotate around the rod, which will allow maximal pressure distribution on the middle phalanx as passive extension improves.
10. Wrap the adhesive hook Velcro around the ulnar rod next to the PIP joint and stick both wings against each other to rest dorsal to the finger (see Fig. 12.20 L).
11. Attach the loop Velcro on the internal side of the hook Velcro (see Fig. 12.20M). Pass it over the PIP joint, and slip it between the finger and the radial rod. Wrap it around this rod, and pass it again over the PIP joint to end its attachment on the external side of the hook Velcro (see Fig. 12.20N). Apply the appropriate tension over the PIP joint to lever the middle phalanx into extension (see Fig. 12.20O)."

Technical Tips for Proper Fit of the Three-Point Extension Orthosis

1. Follow-ups should be scheduled 2 or 3 days after the first visit. If skin redness is noted, a piece of Neoprene or other padding can be added over the PIP joint under the Velcro strap.[1]
2. It is therefore preferable to begin with gentle tension and progressively increase the tension as the tissue allows.[1]
3. The splint should be worn continuously for approximately 3 to 5 days. If full range of motion is not gained at this point, the patient is instructed to wear the splint for an additional 2 to 3 days if skin redness is absent.[1]

PREFABRICATED PROXIMAL INTERPHALANGEAL EXTENSION ORTHOSES

The LMB spring wire, Reverse Knuckle Bender, Joint Jack, Capener splint, and the Dynasplint are prefabricated mobilizing orthotics that aid in PIP extension. Remember that prefabricated orthoses do not always fit well or accommodate edema. Also, there can be problems with distribution of pressure, skin tolerance, and excessive joint forces.

Safety Tips for Three-Point Proximal Interphalangeal Extension Orthosis

1. Instruct client not to tighten the strap too much because this will compromise circulation.

IMPACT OF PROXIMAL INTERPHALANGEAL FLEXION CONTRACTURES ON OCCUPATIONS

PIP flexion contractures often cause difficulty with hand opening. The client may have difficulty reaching his or her hand into narrow spaces and may report jarring the joint. A PIP extension orthosis should improve the client's hand function by allowing the PIP joint to fully extend, enabling the ability to fully open hand.

FABRICATION OF A FINGER-BASED TRIGGER FINGER ORTHOSIS

1. Mark the length of the finger from the web space to the DIP joint.
2. Measure the circumference of the finger, adding approximately ½ inch.
3. Mark the width of the finger, adding approximately ¼ inch on each side.
4. Cut out the pattern, and round the four edges (Fig. 12.21A).
5. Trace the pattern on a sheet of thermoplastic material.
6. Cut the pattern out of the thermoplastic material. Cutting thin material does not require heating of the plastic first.

*Boccolari, P., & Tocco, S. [2009]. Alternative splinting approach for proximal interphalangeal joint flexion contractures: No-profile static progressive splinting and cylinder splint combo. *Journal of Hand Therapy* 22[3], 290-292.

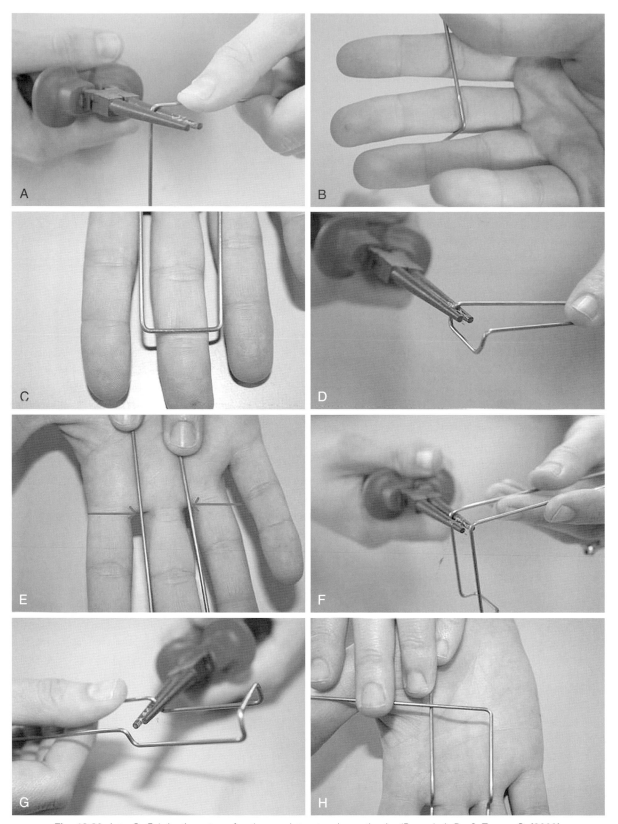

Fig. 12.20 A to O, Fabrication steps for three-point extension orthosis. (Boccolari, P., & Tocco, S. [2009]. Alternative splinting approach for proximal interphalangeal joint flexion contractures: No-profile static progressive splinting and cylinder splint combo. *Journal of Hand Therapy 22*[3], 289–293.)

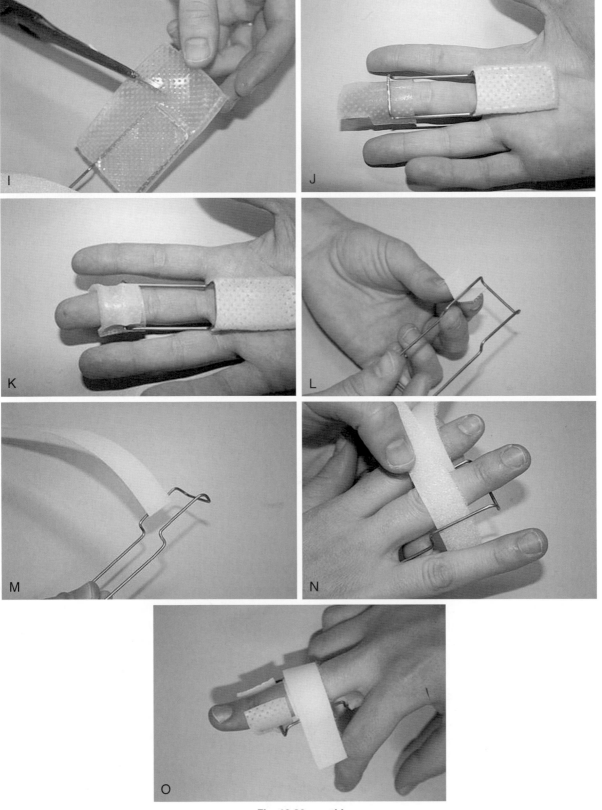

Fig. 12.20, cont'd

7. Apply a light amount of lotion to the finger to enable the material to slide over the finger easily.
8. Heat the thermoplastic material.
9. Lay the material over the volar surface of the finger, wrapping the "tails" completely around the finger and attaching to the back surface of the device (see Fig. 12.21B–C).
10. The dorsal surface of the PIP joint should be free (see Fig. 12.21D).
11. As the orthosis is formed on the finger, keep the PIP in extension.
12. Roll the edges of the volar thermoplastic bar as needed to allow unrestricted DIP and MP flexion.
13. Allow the material to cool completely before removing the orthosis.
14. Ensure proper fit of the orthosis. The orthosis should be loose enough to slide over the PIP joint yet snug enough to not migrate or twist on the finger.
15. Trim the edges as needed.
16. Smooth all edges completely.

Technical Tips for Proper Fit of the Trigger Finger Orthosis

1. If the PIP joint is enlarged or swollen, it may be very difficult to slide the orthosis off the finger once it is made. This can be avoided by gently sliding the orthosis back and forth over the PIP joint a few times before the thermoplastic material is fully cooled.
2. Because this orthosis is meant to enable function, make sure to minimize orthotic bulk by flattening the orthotic material as much as possible so that the device is not too bulky on the finger and rubbing on the adjacent fingers.

Safety Tip for a Trigger Finger Orthosis

1. Ensure that the device is not too tight and that it can be slid on and off and that it has not compromised circulation.

PREFABRICATED TRIGGER FINGER ORTHOSIS

Swan neck orthoses can be used if they are positioned on the PIP joint "upside down" (two bands on the volar surface of the finger). These orthoses are commercially available.

IMPACT OF TRIGGER FINGER ON OCCUPATIONS

Trigger finger often cause difficulty with grasping and manipulating of fine objects. The finger may lock into flexion after composite flexion of the digit. A finger-based orthosis should improve the client's hand function by allowing the palm to be free and immobilizing only one joint.

FABRICATION OF THE DISTAL INTERPHALANGEAL STABILIZATION ORTHOSIS

1. Cut a 6-inch piece of 1-inch blue Orficast tape (Fig. 12.22A).
2. Heat the material.

3. Wrap the material around the DIP joint (see Fig. 12.22B–C).
4. As the orthosis is formed on the finger, keep the PIP in slight flexion or extension.
5. Allow the material to cool completely before removing the orthosis.
6. Ensure proper fit of the orthosis. The orthosis should be loose enough to slide over the DIP joint yet snug enough to not migrate or twist on the finger.
7. Trim the edges as needed.

Technical Tips for Proper Fit of the Distal Interphalangeal Stabilization Orthosis

1. Make sure to minimize orthotic bulk by flattening the orthotic material as much as possible so that the device is not too bulky on the finger.
2. Ensure that the patient can slip the device on and off the finger.

Safety Tip for a Distal Interphalangeal Stabilization Orthosis

1. Ensure that the device is not too tight and that it can be slid on and off and that it has not compromised circulation.

PREFABRICATED DISTAL INTERPHALANGEAL STABILIZATION ORTHOSIS

Swan neck orthoses can be used if they are positioned on the PIP joint "upside down" (two bands on the volar surface of the finger). They are commercially available. If the joint is laterally deviated, the device can be placed "sideways" on the finger with the two-band side placed on the same side of the finger that the deviation is. If the finger is severely deviated, a prefabricated device should not be used.

IMPACT OF DISTAL INTERPHALANGEAL OSTEOARTHRITIS ON OCCUPATIONS

Pain, joint deformity, and loss of extension lag lead to both functional and cosmetic issues for clients with OA. Clients may experience loss of sleep due to pain. Some individuals are concerned about the appearance of the deformed joint. The DIP immobilization orthosis is a safe and inexpensive intervention that reduces DIP joint pain and improves joint extension.

CONCLUSION

There is emerging research and strong clinical support for the use of finger orthoses as a mainstay of care for many common finger problems. Finger biomechanics are very complicated. Added to this, there are multiple custom and prefabricated orthotics to select from. These challenges can understandably confuse decision making, particularly for novice therapists. Hopefully this chapter helps therapists use sound clinical reasoning to work collaboratively with clients. Application of clinical reasoning ensures that the best orthosis is selected based on each client's clinical needs and occupational demands.

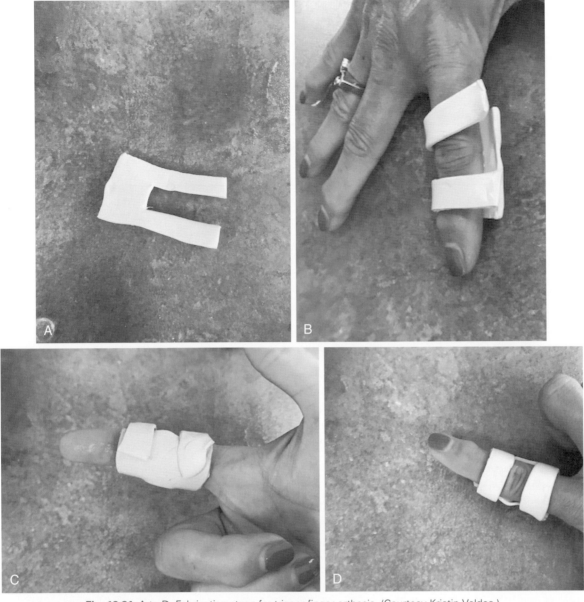

Fig. 12.21 A to D, Fabrication steps for trigger finger orthosis. (Courtesy Kristin Valdes.)

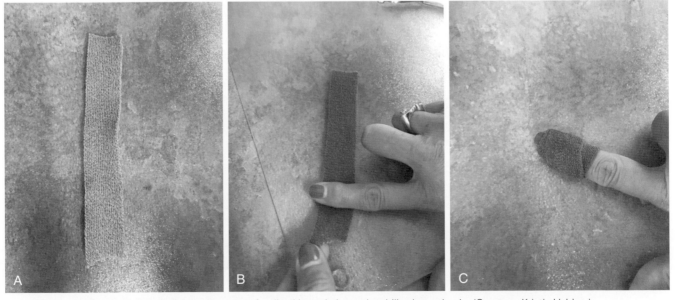

Fig. 12.22 A to C, Fabrication steps for distal interphalangeal stabilization orthosis. (Courtesy Kristin Valdes.)

REVIEW QUESTIONS

1. What is a mallet finger?
2. What is the posture of a finger with a boutonnière deformity?
3. What is the posture of a finger with a swan neck deformity?
4. What is fusiform swelling?
5. What structures provide joint stability and restraint against PIP deviation forces?
6. What is the difference between an extensor lag and a flexion contracture?
7. What type of finger orthosis is typically used for a swan neck deformity?
8. How is the DIP positioned when providing an orthosis for a mallet finger?
9. What position should the PIP be in when providing an orthosis for a boutonnière deformity?
10. What position should the PIP be in when providing an orthosis for a swan neck deformity?

REFERENCES

1. Boccolari P, Tocco S: Alternative splinting approach for proximal interphalangeal joint flexion contractures; no-profile static progressive splinting and cylinder splint combo, *J Hand Ther* 22(3):289–293, 2009.
2. Cantero-Téllez R, Cuesta-Vargas A, Cuadros-Romero M: Treatment of proximal interphalangeal joint flexion contracture: combined static and dynamic orthotic intervention compared with other therapy intervention: a randomized controlled trial, *J Hand Surg* 40(5):951–955, 2015.
3. Glasgow C, Fleming J, Tooth LR, Peters S: Randomized control trial of daily total end range time (TERT) for capener splinting of the stiff proximal interphalangeal joint, *Am J Occup Ther* 66(2):243–248, 2012.
4. Glasgow C, Fleming J, Tooth L, Hockey R: The long-term relationship between duration of treatment and contracture resolution using dynamic orthotic devices for the stiff proximal interphalangeal joint: a prospective cohort study, *J Hand Ther* 25(1):38–47, 2011.
5. Hodkinson B, Maheu E, Michon M, et al.: Assessment and determinants of aesthetic discomfort in hand osteoarthritis, *Ann Rheum Dis* 71(1):45–49, 2012.
6. Ikeda M, Ishii T, Kobayashi Y, Mochida J, Saito I, Oka Y: Custom-made splint treatment for osteoarthritis of the distal interphalangeal joints, *J Hand Surg* 35(4):589–593, 2010.
7. Kjeken I, Dagfinrud H, Slatkowsky-Christensen B, et al.: Activity limitations and participation restrictions in women with hand osteoarthritis: clients' descriptions and associations between dimensions of functioning, *Ann Rheu Dis* 64(11):1633–1638, 2005.
8. Leibovic SJ, Bowers WH: Anatomy of the proximal interphalangeal joint, *Hand Clin* 10(2):169–178, 1994.
9. Makkouk AL, Oetgen ME, Swigart CR, Dodds SD: Trigger finger: etiology, evaluation, and treatment, *Curr Rev Musculoskelet Med* 1(2):92–96, 2008.
10. Tocco S, Boccolari P, Landi A, et al.: Effectiveness of cast immobilization in comparison to the gold-standard self-removal orthotic intervention for closed mallet fingers: a randomized clinical trial, *J Hand Ther* 26(3):191–201, 2013.
11. Valdes K: A retrospective review to determine the long-term efficacy of orthotic devices for trigger finger, *J Hand Ther* 25(1):89–96, 2012.
12. Valdes K, Naughton N, Algar L: Conservative management of mallet finger: a systematic review, *J Hand Ther* 28(3):237–246, 2015.
13. Watt FE, Kennedy DL, Carlisle KE, et al.: Night-time immobilization of the distal interphalangeal joint reduces pain and extension deformity in hand osteoarthritis, *Rheumatology (Oxford)* 53(6):1142–1149, 2014.

APPENDIX 12.1 CASE STUDIES

Case Study 12.1[a]

Read the following scenario, and use your clinical reasoning skills to answer the questions based on information in this chapter.

Marge is a 74-year-old right-hand-dominant woman who is retired from her job. She likes to crochet and knit. She has pain and swelling of her index and small finger DIP joints. Her physician diagnosed her with osteoarthritis of the fingers and sent her to occupational therapy for evaluation and treatment. At her initial evaluation she reports night DIP joint pain that interferes with her sleep.

1. What joint(s) should her finger orthoses cross?

   _____

   _____

2. When does Marge need to wear the orthoses in a 24-hour cycle?

   _____

   _____

   _____

3. How long is Marge likely to need to wear her orthoses?

   _____

   _____

   _____

Case Study 12.2[a]

Read the following scenario, and use your clinical reasoning skills to answer the questions based on information in this chapter.

Ryan is a 23-year-old right-hand–dominant man who jammed his right middle finger while playing softball. He developed pain and swelling of the distal finger, along with a droop of the DIP joint. His physician diagnosed a mallet injury and sent him to occupational therapy for orthotic fabrication.

1. What joint(s) should his finger orthosis cross?

   _____

   _____

2. What is the recommended orthotic wearing schedule?

   _____

   _____

3. List two different types of orthoses that Ryan could use.

   _____

   _____

4. How long is Ryan likely to need to wear his orthosis?

   _____

   _____

Case Study 12.3[a]

Read the following scenario, and use your clinical reasoning skills to answer the questions based on information in this chapter.

Debbie is a 62-year-old left-hand–dominant woman who fell and developed pain and swelling of her left ring finger PIP joint. She was diagnosed with a PIP joint injury to the radial collateral ligament and VP.

1. Should Debbie have a dorsal or volar finger orthosis?

   _____

   _____

2. What joint(s) should the orthosis cross, and what position should they be in?

   _____

   _____

   _____

3. Which fingers would be good to buddy tape or buddy strap together and why?

   _____

   _____

4. Debbie loved to play tennis. When she was medically cleared to play again, she experienced recurrence of swelling at the ring finger PIP joint. What might help her manage her pain and swelling so that she could play tennis again?

   _____

   _____

   _____

Case Study 12.4[a]

Read the following scenario, and apply clinical reasoning skills to answer the questions based on information in this chapter.

Alexa is a 41-year-old right-hand–dominant law firm receptionist who has a 3-year history of rheumatoid arthritis. She was referred to occupational therapy for evaluation of orthotic needs. She presents with recent development of bilateral swan neck deformities of all fingers. She can actively flex her PIPs, but it is awkward and effortful to do so. She reports having difficulty with home and work tasks that involve grasping objects.

1. Do you think Alexa would benefit from PIP hyperextension block orthoses? Why or why not?

   _____

   _____

2. How could you and Alexa determine if orthoses will improve her hand function?

   _____

   _____

3. What key client factors and orthotic options would you consider in selecting the best orthoses for Alexa?

   _____

   _____

   _____

---

[a] See Appendix A for the answer key.

[a] See Appendix A for the answer key.

4. When should Alexa wear her orthoses?

    _____

    _____

    _____

APPENDIX 12.2 LABORATORY EXERCISES

Laboratory Exercise 12.1[a]

1. The following picture shows a mallet finger gutter orthosis. What is wrong with this orthosis?

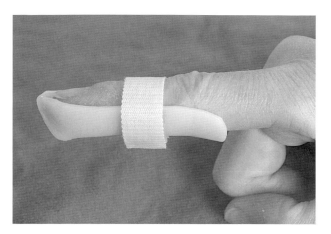

    _____

    _____

    _____

    _____

2. The following picture shows a PIP gutter orthosis. What is wrong with this orthosis?

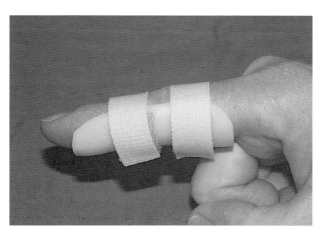

    _____

    _____

    _____

    _____

3. The following picture shows a PIP hyperextension block orthosis. What is wrong with this orthosis?

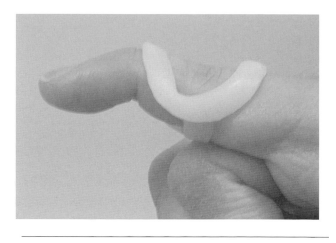

    _____

    _____

    _____

    _____

Laboratory Exercise 12.2

Practice fabricating a dorsal-volar mallet orthosis on a partner with the DIP joint in neutral. Check to be sure that the PIP crease is not blocked and that full PIP active ROM (AROM) is available.

[a] See Appendix A for the answer key.

APPENDIX 12.3 FORM AND GRADING SHEET

Form 12.1 Finger Orthotic

	Name: _____
	Date: _____
After the person wears the orthosis for 30 minutes, answer the following questions. (Mark NA for nonapplicable situations.)	

Evaluation Areas				Comments
Design				
1. The PIP position is at the correct angle.	Yes	No	NA	
2. The DIP position is at the correct angle.	Yes	No	NA	
3. The orthosis provides adequate support and is not constrictive.	Yes	No	NA	
4. The orthotic length is appropriate.	Yes	No	NA	
5. The orthotic width is appropriate.	Yes	No	NA	
6. The orthosis is snug enough to stay in place yet loose enough to apply and remove.	Yes	No	NA	
Function				
1. The orthosis allows full MCP motion.	Yes	No	NA	
2. The orthosis allows full PIP motion.	Yes	No	NA	
3. The orthosis allows full DIP motion.	Yes	No	NA	
4. The orthosis enables as much hand function as possible.	Yes	No	NA	
Straps				
1. The straps are secure, and the terminal edges are rounded.	Yes	No	NA	
Comfort				
2. The orthotic edges are smooth, rounded, contoured, and flared.	Yes	No	NA	
3. The orthosis does not cause pain or pressure areas.	Yes	No	NA	
Cosmetic Appearance				
1. The orthosis is free of fingerprints, dirt, and pencil/pen marks.	Yes	No	NA	
2. The thermoplastic material is free of buckles.	Yes	No	NA	

Therapeutic Regimen				
1. The client or caregiver has been instructed in a wearing schedule.	Yes	No	NA	
2. The client or caregiver has been provided orthotic precautions.	Yes	No	NA	
3. The client or caregiver demonstrates understanding of the orthotic program.	Yes	No	NA	
4. The client or caregiver demonstrates proper donning and doffing of orthosis.	Yes	No	NA	
5. The client or caregiver knows how to clean the orthosis and straps.	Yes	No	NA	

Discuss possible orthotic adjustments or changes you should make based on the self-evaluation. What would you do differently next time?

_____

_____

_____

_____

_____

_____

_____

_____

_____

_____

_____

Discuss possible areas to improve with clinical safety when fabricating the orthosis.

_____

_____

_____

_____

Grading Sheet 12.1 Finger Orthotic

	Name: _____
	Date: _____

Type of finger orthosis:			
Mallet finger	PIP gutter	PIP hyperextension block	Other _____

Grade: _____

1 = Beyond improvement, not acceptable

2 = Requires maximal improvement

3 = Requires moderate improvement

4 = Requires minimal improvement

5 = Requires no improvement

Evaluation Areas						Comments
Design						
1. The PIP position is at the correct angle.	1	2	3	4	5	
2. The DIP position is at the correct angle.	1	2	3	4	5	
3. The orthosis provides adequate support and is not constrictive.	1	2	3	4	5	
4. The orthotic length is appropriate.	1	2	3	4	5	
5. The orthotic width is appropriate.	1	2	3	4	5	
6. The orthosis is snug enough to stay in place yet loose enough to apply and remove.	1	2	3	4	5	
Function						
1. The orthosis allows full MCP motion.	1	2	3	4	5	
2. The orthosis allows full PIP motion.	1	2	3	4	5	
3. The orthosis allows full DIP motion.	1	2	3	4	5	
4. The orthosis enables as much hand function as possible.	1	2	3	4	5	
Straps						
1. The straps are secure and the terminal edges are rounded.	1	2	3	4	5	
Comfort						
1. The orthotic edges are smooth, rounded, contoured, and flared.	1	2	3	4	5	
2. The orthosis does not cause pain or pressure areas.	1	2	3	4	5	
Cosmetic Appearance						
1. The orthosis is free of fingerprints, dirt, and pencil/pen marks.	1	2	3	4	5	
2. The thermoplastic material is free of buckles.	1	2	3	4	5	

Mobilization Orthoses: Serial-Static, Dynamic, and Static-Progressive Orthoses

Paul Bonzani

CHAPTER OBJECTIVES

1. Identify the goals of mobilization orthoses.
2. Define the types of mobilization orthoses.
3. Apply biomechanical principles to mobilization orthoses.
4. Describe common features of mobilization orthoses.

5. Review clinical considerations for mobilization orthoses.
6. Use clinical reasoning skills through a case study presentation applying the principles of mobilization orthotic provision.

KEY TERMS

area of force application
biopsychosocial approach
creep
dynamic orthosis
end feel

finger loops
mechanical advantage
mobilization orthosis
outrigger
serial-static orthosis

stages of tissue healing
static-progressive orthosis
torque

Jay was hiking with his best friend Sam 6 weeks ago. They were having a wonderful time and were descending from the summit when they encountered a group of wet rocks. There seemed to be no way to avoid them so Jay walked over them and promptly tumbled to the ground. In doing so, he landed on his right hand, injuring the proximal interphalangeal (PIP) joint of the small finger.

Upon getting to the bottom of the trail, he wrapped and iced his finger and felt much better.

He awoke the next morning with a stiff and swollen PIP joint but was not worried about it. He tried to treat his finger on his own for 6 weeks; "after all, it is just a little finger." When the finger did not improve, he went to a local physician, who immediately referred Jay to an occupational therapist (OT) to mobilize the PIP flexion contracture that had developed.

The primary goal of every hand orthosis is to enhance the occupational performance of a client with an upper limb impairment. As a top-down approach to intervention, a client-centered, **biopsychosocial approach** to orthotic provision is recommended

as best practice for enhancing occupational performance.[28] This approach considers the thoughts, emotions, behaviors, and social situations of a client as equal concerns to the physical manifestations resulting from a hand injury or disease. This shifts the focus of care from a paternalistic, reductionist, biomedical model to an empowered and holistic approach to recovery.

To further promote the quality of functional outcomes, classifications have been developed with four categories: immobilization, mobilization, restriction, and torque transmission.[1] This chapter focuses on mobilization, including the goals, types, biomechanical principles, and fabrication and design principles specific to the application of mobilization orthoses. Mobilization orthoses are used for a myriad of reasons, including but not limited to joint flexion contractures, intra-articular fractures, limitations in composite finger flexion, tendon repairs, joint implant arthroplasties, peripheral nerve injuries, complex trauma, surgical wounds, second- and third-degree burns, spinal cord injuries, and neurological conditions. Finally, a case study integrates the use of a mobilization orthosis in a client-centered, occupation-based context.

GOALS OF MOBILIZATION ORTHOSES

Mobilization orthoses are selected to move or mobilize a primary or secondary joint.[1] In providing constant or adjustable tension, mobilization orthoses can achieve one of four

---

Acknowledgments: A special thanks to Jean Wilwerding-Peck, OTR/L, CHT, for her contributions in the previous edition and to the staff at Columbus Hand Therapy for their careful review and suggestions.

possible goals: correction of deformities, substitution for loss of muscle function, provision of controlled motion, and facilitation of wound healing.[15] Explanations for each goal are provided. As with any orthosis, it is important that the therapist collaborate with the referring physician on obtaining information about the client's injury, including the interval between the onset of injury, the date of any surgery, surgical intervention, the quality of the repaired structures, and finally, the recommended treatment protocol.

Correction of Deformities

Passive motion limitations in a joint result from multiple factors, including trauma, prolonged immobilization, decreased motion due to pain, and excessive swelling that creates dense scar formation and pericapsular adhesions.[33] A second reason for loss of motion is loss of length of a muscle-tendon unit. The loss of length, through myotatic contracture, creates passive insufficiency that causes the proximal joint position to change to accommodate the shortened muscle-tendon unit.[13,32] When active and passive motions are the same, the goal of intervention begins with decreasing the joint contracture. From there, greater active motion can be gained by incorporating a mobilization orthosis into the client's program.[12] However, if active motion is less than passive motion, or if changes in passive motion occur with changes in digit or wrist position, the focus of intervention shifts from decreasing joint stiffness by means of a mobilization orthosis to improving extrinsic and intrinsic tendon length and excursion.

Optimal results from mobilization orthotic intervention are attained after edema and pain are reduced. A mobilization orthosis applied too early after an injury can result in increased inflammation with resultant increases in scar formation and decreased motion. Furthermore, the best way to remodel tissue is to provide a tolerable force over time. Evidence shows a relationship between the length of time a stiff joint is held at end range and the resulting gain achieved with passive motion.[10,17,18] Therefore mobilization orthotic intervention appears to be more effective when orthoses are worn over longer periods of time compared with shorter periods of time using increased levels of force. This approach to mobilization of stiffness is called *low load, prolonged stress*,[10] and positive results are related to total end-range time (TERT).[17]

Application of external forces necessitates careful monitoring of the skin in case excessive levels of pressure and/or poor distribution of forces are present. A general goal for a **mobilization orthosis** is to increase passive joint motion by 10 degrees per week.[4] Should passive motion not improve following 2 weeks of orthotic intervention, a reevaluation of the orthosis, home program, and intervention adherence should be completed.[14] In this chapter, fabrication of a serial cast, composite finger flexion orthosis, and a hand-based proximal interphalangeal (PIP) extension orthosis are described as examples of the use of mobilization orthoses to resolve joint stiffness.

Substitution for Loss of Muscle Function

The principle of substitution for loss of muscle function is applicable to central nervous system (CNS), peripheral

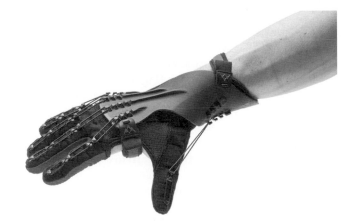

Fig. 13.1 SaeboGlove. (Courtesy of Saebo, Inc.)

nervous system (PNS), and musculoskeletal system (MS) disorders. CNS disorders often have the added variable of increased muscle tone, making dynamic orthotic intervention challenging. For clients with either CNS or PNS impairment, a mobilization orthosis can improve hand function.[15,21] This is readily seen in the application of Saebo orthoses, which are specifically designed to substitute for the loss of digital extensor function typically associated with multiple neurological conditions (Fig. 13.1).

The need to substitute for weak or absent muscle action occurs commonly in conditions such as cerebral vascular accident, traumatic brain injuries, peripheral nerve injuries, spinal cord injuries, and other debilitating neurological conditions. Therefore the goals of orthotic intervention in these cases are to substitute for loss of motor activity, to prevent overstretching of nonfunctional muscles, and to prevent joint deformity.

One common PNS injury is a high-level radial nerve palsy. The functional use of the hand is limited in part due to loss of muscle function for wrist and finger metacarpophalangeal (MCP) joint extension and radial abduction and extension of the thumb. An orthosis that provides passive assistance for loss of extrinsic muscle function greatly increases the functional use of the hand (see Chapter 14, Fig. 14.8). Similar applications for mobilization orthoses are recommended for clients with low-level median and ulnar nerve injuries where the absence or weakness of intrinsic muscles to the thumb and fingers limits hand use significantly.[21] The low-level ulnar nerve injury can present with a strong claw deformity, creating a hook grasping pattern (Fig. 13.2). This substitution of a hook grasp for cylindrical grasp markedly reduces the ability of the client to participate in valued occupations. Dynamic orthoses are one option to rebalance the hand and restore cylindrical grasp.[41] The fabrication of a dynamic anticlaw orthosis is described as one approach to substitute for the loss of muscle function, resulting in improved occupational performance.

Another example of substitution for loss of motor function involves clients with spinal cord injuries. A client with a C6 and/or C7 lesion may also benefit from mobilization orthotic provision. Because of the anatomical or biomechanical effect that wrist extension has on finger flexion, a client's active wrist extension becomes the force to generate pinch using a tenodesis orthosis (Fig. 13.3). A training tenodesis orthosis can be fabricated using thermoplastic. The therapist fabricates a static thumb post and finger flexion dorsal gutter and connects them with an inelastic line. Wrist extension becomes the mobilizing force; however, the client will require significant practice to learn to control the tensile forces effectively. Tenodesis orthoses are often used to assist with eating, dressing, and other self-care tasks requiring prehension.

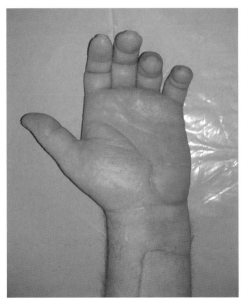

Fig. 13.2 Low ulnar nerve with claw deformity.

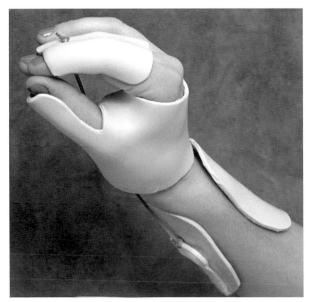

Fig. 13.3 A tenodesis orthosis uses active wrist extension to aid passive finger flexion.

Clients with neurological disorders resulting from degenerative conditions (such as Guillain-Barré, amyotrophic lateral sclerosis, and multiple sclerosis) experience muscle weakness, paralysis, and changes in sensation. Specialized mobilization orthoses may be useful in sustaining hand function, although the presence of spasticity and concerns for sensory loss might preclude candidates from this approach (see Chapter 15).

The use of mobilization orthoses may also be appropriate for clients with conditions such as surgically repaired tendon lacerations of the hand. There are three goals for clients following a tendon repair in the hand. The first goal is to increase the flow of nutrient-rich synovial fluid to enhance healing of the repaired tendon. This is typically accomplished through an exercise regimen. The second goal is to increase the tensile strength of repaired tendons. Tendons that are allowed early protected mobilization have increased tensile strength compared with immobile tendons. Third, tendon excursion reduces edema, and therefore adhesion formation is minimized between tendons and surrounding structures.[32,37] Mobilization orthoses for tendon repairs can assist in attaining these goals by positioning the wrist and fingers appropriately to remove tension from the repaired tendon and in a protected position (i.e., tendon is on slack). A passive assist from the orthosis substitutes for the loss of muscle function during the required healing period.[32]

In this chapter, fabrication of a dynamic anticlaw orthosis is described as one approach to substitute for the loss of muscle function resulting in improved occupational performance.

Provision of Controlled Motion

Occasionally mobilization orthoses are used to control motion after reconstructive surgeries, such as joint implant arthroplasties[42] and complex intra-articular fractures.[33] Mobilization orthoses assist with controlling motion and precise alignment of the repaired tissues while minimizing soft-tissue deformity. For example, a mobilization orthosis with an outrigger provides traction forces to a finger, allowing fracture alignment and maintenance of joint spaces. A second function of a mobilization orthosis is to allow guarded movements of the fingers during rehabilitative exercises.[31] In this chapter, fabrication of a dynamic traction orthosis is used as an example to describe an approach to controlled motion.

Facilitation of Wound Healing

The use of mobilization orthoses facilitates parallel collagen alignment and scar formation that occurs in later stages of wound healing.[7] It is during the proliferative stage, as leukocyte activity decreases and fibroblasts begin the process of collagen deposition, that mobilization orthoses are used to apply controlled stress for scar modeling in a lengthened position. This is accomplished through serial static, static-progressive, or dynamic orthotic application.[7] During the remodeling stage, when the cells are realigned and the joint response to stress is a firm end feel, collagen continues to remodel and reorganize based on the amount of stress applied to the wound. During this stage, tensile strength increases exponentially, and there is a complex system of collagen deposition and collagen lysis, resulting in a firm scar. Mobilization orthoses are particularly important in the proliferative and remodeling stages of healing, especially following complex trauma, surgical wounds, or second- or third-degree burns.[39]

In this chapter, fabrication of a composite flexion orthosis is used as an example of one approach to aid in scar remodeling.

TYPES OF MOBILIZATION ORTHOSES

Mobilization orthoses are divided into three types: serial-static, dynamic, and static-progressive.[40] Each type provides unique advantages for clients with limited passive motion and can be recommended for specific diagnostic groups of clients. A review of each orthosis type follows.

Serial-Static Orthotic Prescription

The purpose of a static orthosis is to immobilize a joint. However, interpretations that the same orthosis is always static in its function are misleading.[19] Tissue lengthening occurs when tissue is held under constant tension that is greater than its resting tension (see Chapter 1).[3] Therefore serial-static orthoses are a type of mobilization orthosis that positions a joint near its elastic limits to overcome a loss in passive motion.[40] A **serial-static orthosis** is well tolerated over long periods of time as the low-load, end-range positioning is applied over a large surface area. This is called the **area of force application.** Fig. 13.4 provides a schematic of the appropriate types of orthoses to use based on the three stages of healing.[13] Although a serial-static orthosis is the only orthotic type recommended across the continuum of healing, it is particularly useful for contractures with a hard end feel[39] or when joint tightness is due to muscle-tendon unit shortening. In this chapter, fabrication of a serial-static orthosis is discussed.

Dynamic Orthotic Prescription

An orthosis is dynamic when it uses a stable static base and an elastic mobilizing component.[1,19] A variety of self-adjusting dynamic components can be used as the mobilizing force, including rubber bands, springs, coils, Lycra, elastic thread, or cord. The purpose of a **dynamic orthosis** is to apply sufficient tension that does not overpower the joint and allows the client to overcome the resistance with active motion in the opposite direction of the line of pull. In this way, active motion with a dynamic orthosis assists in lubrication of joints, flexibility of ligaments, activating muscle fibers, and maximizing tendon gliding.

A dynamic orthosis is recommended primarily during the proliferative stage of healing when collagen is forming.[7] Dynamic orthoses take advantage of tissue elasticity, where tissue is stretched at a constant load, even when it reaches its elastic limit and the passive joint end range has a "soft end feel." More progress can be expected when using a dynamic orthosis for joints with less pretreatment stiffness, shorter time since surgery (<12 weeks), and in flexion rather than extension deficits.[19] For these reasons a dynamic orthotic design may be selected over a static orthosis when active motion is preferred or when the client is developing contractures early in the treatment program. Larger joints such as the elbow and wrist have useful commercial options available to the clinician. These may be reasonable options for conditions such as postfracture elbow flexion contracture,[24,43,44] distal radius fractures[6] with wrist contracture, and post stroke.[23] In this chapter, fabrication of a dynamic orthosis is used as an example for the management of PIP flexion contractures, and this is contrasted with serial-static orthoses.

A final consideration for prescribing a dynamic orthosis is its use with repaired tendons. Although this is not using the orthosis for stiffness management, it is using dynamic traction to reduce strain on repaired tendons and thereby substituting a dynamic action for active function of the repaired tendon (Fig. 13.5).

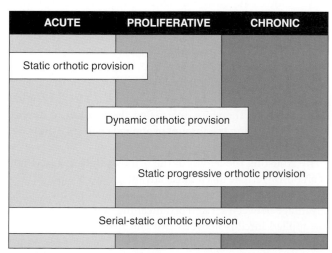

Fig. 13.4 The stage of healing helps to determine the most appropriate type of orthosis.

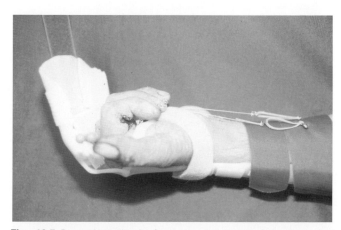

Fig. 13.5 Dynamic orthosis for use with repaired tendons that substitutes for active function of the repaired tendon.

Static-Progressive Orthotic Prescription

A static-progressive orthosis includes a static orthotic base that uses inelastic components to apply **torque** to a joint. The goal is to position the joint as close as possible to the available end range[35] and sustain it in that position for a specific period. Inelastic components may include Velcro tabs, progressive hinges, screws, tuners/turnbuckles, nylon cord, and strapping materials[24,40,43] (Fig. 13.6). Serial adjustments are performed by the therapist or client as the tissue lengthens. The stretch should be perceived by the client as comfortable.[35] A static-progressive orthosis is recommended during the proliferative, remodeling, and chronic **stages of tissue healing**, when collagen is forming, remodeling, and reorganizing. Static-progressive orthoses are considered when there is a decrease in tissue elasticity, where tissue is stretched at a constant length, whereby the force continues until the tissue accommodates and does not stress the tissue beyond its elastic limit. Generally the passive joint end range has a "hard end feel."[19,26] Indications include but are not limited to posttraumatic elbow stiffness,[11,34,46] forearm rotational stiffness,[27] wrist stiffness following distal radius and intercarpal injuries,[25,38,44] and in the management of digital stiffness.[5] In this chapter, fabrication of a static-progressive orthosis is used as an example for increasing composite finger flexion.

BIOMECHANICAL PRINCIPLES

The successful fabrication and use of an orthosis demands that the clinician has a basic mastery of the biomechanical principles that govern orthotic intervention.[14] To safely benefit the client the therapist must consider the force applied (magnitude) and the direction of the force. An important point for the novice to remember is that the purpose of a mobilization orthosis is to direct force to a target tissue.[4] Therefore the goals for mobilization orthotic intervention (e.g., correcting deformities, substituting for loss of muscle function, providing controlled motion, and aiding in wound healing) are accomplished through proper application of

force. Knowledge of complicated mechanical calculations is not required to have a basic understanding of how to fabricate a mobilization orthosis. However, several concepts for mobilization orthotic fabrication are presented that build on the biomechanical principles discussed in Chapter 3. They include anatomical considerations, mechanical advantage and torque, and application of force.

Anatomical and Biomechanical Considerations

Application of an external force to healing tissues poses several clinical questions regarding the timing, the magnitude, and the direction of the force. These questions include, what is the stage of healing,[7] what should be the magnitude of the force, in what direction should the force be applied, and what is the targeted tissue?[8] When applying force to a contracted joint, ongoing assessment of inflammation and pain is essential before and after an orthosis is applied. Connective tissue responds to excessive force by increasing pain and prolonging or restarting the inflammatory process.[16] Mild inflammation is acceptable, but edema should not increase significantly. Connective tissue responds to prolonged stress by changing or reforming in a lengthened or shortened position. This property of connective tissue is called **creep** and results from the application of prolonged force.[8] Through the application of controlled stress, the therapist introduces gentle tension to the connective tissue, thereby facilitating creep without causing tissue injury. Further, by skillfully applying tension within the tissue's elastic limits during the proliferative phase of wound healing, the therapist can improve tissue tensile strength. These results are also seen during the collagen maturation phase but to a lesser extent.[13]

Mechanical Advantage and Torque

Mastery of a few biomechanical principles is necessary for proper application of a dynamic orthosis. One such principle is **mechanical advantage.** This principle is defined as the capacity to balance and overcome resistance using force and resistance lever arms.[30] The two lever arms represent the forces applied by the orthotic base and the dynamic portion of the orthosis. As shown in Fig. 13.7, *applied force (F_a)* refers to the lever that applies force, and *force resistance (F_r)* refers to the lever that applies resistance. The magnitude of the middle opposing force, *force magnitude (F_m)*, is determined by summing the opposing forces: $F_a + F_r$.[16] To calculate mechanical advantage, a ratio of the lever arm length (l_a) for the *applied force (F_a)* is divided by the lever arm length (l_r) for the applied resistance (F_r). Therefore, increasing the amount of applied force or decreasing the amount of applied resistance improves mechanical advantage.

By adjusting the length of the orthosis base or the length of an outrigger, the mechanical advantage can be altered (Fig. 13.8).[36] The goal of the orthosis is to maintain a mechanical advantage between 2:1 and 5:1, meaning that the lever arm of the applied force is between two and five times longer than the lever arm of the applied resistance.[1] An orthosis with a greater mechanical advantage will be more comfortable and durable.[14] A mobilization orthosis for MCP flexion that is

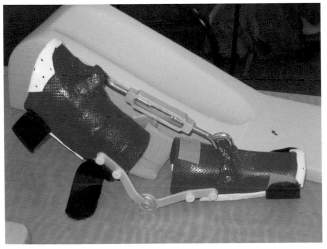

Fig. 13.6 Elbow turnbuckle orthosis.

forearm based disperses pressure more effectively, thereby providing greater mechanical advantage than a mobilization orthosis that is only hand based. The mechanical advantage is due to the longer lever arm of the applied force.

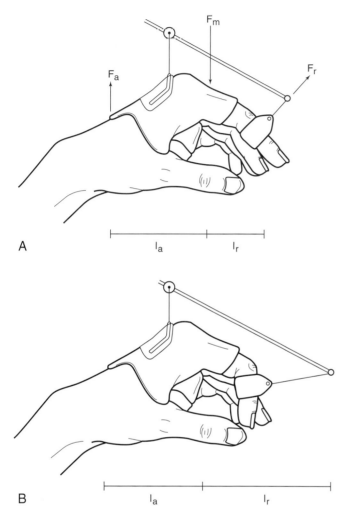

A

B

Fig. 13.7 Mechanical advantage is demonstrated in two dynamic orthoses. Orthosis A has a better mechanical advantage than orthosis B.

Torque is defined as the effect of force on the rotational movement of a joint.[15] The amount of torque is calculated by multiplying the applied force by the length of movement around a pivot point or joint axis. A proportional relationship exists between the distance from a joint axis and the amount of force required to move the joint. To achieve the same rotational result a force applied close to the axis creates a short moment arm. A short moment arm requires a higher force than a longer moment arm to achieve the same motion. Therefore, orthoses with longer moment arms require less force to attain the desired motion.

Clinically the force should be placed as far as possible from the mobilized joint without affecting other joints.[9] For example, a forearm-based dynamic wrist extension orthosis should be constructed so that its mobilizing force is on the most distal aspect of the palm, while not affecting MCP movement. An exception to placing the force as far from the mobilized joint as possible occurs with rheumatoid arthritis. If the joint is unstable, a force applied too far from the joint will result in a tilt rather than a gliding motion of the joint. This results in increasing subluxation deformities rather than increasing motion (Fig. 13.9).[20] Therefore, when fabricating an orthosis for the hand of a person with rheumatoid arthritis, the force should be applied as close to the mobilizing joint as possible.

Application of Force

Force application is a critical consideration for safe and effective application of a dynamic orthosis. When the goal of the intervention is to increase passive joint motion, the linear direction of pull must be at a 90-degree angle to the axis of the joint and perpendicular to the axis of rotation.[22] As the motion increases, adjustments are needed to the outrigger to maintain the 90-degree angle (Fig. 13.10).[15] Furthermore, extension outrigger lines should maintain neutral finger position in radial and ulnar deviation to preserve collateral ligament integrity. A variant of this alignment is when dynamic mobilization is used following MCP implant arthroplasty or extensor tendon centralization.[42] In these cases the 90-degree angle is maintained; however, the lines are set in slight radial deviation to counteract the natural pull into ulnar deviation

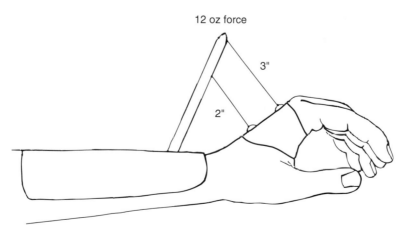

Fig. 13.8 The 2-inch moment arm produces 24-inch ounces of torque. The 3-inch moment arm produces 36-inch ounces of torque.

(Fig. 13.11). Mobilization into finger flexion is based on the number of fingers being mobilized. When one finger is mobilized, the tip of the digits should touch the palm in line with the scaphoid tuberosity[15] (Fig. 13.12). When multiple fingers are mobilized simultaneously, the convergence point shifts to the radial middle third of the forearm (Fig. 13.13).[15]

Other important considerations include the magnitude of force and the duration of the orthotic application. When excessive force is applied to the skin for a prolonged period, motion can be lost and tissue damage can occur. The amount of pressure that the skin can tolerate dictates the maximum tolerable force. A commonly accepted amount of appropriate pressure or force per unit area is 50 g/cm.[2,4,8] This force approximates the same force as the weight of a banana resting on one's palm. As the area of application where force is applied becomes larger, the force is dispersed, and the pressure per unit area becomes less. A smaller sling with less skin contact area concentrates the pressure and is less tolerable.[4] Skin grafts, immature scar tissue, and fragile skin of older clients have less tolerance for sling pressure. The client's tolerance

ultimately determines the amount of force. The client should report the sensation of a *gentle* stretch, not pain.[22] To avoid harm a new orthosis should be monitored for the first 20 to 30 minutes of wear and at every treatment session thereafter. Education is critical for a client to monitor his or her orthosis for signs of pressure areas and skin breakdown, as well as how to don and doff the orthosis properly.

The issue of duration or wearing time remains controversial, and research has not determined the precise amount of wear needed to effect changes in motion. However, Glasgow[19] indicates that the most effective duration is 6 to 8 hours per day. McClure's algorithm[26] for dynamic orthotic interventions indicated that a dynamic orthosis may need to be used for up to 2 months before change is noted in passive motion. However, Prosser[34] reported that resolving difficult contractures can take up 4 months of dynamic mobilization.

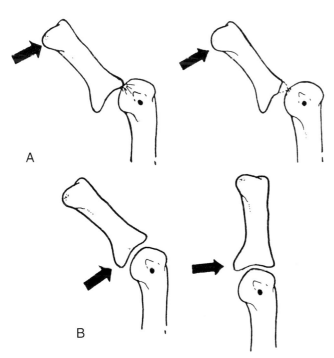

Fig. 13.9 A force applied too far from an unstable joint result in "tilt" (A) rather than glide (B).

SELF-QUIZ 13.1[a]

For the following question, circle either true (T) or false (F).
1. T F When applying a force to the body, the most important consideration is the magnitude or amount of force.
2. T F Creep occurs when soft tissue adapts through application of a prolonged force.
3. T F Dynamic mobilization orthoses are used only to resolve joint stiffness.
4. T F The focus of mobilization orthotic provision should be on increasing tension rather than increasing the amount of time that the orthosis is worn.
5. T F A general goal for mobilization orthotic provision is to increase passive motion by 10 degrees per week.
6. T F Joint end feel is an important consideration when determining whether to use static or dynamic tension.

[a]See Appendix A for the answer key.

COMMON FEATURES OF MOBILIZATION ORTHOSES

Mobilization orthoses often use outriggers to direct force appropriately to the target tissue. The **outrigger** is a projection from the orthotic base and can be custom fabricated or a commercially available kit can be used. The amount and direction of the force needed determines the type of outrigger selected. The outrigger must be securely attached to the

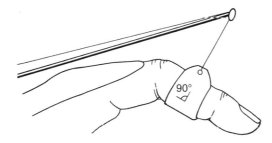
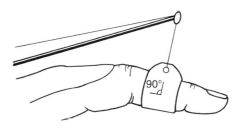

Fig.13.10 The line of tension must be maintained at 90 degrees from the long axis of the bone.

base of the orthosis to ensure that the direction of the force is correct.[11]

An outrigger is classified as either high or low profile (Fig. 13.14). Each type has advantages and disadvantages. It appears that both high- and low-profile outriggers respond in a similar manner to changes in range of movement.[15] Therefore clients are seen in the clinic frequently enough so that increases in motion can be accommodated by outrigger adjustments, which subsequently maintain the 90-degree angle of pull.[2,8,16] It should be noted that high-profile outriggers are bulky and may decrease the client's compliance with wearing the orthosis (Fig.13.15). A low-profile outrigger is more aesthetically pleasing and less cumbersome. Low-profile outriggers are more readily worn with clothing, potentially improving compliance. However, because low-profile outriggers are closer to the base surface, their force distribution is decreased and can increase discomfort during wearing times (Fig 13.16).

Outriggers are made from a variety of materials. Scraps of the thermoplastic material can be rolled to form a strong tubular outrigger that can be easily adjusted and adheres well to the orthotic base. Some thermoplastic outriggers are made from commercially available tubes that are easily formed and provide a more uniform look.

Copper wire is a commonly used material for outrigger construction (Fig. 13.17). Two thicknesses are available, a ⅛-inch wire rod used for its durability and ability to transmit high forces and a ³⁄₃₂-inch rod, which is more flexible and versatile and can be used in low-profile, low-force circumstances. These rods are easy to form with pliers or a bending jig, although, it takes practice to bend the wire into the desired shape. There are several different commercially available outrigger kits that add cost to the fabrication of the orthosis. Orthotic costs are based on the cost of the materials and the fabrication time. Although prefabricated outriggers are initially expensive, they require less fabrication and adjustment time. Further, they are generally lower in profile and have high acceptance rates by clients. Therefore, the therapist should make a cost-benefit assessment before their use.

The therapist uses various methods for applying dynamic force to a joint. **Finger loops** made from strong pliable material are usually best because of the increased conformability to the shape of the finger.[19] The therapist can supply force by using rubber bands, springs, or elastic thread. Although rubber bands are more readily available and easy to adjust, springs offer more consistent tension throughout the range. A long rubber band stretched over the maximum length of the orthosis provides more constant tension than a short rubber band.[6] Rubber bands also lose tension over time due to repeated lengthening and shortening.[14] Elastic thread is the easiest to apply and adjust, thereby saving time in the fabrication process. Its unique properties prevent wear even after 6 weeks of maximum stretch, making it useful for persistent finger contractures. A nonstretchable string or monofilament line is necessary to connect the finger loop to the source of the force (Fig. 13.18). The choice is usually based on clinical experience and preferences, as all accomplish the same goals.

Another method of applying force is through static-progressive orthoses. Rather than providing the variable tension of a serial-static or dynamic orthosis, a **static-progressive orthosis** uses nonelastic tension to provide a constant force.

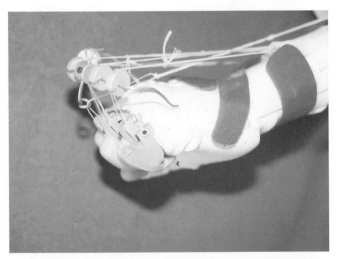
Fig. 13.11 Metacarpophalangeal (MCP) arthroplasty orthosis.

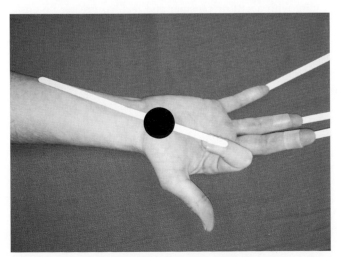
Fig. 13.12 Line of pull for one digit.

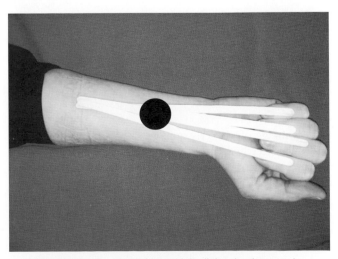
Fig. 13.13 Line of pull for multiple digits simultaneously.

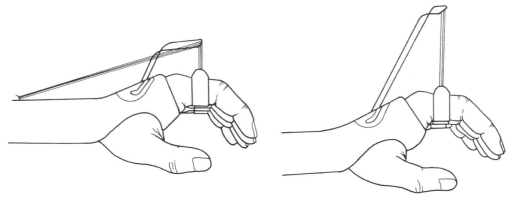

Fig. 13.14 A low-profile outrigger *(left)* versus a high-profile outrigger *(right)*.

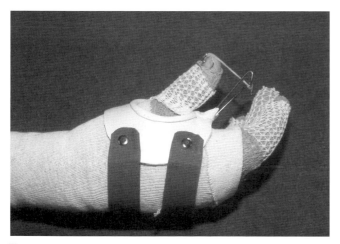

Fig. 13.15 A high-profile outrigger dynamic traction on replanted thumb.

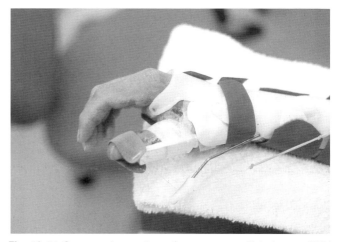

Fig. 13.17 Copper wire outrigger for extensor pollicis longus (EPL) repair.

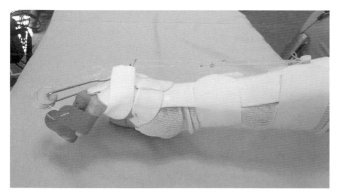

Fig. 13.16 A low-profile proximal interphalangeal (PIP) extension outrigger for Charcot-Marie Tooth polyneuropathy.

An advantage of properly applied static tension is that tissue is not stretched beyond its elastic limit.[36] In place of the rubber band or spring the therapist may use a Velcro tab, a turnbuckle, or commercially available static-progressive components to apply the force. Tension is increased by gradually moving the Velcro tab more proximally on the orthotic base or adjusting the turnbuckle (Figs. 13.19, 13.20, 13.21). The force is static rather than dynamic but is readily adjustable by the client throughout the wearing time. Because the client

has control over the amount of applied tension, the static-progressive orthosis is more tolerable to wear than a dynamic tension orthosis.[36]

Clinical decision making about the type of mobilization force used is typically based on the joint end feel. **End feel** is assessed by passively moving a joint to its maximal end range and is indicative of the potential for regaining motion. A joint with a soft or capsular end feel has greater potential for regaining movement than a joint with a firm end feel. An orthosis with static-progressive or dynamic tension is appropriate for a joint with a capsular end feel; however, a joint with a hard end feel may respond only to static-progressive mobilization.[36]

Another determinant in selecting the type of tension to be used with mobilization orthotic intervention is the stage of tissue healing. Thus different types of orthoses are indicated at different stages of healing (see Fig. 13.4) and can assist with safe mobilization of hand structures.

The common features of mobilization orthoses and their ability to apply forces through serial-static, dynamic, and/or static-progressive methods have been described. The following sections provide technical tips, materials and equipment, and precautions that assist in the fabrication of these orthoses.

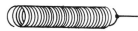

Fig. 13.18 The therapist uses inelastic nylon string to attach finger loops to the source of tension.

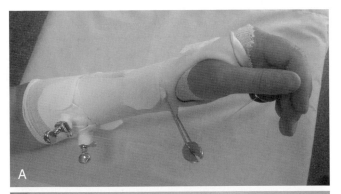

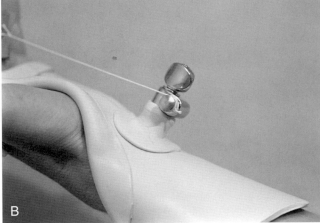

Fig. 13.19 A, Metacarpophalangeal (MCP) flexion static-progressive turnbuckle. B, A turnbuckle can be easily adjusted to provide static tension.

TECHNICAL TIPS FOR DYNAMIC ORTHOTIC FABRICATION

- To apply a thermoplastic outrigger to the orthotic base, which is commonly applied to a wrist or hand immobilization orthosis, both surfaces need to be clean and smooth.
- Most thermoplastic materials are treated or coated to minimize self-adherence when accidentally touched to itself. The coating can be scratched off; however, a bonding agent should be used to increase the self-adherence.
- After determining where the outrigger should be placed, heat both surfaces (with a heat gun, or immerse in hot water. If hot water is used, dry the surfaces thoroughly before pressing them together firmly and smoothing out the edges.
- Using cold spray speeds the hardening process. Alternatively, the orthosis and outrigger can be held under cold water at the sink to hasten hardening. Be aware that rapid cooling with cold spray or cold water can increase material shrinkage, changing the fit of the underlying base.
- To apply a wire outrigger, use a small patch of thermoplastic material. Wire conducts heat more easily than the thermoplastic material and will burn skin if touched accidentally.
- Heat the orthotic base and the thermoplastic patch, and lightly heat the end of the wire. The wire heating allows the wire outrigger to lightly "melt" into the orthotic base while the thermoplastic patch is placed over the ends of the outrigger wire and smoothed into place.

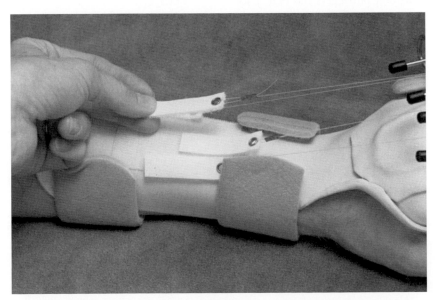

Fig. 13.20 The person may adjust Velcro tabs used for static-progressive tension.

- Be careful that the wire does not deform the base or push through the thermoplastic patch.
- If the orthotic base is curved, the wire needs to be contoured to that shape before it is attached.
- The warm thermoplastic material will adhere to postoperative bandages, dressings, or stockinette. Use a stockinette covering over such dressing to avoid adherence.
- If the client's skin is sensitive to the heat from the thermoplastic material, use a damp paper towel or apply the stockinette to the body part before applying the thermoplastic material. When the orthosis has cooled and is removed, the adhering stockinette can be cut off the arm and pulled from the orthosis.
- Check the line of pull so that a 90-degree angle is present on the finger loops when axial and lateral views are observed.
- Check all joints from various angles to ensure that joints are not pulled into hyperextension, ulnar or radial deviation, or torque/rotational forces to ensure proper direction of force application.

MATERIALS AND EQUIPMENT NEEDED TO FABRICATE A DYNAMIC ORTHOSIS

In addition to the equipment necessary to fabricate a static orthosis, a variety of items are used to fabricate a dynamic orthosis. The following is a list of materials and equipment most commonly used, although not all items are used for every orthosis.

- Thermoplastic materials of choice
- Finger loops/slings
- Nail hooks, an emery board, superglue, and superglue remover, such as acetone or fingernail polish remover
- Solvent
- Inelastic nylon string (e.g., outrigger line—monofilament/fishing line)
- An outrigger kit
- Wire rod (⅛ inch for high-force outriggers and ³⁄₃₂ inch for lighter duty outriggers)

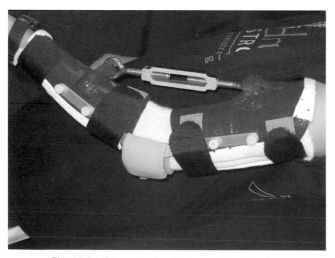

Fig. 13.21 Elbow turnbuckle to regain extension.

- Rubber bands, springs, elastic string, Velcro tabs, turnbuckles, or commercially available static-progressive components, rubber band posts
- Safety pins, paper clips, other material to make a hook or pulley, eyelets
- Pliers, wire bender, wire cutters, scissors to assist with wire bending

Fabrication of mobilization orthoses can be challenging, fun, and very rewarding, particularly when clients' function improves due to the therapists' skilled and creative intervention.

PRECAUTIONS FOR A MOBILIZATION (DYNAMIC) ORTHOSIS

Specific precautions are needed when applying mobilization orthoses. The first rule of mobilization orthoses is to do no harm. Several guidelines are provided for following this rule.[31]

- The client must be responsible enough to care for the orthosis and to follow a guided wearing schedule. A mobilization orthosis is contraindicated for clients with compromised mentation.
- Apply minimal force. The force used should provide a low-grade stretch that is tolerable over a long period of time.[13] Clinical signs of excessive force include reddened pressure areas, cyanosis of the fingertips, and complaints of pain or numbness. A client will likely not wear an orthosis that causes discomfort.
- Consider the risks posed by an ill-fitted orthosis. These include pressure areas, skin breakdown, and prolonged immobilization of noninvolved structures.
- Remember aesthetics. A client is more likely to wear an orthosis that has a finished, professional appearance. An orthosis with a low-profile outrigger is less cumbersome and may be more aesthetically pleasing than a high-profile outrigger.
- Monitor and adjust the orthosis frequently for accurate fit.
- Listen to the client. Complaints by the client require reevaluation of the orthotic fit.
- Caution must be used when applying a mobilization orthosis to an insensate hand. The lack of sensory feedback increases the risk of skin breakdown.
- Dynamic mobilization is generally not indicated for the conservative management of clients with collagen vascular diseases such as rheumatoid arthritis and systemic lupus erythematosus. They may be used in postoperative management following implant arthroplasty or soft tissue reconstruction.

CLINICAL CONSIDERATIONS FOR MOBILIZATION ORTHOSES

Four selected orthoses represent the four types of mobilization orthoses. The fabrication procedure is described for each orthosis.

Serial-Static Casting (Orthosis) for Proximal Interphalangeal Flexion Contractures

Serial casting is an excellent way to correct PIP flexion contractures through low-load, prolonged stress. Serial casts are effective when the contracture is greater than 45 to 50 degrees or less than 20 degrees (Fig. 13.22A and B). Although a cast is worn full time, it does not interfere with function of the hand as the MCP and distal interphalangeal (DIP) joints remain free. The following steps are instructions for creating a serial-static orthosis

1. Cut plaster casting tape into 1 × 8 inch lengths. A product called Specialist Extra-Fast Plaster, Green Label sets in 2 to 4 minutes.
2. Roll plaster strips into rolls.
3. Fill the small bowl with hot water. The hotter the water, the faster the plaster sets.
4. Dip one plaster roll into the hot water, squeeze the excess water from the roll, and begin wrapping the finger with no tension from the DIP crease to the MCP crease while the client extends the finger straight and the therapist applies gentle traction to the fingertip. Be careful not to pull plaster tight during rolling.
5. Smooth the plaster with wet fingers while rolling to laminate layers of plaster together (see Fig. 13.22B).

6. Be sure to smooth the edges at the MCP and DIP joints so that the client can flex these joints.
7. Do not push down on the PIP joint to straighten finger; instead, smooth, roll, and pull along the finger to straighten the finger while the plaster is setting.
8. The plaster cast should be changed every 3 to 5 days or a maximum of 7 days if necessary.[17]
9. To remove the cast, soak the hand in warm water for approximately 5 to 10 minutes, and cut it off with small cast scissors, which are commercially available.
10. Casts are durable and usually hold up during hand washing and showers, but clients may want to wrap the finger in plastic wrap (or Press'n Seal) to maintain the integrity of the cast.
11. Fig. 13.23A and B show completed casts in various stages of extension.

Dynamic Proximal Interphalangeal Extension Orthosis: Fabrication Instructions

A hand-based PIP extension orthosis corrects deformities caused by muscle-tendon tightness or joint contractures. A dynamic orthosis with an outrigger is easily adjusted as the client's motion increases. There are several commercially available outriggers that include the components necessary

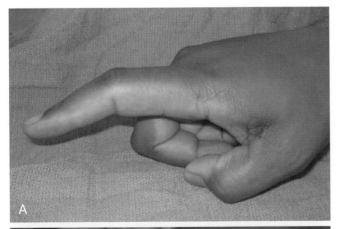

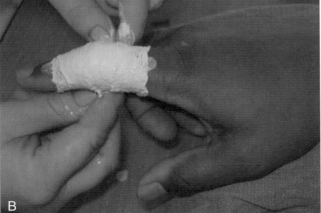

Fig. 13.22 A and B, Demonstration of a serial cast being applied to a finger with a proximal interphalangeal (PIP) flexion contracture.

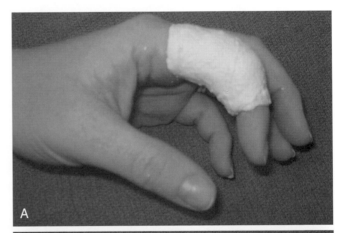

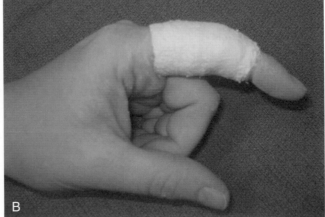

Fig. 13.23 A and B, Examples of finished plaster casts for different proximal interphalangeal (PIP) flexion contractures.

to attach, assemble, and adjust as needed, for one or multiple fingers Fig. 13.24. As previously noted, these kits do add cost but reduce fabrication and adjustment time. Outriggers can be fabricated with the common materials available in the clinic, such as thermoplastic material, outrigger wire, rubber bands, and paper clips.

To fabricate a dynamic PIP extension orthosis, begin by using the pattern for a dorsal-based hand-based orthosis as the base Fig. 13.25A and B. Immobilize the MCP joint of the involved finger(s) in 45 to 50 degrees of flexion. Conform around the thumb web space and ulnar side of the hand to provide a stable base with appropriate force distribution. Clear the distal wrist crease adequately to ensure comfortable wrist motion. Finally, roll all edges to permit motion of the uninvolved digits.

1. The distal edge should extend the length of the proximal phalanx but not impede PIP motion. The edges should be flared. Soft adhesive-backed padding extending over the edges may be added for comfort along the dorsum of the proximal phalanx.
2. If an outrigger kit or wire outrigger is not used, the outrigger can be made from a rolled rectangular piece of thermoplastic materials or tubes that are approximately twice the length of the MCP and finger.

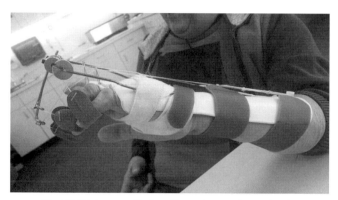

Fig. 13.24 Low-profile hand-based extension orthosis.

3. With the thermoplastic outrigger warm and pliable, find the center. Shape into a half square that is the width of the finger and cool. The outrigger's end should center on the middle phalanx. Using a hole punch, "cut" a half hole or notch to act as a pulley when the finger loop is attached. Immediately proximal to the metacarpal, the outrigger should bend to attach to the base of the orthosis. This angle should be approximately 45 to 50 degrees (Fig. 13.26A). Mark the base where the outrigger will attach with a grease marker or pencil; the marking should follow the metacarpal of the involved finger(s).
4. Remove the orthosis from the hand to attach the outrigger. To create a low-profile outrigger, the outrigger should rise approximately 1 inch above the distal end of the orthosis at the proximal phalanx. Spot heat the ends of the outrigger and the base of the orthosis with a heat gun and attach the outrigger. A bonding solvent is needed for a strong, permanent bond.
5. When cool, reapply the orthosis, and add strapping to secure the orthosis and prevent distal migration. This can be accomplished by placing a strap around the base of the thumb and through the palm.
6. A finger loop is made from soft leather or strapping material. Commercial finger loops are typically used, although loops can be fabricated from moleskin or Molefoam. The loop should be 3 to 4 inches long and as wide as the middle phalanx. Trim the width of the finger loops if they cover the DIP and PIP flexion creases. If holes are punched on both ends of the loop, they should be reinforced with grommets to prevent the line from pulling through the material. The holes are threaded with monofilament line, and this is attached to a force generator, which can be elastic or static progressive (see Fig. 13.26B).
7. If using the Velcro tab, the Velcro hook is attached to the base of the orthosis. If using the dynamic traction, use a needle-nosed pliers to fold a paper clip (see Fig. 13.26C). The paper clip is secured with a small piece of thermoplastic material.

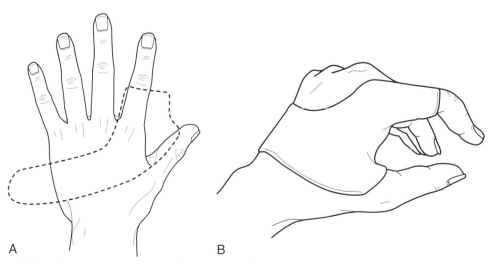

A   B

Fig. 13.25 A, Orthotic pattern for a hand-based proximal interphalangeal (PIP) extension orthosis. B, Orthosis formed on the hand.

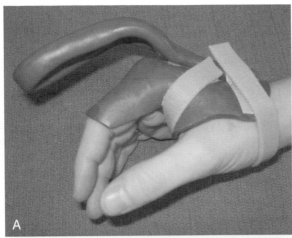

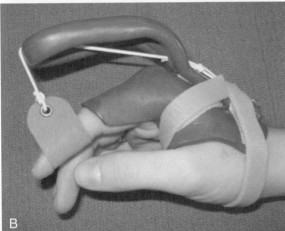

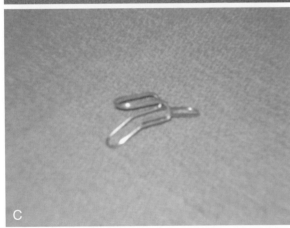

Fig. 13.26 A, The outrigger attaches to the base and extends out over the finger. B, The finished orthosis, with the finger loop extending the finger while maintaining a 90-degree angle of pull. C, Folding the center of the paper clip while curving the ends with needle-nose pliers makes a good anchor for dynamic attachments. The loop can be threaded through the hook and then adjusted by wrapping around the hook. (From Sousa, G.G.Q. & Macêdo MP [2015]. Effects of a dynamic orthosis in an individual with claw deformity, *Journal of Hand Therapy*, 28[4], 425-428.)

8. While the client wears the orthosis, a rubber band is threaded through the paper clip hook. The therapist pulls the finger loop over the top of the distal end of the outrigger into the notch and loop(s) around the finger. Make sure to have a 90-degree angle of pull from anterior and lateral perspectives.

9. The therapist experiments to determine the appropriate length of elastic thread or rubber band. After wearing the orthosis for 20 to 30 minutes, patients should not complain of their finger getting cold, going numb, or turning "blue." Patients should describe feeling gentle tension at the end range.

10. This orthosis is worn 2 hours three to four times per day. Total wearing time may take up to 4 months.[26]

Comparison of the serial-static and dynamic mobilization approaches to PIP flexion contracture management suggest that serial-static casts have significant advantages (see Chapter 19). Serial-static casting is more cost-effective than dynamic orthotic interventions. Further, it is simple to apply, has no moving parts, and is readily removed with hot water soaks. Finally, it is effective in all stages of contracture formation. Problems with casting include an inability to measure the corrective force accurately and patient acceptance of a device that cannot be removed. A dynamic orthosis permits precise measurement of the magnitude and direction of force application; however, these orthoses are expensive, have multiple moving parts, and require the client's compliance with a complicated wearing schedule. Further, they have limited value when joint contractures are firm or chronic in nature.

Fabrication for Dynamic Anti–Claw-Hand Orthosis: Substitution for Weak or Absent Muscles

One of the major problems that occurs when a client sustains a low-level peripheral nerve injury is muscle imbalance. Muscle imbalances create characteristic deformities in the hand due to the loss of intrinsic muscle function while extrinsic function remains intact. This creates abnormal force generation by the intact extrinsic muscles. The result is that movement occurs in line with the intact muscle. If the agonist of that movement is absent, synergistic muscles will act as prime movers. Further, if there is loss of an antagonist, the power of the agonist is unbalanced. The classic presentation of this issue is the muscle imbalance in the low, or wrist level, ulnar nerve injury. (Refer to Chapter 14 for further discussion of these nerve injuries and other orthotic options.)

The claw deformity in the low ulnar nerve injury is a result of the imbalance that occurs when the volar and dorsal interosseous and the third and fourth lumbrical are paralyzed. These muscles flex the MCP joints and extend the PIP and DIP joints. When they are lost and the flexor digitorum profundus and the extensor digitorum remain intact, the small and ring fingers are imbalanced. The functional deficit is that MCP joint flexion occurs only after the PIP and DIP are completely flexed. This causes the fingertips to be rolled into the palm from a hook position. The functional result is that items are pushed out of the palm and the client loses the ability to use cylindrical or spherical grasping patterns.[45] A static lumbrical blocking orthosis can be used to address this issue (Fig. 13.27). However, some of these orthoses are uncomfortable, are difficult to don, and limit the grasping surface by restricting MCP extension, and they create areas of high force concentration on the dorsum of the proximal phalanx.[46] An alternative is the dynamic lumbrical block orthosis as described by Sousa and Pereira de Macêdo.[41] This orthosis has been shown to rebalance the third and fourth digits without causing difficulty in donning the orthosis and skin issues. Orthosis construction instructions follow.

1. Fabricate a semilunar volar base from any thermoplastic material. The orthotic base is the forearm, and it extends to the level of the proximal wrist crease. The orthotic base is secured with a Velcro strap.
2. Attach a hook to secure the rubber bands just proximal to the scaphoid tubercle. Options here include a band post, a paper clip, or a secured thermoplastic hook.
3. Finger slings/cuffs are attached to rubber bands. The small and ring fingers are always secured with the middle finger being optional.
4. A sling is also extended to the MCP joint of the thumb to act as an adduction assist during pinch[41] (Fig. 13.28A–D).

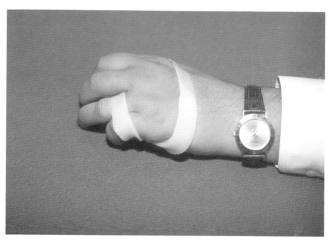

Fig. 13.27 Static lumbrical block orthosis.

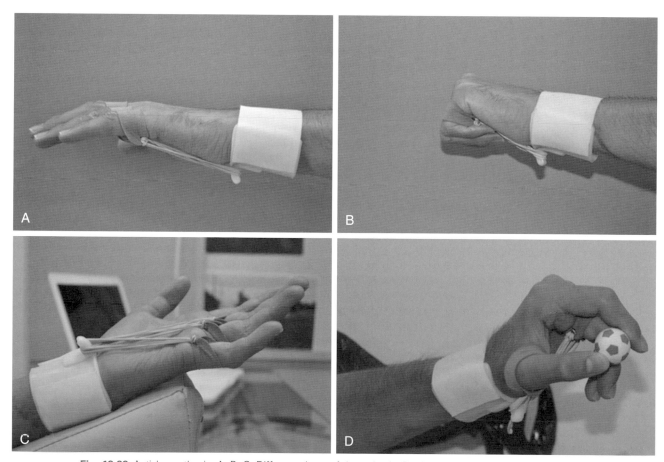

Fig. 13.28 Anticlaw orthosis. A, B, C, Different views of the orthosis. D, Using the orthosis functionally. (From Sousa, G.G.Q. & Macêdo MP [2015]. Effects of a dynamic orthosis in an individual with claw deformity, *Journal of Hand Therapy*, 28[4], 425-428.)

This simple but biomechanically sound design is inexpensive, well tolerated by the client, and can create improved pinch and grasp in the selected client.

Traction Orthosis for Complex Proximal Interphalangeal Fracture: Application of Controlled Motion

The traction orthosis has a long history as a primary intervention for the management of complex intra-articular fracture of the PIP joint.[47,48] Many designs have been advocated, and many of these have had a high profile with poor patient compliance and patient acceptance.[32] Further, clients did not appreciate the need for a complex orthotic regimen for what was perceived to be a relatively minor injury.[32] Technological advancements led to the creation of lower-profile devices, which has improved the application and acceptance by some clients.[32] Further, these devices often are used in lieu of surgical intervention with similar outcomes in motion and functional use.[32,33] This intervention requires careful coordination with the hand surgeon to determine both the clinical fracture need and the client's ability to accept this intervention and comply with a complex rehabilitation regimen. However, the results can be rewarding when the intervention is planned and executed effectively. Fabrication directions and rehabilitation program are as follows:

1. A static base is fabricated. This forearm-based dorsal orthosis positions the involved MCP joint in 70 degrees of flexion. The MCP block extends to the level of the PIP joint. The block is an open cylinder, which provides adequate support while allowing access to the involved digit (Figs. 13.29 A and 13.29B).
2. The physician drills a K-wire through the head of the middle phalanx (Fig. 13.30).
3. The copper wire or spring wire outrigger is contoured to the digit. This is more difficult with the middle and long finger as an over-top approach must be used (Fig. 13.31). The lateral outrigger can be used for the small finger. It is easier to fabricate, but it is more cumbersome (see Fig 13.29A).
4. The end of the outrigger is curled to form a circle, and it is riveted to the base at the level of the PIP joint. Care is taken to ensure that this aligns with the PIP axis of rotation.
5. The traction orthosis is then placed, and volar support is provided to the digit as needed (Fig. 13.32).
6. Rubber band traction is applied by hooking the rubber bands to the K-wire and adhering them to the distal component of the outrigger (see Fig. 13.29).
7. Tape the end of the outrigger to prevent the rubber bands from sliding laterally.
8. Add traction force through the rubber bands. This force should measure 200 g of force using a strain gauge. Occasionally, greater traction forces are necessary; however, no more than 300 g should be applied to prevent soft-tissue complications.
9. The client will move the distracted joint through a passive motion, 10 to 15 repetitions, five times per day for 6 weeks.

10. The client is seen frequently to ensure proper outrigger placement and orthotic fit and to carefully monitor the skin for potential breakdown.

Completed traction splinting programs typically have good results as seen in Fig. 13.33A–C.

Static-Progressive Approach for Composite Finger Flexion

It is common for the fingers to become stiff after trauma to the hand or wrist. Stiffness may be due to joint pain or swelling, which prevents an ability to achieve full finger flexion. Although clients may be actively participating in a therapy program that focuses on edema control, range of motion, and tendon gliding to achieve full composite finger flexion, an orthosis that aids in wound healing or tissue remodeling

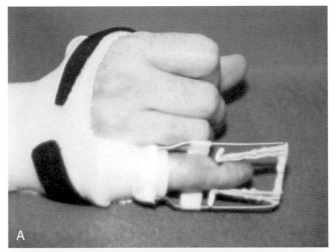
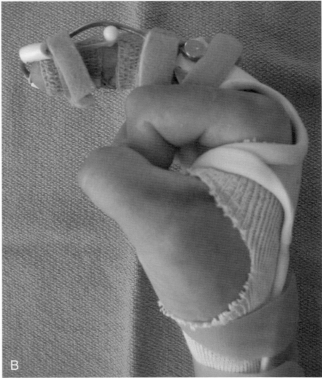

Fig. 13.29 A, Small finger traction orthosis. B, Middle finger traction orthosis.

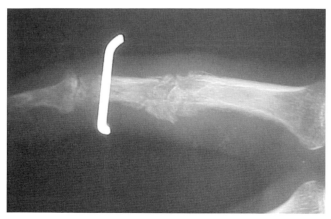

Fig. 13.30 Proximal interphalangeal (PIP) fracture with K-wire placement.

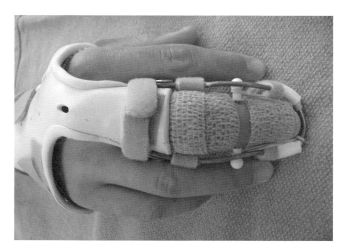

Fig. 13.31 Traction outrigger conforming to digit.

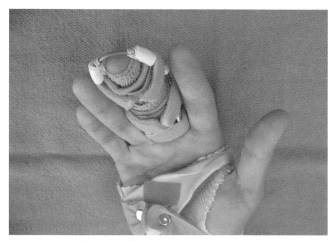

Fig. 13.32 Traction with volar support.

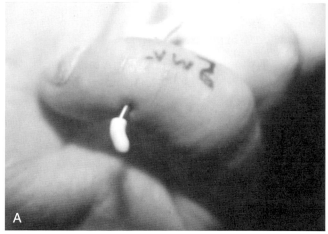

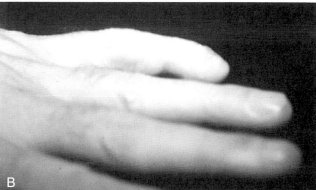

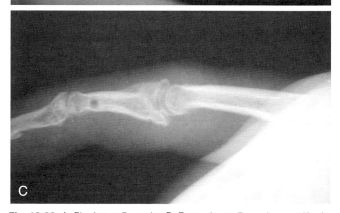

Fig. 13.33 A, Flexion at 5 weeks. B, Extension at 5 weeks post K-wire removal. C, Posttreatment x-ray image (compare to Fig. 13.30).

through low-load prolonged stress to the joints can maximize return to function.

For the hand to function optimally, the PIP joint needs to extend and flex to the palm. Different types of grasps are important for occupational activities, such as the ability to slip the hand into a pocket, to put on a glove, to grasp coins, or to hold a wrench. The PIP joint can lose extension from the following:

- Crush injury
- Burn or fracture around the PIP joint
- Flexor tendon injury
- Ligament injury
- Excessive swelling of the hand following injury elsewhere
- Immobilization and disuse

There are several different ways to mobilize PIP joints to gain passive flexion with either custom-fabricated or prefabricated orthoses. The following steps are instructions for creating a custom-fabricated static-progressive orthosis for the hand. Static-progressive tension allows the person to maintain the tissue at a maximum tolerable stretch.[35]

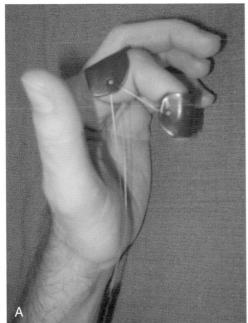

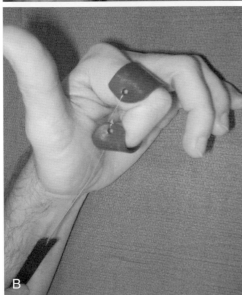

Fig. 13.34 The fishing line should start from the distal cuff through both holes on the proximal cuff before ending on the other side of the distal cuff, leaving enough fishing line to loop through the Velcro tab and reach midway down the forearm.

1. Fabricate a volar-based wrist immobilization orthosis with the wrist in 30 to 45 degrees extension to maximize finger flexion (refer to Chapter 7 for instructions).
2. To fabricate the finger cuff, use a thinner (1/16 inch) thermoplastic material. Cut two pieces 1/2 inch to 3/4 inch wide and 1 1/2 to 2 inches long. Mold one cuff halfway around the dorsum of the proximal phalanx and the other cuff over the distal phalanx.
3. Punch small holes using a hole punch on either side of the two cuffs. Cut a piece of monofilament line approximately 10 to 12 inches long. Tie the start of the monofilament line

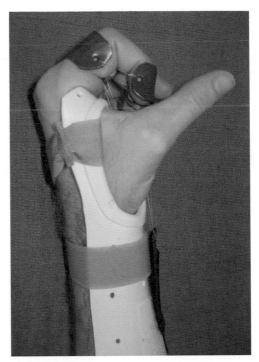

Fig. 13.35 When completed, the fingers can be pulled into a composite fist position, adjusting the Velcro loop as tolerated every 5 minutes with a goal of wearing the orthosis 30 minutes at a time.

on one side of the distal cuff. Thread it through one side of the proximal cuff, and then through the other side of the proximal cuff. Tie off on the other side of the distal cuff.
4. Find the center of the monofilament line, and slip it through the small hole at one end of a Velcro loop 1/2 × 2 inches to create a completed flexion cuff.
5. Repeat this for additional fingers as needed.
6. This cuff is applied to the stiff finger(s) when pulled toward the forearm. The tension should cause the finger to flex first at the DIP, then at the PIP, and finally at the MCP into the palm (composite fist).
7. Replace the volar orthosis, and apply straps across the dorsum of the hand, at the wrist and forearm.
8. Fit the individual finger flexion cuffs, and gently pull them toward the forearm. The fishing line should start from the distal cuff through both holes on the proximal cuff before ending on the other side of the distal cuff, leaving enough fishing line to loop through the Velcro tab and reach midway down the forearm (Fig. 13.34).
9. Determine where to place the Velcro hook on the volar aspect of the wrist orthosis
10. The cuffs should be pulled tight enough to provide gentle tension to the fingers (Fig. 13.35. After a 5-minute iterval, attempt to tighten the tension as tolerated. Repeat this every 5 minutes with the goal of wearing the orthosis 30 minutes five to six times per day.

There are other options for finger cuffs, including leather, commercially available finger loops, or strapping material.

REVIEW QUESTIONS

1. What are four possible goals of mobilization orthotic provision?
2. What criteria determine the use of static-progressive or dynamic tension?
3. What is the angle of pull between the long axis of the bone and the outrigger line that must be maintained?
4. What are the complications associated with a mobilization orthosis that uses excessive force?
5. What is the acceptable force per unit area for sling pressure?
6. What information should the therapist gather before considering fabrication of a mobilization orthosis?
7. What is the difference between a high- and a low-profile outrigger? What are the advantages and disadvantages of each?
8. What are three methods of force application?
9. What are the steps for attaching a wire outrigger to the base of an orthosis?
10. What are three precautions when using a mobilization orthosis?

REFERENCES

1. Austin G, Slamet M, Cameron D, et al.: A comparison of high-profile and low-profile mobilization splint designs, *J Hand Ther* 17(3):336–343, 2004.
2. Bailey J, Cannon N, Colditz J, et al.: *Splint classification system*, Chicago, 1992, American Society of Hand Therapists.
3. Bell-Krotoski JA, Figarola JH: Biomechanics of soft-tissue growth and remodeling with plaster casting, *J Hand Ther* 8(2):131–137, 1995.
4. Bell-Krotoski JA, Stanton DB: The forces of dynamic splinting. Ten questions before applying a dynamic splint to the hand. (Archived chapter). In Skirven T, Osterman A, Fedorczyk J, Amadio P, editors: *Rehabilitation of the hand and upper extremity*, Philadelphia, 2011, Elsevier.
5. Benaglia PG, Sartorio F, Franchignoni F: A new thermoplastic splint for proximal interphalangeal joint flexion contractures, *J Sports Med Phys Fitness* 39(3):249–252, 1999.
6. Berner SH, Willis FB: Dynamic splinting in wrist extension following distal radius fractures, *J Orthop Surg Res* 5:53, 2010.
7. Bernstein RA: Tissue healing. In Jacobs MA, Austin NM, editors: *Orthotic intervention for the hand and upper extremity: splinting principles and process*, Philadelphia, 2014, Lippincott.
8. Brand PW: Hollister AM: Terminology, how joints move, mechanical resistance, and external stress: effect at the surface. In Brand PW, Hollister AM, editors: *Clinical mechanics of the hand*, St. Louis, 1993, Mosby.
9. Brand PW, Hollister A: External stress: effects at the surface. In Brand PW, Hollister AM, editors: *Clinical mechanics of the hand*, St. Louis, 1993, Mosby.
10. Brown C: Experimental joint contracture correction with low-torque long-duration repeated stretching, *J Hand Ther* 1(22):93, 2009.
11. Chinchalkar SJ, Pearce J, Athwal GS: Static progressive versus three-point elbow extension splinting: a mathematical analysis, *J Hand Ther* 22(1):22–37, 2009.
12. Coldiz JC: Low profile dynamic splinting of the injured hand, *Am J Occup Ther* 37(3):182–188, 1983.
13. Colditz JC: Therapist's management of the stiff hand. In Skirven T, Osterman A, Fedorczyk J, Amadio P, editors: *Rehabilitation of the hand and upper extremity*, Philadelphia, Elsevier, pp. 905–909.
14. Fess EE: Splints: mechanics versus convention, *J Hand Ther* 8(2):124–130, 1995.
15. Fess EE, Gettle K, Philips C, et al.: *Hand and upper extremity splinting: principles and methods*, ed 3, St. Louis, 2005, Mosby.
16. Fess EE, McCollum M: The influence of splinting on healing tissues, *J Hand Ther* 11:125–130, 1998.
17. Flowers K, LaStayo P: Effect of total end range time on improving passive range of motion, *J Hand Ther* 7:150–157, 1994.
18. Glasgow C, Fleming J, Tooth LR, Hockey RL: The long-term relationship between duration of treatment and contracture resolution using dynamic orthotic devices for the stiff proximal interphalangeal joint: a prospective cohort study, *J Hand Ther* 25(1):38–47, 2009.
19. Glasgow C, Tooth L, Fleming J, et al.: Dynamic splinting for the stiff hand after trauma: predictors of contracture resolution, *J Hand Ther* 24:195–206, 2011.
20. Hollister A, Giurintano D: How joints move: clinical mechanics of the hand, St. Louis, 1993, Mosby.
21. Jacobs ML: Mechanical principles. In Jacobs MA, Austin NM, editors: *Orthotic intervention for the hand and upper extremity: splinting principles and process*, Philadelphia, 2014, Lippincott.
22. Jacobs ML: Peripheral nerve injuries. In Jacobs MA, Austin NM, editors: *Orthotic intervention for the hand and upper extremity: splinting principles and process*, Philadelphia, 2014, Lippincott.
23. Lai JM, Francisco GE, Willis B: Dynamic splinting after treatment with botulinum toxin type-A: a randomized controlled pilot study, *Advanced Ther* 26(2):241–248, 2009.
24. Lindeenhovius ALC, Doornberg NJ, Brouwer KM, et al.: A prospective randomized controlled trial of dynamic versus static-progressive splinting for posttraumatic elbow stiffness, *J Bone Joint Surg* 94:694–700, 2012.
25. Lucado AM, Li Z: Static progressive splinting to improve wrist stiffness after distal radius fracture: a prospective case series study, *Physiother Theory Pract* 25(4):297–309, 2009.
26. McClure PW, Blackburn LG, Dusold C: The use of splints in the treatment of joint stiffness: biological rationale and an algorithm for making clinical decisions, *Physical Ther* 74(12):1101–1107, 1994.
27. McGrath MS, Ulrich SF, Bonutti PM, et al.: Static progressive splinting for restoration of rotational motion of the forearm, *J Hand Ther* 22(1):3–8, 2009.
28. McKee PR, Rivard A: A biopsychosocial approach to orthotic intervention, *J Hand Ther* 24:155–163, 2011.
29. Means KR, Saunders RJ, Graham TJ: Pathophysiology and surgical management of the stiff hand. In Skirven T, Osterman A, Fedorczyk J, Amadio P, editors: *Rehabilitation of the hand and upper extremity*, Philadelphia, 2011, Elsevier, pp 885–886.
30. Morgan J, Gordon D, Klug M, et al.: Dynamic digital traction for unstable comminuted intra-articular fracture-dislocations of the proximal interphalangeal joint, *J Hand Surg* 20(4):565–573, 1995.

31. O'Brien L, Presnell S: Patient experience of distraction splinting for complex finger fracture dislocations, *J Hand Ther* 23(3):249–260, 2010.

32. O'Brien LJ, Simm AT, Loh IWH, et al.: Swing traction versus no-traction for complex intra-articular proximal inter-phalangeal fractures, *J Hand Ther* 27(4):309–316, 2014.

33. Packham TL, Ball PD, MacDermid JC, et al.: A scoping review of applications and outcomes of traction orthoses and constructs for the management of intra-articular fractures and fracture dislocations in the hand, *J Hand Ther* 29:246–268, 2016.

34. Prosser R: Splinting in the management of proximal interphalangeal joint flexion contracture, *J Hand Ther* 9(4):378–386, 1996.

35. Recor CJ, Johnson CW: Hand therapy. In Trumble T, Rayan GM, Budoff JE, editors: *Principles of hand surgery and therapy*, ed 2, Philadelphia, 2010, Saunders.

36. Sandaval BK, Kuhlman-Wood K, Recor C, et al.: Flexor tendon repair, rehabilitation, and reconstruction, *Plast Reconstr Surg* 132:1493–1508, 2013.

37. Schultz-Johnson K: Static progressive splinting, *J Hand Ther* 15(2):163–178, 2002.

38. Seu M, Pasqualetto M: Hand therapy for dysfunction of the intrinsic muscles, *Hand Clin* 28(1):87–100, 2012.

39. Shanesy RR, Miller CP: Dynamic versus static splints: a prospective case for sustained stress, *J Burn Care Rehabil* 16 (3 Pt 1):284–287, 1995.

40. Smith LK, Weiss EL, Lehmkuhl DL: *Brunnstrom's clinical kinesiology*, ed 5, Philadelphia, 1996, FA Davis.

41. Sousa GGQ, Pereira de Macêdo M: Effects of a dynamic orthosis in an individual with claw deformity, *J Hand Ther* 28:425–428, 2015.

42. Stern P, Roman R, Kiefhaber T, et al.: Pilon fractures of the proximal interphalangeal joint, *J Hand Surg* 16(5): 844–850, 1991.

43. Sueoka SS, Detemple K: Static-progressive splinting in under 25 minutes and 25 dollars, *J Hand Ther* 24(3):280–286, 2011.

44. Thomsen NO, Boeckstyns MEH, Leth-Epsensen P: Value of dynamic splinting after replacement of the metacarpophalangeal joint in patients with rheumatoid arthritis, *Scand J Plast Reconstr Surg Hand Surg* 37:113–116, 2003.

45. Trumble TE, Rayan GM, Budoff JE, et al.: *Principles of hand surgery and therapy*, ed 2, Philadelphia, 2010, Saunders.

46. Veltman E, Doornberg J, Evgendaal D, Static progressive versus dynamic splinting for posttraumatic elbow stiffness: a systematic review of 232 patients, *Arch Orthop Trauma Surg* 135(5):613–617, 2015.

47. Woo A, Bakri K, Moran SL: Management of ulnar nerve injuries, *J Hand Surg* 40(1):173–181, 2015.

48. Wu FY, Tang JB: Tendon healing, edema and resistance to flexor tendon gliding, *Hand Clin* 29(2):167–178, 2013.

APPENDIX 13.1 CASE STUDY

Case Study 13.1[a]

Joseph is a 27-year-old right-handed man who was out late with his friends after work. When he awakened the next morning, he was surprised to find that he was unable to move his right wrist and fingers. He became alarmed and went to the local emergency department and was diagnosed with a radial nerve palsy. He was given an elastic wrist splint and was told to see an orthopedic physician if it did not resolve in a few weeks. After 4 weeks, things were no better, and he saw a local hand surgeon. The surgeon was not considering therapy until Joseph began to talk about his inability to use his right (dominant) hand for work activities (he is a video-terminal worker) and simple daily living tasks such as preparing meals. He also reported difficulty putting his hand in his pocket and in donning gloves, which is an important skill for Joseph in his environment. He is now 6 weeks' post injury, and your referral includes the option for orthotic fabrication as indicated in addition to functional retraining to attain activities of daily living (ADLs) independence with a full return to work goal.

1. What clinical evaluation is required before fabrication of the orthosis? Circle yes (Y) or no (N) to the following options:
   a. Y N Evaluation of active and passive motion of the wrist and fingers
   b. Y N Manual muscle testing of the elbow, wrist, and hand
   c. Y N Evaluation of sensibility
   d. Y N ADLs evaluation
   e. Y N Occupational performance measure

2. Which of the following is the appropriate orthosis for this client?
   a. Hand-based digital extension
   b. Forearm-based low-profile wrist and digital extension
   c. Anticlaw
   d. Static-progressive digital flexion

3. What is the primary purpose of this orthosis?
   a. To increase active extension of the fingers
   b. To protect damaged nerves in the hand
   c. To provide controlled stress or motion to the involved digits
   d. To substitute for weak or absent muscles

4. What is the most desirable source of finger traction for this orthosis?
   a. Rubber band traction
   b. Spring wire
   c. Turnbuckle
   d. Static Velcro tabs

5. How often should Joseph wear the orthosis?
   a. 60 minutes, four times a day
   b. 30 minutes, two times a day
   c. As needed for occupational performance improvement
   d. 4 hours at a time

[a] See Appendix A for the answer key.

APPENDIX 13.2 FORM AND GRADING SHEET

Form 13.1 Static-Progressive Finger Flexion Orthosis

After the person wears the orthosis for 30 minutes, answer the following questions.
(Mark NA for nonapplicable situations.)

Evaluation Areas				Comments
Design				
1. The orthotic trough is the proper length and width.	Yes	No	NA	
2. The orthotic trough supports, does not push on the arches.	Yes	No	NA	
3. The orthotic trough allows full motion of the finger MCP and thumb joints.	Yes	No	NA	
4. Adequate Velcro hooks are used on the orthotic trough to secure the number of monofilament straps.	Yes	No	NA	
Function				
1. The fit of the orthotic trough and straps prevents migration.	Yes	No	NA	
2. The monofilament allows full composite flexion when pulled.	Yes	No	NA	
3. Each finger cuff maintains its position on the digit with finger flexion and extension.	Yes	No	NA	
Straps				
1. All straps are rounded at the ends.	Yes	No	NA	
2. The Velcro hooks on the orthotic trough are covered to prevent snagging clothes.	Yes	No	NA	
3. The correct width of straps is used to increase the surface area, to diffuse pressure, and to prevent pockets of swelling.	Yes	No	NA	
Comfort				
1. The proximal, distal, and thenar edges of the orthotic trough are smooth and slightly flared.	Yes	No	NA	
2. The orthotic trough is free of impingement and pressure areas.	Yes	No	NA	
3. The edges of the finger cuffs are smooth.	Yes	No	NA	
4. The width of the finger cuffs disperses the application of forces.	Yes	No	NA	
5. The direction of pull for each finger cuff is accurate.	Yes	No	NA	
6. The tension from the finger cuffs can be adjusted to provide appropriate levels of force.	Yes	No	NA	
Cosmetic Appearance				
1. The orthotic trough is free of fingerprints, dirt, pencil or pen marks.	Yes	No	NA	
2. The orthotic trough is smooth and free of buckles or wrinkles.	Yes	No	NA	
Therapeutic Regimen				
1. The client is able to demonstrate correct application of the orthotic trough and to adjust finger cuffs as instructed.	Yes	No	NA	
2. The client is instructed in the orthotic wearing schedule.	Yes	No	NA	
3. The client is aware of orthotic precautions.	Yes	No	NA	
4. The client is knowledgeable of how to clean and care for the orthosis.	Yes	No	NA	

Discuss possible adjustments or changes you would make based on the self-evaluation.
What would you do differently next time?

_____

_____

_____

Discuss possible areas to improve with clinical safety when fabricating the orthosis.

_____

_____

_____

Grading Sheet 13.1 Static-Progressive Finger Flexion Orthosis

	Name: _____			
	Date: _____			
Wrist position at rest:				
Grade: _____ 1 = Beyond improvement, not acceptable 2 = Requires maximal improvement 3 = Requires moderate improvement 4 = Requires minimal improvement 5 = Requires no improvement				

Evaluation Areas						Comments
Design						
1. The orthotic trough is the proper length and width.	1	2	3	4	5	
2. The orthotic trough supports, does not push on the arches.	1	2	3	4	5	
3. The orthotic trough allows full motion of the finger MCP and thumb joints.	1	2	3	4	5	
4. Adequate Velcro hooks are used on the orthotic trough to secure the number of monofilament straps.	1	2	3	4	5	
Function						
1. The fit of the orthotic trough and straps prevents migration.	1	2	3	4	5	
2. The monofilament allows full composite flexion when pulled.	1	2	3	4	5	
3. Each finger cuff maintains its position on the digit with finger flexion and extension.	1	2	3	4	5	
Straps						
1. All straps are rounded at the ends.	1	2	3	4	5	
2. The Velcro hooks on the orthotic trough are covered to prevent snagging clothes.	1	2	3	4	5	
3. The correct width of straps is used to increase the surface area, to diffuse pressure, and to prevent pockets of swelling.	1	2	3	4	5	
Comfort						
1. The proximal, distal, and thenar edges of the orthotic trough are smooth and slightly flared.	1	2	3	4	5	
2. The orthotic trough is free of impingement and pressure areas.	1	2	3	4	5	
3. The edges of the finger cuffs are smooth.	1	2	3	4	5	
4. The width of the finger cuffs disperses the application of forces.	1	2	3	4	5	
5. The direction of pull for each finger cuff is accurate.	1	2	3	4	5	
6. The tension from the finger cuffs can be adjusted to provide appropriate levels of force.	1	2	3	4	5	
Cosmetic Appearance						
1. The orthotic trough is free of fingerprints, dirt, pencil or pen marks.	1	2	3	4	5	
2. The orthotic trough is smooth and free of buckles or wrinkles.	1	2	3	4	5	

Comments:

Orthotic Intervention for Nerve Injuries

Helene L. Lohman
Brenda M. Coppard

CHAPTER OBJECTIVES

1. Identify the components of a peripheral nerve.
2. Describe a peripheral nerve's response to injury and repair.
3. Describe the operative procedures used for nerve repair.
4. Explain the three purposes for orthotic intervention of nerve palsies.
5. Describe nerve injury classification.
6. Identify the locations for low and high peripheral nerve lesions.
7. Explain common causes of radial, ulnar, and median nerve lesions.
8. Review the sensory and motor distributions of the radial, median, and ulnar nerves.
9. Explain the functional effects of radial, ulnar, and median nerve lesions.
10. Identify the orthotic intervention approaches and rationale for radial, ulnar, and median nerve injuries.
11. Use clinical judgment to evaluate a problematic orthosis for a nerve lesion.
12. Use clinical judgment to evaluate a fabricated hand-based ulnar nerve orthosis.
13. Apply documentation skills to a case study.
14. Summarize the importance of evidence-based practice with provision of orthoses for nerve conditions.

KEY TERMS

axonotmesis
cubital tunnel syndrome
cumulative trauma disorder (CTD)
median nerve
neurapraxia

neurotmesis
posterior interosseous nerve
   syndrome
pronator tunnel syndrome
radial nerve

radial tunnel syndrome
ulnar nerve
wallerian degeneration
Wartenberg neuropathy

Your friend, Madison, is an avid bicyclist. She bikes almost every day to work and weekly with members of several bicycling clubs. After completing a particularly rigorous event biking across the state, Madison developed pain and a "pins and needles" feeling in the ring and little fingers of both hands. Over the next several months, she began complaining of feeling clumsy picking up objects and spreading her fingers apart to grasp items. Madison approached you about her hand problems stating, "I believe that I might have carpal tunnel syndrome!" From listening to her symptoms and how they developed, you suspect compression of the ulnar nerve at the wrist and suggest that she go to an orthopedic physician for a diagnosis. After her appointment she shares with you that she did have an ulnar nerve compression at the wrist called Guyon canal syndrome, and she received an order for therapy and an orthosis.

Orthotic interventions for nerve lesions require therapists to possess a thorough knowledge of static (immobilization) and dynamic (mobilization) principles as well as sound critical-thinking skills. Comprehension of kinesiology, physiology, and anatomy is paramount to understanding the motor, sensory, and vasomotor implications of a nerve injury. Competence in manual muscle-testing skills is also necessary to evaluate affected muscles as nerves recover from injuries.[18] This chapter addresses peripheral nerve anatomy; nerve injury classifications; nerve repair; and types, effects, and interventions for radial, ulnar, and median nerve injuries. The focus is orthotic intervention with these peripheral nerves. Beyond the foundational information provided, therapists should always remember the huge impact that a nerve

---

NOTE: This chapter includes content from previous contributions from Mackenzie Raber.

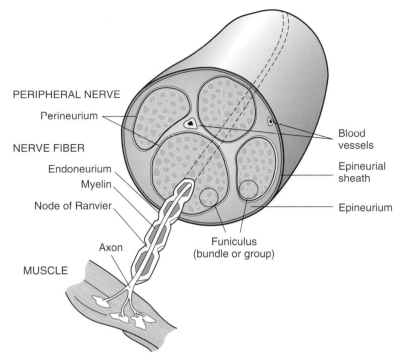

PERIPHERAL NERVE
Perineurium

NERVE FIBER
Endoneurium
Myelin
Node of Ranvier

Axon

MUSCLE

Blood vessels

Epineurial sheath

Epineurium

Funiculus (bundle or group)

Fig. 14.1 Components of a peripheral nerve: epineurium, perineurium, endoneurium, funiculi, axons, and blood vessels.

condition has on function and ultimately the quality of a person's life.[54] As realistically as possible, therapists must address occupation with intervention. Finally, although this chapter focuses on nerve conditions, therapists must be aware that nerve conditions do not always appear in isolation and can be quite complicated as traumatic nerve injuries are often accompanied by bone, tendon, ligament, vessel, and soft tissue conditions.

The following sections provide foundational education about nerve anatomy and classification. An understanding of this information is essential for effective intervention.

PERIPHERAL NERVE ANATOMY

A peripheral nerve consists of the epineurium, perineurium, endoneurium, funiculi, axons, and blood vessels (Fig. 14.1).[41] The epineurium is made of loose collagenous connective tissue. There are external and internal types of epineurium. The external epineurium contains blood vessels. The internal epineurium protects the funiculi from pressure and allows for gliding of fascicles. The amount of epineurium varies among persons and nerve types and along each individual nerve. The perineurium surrounds funiculi, and the endoneurium surrounds the axons. A funiculus, or fascicle, consists of a group of axons that is surrounded by endoneurium and is covered by a sheath of perineurium. An individual fascicle contains a mix of myelinated and unmyelinated fibers. The myelin sheath encapsulates the axon. Myelin is a lipoprotein, which allows for conduction of fast impulses. Each nerve contains a varied number and varied sizes of funiculi.

Nerves are at risk for injury when laceration, avulsion, stretch, crush, compression, or contusion occurs.[11] Peripheral

nerves can also be attacked by viruses, bacteria, or the body's immune system.[11] Accompanying conditions such as tendon lacerations increase the complexity that therapists manage with intervention.

NERVE INJURY CLASSIFICATION

Nerve injuries are categorized by the extent of damage to the axon and sheath.[11] Nerve compression lesions often contribute to peripheral neuropathies. When a specific portion of a peripheral nerve is compressed, the peripheral axons within that nerve sustain the greatest injury. Initial changes occur in the blood/nerve barrier followed by subperineural edema. This edema results in a thickening of the internal and external perineurium.[59] As the compression worsens, the motor, proprioceptive, light touch, and vibratory sensory receptor specific functions are compromised.[86] All the nerve fibers may be paralyzed after enduring severe and prolonged compression. Seddon[80] originally described three levels of nerve injury (Fig. 14.2):

1. **Neurapraxia**
2. **Axonotmesis**
3. **Neurotmesis**

Neurapraxia, often occurring from compression or crush injuries, impairs conduction because of damage to the myelin. With neurapraxia (see Fig. 14-14.2), spontaneous recovery occurs in approximately 3 to 6 weeks.[31] As illustrated by Fig. 14.2, axonotmesis results in complete interruption of the axon. With this level and higher **wallerian degeneration** occurs. Wallerian degeneration occurs when a nerve is completely severed or the axon and myelin sheath are damaged. The segment of axon and the motor and sensory end receptors

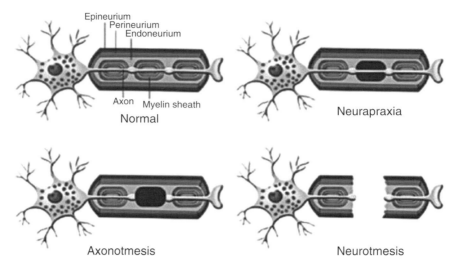

Fig. 14.2 The three classifications of nerve injuries are (1) neurapraxia, (2) axonotmesis, and (3) neurotmesis. (From Duffy, B. & Tubog, T. [2017]. The prevention and recognition of ulnar nerve and brachial plexus injuries, *Journal of PeriAnesthesia Nursing,* 32[6], 636–649. Copyright Elsevier [Figure 2]).

distal to the lesion become ischemic and begin to degenerate, thus preparing the nerve for regeneration.[41,57] The third level, neurotmesis (see Fig. 14.2), results in complete transection of the axon and other tissues. Penetrating and gunshot wounds, fractures, high-energy blunt trauma, traction, and crush are examples of injuries that can lead to axonotmesis or neurotmesis types of injury.[31]

Later in 1968 Sunderland[87] extended the classification to five levels, which are termed first- through fifth-degree injuries. Mackinnon and Dellon[47] describe an added sixth-degree injury, which addresses mixed grades of nerve injuries. Although it is helpful to learn the Sunderland classifications, therapists must recognize that most nerve injuries do not exactly fit into these categories due to being mixed-grade types of injuries. Furthermore, there is no specific discriminatory test for Sunderland grades II and IV, especially during the initial 6 weeks after a nerve injury.[32] Early physician diagnosis occurs with clinical and or surgical examination. Nerve conduction studies (NCSs) and electromyograms (EMGs) are beneficial diagnostic measures at 6 weeks post injury, when nerve fibrillation occurs. Thus nerve recovery can be charted over time.[32]

First-Degree Injury

A first-degree injury usually occurs from compression[32] and involves the demyelination of the nerve, which temporarily blocks conduction.[8,60] This level of injury corresponds to the neuropraxia level with axonal integrity remaining.[31] The prognosis for persons with this injury is extremely good; recovery is usually spontaneous within 3 months,[86] although maximum outcome can take as long as 7.15 months.[77]

Second-Degree Injury

A second-degree injury corresponds to the axonotmesis level with the axon severed and the sheath remaining intact.

A typical cause of this degree of injury is from a crush.[32] At this level wallerian degeneration can occur. However, the intact endoneurial tube allows for potential regrowth for the proximal part of the nerve to regenerate. With the ideal scenario the rate of regeneration is approximately 1 inch per month. Complete recovery usually occurs if regeneration happens in a timely manner before muscle degeneration,[60] but it is not unusual to have incomplete recovery.[32] Research indicates a recovery time up to 10.69 months.[77]

Third-Degree Injury

A third-degree injury varies from a second-degree injury in that the "continuity of the endoneurial tube [is] destroyed from a disorganization of the internal structures of the nerve bundles,"[87] and scarring is present within the tube.[27] This level corresponds to axonotmesis or neurotmesis levels. Recovery is more complicated with possible delayed or incomplete axonal growth.[87] Because fibers are often mismatched, clients benefit from motor and sensory reeducation.[60] Research indicates a maximum recovery time up to 14.08 months for this level.[77]

Fourth-Degree Injury

With the fourth-degree injury "the involved segment is ultimately converted into a tangled strand of connective tissue, Schwann cells, and regenerating axons which can be enlarged to form a neuroma."[87] Fourth-degree injuries correspond to the neurotmesis level. The effects are more severe than a third-degree injury with increased neuronal degeneration, misdirected axons, less axon survival,[87] and more scar tissue.[27] Complete "distal loss of function" occurs with this level of injury.[27] Surgical intervention is necessary to remove a neuroma (tumor of nerve fibers and cells). Research indicates a maximum recovery time up to 17.66 months for this level.[77]

Fifth-Degree Injury

A fifth-degree injury corresponding to the neurotmesis level results in partial or complete severance of the axon and the sheath with loss of motor, sensory, and sympathetic function.[87] Without the directional guidance from an intact endoneurial tube, malaligned axon growth may lead to a complicated recovery. Microsurgery is required as the person will not restore distal functioning without surgery.[27] Occasionally grafting is necessary if the severance gap is too large for approximation of the two nerve ends.[86] Research indicates a maximum recovery time up to 19.03 months for this level.[77]

Sixth-Degree Injury

A sixth-degree injury is a mixed injury involving a "neuroma-in-continuity."[27] This type of injury involves many of the aspects of the earlier five degrees to varying degrees.[47] Surgery needs will vary according to the specific condition, and in some cases surgery may not be required.

SURGICAL NERVE REPAIR

Peripheral nerve lesions often occur to the median, radial, and ulnar nerves. The location of the lesion determines the impairment of sudomotor, vasomotor, muscular, sensory, and functional involvement.[8] Sometimes nerves can be compressed at more than one site, and this is known as double crush syndrome.[72,89] Although the concept is controversial, it is believed that proximal compressions in the upper arm predispose the distal portions of the arm to developing additional nerve compressions[40] due to decreased blood flow.[57] For example, a therapist might be treating a client for carpal tunnel syndrome at the wrist and may recognize symptoms of a higher-level median nerve condition called C6 radiculopathy. Therefore it is important to be aware of key diagnostic procedures (e.g., cervical nerve root rule out) to determine the extent and placement of compressions, and such rule outs might be considered with all peripheral nerve injuries.

Operative Procedures for Nerve Repair

There are five procedures used to surgically repair nerves[74]:
1. Decompression
2. Repair
3. Neurolysis
4. Grafting (conduits)
5. Nerve transfers

Nerve decompression is the most common surgery performed on nerves. An example of surgical decompression is the transection of the transverse carpal ligament to decompress the **median nerve** or release the carpal tunnel.

Surgical nerve repairs involve microsurgical sutures to fix the epineurium, which is the current standard of care for lacerations.[31] End-to end repairs completed with little tension result in more predictable results.[31] Surgical nerve repairs are classified as primary, delayed primary, or secondary.[14] A primary repair occurs within hours of the injury. A delayed primary repair occurs within 5 to 7 days after the injury. Any surgical repair performed beyond 7 days is considered a secondary repair.[14]

Neurolysis is a procedure performed on a nerve that has become encapsulated in dense scar tissue. The scar tissue compresses the nerve to surrounding soft tissues and prevents it from gliding. When the client attempts to move in a way that would normally glide the nerve, the movement instead stretches the nerve, affecting circulation and chemical balance. Scars may also physically interfere with the axon regeneration.

Nerve grafting and nerve conduits are necessary when there is a large gap in a nerve and an end-to-end tensionless nerve repair is not possible. Nerve conduits serve as scaffolds and guides to provide structure for nerve regeneration.[52] Autografts from donated nerves such as the sural nerve are commonly performed surgically to fill a large gap. Risks exist with autografts for donor site morbidity with sensory and functional loss, neuroma, and infection.[29,65]

Nerve Transfers

A relatively recent surgical approach for peripheral nerve injuries is nerve transfers to the elbow, forearm, and hand.[56] Nerve transfers involve moving a healthy innervated nerve or nerve fascicles to a denervated nerve to facilitate nerve regeneration.[56,88] Post surgery, provision of orthotic intervention is variable. However, in some cases, after the bulky dressing is removed, application of an orthosis may be an option as prescribed by the surgeon. Nerve transfers for elbow flexion and forearm are typically immobilized briefly for 7 to 10 days.[56] Transfers for the wrist and hand are also surgically performed. For example, the flexor carpi radialis can be transferred to the extensor carpi radialis brevis to facilitate wrist extension.[88]

Following surgical repair, orthoses may be ordered by the physician. However, there are various reasons for orthotic provision with nerve conditions, which are summarized in the next section.

PURPOSES OF ORTHOTIC INTERVENTION FOR NERVE INJURIES

The three purposes for orthotic intervention of an extremity that has nerve injury are protection, prevention, and assistance with function.[3,50] If a nerve has undergone surgical repair, the physician may order application of a cast or an orthosis to place the hand, wrist, or elbow in a protective position, thus reducing the amount of tension on the repaired nerve. Avoiding tension on a repaired nerve is extremely important because outcomes of nerve repairs are directly related to the amount of tension across the repair site.[83]

Prevention of contractures is important because nerve lesions result in various degrees of muscle denervation. For example, a short opponens orthosis prevents contracture of the thumb web space after a median nerve injury.[26] Sometimes a client does not seek immediate medical attention after nerve injury, resulting in contracture development in which an orthosis is required for contracture correction. For example, a client with a claw hand deformity from an ulnar nerve injury may require a mobilizing ulnar gutter orthosis. This orthosis helps remodel the soft tissues to increase passive extension of the ring and little fingers' proximal interphalangeal (PIP) joints[11] by placing the metacarpophalangeal (MCP) joints in a flexed position. Concurrently intervention focuses on regaining maximum passive range of motion (PROM). After normal PROM is regained, orthotic interventions for the muscle imbalance becomes an option.[25]

Often function after a nerve injury can require or be enhanced by orthotic intervention. For example, a client may be better able to grasp and release objects after a radial nerve injury while wearing an orthosis that reestablishes the tenodesis action of the hand and wrist. This orthosis assists the wrist and MCP joints with extending to open the hand for grasp and release. Without the orthosis the wrist and MCP joints are unable to extend, resulting in difficulty with grasp and grasp release activities.

GENERAL GUIDELINES FOR ORTHOTIC PROVISION WITH NERVE INJURIES

Every nerve condition requires specific positioning to address nerve deficits. Obtaining the right position with orthotic intervention can be challenging because of issues with denervated muscles and insensate areas. Selection of a custom versus a prefabricated orthosis is based on the condition and therapeutic objectives. With orthotic fabrication, extreme care is taken to protect insensate areas from further damage and for general patient safety (see Patient Safety Tips and Precautions Box). Thus selecting conforming and drapable thermoplastic materials and recognizing areas to round, pad, or push out to prevent pressure are important considerations.

The next section summarizes various nerve conditions that therapists encounter. A brief overview of cumulative trauma disorders (CTDs) is provided.

Nerve injuries occur either from trauma (e.g., lacerations, gunshot, crush) or from compressions with CTDs. During therapy the therapist must note any substituted motions to prevent further muscle imbalance. Knowing the challenges, location, and prognoses for nerve conditions helps the therapist be realistic with setting objectives for intervention and collaborating with client goals.

UPPER EXTREMITY COMPRESSION NEUROPATHIES

Cumulative trauma disorder (CTD) is not a medical diagnosis but an etiological label for a range of disorders.[53] The cause of CTD is not solely from engaging in work activities. Social activities, activities of daily living (ADLs), and leisure pursuits may enhance the development and exacerbation of CTD.[53] Most CTDs are classified as neuropraxia or Sunderland grade 1 injuries. They can further be characterized as acute or chronic conditions. An example of an acute CTD is a radial nerve compression in the upper arm sometimes nicknamed Saturday night palsy. An example of a chronic condition may be long-standing carpal tunnel syndrome condition.[54] The

first step in managing the CTD derives from understanding the compressive neuropathies of the upper extremity.[90] Table 14.1 outlines the nature and intervention of compressive neuropathies that occur at the wrist, elbow, and forearm. The compressive neuropathies are discussed in more detail later in this chapter.

LOCATIONS OF NERVE LESIONS

The location of a nerve lesion determines the sensory and motor involvement. Lesions are referred to as low or high. Low lesions occur distal to the elbow, and high lesions occur proximal to the elbow.[5] High lesions affect more muscles and may influence a larger sensory distribution than low lesions. Therefore knowledge of relevant anatomy is important for determining physical and functional implications of nerve injuries.

SUBSTITUTIONS

When a nerve lesion occurs, "there is no opposing balancing force to the intact active muscle group."[18] If a person with a nerve lesion does not receive orthotic intervention, the intact musculature overpowers the denervated muscles. Intact musculature takes over and produces movement normally generated by the denervated muscles.[15] The person learns to adapt to the imbalance through substitutions and compensation.[18,71] An example of a substitution or trick movement is the pinch that develops after a low-level median nerve injury. With the help of the adductor pollicis, the flexor pollicis longus pinches objects against the radial side of the index finger. A therapist may mistakenly think that motor return has occurred for the abductor pollicis brevis, flexor pollicis brevis, opponens pollicis, and the first and second lumbricals. However, the pinch movement observed is actually a substitution.

PROGNOSIS

Many factors affect the prognosis for recovery from nerve injuries, particularly following surgical repair. Full motor and/or sensory recovery may not always occur. Less than half of people undergoing surgical repair have good to excellent results.[32] Prognostic factors include the extent and location of the injury, cleanliness of the wound, method of repair, timing of repair and the client's age.[11,83] Other factors that impact recovery from nerve repair include the person's general health and cognitive capacities and whether the person smokes or has a concurrent diagnosis such as diabetes.

Extensive injuries, such as from a crush mechanism, add challenges to the repair and generally have less positive prognoses. In contrast, injuries that are solely a motor or sensory fiber repair have a better prognosis.[46] Generally, proximal nerve injuries have worse prognoses than distal injuries because regeneration takes longer to reach the hand, resulting in irreversible nerve end plate damage.[46] Proximal wounds at the level of the brachial plexus can take as long as 2 to 3 years to regenerate to the hand.[32] It is postulated that the rate of axonal regeneration is 1 to 2 mm per day.[73] Because nerve

TABLE 14.1　Upper Extremity Compression Neuropathies

	Presentation	Orthotic Intervention
Wrist		
Radial sensory entrapment (Wartenberg neuropathy)	Compression of the superficial radial nerve usually includes numbness, tingling, and pain of the dorsoradial aspect of the forearm, wrist, and hand. Symptoms occur during ulnar deviation of the wrist, thumb composite flexion, and forceful pronation of the forearm.	Conservative intervention involves avoidance of wrist and forearm motions. Fabricate a wrist immobilization orthosis with the wrist in 20 to 30 degrees of extension. If pain occurs with thumb motion, the thumb should also be incorporated into the orthosis.
Ulnar nerve entrapment at the wrist (ulnar tunnel syndrome)	Entrapment of the ulnar nerve usually occurs in the Guyon canal. Sensory or motor changes involve the fifth digit and ulnar side of the fourth digit. True ulnar nerve entrapment is not common.	Wrist immobilization orthosis in a neutral wrist position. Or, with more involvement orthotic provision may include a dorsal hand-based orthosis or a figure-eight orthosis with fourth and fifth digits in 30 to 45 degrees of flexion at the MCP joint to block MCP hyperextension. Orthosis can be dynamic (mobilization) or static. Orthosis is worn until the nerve regenerates.
Carpal tunnel syndrome (CTS)	Complaints of numbness, tingling, and paresthesias in the median nerve distribution. Persons may complain of dropping objects or cramping and aching in the wrist and hand, especially during sleep and driving. In severe cases, thenar atrophy or loss of strength of palmar abduction of the thumb are present. Positive Phalen and Tinel signs and night pain are present.	Orthotic provision involves custom-made or prefabricated wrist orthosis with the wrist in neutral. The MCPs may be included in the orthosis to alleviate the pressure in the carpal tunnel (see Chapter 7) Orthotic regimens vary, but most include nighttime wear.
Elbow and Forearm		
Radial tunnel syndrome	True radial tunnel syndrome is rare and often misdiagnosed as lateral epicondylitis. Radial tunnel syndrome presents with pain and discomfort in the extensor-supinator muscle mass in the proximal forearm. Radial tunnel syndrome has pain as the presenting symptom, not motor dysfunction.	Currently the trend is to immobilize only as much as needed to resolve the symptoms. Conservative management may involve immobilization in a volar wrist immobilization orthosis in slight extension and/or Kinesio taping[70] when the area is irritated to reduce tension. Another suggestion is a "yoke orthosis" for support of the middle finger MCP joint.[70]
Posterior interosseous nerve syndrome	Presentation is similar to radial tunnel syndrome. However, posterior interosseous syndrome includes weakness or paralysis of any muscles innervated by the posterior interosseous nerve and does not involve sensory loss. The ability to extend the wrist in radial deviation is present, but extension of the wrist is impaired in neutral or ulnar deviation. Loss of thumb extension and abduction and active extension of the MCP joints are also present.	It is important to provide orthotic intervention as much as possible for this condition to prevent stretch of structures innervated by the radial nerve. Various orthotic options are suggested for posterior interosseous nerve syndrome. Several options are presented in this chapter for the condition, including mobilization orthoses typically with the wrist in some degree of extension (e.g., 30 to 40 degrees of extension) and MCPs in neutral degree or 0-degree extension. With muscle return at the wrist a hand-based orthosis may be all that is necessary.
Cubital tunnel syndrome	Presents with localized pain to the medial side of the proximal forearm and elbow. There is numbness and tingling of the fifth digit and the medial side of the fourth digit. Advanced compression presents with hypothenar eminence atrophy. A positive Froment sign may accompany this syndrome.	Conservative intervention includes avoidance of direct pressure on the medial aspect of the elbow and on the flexor carpi ulnaris. An elbow pad may help to protect the nerve from direct pressure. During the daytime, prolonged elbow flexion should be avoided to prevent compression of the ulnar nerve, and orthotic provision is usually not necessary. Orthotic provision for nighttime includes positioning the elbow in 30 to 45 degrees of flexion. If the wrist is included, it is positioned in 20 degrees of extension.

Continued

TABLE 14.1   Upper Extremity Compression Neuropathies—cont'd

	Presentation	Orthotic Intervention
Pronator syndrome	Compression of the median nerve as it crosses the elbow at the origin of the pronator teres. It is associated with pain in the proximal forearm and is aggravated by resisted forearm pronation when the elbow is flexed.	One orthotic option is to place the elbow in 90 degrees flexion and forearm in neutral rotation (between supination and pronation).[64]
Anterior interosseous syndrome	Compression of the anterior interosseous branch of the median nerve is associated with pain in the proximal volar forearm followed by loss of ability to flex the IP joint of the thumb and the DIP joint of the second and third digits. There are usually no sensory complaints.	Orthotic provision may include immobilizing the elbow in 90 degrees of flexion with the forearm in neutral. Another option is to fabricate small orthoses to block index DIP and thumb IP extension or hyperextension (see Fig. 14.18).
Upper Arm		
Radial nerve palsy (Saturday night palsy)	Presents as sensory hypesthesia on dorsal forearm and hand and some degree of wrist, digit, and thumb extension loss.	With diminished extension various options are presented in the chapter for mobilization orthoses (e.g., low-profile design with an outrigger, tenodesis orthosis, low-profile radial nerve palsy orthosis with radial and ulnar deviation) and a wrist or hand immobilization orthosis can be used for nighttime wear. Generally, the wrist is positioned in 30 to 45 degrees extension and MCPs are in neutral extension or 0 degree extension. With muscle return at the wrist a hand-based orthosis that supports the thumb in extension and the MCPs in neutral extension may be all that is necessary (see Fig. 14.11).

DIP, Distal interphalangeal; *IP,* interphalangeal; *MCP,* metacarpophalangeal.

regeneration is slow, the therapist conducts periodic monitoring; furthermore, orthotic intervention is often part of the intervention protocol. Correct alignment of axons and avoidance of tension on the damaged nerve improve the prognosis. However, regardless of surgical technique, axonal mismatching occurs as surgeons cannot repair individual Schwann tubes or axons.[46] A clean wound has a better prognosis than a dirty wound.[8] Sharply severed nerves, such as from a laceration, recover better than frayed nerves resulting from a gunshot wound.[28] Early surgical repair is associated with better outcomes,[11,45] and delayed repairs usually require grafts because of scarring and nerve retraction.[46] Age is also a critical factor in the speed and extent of recovery. A child's potential for nerve regeneration is greater than an adult's.[11] Adults rarely fully recover from a nerve injury.[45] As with any injury, a person's general health is related to recovery, and cigarette smoking is linked to poorer results.[9]

The following section summarizes radial, ulnar, and median peripheral nerve injuries. Accompanying each type of nerve injury is a discussion of the causes, muscles involved, functional implications, and orthotic intervention.

RADIAL NERVE INJURIES

Radial nerve palsies are very common with the most prevalent causative factor being midhumeral fractures or

compressions.[3,13,17] Other causes of superficial radial nerve palsies at the wrist include pressure, edema, and trauma on the nerve from crush injuries; de Quervain tendonitis; handcuffs; and a tight or heavy wristwatch.[22] The location of the radial nerve injury determines which muscles are affected (Fig. 14.3).

Three types of lesions are possible when the **radial nerve** is injured.[18] The first type of lesion involves a high-level injury at the humerus resulting in wrist drop and lack of finger MCP extension (Fig. 14.4). With this type of lesion the triceps are rarely affected unless the injury is extremely high. Radial nerve palsy, sometimes known as Saturday night palsy, is a sensory and motor compression of the radial nerve in the upper arm. The term *Saturday night palsy* refers to a person who is drinking and falls asleep with his or her arm over a chair, putting pressure on the upper arm and causing hyperesthesia or diminished sensation on the dorsal forearm and hand and weak or absent wrist, digit, and thumb extensors.[69] Radial nerve palsy usually presents as a neuropraxia type of nerve injury that spontaneously resolves in a few months.[57]

The second type of lesion involves the posterior interosseous nerve. After spiraling around the humerus and crossing the elbow, the radial nerve divides into a motor and a sensory branch.[22] The motor branch is the posterior interosseous nerve, and the sensory branch is the superficial branch of the radial nerve. Compression usually causes the posterior interosseous

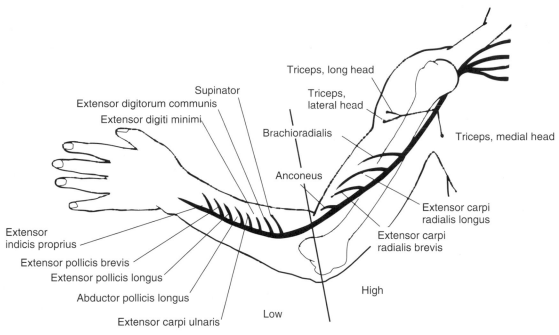

Fig. 14.3 Radial nerve motor innervation.

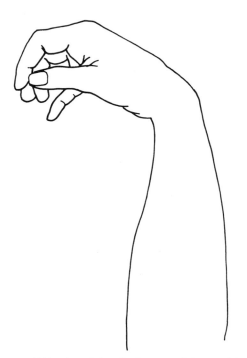

Fig. 14.4 Wrist drop deformity from a radial nerve injury.

nerve injury, but lacerations or stab wounds can be sources of lesions to the posterior interosseous nerve. Radial tunnel syndrome and posterior interosseous nerve compression are two distinct types of compression syndromes described in the literature that occur in the same tunnel with the same nerve. As Gelberman and colleagues[30] stated, "It is difficult for the conscientious diagnostician to accept the reality that the same nerve compressed in the same anatomical site can result in two entirely different symptom complexes." Radial tunnel syndrome refers to compression of the radial nerve just distal to the elbow

between the radial head and the supinator muscle,[69,83] and it is linked to repetitive forearm rotation.[16] With radial tunnel syndrome, complaints of pain occur usually at night in the radial nerve distribution of the distal forearm,[38] and the condition involves pain without muscle weakness.[20,22,30] Radial tunnel syndrome is controversial because it is complicated to diagnose a pain syndrome that does not have motor components. The condition needs to be differentiated from lateral epicondylitis, which is close to the same area.[20]

Posterior interosseous nerve compression results in rapid motor loss[30] with no sensory loss.[22,30,42] This compression is characterized by aching on the lateral side of the elbow, weakness in supination, difficulty with MCP finger and thumb extension, and difficulty with thumb abduction. Wrist extension is intact, but the wrist tends to radially deviate due to muscle imbalance.[42]

The third type of lesion is damage to the sensory branch of the radial nerve. Compression of this superficial branch is called *Wartenberg syndrome.*[61] Compression can occur between the brachioradialis and extensor carpi radialis longus. The condition is caused by repetitive pronation and at the distal forearm, repetitive wrist flexion and ulnar deviation, and tight wrist bands.[69] Wartenberg syndrome does not result in functional loss. However, symptoms include numbness, tingling, burning, and pain over the dorsoradial surface of the forearm and in the areas of the thumb and index finger.[84]

Functional Involvement From Radial Nerve Lesions

Table 14.2 outlines lesion locations and the muscles and motions that are affected in radial nerve lesions. After crossing the elbow and dropping below the supinator, the radial nerve divides and forms the posterior interosseous nerve.[18] Refer to Table 14.2 for a list of muscles affected with the posterior interosseous nerve at the forearm level. Loss of these muscles

TABLE 14.2   Radial Nerve Lesions

Affected Muscles	Weak or Lost Motions
Forearm Level (Posterior Interosseous Nerve)	
Extensor digitorum communis	MCP extension of digits 2 through 5
Extensor carpi ulnaris	Wrist extension and wrist ulnar deviation
Extensor indicis proprius	Extension of the MCP of the second digit
Extensor digiti minimi	Extension of the MCP of the fifth digit
Abductor pollicis longus	Thumb abduction
Extensor pollicis longus	Thumb extension at the IP and MCP joints
Extensor pollicis brevis	MCP extension and assist CMC extension
Elbow Level	
Extensor carpi radialis longus	Radial wrist extension
Extensor carpi radialis brevis	Neutral wrist extension
Supinator	Supination
Extensor digitorum communis	MCP extension of digits 2 through 5
Extensor carpi ulnaris	Wrist extension and wrist ulnar deviation
Extensor indicis proprius	Extension of the MCP joint of the second digit
Extensor digiti minimi	Extension of the MCP joints of the fifth digit
Abductor pollicis longus	Thumb abduction
Extensor pollicis longus	Thumb extension of the MCP and IP joints
Extensor pollicis brevis	Thumb extension and abduction at the CMC and MCP joints
Axilla Level	
Brachioradialis	Elbow flexion in neutral forearm position
Triceps	Elbow extension
Extensor carpi radialis longus	Radial wrist extension
Extensor carpi radialis brevis	Neutral wrist extension
Supinator	Supination
Extensor digitorum communis	MCP extension of digits 2 through 5
Extensor carpi ulnaris	Wrist extension and wrist ulnar deviation
Extensor indicis proprius	Extension of the MCP of the second digit
Extensor digiti minimi	Extension of the MCP of the fifth digit
Abductor pollicis longus	Thumb abduction
Extensor pollicis longus	Thumb extension at the MCP and IP joints
Extensor pollicis brevis	MCP extension and assist CMC extension

CMC, Carpometacarpal; *IP,* interphalangeal; *MCP,* metacarpophalangeal.

results in absent MCP extension of all digits, thumb radial abduction, and thumb extension. With attempts at wrist extension, strong wrist radial deviation is present. With attempts at finger extension, the MCPs flex and the PIPs extend because the extensor digitorum muscle is affected. In addition to the muscles previously indicated, a radial nerve injury at the elbow level can affect the supinator and extensor carpi radialis longus and brevis. Along with motions lost at the forearm level, an injury at the elbow level involves inability to produce radial wrist extension, MCP joint extension, thumb extension, thumb radial abduction, and weakened forearm supination.

With a high-level lesion or compression in the upper arm (i.e., axilla level), the injury affects the triceps and brachioradialis muscles. Loss of these muscles results in lost elbow extension, weak supination, absent wrist and finger extensors, and lost thumb extension and abduction.

The functional results of an axilla-level lesion include an inability to stabilize the wrist in an extended position, extend fingers and thumb, and abduct the thumb. For example, a client with a high radial nerve lesion has poor grip and

coordination because of the lack of wrist extensor opposition to the flexors.[8,25] The resulting deformity is called *wrist drop* (see Fig. 14.4).

Significant impairment of sensation is not present with radial nerve injuries. The superficial sensory branch of the radial nerve supplies sensation to the dorsum of the index and middle fingers and half of the ring finger to the PIP joint level (Fig. 14.5). Laceration or contusion to the sensory branch of the radial nerve can be bothersome to a client. This often occurs in conjunction with de Quervain release. Sensory compromise over the dorsum of the thumb may result in hypersensitivity. An orthosis or padded device can protect the area while a desensitization program is implemented.[79]

Orthotic Intervention for Radial Nerve Injury

The client with a radial nerve injury benefits from orthotic intervention and a therapeutic program. There are several orthotic options for radial nerve injuries. Orthoses specific for diagnoses are discussed first, followed by various orthotic design options.

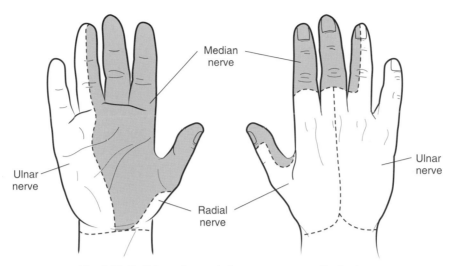

Fig. 14.5 Radial, median, and ulnar nerve sensory distribution.

Orthotic Intervention for Radial Nerve Palsy

Forearm-level orthoses promote function usually with the wrist positioned in 30 to 45 degrees of extension.[69] Many options exist, such as a traditional low-profile design as illustrated in Fig. 14.7, a tenodesis orthosis as illustrated in Fig. 14.8, a low-profile radial nerve palsy orthosis with radial and ulnar deviation as illustrated in Fig. 14.9, or a low-profile static wrist extension and MCP mobilization extension orthosis as illustrated in Fig. 14.14. A hand immobilization orthosis to support the MCPs in extension with the wrist in neutral to slight extension can be provided for nighttime wear to promote a functional hand position that prevents "shortening of the flexors and overstretching of the extensors"[21] (see Chapter 9.) As wrist function returns, a hand-based orthosis can be fabricated to promote wrist and finger extension. For example, the hand portion of the low-profile static wrist extension and MCP extension orthosis (see Fig. 14.11) can be solely used with wrist musculature return and if only the MCPs and thumb need support.

Orthotic Intervention for Radial Tunnel Syndrome

Currently the trend for orthotic intervention for **radial tunnel syndrome** is to immobilize only to the extent needed to relieve symptoms. Conservative management may involve immobilization when symptomatic in a volar wrist immobilization orthosis in slight extension and/or Kinesio taping[70] to reduce tension. Another conservative suggestion is a yoke orthosis to support the middle MCP joint to allow functional activities (Fig. 14.6).[70]

Orthotic Intervention for Posterior Interosseous Nerve Syndrome

It is important to apply orthotic intervention as much as possible for **posterior interosseous nerve syndrome** to prevent stretch of structures innervated by the radial nerve. The same various orthotic options are suggested for posterior interosseous nerve syndrome as for radial nerve palsy.

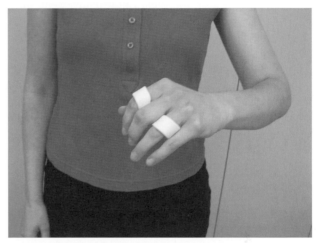

Fig. 14.6 Yoke orthosis for support of the middle metacarpophalangeal (MCP) joint with radial tunnel syndrome. (From Porretto-Loehrke, A., & Soika, E. [2011]. Therapist's management of other nerve compressions about the elbow and wrist. In T. M. Skirven, A. L. Osterman, J. M. Fedorczyk, et al. [Eds.], *Rehabilitation of the hand and upper extremity* [6th ed.]. Philadelphia, Elsevier.)

Orthotic Intervention for Wartenberg Neuropathy

For **Wartenberg neuropathy** a wrist immobilization orthosis is fabricated with the wrist in 20 to 30 degrees of extension. If pain occurs with thumb motion, the thumb is also incorporated into the orthosis. Padding or other ways to relieve pressure over the aggravated areas, especially over the radial styloid, is helpful with orthotic fabrication.[24,57,69] (See Chapter 8 for information on thumb orthoses.)

The next section summarizes the two types of orthoses for radial nerve conditions: immobilization and mobilization orthoses.

Immobilization and Mobilization Orthoses

Immobilization orthoses. The therapist applies a wrist immobilization orthosis to place the wrist in a functional position of 30 degrees of extension.[12] When wearing a wrist

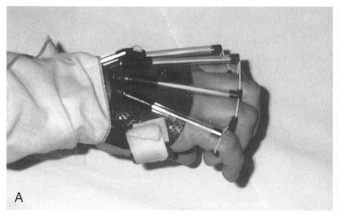
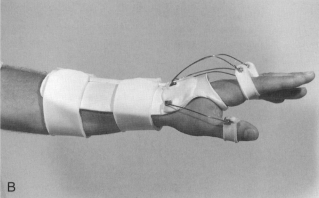

Fig. 14.7 Low-profile designs with pre-purchased outrigger parts. (From Fess EE, Gettle KS, Philips CA, et al: *Hand and upper extremity splinting: principles and methods*, ed 3, St Louis, 2005, Elsevier/Mosby.)

immobilization orthosis, the client can usually extend the IP joints of the fingers to release an object by using the intrinsic hand muscles.[8] The therapist keeps in mind the advantages, disadvantages, and patterns of volar and dorsal wrist orthoses (see Chapter 7). A wrist immobilization orthosis is appropriate to wear on occasions when the client desires a more inconspicuous design than a mobilization orthosis. A wrist or hand/thumb immobilization orthosis (see Chapter 9) may also be more appropriate for nighttime wear than a mobilization orthosis with an outrigger. Wearing a traditional mobilization orthosis with an outrigger at night may result in damage to the outrigger and injury to the client. Some people who have heavy demands on their hands prefer the simple wrist immobilization orthoses to the more fragile outrigger-mobilization designs. A therapist may offer both a wrist immobilization orthosis and a wrist mobilization orthosis to the person. Alternating the orthoses is another solution that may maximize function. The low-profile mobilization orthoses discussed later in this chapter is an alternative for the client to wear both day and night because it is less cumbersome and allows for functional movements.

Mobilization orthoses. Mobilization orthotic intervention for a radial nerve injury promotes functional hand use,[7] and several options exist. One traditional option involves fabricating a dorsal wrist immobilization orthosis as the base for a mobilization extension finger/thumb orthosis (using elastic for the source of tension).[3] The dynamic component for this orthosis positions the MCPs in neutral (extension). Several low-profile options exist that can be made with purchased outrigger parts (Fig. 14.7). The costs of using purchased outrigger parts should be considered. Alternatively, the therapist can use wire or thermoplastic material to fabricate an outrigger. (See Chapter 13 for more information on outriggers).

A mobilization MCP extension orthosis for radial nerve injury substitutes for the absent muscle power by assisting the MCP extensors. This orthosis is worn throughout the day until the impaired musculature reaches a manual muscle testing (MMT) grade of fair (3).[10] Colditz[18] cautions that "the

powerful unopposed flexors often overcome the force of the dynamic splint during finger flexion." A client who shows no clinical improvement in 3 months should return to the physician for consideration of surgical intervention.[22] Because wrist control usually returns first, the therapist closely monitors and modifies the orthotic design and uses a hand-based mobilization orthosis after the forearm-based mobilization orthosis has been worn and improvement in wrist control is demonstrated.[3,93] If only one finger is lagging in extension, the therapist dynamically incorporates that finger into the orthosis.[93]

Another type of mobilization orthosis for radial nerve injuries is a mobilization orthosis that reestablishes the tenodesis action of the hand.[17-19] A tenodesis action occurs when the client flexes the wrist and the fingers extend. When the client extends the wrist, the fingers flex (Fig. 14.8). The tenodesis orthosis includes a dorsal base with a low-profile outrigger that spans from the wrist to each proximal phalanx. This orthosis is sometimes called a *dynamic tenodesis suspension orthosis.*[34] Finger loops are worn on each proximal phalanx, and a nylon cord attaches the finger loops to the dorsal base.

The tenodesis orthosis has many advantages. First, the design allows the palmar surface of the hand to be relatively free for sensory input and normal grasp.[18] The wrist is not immobilized and moves only with the natural tenodesis effect, whereas the thumb can move independently.[17] In addition, the hand arches are maintained.[18] The components of the tenodesis orthosis "follow the contours of the hand and take up less space."[51] As wrist extension returns, the client continues to wear the orthosis because it does not immobilize the wrist and it enhances the strength of the wrist extensors for functional tasks.[18] Therefore a hand-based orthosis is not required. The low-profile design enhances the performance of functional tasks.

There are some disadvantages with the tenodesis orthosis. Because finger MCP flexion and extension mobilize as a group, independent finger motion is not achieved. An additional orthotic component is added if the thumb is to be included in the orthosis. Because the orthotic design supports the weight of the hand through the finger cuffs, wearing the

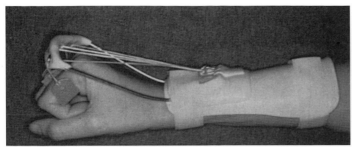
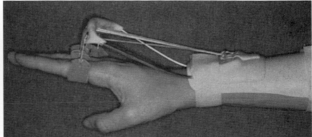

Fig. 14.8 A tenodesis orthosis for a high-level radial nerve injury. (From Colditz, J. C. [2002]. Splinting the hand with a peripheral nerve injury. In E. J. Mackin, A. D. Callahan, T. M. Skirven, et al. [Eds.], *Rehabilitation of the hand and upper extremity* [5th ed., pp. 622–634]. St. Louis, MO: Mosby.)

orthosis can be fatiguing.[50] The tenodesis orthotic design is usually not sturdy enough for people with high load demands on their hands.[79] Newer options for mobilization orthoses for the radial nerve continue to be developed. The next section provides two pattern options for mobilization orthoses for radial nerve palsy.

Fabrication of a Low-Profile Radial Nerve Palsy Orthosis With Radial and Ulnar Deviation

This low-profile radial nerve palsy orthosis allows for radial and ulnar deviation. The orthosis is very comfortable to wear as the client can use the hand functionally.[67] A beneficial aspect of the design is that the hand piece can be separated from the forearm piece for use with radial nerve functional return. This orthotic adaption was first conceived by Sally Fistler Desilva, OTR, CHT.[67]

Before fabrication, assemble the following materials: 3 mm thermoplastic material, adhesive hook, nonadhesive loop, ½-inch (1.9-cm) elastic band that adheres to Velcro, 3-mm elastic cord, screw rivet, piece of stockinette, and hard-grade Theraputty. Fig. 14.9 illustrates the finished orthosis, and Fig. 14.10 provides the pattern for the orthosis.

PROCEDURE FOR LOW-PROFILE MOBILIZATION ORTHOSIS FOR RADIAL NERVE PALSY

1. Place a piece of Theraputty over the dorsal aspect of the wrist to protect the skin surface from the hinge. Secure the Theraputty with the piece of stockinette wrapped around the extremity.
2. Position the thumb between palmar and radial abduction and the wrist in 20 to 30 degrees extension to mold the hand section of the orthosis. Cut out an open area on the dorsal surface of the orthosis to align with the MP joints of the index through small finger (Fig. 14.11).
3. Over the distal aspect of the hand piece of the orthosis put a damp paper towel where the two thermoplastic pattern pieces will overlap. This damp towel prevents the two pieces from sticking together (Fig. 14.12).
4. Fabricate the forearm piece, making sure to overlap it on top of the distal hand piece by approximately 2 cm. Make sure that the forearm piece is two-thirds the length and one-half the circumference of the forearm.
5. Remove the paper towel, Theraputty, and stockinette. Remove the thermoplastic pattern pieces.
6. Mark the forearm section of the orthosis for the pivot point where the screw rivet will be placed directly over the capitate bone, which is located proximal to the base of the middle metacarpal.
7. Punch the correct size hole with a hole punch for the screw rivet.
8. After positioning the hand piece beneath the forearm piece, mark the corresponding pivot placement, and punch a second hole.
9. Check for adequate ulnar and radial deviation with the two pieces positioned on the client.
10. For MP finger extension, place the ¾-inch piece of elastic on the hand portion distal to the cutout hole. The elastic piece will fit beneath the proximal phalanges of the index through middle fingers. Cut a smaller piece of elastic to secure the thumb at the proximal phalanx. Secure the elastic pieces with Velcro.
11. On the dorsal surface of the hand piece mark two parallel vertical points between the PIP and MP joints of the fingers above the three locations of the finger web spaces. Then punch out two small holes. Refer to Figs. 14.9 and 14.11 for placement.
12. To create the slings to position the MP joints in extension, loop the elastic thread through the holes, and tie them on top (Fig. 14.13; see Figs. 14.9 and 14.11).
13. Place the forearm piece of thermoplastic material over the hand piece to secure the screw rivet at a tightness that allows for ulnar and radial deviation.
14. Complete the orthosis by securing it with two straps on the forearm.

MP, Metacarpophalangeal; *PIP*, proximal interphalangeal.
Instructions were modified and reprinted with permission from Peck, J., & Ollason, J. (2015). Low profile radial nerve palsy orthosis with radial and ulnar deviation. *Journal of Hand Therapy, 28*(4), 421–424.

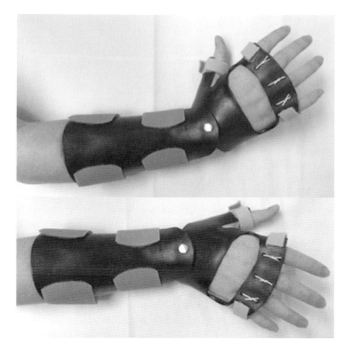

Fig. 14.9 A low-profile radial nerve palsy orthosis with radial and ulnar deviation. (From Peck, J., & Ollason, J. [2015]. Low profile radial nerve palsy orthosis with radial and ulnar deviation. *Journal of Hand Therapy, 28*[4], 421–424.)

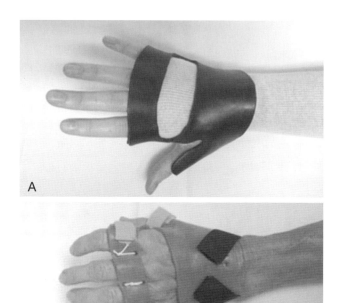

Fig. 14.11 A, Molding of the hand section of the orthosis. B, Completed hand product by itself. (From Peck, J., & Ollason, J. [2015]. Low profile radial nerve palsy orthosis with radial and ulnar deviation. *Journal of Hand Therapy, 28*[4], 421–424.)

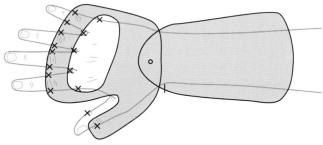

Fig. 14.10 Pattern for the low-profile radial nerve palsy orthosis with radial and ulnar deviation. (Modified from Peck, J., & Ollason, J. [2015]. Low profile radial nerve palsy orthosis with radial and ulnar deviation. *Journal of Hand Therapy, 28*[4], 421–424.)

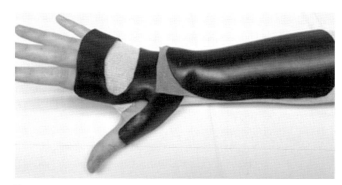

Fig. 14.12 Placement of damp paper towel where the pieces overlap to prevent sticking. (From Peck, J., & Ollason, J. [2015]. Low profile radial nerve palsy orthosis with radial and ulnar deviation. *Journal of Hand Therapy, 28*[4], 421–424.)

Fabrication of a Low-Profile Mobilization Orthosis for Radial Nerve Palsy

A unique mobilization orthosis for radial nerve palsy is a static wrist extension and dynamic MCP extension orthosis, which was originally designed by Mark Walsh and Sue Blackmore with adaptations by the Philadelphia Hand Center Therapy Department. Besides radial nerve palsy, this orthosis may be used with other conditions that require immobilization, such as post cerebrovascular accidents (CVAs).[92] The instructions are based on an adaptation for making the orthosis with moleskin loops. The original design by Walsh and Blackmore is fabricated slightly differently. Walsh and Blackmore's design includes

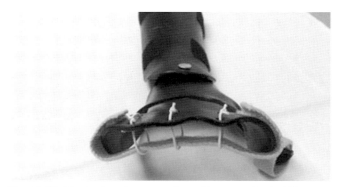

Fig. 14.13 Elastic thread creates sling effect to maintain MP extension. (From Peck, J., & Ollason, J. [2015]. Low profile radial nerve palsy orthosis with radial and ulnar deviation. *Journal of Hand Therapy, 28*[4], 421–424.)

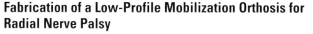

PROCEDURE FOR MOBILIZATION LOW-PROFILE ORTHOSIS FOR RADIAL NERVE PALSY

1. Position the person's hand palm-side up on a piece of paper. The wrist should be as neutral as possible with respect to radial and ulnar deviation. The fingers are abducted, and the thumb is radially abducted.
2. Trace the hand and forearm. With the person's hand still on the paper, mark X's corresponding to (Fig. 14.15):
   - Each web space between the fingers
   - PIP joints (both ulnar and radial sides) of all four fingers
   - IP joints (both ulnar and radial sides) of the thumb
   - Two-thirds the length of the forearm
   - ¼ to ½ inch lateral and parallel from the side of the little finger PIP joint on the ulnar side of the hand
   - ¼ to ½ inch lateral and parallel from the ulnar side of the thumb IP joint
3. Draw the pattern (see Fig. 14.15). Start with the PIP joint of the index finger radial side, and draw a straight line across the joint to the ulnar side. Draw a straight line down from the ulnar side of the PIP joint to the marking at the web space between the index and middle fingers. Continue the same process of drawing lines across the PIP joints and connecting them to a line down to the marking at the base of the web space for all digits. Connect the line from the little finger to the marking ¼ to ½ inch outside of the PIP joint and continue the line down the side of the forearm, curving it to adjust to the forearm muscle bulk. End the line at the two-thirds marking. Connect the line that is ¼ to ½ inch parallel to the index finger to the middle of the thumb IP joint, curving it to follow the C shape of the index and thumb. From the middle of the thumb, cross the IP joint and curve the line down the side of the forearm, ending it at the two-thirds marking. Connect the two lines at the two-thirds marking.
4. Cut out the pattern, making certain to completely cut through web space marks.
5. Trace the pattern onto the sheet of thermoplastic material.
6. Heat the thermoplastic material.
7. An option is to place padding on the dorsal MCPs and on the ulnar styloid during orthotic formation and later adhere the padding to the orthosis.
8. Cut the pattern out of the thermoplastic material. Wait until later to cut out the markings between the web spaces so that they do not adhere together. Another approach is to cut the area between the web space as a V shape to prevent the thermoplastic material from sticking together.
9. Position the person's upper extremity on a table with the elbow resting on a pad (folded towel or foam wedge) and the forearm in pronation. Place the wrist and hand in the following position:
   - Wrist: Approximately 10 to 20 degrees extension
   - Index through small MCPs: Neutral
   - Thumb: Functional position of palmar abduction
10. Reheat the thermoplastic material, and cut out the markings between the web spaces.
11. Mold the warmed thermoplastic material over the dorsum of the wrist and hand, making sure to conform the orthosis around the proximal phalanx of each finger and thumb. Push out the material at the area of the ulnar styloid, or use Theraputty over the styloid.
12. Make any adjustment for proper fit, and position the orthosis on the person.
13. Once the orthosis is formed, cut a piece of ½-inch to ¾-inch elastic to comfortably fit over and around each proximal phalanx within the orthosis. Allow the elastic material to overlap ½ inch to ¾ inch. After the size of loop is determined, using a small stapler, place two staples in the elastic to secure each loop.
14. Remove the orthosis; be careful that the elastic pieces stay in the proper place for each finger.
15. With strips of moleskin that are approximately ¾ inch × 4 inches, secure loops in place for each finger and thumb.
16. Apply straps to the wrist and forearm. When placing the orthosis on the person, position the staples on the dorsal side of the orthosis.

IP, Interphalangeal; *MCP,* metacarpophalangeal; *PIP,* proximal interphalangeal.

---

slits approximately ½ inch wide and 1 inch long between each of the fingers, leaving enough material distally to heat the area to allow a ³⁄₃₂-inch wire to be pushed into the material. The wire creates a bar to support the elastic between each finger. The elastic is woven through this part of the orthosis (Fig. 14.14).

Steps for fabricating a mobilization orthosis for radial nerve palsy can be found in the following procedure.

ULNAR NERVE INJURIES

Ulnar compression syndromes are the second most common upper extremity compression neuropathies.[71] An ulnar nerve lesion can occur in conjunction with a median nerve lesion[23] and can arise because of compression in many places throughout the extremity. Thoracic outlet syndrome (TOS) is sometimes initially considered as an ulnar nerve injury or a high-level median nerve injury because symptoms can resemble such nerve compressions.[55] Thus it is postulated that for TOS the concept of double crush applies with compression higher up in the arm making lower areas more susceptible to symptoms of nerve compression.[44] Compression with TOS can occur as the brachial plexus passes through the scalene muscles (scalene triangle) in the neck, between the clavicle and first rib (costoclavicular region), or underneath the pectoralis minor muscle (subcoracoid space) due to many reasons such as whiplash, posture, or repetitive motions.[44]

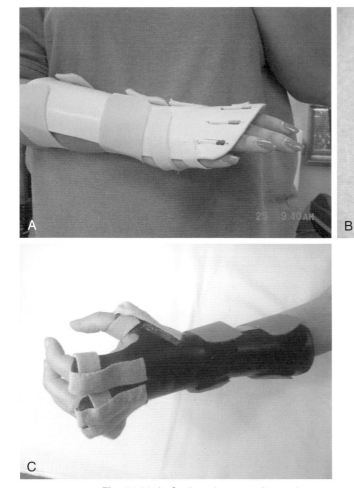

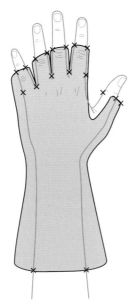

Fig. 14.14 A, Static wrist extension and metacarpophalangeal (MCP) mobilization extension orthosis for radial nerve palsy originally designed by Mark Walsh and Sue Blackmore. B and C, Adapted static wrist extension and MCP mobilization extension orthosis using moleskin and elastic finger loops.

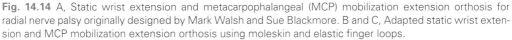

Fig. 14.15 Pattern for dorsal base of static wrist extension and metacarpophalangeal (MCP) mobilization extension orthosis. (Redrawn from Coppard, *Introduction to Orthotics*, 4th edition.)

Lesions to the **ulnar nerve** often result from a fracture of the medial epicondyle of the humerus, a fracture of the olecranon process of the ulna, or a laceration or ganglia at the wrist. Typically the site of ulnar nerve compression at the elbow is the epicondylar groove, or where the ulnar nerve courses between the two heads of the flexor carpi ulnaris muscle.[71]

Ulnar nerve compressions at the wrist level within the Guyon canal are less common.[37,71] Those that develop from downhill bike riding are also known as "cyclist or handle bar palsy."[37,58] The Guyon canal is a small tunnel, and it is also called the ulnar tunnel. It consists of several key structures on the ulnar side of the hand, including the roof–palmar carpal ligament, medial wall–pisiform bone, lateral wall–hook of hamate, and floor–transverse carpal ligament.[37] Symptoms can be motor or sensory depending on the location of the compression.[37] Wrist-level injuries usually result from compression because of the superficial nature of the ulnar nerve within the Guyon canal (see Table 14.1).[71]

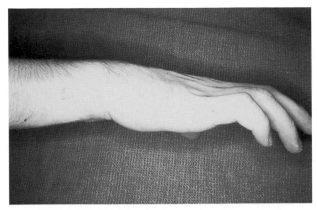

Fig. 14.16 A claw hand deformity caused by an ulnar nerve injury. (From Seftchick, J. L., Detullio, L. M., Fedorczk, J. M., et al. [2011]. Clinical examination of the hand. In T. M. Skirven, A. L. Osterman, J. M. Fedorczyk, et al. [Eds.], *Rehabilitation of the hand and upper extremity* [6th ed.]. Philadelphia, Elsevier. Photo by Mark Walsh, PT, DPT, MS, CHT, ATC.)

McGowan[49] developed a grading system for ulnar nerve conditions: grade I manifests with paresthesias and clumsiness, grade II exhibits interosseous weakness and some muscle wasting, and grade III involves paralysis of the ulnar intrinsic muscles. Ulnar nerve injuries at the elbow are classified as acute, subacute, or chronic.[71] Acute injuries result from trauma. Subacute injuries develop over time and involve continual elbow compression, such as a factory worker whose elbow is continuously positioned on a table while doing work. Both acute and subacute injuries respond to conservative interventions, such as reducing elbow flexion during tasks and/or orthotic intervention.

Chronic conditions require surgery, especially if daily living tasks are severely impacted.[71] Clinically a person with an ulnar nerve compression at the elbow (**cubital tunnel syndrome**) complains of discomfort on the medial side of the arm and numbness and tingling in digits 4 and 5.[36] Prolonged flexion and force from occupations or sports such as baseball and tennis are common causes of ulnar nerve compression and irritation.[26]

Regardless of the cause or location, if a deformity results from an ulnar lesion it is called a *claw hand*. Anatomically this deformity occurs because the MCP joints of the ring and little fingers are positioned in hyperextension. This position, which is more pronounced in lower-level ulnar nerve injuries,[68] occurs because the lumbricals and the intrinsic muscles responsible for interphalangeal (IP) extension are paralyzed.[8] The fourth and fifth digits are incapable of fully extending the PIP and distal interphalangeal (DIP) joints because of the unopposed action of the extensor digitorum communis and the extensor digiti minimi (Fig. 14.16). In the early stages of an ulnar nerve injury, a person may have difficulty performing ADLs and may experience hand fatigue. Muscle weakness is not usually evident until after the condition progresses.[71] Table 14.3 identifies the muscles that the ulnar nerve innervates in a low-level or wrist lesion and a high-level lesion that occurs at or above the elbow. If an ulnar nerve lesion occurs just distal to the elbow, the extrinsic muscles of the hand are lost because they are innervated distal

TABLE 14.3 **Ulnar Nerve Lesions**	
Affected Muscles	**Weak and Lost Motions**
Low Level (Wrist Level)	
Abductor digiti minimi	MCP abduction of the fifth digit
Flexor digiti minimi	MCP flexion of the fifth digit and opposition
Opponens digiti minimi	Opposition of the fifth digit
Lumbricals to the fourth and fifth digits	MCP finger flexion and IP extension to the fourth and fifth digits
Dorsal interossei	MCP abduction of the digits
Palmar interossei	MCP adduction of the digits
Flexor pollicis brevis (deep head)	MCP and CMC flexion of the thumb and opposition
Adductor pollicis	Adduction of the CMC joint and MCP flexion
High Level (At or Above the Elbow Level)	
Flexor carpi ulnaris	Wrist flexion and ulnar deviation
Flexor digitorum profundus of the fourth and fifth digits	Flexion of the DIP and PIP joints of the fourth and fifth digits
Abductor digiti minimi	MCP abduction of the fifth digit
Flexor digiti minimi	MCP flexion of the fifth digit and opposition
Opponens digiti minimi	Opposition of the fifth digit
Lumbricals to the fourth and fifth digits	MCP flexion and IP extension to the fourth and fifth digits
Dorsal interossei	MCP abduction of the digits
Palmar interossei	MCP adduction of the digits
Flexor pollicis brevis (deep head)	MCP and CMC flexion of the thumb and opposition
Adductor pollicis	Adduction of the CMC joint and MCP flexion

CMC, Carpometacarpal; *DIP*, distal interphalangeal; *IP*, interphalangeal; *MCP*, metacarpophalangeal.

to the elbow. At the wrist level, compression of the ulnar nerve in the distal part of the ulnar tunnel results in different functional effects based on the zone location of the nerve.[33,71]

Generally the functional result from a high- or low-level ulnar nerve lesion is loss of pinch and power grip strength.[11,25] The client is unable to grasp an object fully because of the denervation of the finger abductors, atrophy of the hypothenar eminence, inability to oppose the little finger to the thumb, and ineffective pinch with the thumb.[8,76] The loss of the first dorsal interosseous and the adductor pollicis leads to unstable pinching of the thumb and index finger.[8] Loss of lateral finger movements and diminished sensory feedback can affect functional occupational activities, such as typing on a computer[76] and other daily tasks. With a high lesion the loss of the flexor digitorum profundus of the ring and small fingers further compromises hand grasp.[11] In addition, the client presents with weakened wrist ulnar deviation.

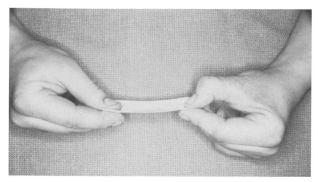

Fig. 14.17 Froments sign with flexion of the thumb IP joint and Jeanne's sign with hyperextension of the thumb MP joint. (From Seftchick, J. L., Detullio, L. M., Fedorczk, J. M., et al. [2011]. Clinical examination of the hand. In T. M. Skirven, A. L. Osterman, J. M. Fedorczyk, et al. [Eds.], *Rehabilitation of the hand and upper extremity* [6th ed.]. Philadelphia, Elsevier.) Photo by Mark Walsh, PT, DPT, MS, CHT, ATC.

Three abnormal postures can develop from ulnar nerve injuries: Froment sign,[10] Jeanne sign,[91] and Wartenberg sign.[57] The Froment sign functionally results in flexion of the thumb IP joint during pinching activities.[10] The Froment sign is apparent because the adductor pollicis, the deep head of the flexor pollicis brevis, and first dorsal interosseous muscle are not working. Because of these losses, performance of the fine dexterity tasks of daily living is remarkably affected. The Jeanne sign occurs with the advancement of ulnar nerve conditions. In addition to displaying a positive Froment sign, with Jeanne sign (Fig. 14.17) the MP joint of the thumb becomes hyperextended with pinch secondary to weakness of the flexor pollicis brevis muscle.[91] The Jeanne sign can be managed with a thumb orthosis placing the MP joint in a functional position with slight flexion to counterbalance the hyperextension.[39] The Wartenberg sign develops because of interossei weakness resulting in the fifth digit abducted from the other fingers.[57] Often, buddy taping the last two digits with Coban helps this interossei weakness.

The sensory distribution of the ulnar nerve typically innervates the little finger and the ulnar half of the ring finger on the volar and dorsal surfaces of the hand (see Fig. 14.5). Clients who have ulnar nerve compression can experience numbness, tingling, and paresthesia in this nerve distribution. When designing an orthosis for ulnar nerve lesions, the therapist monitors the areas of decreased sensation for pressure sores and skin irritation. Fig. 14.18 illustrates the muscles an ulnar nerve lesion affects.

Orthotic Interventions for Ulnar Nerve Injury

The client with an ulnar nerve injury benefits from orthotic intervention and a therapeutic program. There are several orthotic options for ulnar nerve injuries. Orthoses specific for diagnoses are discussed first, followed by various orthotic design options.

Orthotic Intervention for Ulnar Nerve Compression at the Elbow

A common intervention for compression at the cubital tunnel is an elbow orthosis with the elbow typically flexed 30 to

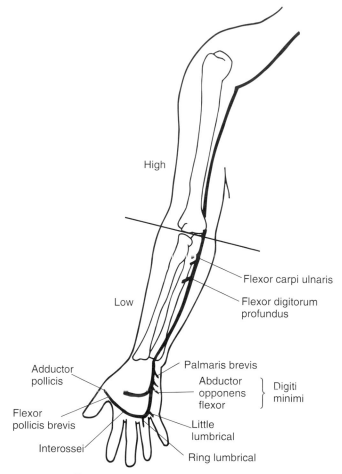

Fig. 14.18 Ulnar nerve motor innervation.

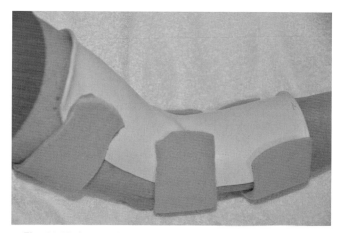

Fig. 14.19 An anterior-based elbow orthosis for cubital tunnel.

45 degrees[1,35] with a maximal flexed position of 70 degrees.[45] (Refer to Chapter 10 for elbow orthoses.) Fig. 14.19 illustrates an anterior elbow orthosis for cubital tunnel. Thermoplastic material with conformability and drapability works well for this anterior-based orthosis. Sometimes the wrist is included with the elbow design. The wrist is positioned in neutral to 20 degrees of extension. Incorporating the wrist into the orthotic design decreases the effects from flexor carpi ulnaris contraction[71] (Fig. 14.20).

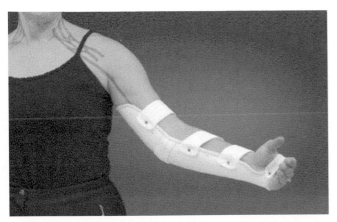

Fig. 14.20 A long arm orthosis for cubital tunnel that includes the hand and wrist. (From Lund, A. T., & Amadio, P. C. [2006]. Treatment of cubital tunnel syndrome: Perspectives for the therapist. *Journal of Hand Therapy, 19*[2], 174.)

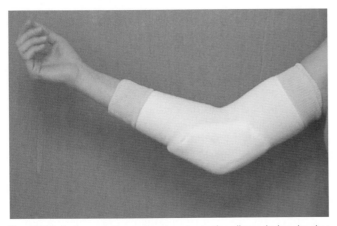

Fig. 14.21 A sleeve with a gel pad protects the elbow during the day. (From Porretto-Loehrke, A., & Soika, E. [2011]. Therapist's management of other nerve compressions about the elbow and wrist. In T. M. Skirven, A. L. Osterman, J. M. Fedorczyk, et al. [Eds.], *Rehabilitation of the hand and upper extremity* [6th ed., p. 702]. Philadelphia, Elsevier.)

The elbow orthosis helps prevent repetitive or prolonged elbow flexion. Prolonged elbow flexion can stress the ulnar nerve via traction[35,81] and increase pressure in the cubital tunnel.[48] This flexed position commonly occurs during sleep or with computer usage.[81] For sporadic or mild symptoms the elbow orthosis may be worn during the night for approximately 3 weeks.[6] If demonstrating dysthesia, decreased sensibility, and continuous symptoms, the client may wear the elbow orthosis all the time.[6,12,71] However, it is generally recommended that instead of daytime elbow orthosis wear, the patient is educated to avoid flexing the elbow and/or resting the elbow on a surface during activities. A sleeve with a gel pad (Heelbo pad) is an option for day protection (Fig. 14.21).[70]

Many therapists recommend a soft elbow orthosis for comfort. Commercial soft elbow orthoses allow some movement but limit flexion to less than 45 degrees. Fig. 14.22 provides options for commercial soft orthoses. Other options are pictured in Chapter 10. If finances are tight, simply securing a towel with the arm correctly positioned can work for comfort.[70]

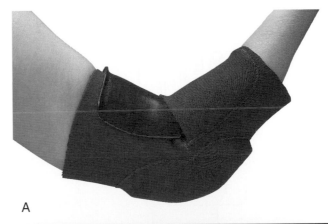

A

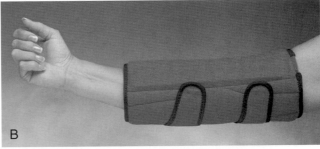

B

Fig. 14.22 Two prefabricated options for cubital tunnel. A, A soft pre-fabricated orthosis (IMAK ® Elbow Support). B, Comfort Cool ® Ulnar Nerve Elbow Orthosis. (Orthosis from North Coast Medical & Rehabilitation Products.)

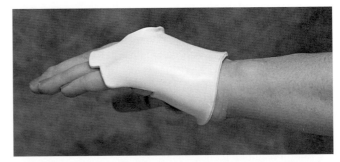

Fig. 14.23 The hand position for orthotic intervention of an ulnar nerve injury in a static orthosis.

Wrist- and Hand-Based Orthotic Intervention for Ulnar Nerve Injury

In recent published treatment guidelines for Guyon canal syndrome (based on a European Delphi consensus strategy), experts suggested a neutral wrist orthosis for nonsurgical treatment.[37] Another option for some ulnar nerve conditions, including Guyon canal syndrome, with potential for developing a claw deformity is a hand-based orthosis. The orthosis (Fig. 14.23) positions the ring and little fingers in 30 to 45 degrees of MCP flexion[11] as a counterforce to prevent a claw hand deformity.[11] Fig. 14.24 depicts the pattern for this orthosis. This position (30 to 45 degrees of MCP flexion) prevents attenuation of the denervated intrinsic muscles and the MCP volar plates of the ring and little fingers[18] and corrects the claw hand deformity of MCP hyperextension and PIP flexion. With the MCPs blocked in flexion, the power of the extensor digitorum communis is transferred to the IP joints

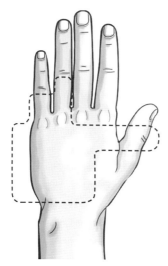

Fig. 14.24 A hand-based pattern for an ulnar nerve orthosis.

and allows them to extend in the absence of the intrinsic muscles. Ultimately, the orthosis facilitates functional grasp.[11] A client usually wears an immobilization orthosis continuously with removal only for hygiene and exercise. Some therapists recommend daytime use only.[66]

Colditz[18] suggests the fabrication of a less bulky orthosis to keep from impeding the palmar sensation and function of the hand. One such orthosis is the figure-eight orthotic designed by Kiyoshi Yasaki and developed at the Hand Rehabilitation Center in Philadelphia, Pennsylvania (Fig. 14.25).[11] The instructions in the following procedure include one method to fabricate a figure-eight hand-based orthosis for an ulnar nerve injury.

PROCEDURE FOR FABRICATION OF AN ORTHOSIS FOR ULNAR NERVE INJURY

1. Cut a ½-inch strip of thermoplastic material approximately 12 to 14 inches.
2. Heat the strip of thermoplastic material.
3. Position the arm with the elbow resting on a towel on a table and the hand in an upright position. Position the ring and small fingers in 30 to 45 degrees of MCP flexion. (IPs are in extension.)
4. Determine the midpoint of the strip, and place it midway between the ring and little fingers on the dorsal side of the fingers at the level of the MCP joints over the proximal phalanx.
5. Wrap one end of the strip around the ulnar side of the little finger to the volar surface and one end of the strip around the radial side of the ring finger to the volar (palmar) surface.
6. On the volar surface, cross straps (proximal to the MCP joints) over each other at the level of the metacarpals circling the ring and little finger.
7. Bring the straps back around to the dorsal surface proximal to the heads of the MCP joints. Overlap the straps approximately 1 inch, and adhere the pieces together.
8. Roll any areas that could interfere with function, such as rolling the area on the volar surface distal to the second and third digits and around the thenar crease.

IP, Interphalangeal; *MCP,* metacarpophalangeal.

Mobilization Orthoses for Ulnar Nerve Injuries

With a mobilizing (dynamic) orthosis, the therapist places the hand in the same position with the fourth and fifth digits in 30 to 45 degrees of MCP flexion. The therapist uses a mobilization orthotic design that includes finger loops attached to the ring and little fingers' proximal phalanges (Fig. 14.26). The rubber band is connected to a soft wrist cuff and uses traction to pull the two fingers into MCP flexion. The client wears the orthosis throughout the day with removal for hygiene and exercise. Physicians usually prescribe this type of orthosis when there is a need for a strong force to prevent hyperextension contractures at the MCP joints. To supplement this orthosis, a positioning (immobilization) nighttime orthosis may be necessary.

Another mobilization option for orthotic intervention of the ulnar nerve lesion is a spring-wire-and-foam orthosis, which is available commercially or can be custom made. Clients appreciate the low-profile design of the spring-wire-and-foam orthosis, and adherence tends to be high.[79]

MEDIAN NERVE LESIONS

Traumatic median nerve lesions result from humeral fractures, elbow dislocations, distal radius fractures, dislocations of the lunate into the carpal canal, and lacerations of the volar wrist.[11] The median nerve innervates the muscles depicted in Fig. 14.27 (Table 14.4) in a low-level or wrist lesion and a high-level lesion involving the elbow or neck area.

Functional Implications of Median Nerve Injuries

The impact on function from a median nerve lesion results in clumsiness with pinch and a decrease in power hand grip.[8] Power grip is affected because the thumb is no longer a stabilizing force due to the loss of the abductor pollicis brevis, flexor pollicis brevis, and the opponens pollicis. Weakness in the lumbricals of the index and middle fingers further affects skilled movements of the hand.[7] The sensory areas innervated by the median nerve are used for identifying objects, temperature, and texture.[3] With lack of sensation in the fingers, skilled functions are difficult to perform with the hand.

Locations and Types of Median Nerve Injuries

The classic deformity associated with low-level median nerve damage is called an *ape* (or *simian*) *hand* because the thenar eminence appears flattened due to denervation. A loss of thumb opposition occurs (Fig. 14.28). The thumb is positioned in extension and adduction next to the index finger because of the unopposed action of the extensor pollicis longus and the adductor pollicis.[8] The thumb web space may contract, and the fingers may show trophic changes. In addition, a slight claw deformity of the index and middle fingers may occur because of the loss of lumbrical innervation.[76]

The most common type of lower-level median nerve compression is carpal tunnel syndrome (CTS). Compression

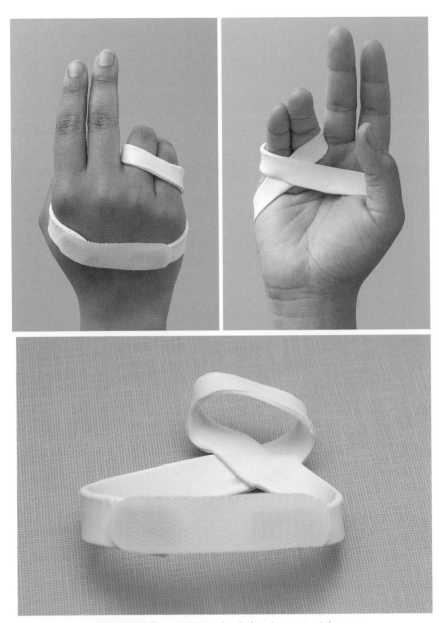

Fig. 14.25 Figure-eight orthosis for ulnar nerve injury.

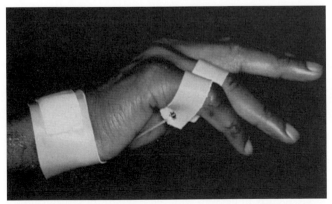

Fig. 14.26 A flexion mobilization orthosis for an ulnar nerve injury. (From Colditz, J. C. [2002]. Splinting the hand with a peripheral nerve injury. In E. J. Mackin, A. D. Callahan, T. M. Skirven, et al. [Eds.], *Rehabilitation of the hand and upper extremity* [5th ed., pp. 622–634]. St. Louis, MO: Mosby.)

at the wrist occurs because of a discrepancy in the volume of the rigid carpal canal and its contents, consisting of the median nerve and flexor tendons. Some conditions (such as, diabetes, pregnancy, Dupuytren disease, and carpometacarpal [CMC] arthritis) are associated with CTS. Home, leisure, and occupational activities involving repetitive or sustained wrist flexion, extension, and ulnar deviation; forearm supination; forceful gripping; and pinching all contribute to the development and exacerbation of CTS. Vibration, cold temperatures, and constriction over the wrist can also be contributing factors.[4,24,64,78]

Higher lesions can weaken or impair forearm pronation, wrist flexion, thumb IP flexion, and flexion of the proximal and distal IP joints of the index and middle fingers. Compression syndromes that occur from higher median nerve injuries are pronator syndrome and anterior interosseous syndrome. Pronator syndrome often results from strong

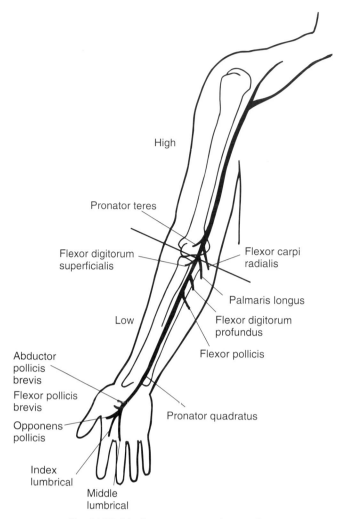

High

Pronator teres

Flexor digitorum
superficialis

Flexor carpi
radialis

Palmaris longus

Low

Flexor digitorum
profundus

Flexor pollicis

Abductor
pollicis
brevis

Flexor pollicis
brevis

Pronator quadratus

Opponens
pollicis

Index
lumbrical

Middle
lumbrical

Fig. 14.27 Median nerve motor innervation.

TABLE 14.4	**Median Nerve Lesions**
Affected Muscles	**Weak and Lost Motions**
Low Level (Wrist Level)	
Abductor pollicis brevis	Abduction of the CMC and MCP joints of the thumb, weak extension of the IP joint, and opposition
Flexor pollicis brevis (superficial head)	Flexion of the MCP and CMC joints and opposition
Opponens pollicis	Thumb opposition
First and second lumbricals	IP extension and MCP flexion of the second and third digits
High Level (Elbow or Neck Level)	
Flexor pollicis longus	IP thumb flexion and weakness with flexion of the MCP and CMC joints
Lateral half of the flexor digitorum profundus to the second and third digits	DIP and PIP flexion of the second and third digits
Pronator quadratus	Forearm pronation
Pronator teres	Forearm pronation and elbow flexion
Flexor carpi radialis	Flexion and radial deviation of the wrist
Palmaris longus	Wrist flexion
Flexor digitorum superficialis	Flexion of the PIP joints second through fifth digits and weak flexion of the MCP joints and wrist flexion
Abductor pollicis brevis	Abduction of the CMC and MCP joints of the thumb, weak extension of the IP joint, and opposition
Flexor pollicis brevis (superficial head)	Flexion of the MCP and CMC joints and opposition
Opponens pollicis	Thumb opposition
First and second lumbricals	IP extension and MCP flexion of the second and third digits

CMC, Carpometacarpal; *DIP,* distal interphalangeal; *IP,* interphalangeal; *MCP,* metacarpophalangeal; *PIP,* proximal interphalangeal.

and repetitive pronation and supination motions, with the most common compression site between the two heads of the pronator teres.[61] Anterior interosseous syndrome is rare and is characterized by a vague discomfort in the proximal forearm. It usually involves compression of the deep head of the pronator teres and results in a motor rather than sensory injury. Clinically the person presents with an inability to make an O with the thumb and index finger because usually there are no sensory losses with this condition.[61]

Because median nerve injuries occur throughout the extremity, it is possible that a person is mistakenly thought to have one type of median nerve injury when he or she has another. Therefore, the astute therapist carefully considers the symptoms present for each person. For example, a person may have pronator syndrome instead of CTS if:[61,72,74]

- Pain is experienced with resisted pronation and passive supination activities
- A positive Tinel sign at the proximal forearm is present
- Tenderness of the pronator muscle is evident
- "Numbness in the thenar eminence in the distribution of the palmar cutaneous branch of the median nerve" is present[72]
- Nocturnal symptoms are absent
- Muscle fatigue is present

- Thenar atrophy is absent
- Phalen test is negative

CTS is a likely diagnosis for persons who have complaints of night pain, symptoms with repetitive wrist movements (especially flexion), weakness in thumb opposition and abduction, a positive Phalen test, and a positive Tinel sign at the wrist.[74] If a person is referred with a diagnosis of CTS and has symptoms of pronator syndrome, it is recommended that the therapist call the referring physician and discusses examination findings.

Frequently in persons with these syndromes, surgical procedures are required to decompress the nerve.[7] On occasion a physician may request an orthosis for conservative management of mild cases. For example, for a mild case of **pronator tunnel syndrome** the physician may prescribe an elbow

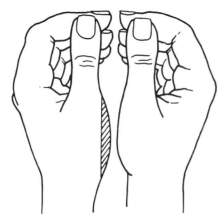

Fig. 14.28 The classic median nerve deformity called an *ape* (or *simian*) *hand*. Note thenar muscle atrophy of the left hand.

TABLE 14.5 Orthotic Interventions for Peripheral Nerve Lesions

Orthosis	Position
Radial	
Wrist immobilization orthosis	Wrist in 30 to 40 degrees of extension
Mobilization dorsal-based MCP extension orthosis	Wrist in 30 to 40 degrees of extension; MCPs in dynamic extension
Tenodesis orthosis (described by Colditz) (Other options for radial nerve orthotic provision are listed within the chapter)	Dorsal base using the tenodesis effect with MCPs in dynamic extension
Low-profile radial nerve palsy orthosis with radial and ulnar deviation	Wrist in 20 to 30 degrees of extension and MCPs in neutral
Low-profile radial nerve palsy orthosis	Wrist in 10 to 20 degrees of extension and MCPs positioned in neutral
Ulnar	
Elbow orthosis	Elbow in 30 to 45 degrees of flexion
Hand-based immobilization anticlaw orthosis	MCPs of fourth and fifth digits in 30 to 45 degrees of MCP flexion
Median	
Dorsal- or volar-based wrist orthosis	Wrist in neutral, MCPs may be included
Ulnar gutter wrist orthosis	Wrist in neutral
Thumb web spacer orthosis or C bar orthosis	Thumb in 40 to 45 degrees of palmar abduction

MCP, Metacarpophalangeal.

orthosis to position the forearm in neutral between pronation and supination and the elbow in flexion (Table 14.5).[10] This elbow position takes tension off the nerve, and the forearm position prevents compression via pronator contraction or stretch.

The median nerve's classic course and sensory distribution include the volar surface of the thumb, index, middle, and radial half of the ring fingers and the dorsal surface of the distal phalanxes of the thumb, index, middle, and radial half of the ring finger (see Fig. 14.5). Clients who have median nerve compression can experience numbness, tingling, and paresthesia in this nerve distribution. Because the area of sensory distribution is large, the therapist monitors and educates clients or caregivers about the associated risks and prevention of skin injury or breakdown.

Orthotic Interventions for Median Nerve Injuries

Understanding the functional effects of the muscular loss resulting from a median nerve injury or compression syndrome is important because it influences the therapist's orthotic provision. With a median nerve lesion, if the therapist can maintain good passive mobility of the joints, extensive orthotic intervention may be unnecessary, and occasional night orthotic intervention may be sufficient.[25]

Orthotic Intervention for Pronator Syndrome

Clients with pronator syndrome should avoid resisted pronation and passive supination.[74] Other than changing activities that contribute to pronator syndrome, the person may benefit from orthotic intervention. One orthotic option is to place the elbow in 90 degrees flexion and forearm in neutral rotation.[85]

Orthotic Intervention for Anterior Interosseous Nerve Compression

Besides the suggestion to avoid elbow extension and extreme forearm pronation and supination, orthotic intervention options are recommended for anterior interosseous nerve compressions. One option is to immobilize the elbow in 90 degrees flexion and the forearm in neutral. As discussed, impairments to the anterior interosseous nerve result in difficulty making an O with the thumb and index finger flexed. To compensate for this deficit, the therapist fabricates a small thermoplastic orthosis to block thumb IP and index DIP extension (Fig. 14.29).[17]

Orthotic Intervention for Carpal Tunnel Syndrome

When manifestations of CTS are primarily sensory and occur from overuse or occupational causes, orthotic intervention of the wrist often reduces pain and symptoms.[7] To accompany the orthotic intervention program for CTS, include interventions as follows: ergonomic adaptations for home, leisure, and work environments; education on prevention; activity modifications; range-of-motion program with emphasis on tendon gliding exercises; and edema control techniques.[75] See Chapter 7 for an overview of efficacy studies on orthoses with carpal tunnel intervention.

Usually, any orthosis for CTS positions the wrist as close to neutral as possible.[62] This neutral position maximizes available carpal tunnel space, minimizes median

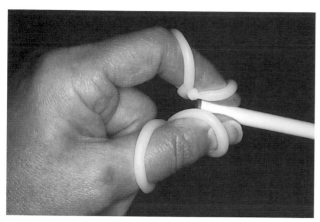

Fig. 14.29 To encourage fingertip to thumb prehension, these small orthoses help someone with anterior interosseus nerve palsy. (From Colditz, J. C. [2002]. Splinting the hand with a peripheral nerve injury. In E. J. Mackin, A. D. Callahan, T. M. Skirven, et al. [Eds.], *Rehabilitation of the hand and upper extremity* [5th ed., pp 622–634]. St. Louis, MO: Mosby.)

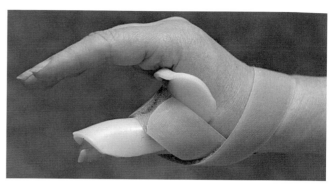

Fig. 14.30 A thumb web spacer for median nerve injuries.

nerve compression, and facilitates pain relief.[43,55] A newer approach to wrist immobilization orthotic design includes the MCP joints to decrease pressure in the carpal tunnel (see Chapter 7). A wrist immobilization orthosis is commonly worn at night and sometimes during home, leisure, or work activities that involve repetitive stressful wrist movements.[63] As discussed in Chapter 7, the wearing schedule can vary. Minimally, nighttime wear is required[63] to prevent extreme wrist flexion postures that often occur during sleep.[75] Immobilization orthotic intervention with CTS has shown to improve long-term nerve conduction outcomes when consistently worn every night.[82] The wearing schedule is carefully monitored to prevent weakening of the muscles as a result of inactivity.[55] The orthosis may exacerbate symptoms if the person fights against the orthosis.[79]

Volar Wrist Immobilization Orthosis

Some clients and therapists prefer volar wrist orthoses, which provide adequate support to the wrist. A volar wrist orthosis with a gel sheet or elastomer putty insert may be beneficial to control scar formation after carpal tunnel release surgery. A disadvantage of the volar wrist orthotic design for CTS is that the orthosis may interfere with palmar sensation.[7] Positioning the wrist in the orthosis is important. A poorly designed wrist orthosis may compress the carpal tunnel area of the wrist. Some people may benefit from a volar wrist orthosis because it also immobilizes the MCP joints (see Chapter 7).

Dorsal or Ulnar Gutter Wrist Immobilization Orthoses

Other orthotic intervention approaches for CTS include fabrication of a dorsal, ulnar gutter, or circumferential wrist orthosis. An advantage of the dorsal wrist orthosis is that there is no thermoplastic material directly over the carpal tunnel, thus avoiding compression as well as no interference with palmar sensation. However, a disadvantage of the dorsal wrist orthosis is that it may not provide as much support and/

or distribute pressure as well as the volar wrist orthosis. Some therapists fabricate the dorsal orthosis with a larger palmar area to increase support. An ulnar gutter wrist orthosis positions the wrist in neutral and is less likely to compress the carpal tunnel. A circumferential wrist orthosis provides a high degree of wrist immobilization (see Chapter 7).

Some clients may be more comfortable with soft prefabricated wrist orthoses that are appropriately sized based on manufacturer recommendations. The therapist must check the orthosis on the client to ensure a correct fit for function and preservation of hand structures based on clinical reasoning.[2] (Refer to Chapter 7 for ideas for prefabricated orthoses.) Clients are educated to avoid pulling the strapping too tightly to avoid inadvertent compression of the median nerve.

Orthotic Intervention for Median Nerve Injuries With Thumb Involvement

For a client who has a median nerve injury involving the thumb, which occurs in the later stages of CTS, the therapist addresses loss of thumb opposition for functional grasp and pinch. The orthosis positions the thumb in opposition and palmar abduction, which assists the thumb for tip prehension. A C bar between the thumb and the index finger helps maintain the thumb web space. The thumb web space is a common site for muscular shortening of the adductor pollicis after median nerve damage. The orthotic design is usually static. A person with a median nerve injury with thumb involvement may benefit from a hand-based thumb orthosis (see Chapter 8).

For a low-level median nerve injury the therapist may fabricate a thumb web spacer orthosis constructed from thermoplastic material or out of other materials, such as out of Neoprene. Prefabricated orthoses that position the thumb can also be provided (Fig. 14.30).

Orthotic Intervention for Combined Median and Ulnar Nerve Injuries

Sometimes with extensive low-level injuries, both median and ulnar nerves are involved and clawing is evident in all fingers due to intrinsic weakness and the loss of the flexor digitorum profundus. In such cases, orthotic intervention to prevent further deformities entails designs that are for a singular nerve injury but with all digits included. The thumb may be incorporated if it is affected (Fig. 14.31).

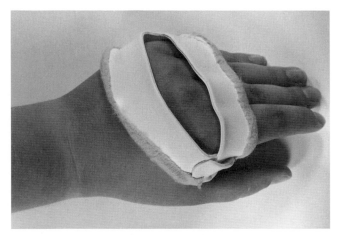

Fig. 14.31 This orthosis inhibits metacarpophalangeal (MCP) extension with a combined median and ulnar nerve. (From Fess, E. E., Gettle, K. S., Philips, C. A., et al. [2005]. *Hand and upper extremity splinting: Principles and methods* [3rd ed.]. St. Louis, MO: Elsevier Mosby.)

SUMMARY

There are various orthotic interventions with general guidelines to consider for nerve injuries. Orthotic intervention for nerve injuries involves comprehensive knowledge of the muscular, sensory, and functional implications for each client.

The therapist must note that there are general guidelines and physicians and experienced therapists may have other protocols for positioning and orthotic intervention.

⚡ PATIENT SAFETY TIPS AND PRECAUTIONS BOX

- Be aware of natural reactions to a nerve injury, including skin changes, muscle imbalance with possible deformity and joint contracture, and circulatory changes such as cold skin.
- Teach patients to regularly inspect their skin, especially with median/ulnar nerve injuries because of sensory loss.
- Avoid heavy lifting or resistance, as well as forceful or repetitive motions.
- Pay attention to potential pressure areas from the orthosis, and pad or push out thermoplastic material over any sensitive areas.
- Pay attention to cleaning the orthosis and wound care management.
- Do not neglect nail care despite orthotic intervention.
- Be aware of protecting versus overprotection. Overprotection of injury while wearing the orthosis may cause decreased motion and put the client at further risk for contractures or deformity.
- Be aware of substitution motions, which are a normal reaction after a nerve injury to protect and decrease pain. These unnatural movements may cause further harm to a recovering nerve and put the client at risk for muscle imbalance.

REVIEW QUESTIONS

1. Which factors are important in the prognosis of a peripheral nerve lesion?
2. What are the common deformities resulting from radial, ulnar, and median nerve lesions?
3. What are the functional implications of radial, ulnar, and median nerve lesions?
4. What are the orthotic intervention options for radial nerve injuries? In which position should the therapist place the hand?
5. What is the proper type, position, and thermoplastic material needed for fabrication of an orthosis for ulnar nerve compression at the elbow?
6. What is the proper orthotic position for a claw hand deformity? Why is this a good position?
7. What are the advantages and disadvantages of the different approaches to wrist orthotic intervention for CTS?
8. What is the appropriate position in which to place a hand with a median nerve lesion that includes thumb symptoms?

👤 SELF-QUIZ 14.1ᵃ

For the following questions, circle either true (T) or false (F).

1. T F With neurapraxia, the prognosis is extremely good because recovery is usually spontaneous.
2. T F Functionally a client diagnosed with a radial nerve injury has a poor grip because of wrist positioning.
3. T F The main purpose of orthotic intervention for a nerve injury is to immobilize the extremity.
4. T F The claw hand deformity is more pronounced with a low-level ulnar nerve injury.
5. T F The therapist should position an elbow orthosis in 110 degrees of flexion for a client who has an ulnar nerve compression at the elbow level.
6. T F For an ulnar nerve orthosis the therapist should position the ring and little fingers in approximately 30 to 45 degrees of MCP flexion.
7. T F An option for orthotic provision for radial nerve injuries is a wrist or hand immobilization orthosis for nighttime use and a mobilization orthosis that places the wrist in extension and the MCPs in neutral extension.
8. T F The therapist should immobilize radial, ulnar, and median nerve injuries only in static orthoses.
9. T F The Froment, Jeanne, and Wartenberg signs are postures indicative of median nerve injuries.
10. T F Functionally a client diagnosed with an ulnar nerve injury has loss of pinch strength and power grip.
11. T F The therapist may use a thumb web spacer orthosis for a median nerve injury.
12. T F Low-level nerve injuries occur only distal to the wrist.

ᵃSee Appendix A for the answer key.

👤 SELF-QUIZ 14.2ᵃ

Match the following nerve conditions with the appropriate upper extremity positions required for conservative orthotic intervention.

1. Ulnar tunnel syndrome
2. Pronator syndrome
3. Anterior interosseous syndrome
4. Radial tunnel syndrome
5. Posterior interosseous nerve syndrome
6. Cubital tunnel syndrome
7. Wartenberg neuropathy
8. Carpal tunnel syndrome (CTS)
   a. 90 degrees elbow flexion and neutral forearm and/or a small orthosis to block index DIP and thumb IP extension or hyperextension
   b. 30 to 45 degrees MCP flexion of the fourth and fifth digits
   c. 20 to 30 degrees wrist extension
   d. 30 to 40 degrees wrist extension and neutral MCP extension
   e. 30 to 45 degrees elbow flexion
   f. 90 degrees elbow flexion and neutral forearm
   g. Slight wrist extension
   h. Neutral wrist

ᵃSee Appendix A for the answer key.

REFERENCES

1. Aiello B: Ulnar nerve compression in cubital tunnel. In Clark GL, Shaw EF, Aiello WB, et al.: *Hand rehabilitation: a practical guide*, New York, 1993, Churchill Livingstone.
2. Apfel E, Sigafoos GT: Comparison of range-of-motion constraints provided by splints used in the treatment of cubital tunnel syndrome: a pilot study, *J Hand Ther* 19(4):384–392, 2006.
3. Arsham NZ: Nerve injury. In Ziegler EM, editor: *Current concepts in orthotics: a diagnosis-related approach to splinting*, Germantown, WI, 1984, Rolyan Medical Products.
4. Barnhart S, Demers PA, Miller M, et al.: Carpal tunnel syndrome among ski manufacturing workers, *Scand J Work Environ Health* 17(1):46–52, 1991.
5. Barr NR, Swan D: *The hand: principles and techniques of splint-making*, Boston, 1988, Butterworth Publishers.
6. Blackmore SM: Therapist's management of ulnar nerve neuropathy at the elbow. In Mackin EJ, Callahan AD, Skirven TM, et al.: *Rehabilitation of the hand*, 5th ed., St. Louis, 2002, Mosby, pp 679–689.
7. Borucki S, Schmidt J: Peripheral neuropathies. In Aisen ML, editor: *Orthotics in neurologic rehabilitation*, New York, 1992, Demos Publications.
8. Boscheinen-Morrin J, Davey V, Conolly WB: Peripheral nerve injuries (including tendon transfers). In Boscheinen-Morrin J, Davey V, Conolly WB, editors: *The hand: fundamentals of therapy*, Boston, 1987, Butterworth Publishers.
9. Bulut T, Akgun U, Citlak A, et al.: Prognostic factors in sensory recovery after digital nerve repair, *Acta Orthop Traumatol Turc* 50(2):157–161, 2016.
10. Cailliet R: *Hand pain and impairment*, 4th ed., Philadelphia, 1994, FA Davis.
11. Callahan A: Nerve injuries. In Malick MH, Kasch MC, editors: *Manual on management of specific hand problems*, Pittsburgh, 1984, American Rehabilitation Educational Network.
12. Cannon NM, editor: *Diagnosis and treatment manual for physicians and therapists*, 3rd ed., Indianapolis, 1991, The Hand Rehabilitation Center of Indiana.
13. Cantero-Téllez R, Gómez-Martínez M, Labrador-Toribio C: Effects on upper-limb function with dynamic and static orthosis use for radial nerve injury: a randomized trial, *J Neurol Disord* 4(2):264, 2016, https://doi.org/10.4172/2329-6895.1000264.
14. Cederna PS: Peripheral nerve injury. In Jebson PJL, Kasdan ML, editors: *Hand secrets*, 3rd ed., Philadelphia, 1998, Hanley & Belfus.
15. Clarkson HM, Gilewich GB: *Musculoskeletal assessment: joint range of motion and manual muscle strength*, Baltimore, 1989, Williams & Wilkins.
16. Cohen MS, Garfin SR: Nerve compression syndromes: finding the cause of upper-extremity symptoms, *Consultant* 37:241–254, 1997.
17. Colditz JC: Splinting for radial nerve palsy, *J Hand Ther* 1:18–23, 1987.
18. Colditz JC: Splinting the hand with a peripheral nerve injury. In Mackin EJ, Callahan AD, Skirven TM, et al.: *Rehabilitation of the hand*, 5th ed., St. Louis, 2002, Mosby, pp 622–634.
19. Crochetiere WJ, Goldstein SA, Granger GV, et al.: The Granger orthosis for radial nerve palsy, *Orthot Prosthet* 29(4):27–31, 1975.
20. Dang AC, Roder CM: Unusual compression neuropathies of the forearm, part I: radial nerve, *J Hand Surg* 34(10):1906–1914, 2009.
21. Duff S, Estilow T: Therapists' management of peripheral nerve injury. In Skirven TM, Osterman AL, Fedorczyk JM, et al.: *Rehabilitation of the hand and upper extremity*, 6th ed., Philadelphia, 2011, Elsevier/Mosby.
22. Eaton CJ, Lister GD: Radial nerve compression, *Hand Clin* 8(2):345–357, 1992.
23. Enna CD: *Peripheral denervation of the hand*, New York, 1988, Alan R. Liss.
24. Feldman RG, Travers PH, Chirico-Post J, et al.: Risk assessment in electronic assembly workers: carpal tunnel syndrome, *J Hand Surg Am* 12(5):849–855, 1987.
25. Fess EE: Rehabilitation of the patient with peripheral nerve injury, *Hand Clin* 2(1):207–215, 1986.
26. Fess EE, Gettle KS, Philips CA, et al.: *Hand splinting principles and methods*, 3rd ed., St. Louis, 2005, Elsevier Mosby.
27. Fox IK, Mackinnon SE: Adult peripheral nerve disorders: nerve entrapment, repair, transfer, and brachial plexus disorders, *Plast Reconstr Surg* 127(5):105e–118e, 2011.
28. Frykman GK: The quest for better recovery from peripheral nerve injury: current status of nerve regeneration research, *J Hand Ther* 6(2):83–88, 1993.
29. Gaudin R, Knipfer C, Henningsen A, et al.: Approaches to peripheral nerve repair: generations of biomaterial conduits yielding to replacing autologous nerve grafts in cranio-maxillofacial surgery, *BioMed Res Int*, 2016. https://doi.org/10.1155/2016/3856262.
30. Gelberman RH, Eaton R, Urbanisk JR: Peripheral nerve compression, *J Bone Joint Surg Am* 75:1854–1878, 1993.
31. Griffin JW, Hogan MV, Chhabra AB, Deal DN: Peripheral nerve repair and reconstruction, *J Bone Joint Surg Am* 95(23):2144–2151, 2013.
32. Grinsell D, Keating CP: Peripheral nerve reconstruction after injury: a review of clinical and experimental therapies, *BioMed Res Int*, 2014. https://doi.org/10.1155/2014/698256.
33. Gross MS, Gelberman RH: The anatomy of the distal ulnar tunnel, *Clin Orthop Relat Res* 196:238–247, 1985.
34. Hannah SD, Hudak PL: Splinting and radial nerve palsy: a single-subject experiment, *J Hand Ther* 14(3):195–201, 2001.
35. Harper BD: The drop-out splint: an alternative to the conservative management of ulnar nerve entrapment at the elbow, *J Hand Ther* 3:199–210, 1990.
36. Hong CZ, Long HA, Kanakamedala V, et al.: Splinting and local steroid injection for the treatment of ulnar neuropathy at the elbow: clinical and electrophysiological evaluation, *Arch Phys Med Rehabil* 77(6):573–576, 1996.
37. Hoogvliet P, Coert JH, Friden J, et al.: How to treat Guyon's canal syndrome? Results from the European handguide study: a multidisciplinary treatment guideline, *Br J Sports Med* 47(17):1063–1070, 2013.
38. Culp Hornbach: Radial tunnel syndrome. In Mackin EJ, Callahan AD, Skirven TM, et al.: *Rehabilitation of the hand*, 5th ed., St. Louis, 2002, Mosby.
39. Jacobs ML: Peripheral nerve injuries. In Jacobs MA, Uastin NM, editors: *Orthotic Intervention for the Hand and Upper Extremity*, 3rd ed., Philadelphia, 2014, Lippincott Williams & Wilkins.
40. Jacoby SM, Eichenbaum MD, Osterman AL: Basic science of nerve compressions. In Skirven TM, Osterman AL, Fedorczyk JM, et al.: *Rehabilitation of the hand and upper extremity*, 6th ed., Philadelphia, 2011, Elsevier Mosby, pp 649–656.

41. Jebson PJL, Gaul JS: Peripheral nerve injury. In Jebson PJL, Kasdan ML, editors: *Hand secrets*, Philadelphia, 1998, Hanley & Belfus.

42. Kleinert MJ, Mehta S: Radial nerve entrapment, *Orthop Clin North Am* 27(2):305–315, 1996.

43. Kruger VL, Kraft GH, Deitz JC, et al.: Carpal tunnel syndrome: objective measures and splint use, *Arch Phys Med Rehabil* 72(7):517–520, 1991.

44. Lucy L, Anthony MS: Thoracic outlet syndrome. In Saunders RJ, Astifidis RP, Burke SL, et al.: *Hand and upper extremity rehabilitation: a practical guide*, 4th ed., St. Louis, 2016, Elsevier.

45. Lund AT, Amadio PC: Treatment of cubital tunnel syndrome: perspectives for the therapist, *J Hand Ther* 19(2):170–179, 2007.

46. Lundborg G, Rosen B: Hand function after nerve repair, *Acta Physiol* 189(2):207–217, 2007.

47. Mackinnon SE, Dellon AL: *Surgery of the peripheral nerve*, New York, 1988, Thieme Medical Publishers, Inc.

48. MacNicol MF: Mechanics of the ulnar nerve at the elbow, *J Bone Joint Surg Br* 62(53):518, 1980.

49. McGowan AJ: The results of transposition of the ulnar nerve for traumatic ulnar neuritis, *J Bone Joint Surg Br* 23:293–301, 1950.

50. McKee P, Nguyen C: Customized dynamic splinting: orthoses that promote optimal function and recovery after radial nerve injury: a case report, *J Hand Ther* 20:73–88, 2007.

51. McKee P, Nguyen C: Low-profile dorsal dynamic wrist-finger-thumb-assistive-extension orthosis for high radial nerve injury-fabrication instructions, *J Hand Ther* 20:70–72, 2007.

52. Meek MF, Coert JH: Clinical use of nerve conduits in peripheral-nerve repair: review of the literature, *J Reconstr Microsurg* 18(2):97–109, 2002.

53. Melhorn JM: Cumulative trauma disorders and repetitive strain injuries: the future, *Clin Orthop Relat Res* 351:107–126, 1998.

54. Menorca RMG, Fussell TS, Elfar JC: Nerve physiology: mechanisms of injury and recovery, *Hand Clin* 29(3):317–330, 2013.

55. Messer RS, Bankers RM: Evaluating and treating common upper extremity nerve compression and tendonitis syndromes …without becoming cumulatively traumatized, *Nurse Pract Forum* 6(3):152–166, 1995.

56. Moore AM, Novak CB: Advances in nerve transfer surgery, *J Hand Ther* 27(2):96–104, 2014.

57. Moscony AMB: Peripheral nerve problems. In Cooper C, editor: *Fundamentals of hand therapy: clinical reasoning and treatment guidelines for common diagnoses of the upper extremity*, 2nd ed., London, 2014, Elsevier.

58. Neal S, Fields KB: Peripheral nerve entrapment and injury in the upper extremity, *Am Fam Physician* 81(2):147–155, 2010.

59. Novak CB, Mackinnon SE: Nerve injury in repetitive motion disorders, *Clin Orthop Relat Res* 351:10–20, 1998.

60. Novak CB, Mackinnon SE: Evaluation of nerve injury and nerve compression in the upper quadrant, *J Hand Ther* 18:230–240, 2005.

61. Nuber GW, Assenmacher J, Bowen MK: Neurovascular problems in the forearm, wrist, and hand, *Clin Sports Med* 17(3):585–610, 1998.

62. Nuckols T, Harber P, Sandin K, et al.: Quality measures for the diagnosis and non-operative management of carpal tunnel syndrome in occupational settings, *J Occup Rehabil* 21(1):100–119, 2011.

63. Ono S, Chapham PJ, Chung KC: Optimal management of carpal tunnel syndrome, *Int J Gen Med* 3:235–261, 2010.

64. Ostorio AM, Ames RG, Jones J, et al.: Carpal tunnel syndrome among grocery store workers, *Am J Int Med* 25:229–245, 1994.

65. Pabari A, Lloyd-Hughes H, Seifalian AM: Nerve conduits for peripheral nerve surgery, *Plast Reconstr Surg* 133(6), 2014. 1420–1430.

66. Peck J: *Personal communication*, March 2013.

67. Peck J, Ollason J: Low profile radial nerve palsy orthosis with radial and ulnar deviation, *J Hand Ther* 28(4):421–424, 2015.

68. Pfaeffle HJ, Waitayawinyu T, Trumble TE: Ulnar nerve laceration and repair, *Hand Clin* 23(3):291–299, 2007.

69. Pitts G, Umansky SC, Foister RD: Radial nerve compression. In Saunders RJ, Astifidis RP, Burke SL, et al.: *Hand and upper extremity rehabilitation: a practical guide*, 4th ed., St. Louis, 2016, Elsevier.

70. Porretto-Loehrke A, Soika E: Therapist's management of other nerve compressions about the elbow and wrist. In Skirven TM, Osterman AL, Fedorczyk JM, et al.: *Rehabilitation of the hand and upper extremity*, 6th ed., Philadelphia, 2011, Mosby.

71. Possner MA: Compressive neuropathies of the ulnar nerve at the elbow and wrist, *Instr Course Lect* 49:305–317, 2000.

72. Rehak DC: Pronator syndrome, *Clin Sports Med* 20(3):531–540, 2001.

73. Rosen B, Lundborg G: Sensory reeducation. In Skirven TM, Osterman AL, Fedorczyk JM, et al.: *Rehabilitation of the hand and upper extremity*, 6th ed., Philadelphia, 2011, Elsevier/Mosby, pp 634–645.

74. Saidoff DC, McDonough AL: *Critical pathways in therapeutic intervention: upper extremities*, St. Louis, 1997, Mosby.

75. Sailer SM: The role of splinting and rehabilitation, *Hand Clin* 12(2):223–240, 1996.

76. Salter MI: *Hand injuries: a therapeutic approach*, Edinburgh, London, 1987, Churchill Livingstone.

77. Scholz T, Krichevsky A, Sumarto A, et al.: Peripheral nerve injuries: an international survey of current treatments and future perspectives, *J Reconstr Microsurg* 25(6):339–344, 2009.

78. Schottland JR, Kirschberg GJ, Fillingim R, et al.: Median nerve latencies in poultry processing workers: an approach to resolving the role of industrial "cumulative trauma" in the development of carpal tunnel syndrome, *J Occup Med* 33(5):627–631, 1991.

79. Schultz-Johnson K: *Personal communication*, October 1999.

80. Seddon HJ: Three types of nerve injury, *J Neurol* 66:237–288, 1943.

81. Seror P: Treatment of ulnar nerve palsy at the elbow with a night splint, *J Bone Joint Surg Br* 75(2):322–327, 1993.

82. Sevim S, Dogu O, Camdeviren H, et al.: Long-term effectiveness of steroid injections and splinting in mild and moderate carpal tunnel syndrome, *Neurol Sci* 25(2):48–52, 2004.

83. Skirven TM, Callahan AD: Therapist's management of peripheral-nerve injuries. In Mackin EJ, Callahan AD, Skirven TM, et al.: *Rehabilitation of the hand*, 5th ed., St. Louis, 2002, Mosby, pp 599–621.

84. Skirven T, Osterman AL: Clinical examination of the wrist. In Mackin EJ, Callahan AD, Skirven TM, et al.: *Rehabilitation of the hand*, 5th ed, St. Louis, 2002, Mosby, pp 1099–1116.

85. Slutsky DJ: New advances in nerve repair. In Skirven TM, Osterman AL, Fedorczyk JM, et al.: *Rehabilitation of the hand and upper extremity*, 6th ed, Philadelphia, 2011, Elsevier Mosby, pp 611–618.

86. Spinner M: Nerve lesions in continuity. In Hunter JM, Schneider LH, Mackin EJ, et al.: *Rehabilitation of the hand*, 3rd ed., St. Louis, 1990, Mosby, pp 523–529.

87. Sunderland S: The peripheral nerve trunk in relation to injury: a classification of nerve injury. In Sunderland S, editor: *Nerves and nerve injuries*, Baltimore, 1968, Williams & Wilkins, pp 127–137.

88. Tung TH: Nerve transfers. In Skirven TM, Osterman AL, Fedorczyk JM, et al.: *Rehabilitation of the hand and upper extremity*, 6th ed., Philadelphia, 2011, Elsevier/Mosby, pp 813–822.

89. Upton AR, McComas AJ: The double crush in nerve entrapment syndromes, *Lancet* 2:359–362, 1973.

90. Vender MI, Truppa KL, Ruder JR, et al.: Upper extremity compressive neuropathies, *Phy Med Rehabil: Stat Art Rev* 12(2):243–262, 1998.

91. Waldman SD: The Jeanne sign for ulnar nerve entrapment at the elbow. In Waldman SD, editor: *Physical diagnosis of pain: an atlas of signs and symptoms*, 3rd ed., St. Louis, 2016, Elsevier, p 132.

92. Walsh M: *Personal communication*, June 2012.

93. Ziegler EM: *Current concepts in orthotics: a diagnosis-related approach to splinting*, Germantown, WI, 1984, Rolyan Medical Products.

APPENDIX 14.1 CASE STUDIES

Case Study 14.1ᵃ

Read the following scenario, and use your clinical reasoning skills to answer the questions based on information in this chapter.

Mark is a 52-year-old man who is employed as a truck driver. During driving his elbow is positioned in flexion, and he often rests his left elbow on the window seal. Mark sleeps with his elbow flexed behind his head. Over time Mark developed compression of the ulnar nerve at the elbow, which manifested by interosseous weakness with a positive Wartenberg sign and a positive Froment sign. He complains of discomfort on the medial side of the arm and continuous numbness and tingling in digits 4 and 5.

1. Functionally, what might Mark have difficulty doing?
2. What is the correct orthosis for his condition?
3. What are the correct positions for his joints in the orthosis?
4. After being fitted with a custom thermoplastic orthosis, Mark complains that he does not like the hard feel of the material. What would you do?
5. What is your suggested wearing schedule?
6. What other lifestyle adjustments would be suggested?

Case Study 14.2ᵃ

Read the following scenario, and use your clinical reasoning skills to answer the questions based on information in this chapter. Indicate all answers that are correct.

Diana sustained a fall breaking the middle third of her right humeral shaft. Diana later reflected that it was a classic beautiful summer evening when the fall happened. She had been taking a leisurely walk with her fiancé, and when walking across a bridge, she turned around to admire the view. In the dark she did not see a pole sticking out of the middle of the bridge. This led to a fall on the hard surface of the bridge. In the emergency department the physician identified not only a fracture of the right humeral shaft, which needed to be set, but a complete transection of the radial nerve. After surgery you (the therapist working with her) have been ordered to provide therapy for Diana and an orthosis for her radial nerve condition.

1. Which of the following motion difficulties would you expect to see with Diana?
   a. Difficulty with abduction of the carpometacarpal (CMC) joint of the thumb, weakness with thumb opposition and with interphalangeal (IP) extension, and weakness with metacarpophalangeal (MCP) flexion of the second and third digits.
   b. Difficulty with MCP extension, wrist extension, thumb abduction and extension, as well as weakness with elbow flexion/extension, wrist extension, and deviation.
   c. Difficulty with wrist flexion and adduction, flexion of the distal interphalangeal (DIP) of the fourth and fifth digit, MCP flexion of the fifth digit and opposition, and abduction and adduction at the MCP joints. Difficulty also with some thumb motions, especially with thumb adduction.
   d. Diana will not have motion difficulties and will experience only sensory difficulties.

2. What is one optional type of orthosis for the condition that you might consider providing?
   a. Volar wrist orthosis
   b. Dynamic tenodesis suspension orthosis
   c. Thumb immobilization orthosis
   d. Elbow extension orthosis

3. What is the functional advantage of this orthosis?
   a. The design allows the dorsal surface of the hand to be relatively free
   b. The wrist and thumb can move
   c. The fingers are not immobilized
   d. The hand is completely free to move

4. What would be your suggested wearing schedule?
   a. Only during painful activities
   b. All the time with removal for hygiene

5. What could be another orthotic option for Diana?
   a. A low-profile orthosis for the condition that allows radial and ulnar deviation
   b. Thumb immobilization orthosis
   c. Static orthosis with fourth and fifth digits in 30 degrees of flexion
   d. Thumb web spacer orthosis

APPENDIX 14.2 LABORATORY EXERCISES

Laboratory Exercise 14.1ᵃ Metacarpophalangeal Extension Hand-Based Orthosis

Read the following scenario, and use your clinical reasoning skills to answer the question based on information from the chapter.

Adena is a 36-year-old right-handed woman who presents with left forearm level posterior interosseous nerve syndrome. The physician referred Adena to a therapist for orthotic fabrication and a home exercise program. The therapist wrote the following SOAP note in an electronic health record system:

S: "I really want to get better fast."

O: Pt. presented with posterior interosseous nerve syndrome. Manual muscle testing (MMT) scores for the extensor digitorum communis, extensor digiti minimi, extensor indicis, abductor pollicis longus, and extensor carpi ulnaris were all 0 (zero). Pt. reports no pain in the left upper extremity (LUE). A left low-profile radial nerve palsy orthosis with radial and ulnar deviation was fabricated and fitted. Pt. was instructed in how to don and doff the orthosis and how to grasp and release objects. Pt. was also instructed verbally and given written information on the wearing schedule, orthotic care, and precautions. Pt. was given a home exercise program to be completed five times daily.

ᵃSee Appendix A for the answer key.

A: Pt. was receptive to the orthosis and home exercise program. Pt. could independently grasp objects while wearing the orthosis. Anticipate compliance with wearing schedule and home exercise program.

P: Will monitor needs for modifications of the orthosis and home exercise program.

Several appointments later the client regained muscle strength with an MMT score of fair (3) wrist extensors. The forearm portion of the orthosis was removed, and the client was instructed to wear the hand component of the orthosis. The therapist encouraged the patient to continue with activities of daily living (ADLs) and the home exercise program and initiated gentle strengthening activities. The orthotic-wearing schedule and home exercise program were modified. The client was instructed to complete the program five times daily. The client had no complaints and was able to independently grasp light objects while wearing the orthosis.

Write the next progress note.

Laboratory Exercise 14.2 Anticlaw Orthosis

On a partner, practice fabricating a hand-based orthosis in the anticlaw position for a client who has an ulnar nerve lesion. Refer to options provided in the chapter (figure-eight orthosis, hand-based static orthosis, or hand-based mobilization orthosis). Before starting, determine the position to place the person's hand. Remember to position the MCP joints of the ring and little fingers in approximately 30 to 45 degrees of flexion. After fitting the orthosis and making all adjustments, use Form 14.1. This check-off sheet is a self-evaluation of the orthosis. Use Grading Sheet 14.1 as a classroom grading sheet.

APPENDIX 14.3 FORM AND GRADING SHEET
Form 14.1 Anticlaw Orthosis

| Name: _____ |
| Date: _____ |
| Answer the following questions after the orthosis has been worn for 30 minutes. (Mark NA for nonapplicable situations.) |

Evaluation Areas				Comments
Design				
1. The orthosis prevents hyperextension of the MCP joints of the ring and little fingers.	Yes ○	No ○	NA ○	
Function				
1. The orthosis allows full wrist motions.	Yes ○	No ○	NA ○	
2. The orthosis allows full function of the middle and index fingers.	Yes ○	No ○	NA ○	
Straps (if used)				
1. The straps avoid body prominences.	Yes ○	No ○	NA ○	
2. The straps are secure and rounded.	Yes ○	No ○	NA ○	
Comfort				
1. The edges are smooth with rounded corners.	Yes ○	No ○	NA ○	
2. The proximal end is flared (if appropriate).	Yes ○	No ○	NA ○	
3. Impingements or pressure areas are not present.	Yes ○	No ○	NA ○	
4. Orthosis pressure is well distributed over the proximal phalanx of the ring and little fingers.	Yes ○	No ○	NA ○	
Cosmetic Appearance				
1. The orthosis is free of fingerprints, dirt, and pencil or pen marks.	Yes ○	No ○	NA ○	
2. The orthosis is smooth and free of buckles.	Yes ○	No ○	NA ○	
Therapeutic Regimen				
1. The person has been instructed in a wearing schedule.	Yes ○	No ○	NA ○	
2. The person has been provided with orthosis precautions.	Yes ○	No ○	NA ○	
3. The person demonstrates understanding of the education.	Yes ○	No ○	NA ○	
4. Client/caregiver knows how to clean the orthosis.	Yes ○	No ○	NA ○	

Discuss possible adjustments or changes you would make based on the self-evaluation.
_____
_____
_____
_____

Discuss possible areas to improve with clinical safety when fabricating the orthosis.
_____
_____
_____
_____
_____

Grading Sheet 14.1 Anticlaw Orthosis

	Name: _____
	Date: _____
Grade: _____ 1 = Beyond improvement, not acceptable 2 = Requires maximal improvement 3 = Requires moderate improvement 4 = Requires minimal improvement 5 = Requires no improvement	

Evaluation Areas						Comments
Design						
1. The orthosis prevents hyperextension of the MCP joints of the ring and little fingers.	1	2	3	4	5	
Function						
1. The orthosis allows full wrist motions.	1	2	3	4	5	
2. The orthosis allows full function of the middle and index fingers.	1	2	3	4	5	
Straps (if used)						
1. The straps avoid body prominences.	1	2	3	4	5	
2. The straps are secure and rounded.	1	2	3	4	5	
Comfort						
1. The edges are smooth with rounded corners.	1	2	3	4	5	
2. The proximal end is flared (if appropriate).	1	2	3	4	5	
3. Impingements or pressure areas are not present.	1	2	3	4	5	
4. The pressure is well distributed over the proximal phalanx of the ring and little fingers.	1	2	3	4	5	
Cosmetic Appearance						
1. The orthosis is free of fingerprints, dirt, and pencil or pen marks.	1	2	3	4	5	
2. The orthosis is not buckled.	1	2	3	4	5	

Orthotic Provision to Manage Spasticity

Salvador Bondoc
Elizabeth Kloczko

CHAPTER OBJECTIVES

1. Define spasticity.
2. Compare the strengths and weaknesses of dorsal and volar forearm platforms.
3. Discuss orthotic design based on a neurophysiological rationale.
4. Discuss orthotic design based on a biomechanical rationale.
5. Differentiate between the elastic and contractile properties of muscle and describe their implications on using an orthosis.
6. Describe the properties of alternative materials to thermoplastics and plaster and fiberglass casts used for neurological orthoses.
7. Successfully fabricate and clinically evaluate the proper fit of a dorsal forearm–volar hand immobilization orthosis.
8. Use clinical judgment to correctly analyze two case studies.

KEY TERMS

biomechanical	neurophysiological	stretch reflex
composite extension	orthosis	submaximal range
contracture	plaster bandage	task-oriented approach
minimalist design	serial casting	
Neoprene	spasticity	

Lucille is a homemaker and a stroke survivor. Three years ago she sustained an infarction to her right middle cerebral artery that resulted in left-sided weakness (hemiparesis) and spasticity. She underwent nearly 4 months of rehabilitation, starting with an intensive inpatient rehabilitation stay followed by home health until she was able to walk with a cane. Although outpatient services were recommended, she did not pursue this due to insurance limitations. During her annual physical she told her primary care provider that she has been experiencing increased pain and stiffness in her left arm and hand, along with fatigue and unsteady balance. Her provider recommended a neurologist to rule out a recurrence of a stroke. After a series of diagnostic procedures, the neurologist determined that what Lucille was experiencing was a syndrome of late effects from her hemiparesis. Her neurologist suggested antispasticity medications and a referral to occupational and physical therapy as an outpatient. During her first therapy session the occupational therapist determined that Lucille could benefit from an orthotic program to prevent further stiffness of her wrist and hand. Both the therapist and Lucille collaborated on priority goals and a plan of care, which includes a mod-

ified form of constraint-induced movement therapy to help her regain as much functional use of her arm and hand while also reducing her pain and stiffness.

Occupational therapy practitioners, throughout the continuum of care, encounter individuals who are developing abnormally or who are recovering from damage to the central nervous system (CNS). Damage and abnormal development of the brain or spinal cord can result in an imbalance of muscle activity. Therapist and client collaborative goals when addressing spasticity must revolve around functional outcomes, pain management, and health and hygiene. In this chapter spasticity will be defined, options for orthotics will be outlined to guide the therapist in critically thinking about the intervention used in an individualized manner, splinting patterns will be provided, and case studies will be applied for clinical learning.

SPASTICITY

Spasticity is defined as a velocity-dependent increase in muscle tone due to hyperactive **stretch reflex**.[5,44] The defining feature of velocity dependence is highlighted when clinicians assess spastic tone by the degree and extent of resistance to passive stretch. Some scholars have expanded on the definition of **spasticity** to highlight other manifestations of impaired motor control, including the loss of normal reciprocal inhibition and abnormal coactivation of agonist and antagonist muscles during active movement.[12,40,46] This definition has important implications for therapy management using a problem-solving and evidence-based approach.

The onset of spasticity is associated with upper motor neuron lesions (UMNLs) seen in many common CNS conditions, such as cerebrovascular accident, cerebral palsy, traumatic brain injury, spinal cord injury, and multiple sclerosis. During the acute stages following the onset of the lesion, spasticity affects motion by restricting active and passive movement in the direction of the agonist (e.g., spasticity in the flexors limits agonistic extension). From acute to chronic stages the loss of upper motor neuron (cortical) inhibition on the reflex arc[72] continues to perpetuate the spasticity, which further exacerbates the loss of motion. Movement restriction brought on by spastic or hypertonic muscles leads to **contracture** formation, or tissue shortening in the immobile muscles. Muscles atrophy, sarcomeres are lost, and muscle fibers undergo fibrotic changes.[20,53,62] This state of shortening of spastic muscle further increases the muscle's sensitivity to stretch[32] and therefore greater resistance to agonist movement and more subsequent loss of motion. In addition to the muscle shortening, contractures may also develop to the soft tissues that surround the joints where the spastic muscles cross, causing joint stiffness, and in severe cases, joint ossification or arthrodesis. Unabated spasticity may cause pain and muscle spasms with either passive or active movement, further leading to immobility. Thus, with the onset of spasticity a negative cycle of neurological and biomechanical pathophysiological processes ensues. Early intervention and ongoing management are key to abating the impairment process.

Given the complexity of spasticity, effective management requires a multidisciplinary effort. Medical management is conducted primarily using pharmacological agents. These agents vary in their pharmacokinetics and therapeutic effects, including a generalized reduction in the excitability of the spinal reflex arc (via oral or intrathecal medications) or localized functional denervation of muscles (via nerve block or neurotoxin injections).[29] Medical management must be complemented by rehabilitative intervention with major considerations to the pathophysiological processes associated with spasticity and their functional consequences.

Rehabilitative intervention for spasticity should be multipronged with the goals of maintaining biomechanics, preventing further musculoskeletal and neuromuscular impairments and pain, regaining motor control, and relearning functional limb use. To achieve these goals the use of multiple techniques or modalities, including orthotics, is necessary, in combination with pharmacological treatment options.[6,8] (A discussion of other modalities or therapeutic procedures goes beyond the scope of this chapter.) Furthermore, the development of an intervention plan should be individualized. Specific to the use of orthoses to manage spasticity, there is no one-size-fits-all approach (Table 15.1). The therapist's challenge is to use clinical reasoning to problem solve the issues

brought on by spasticity and minimize their negative impact on function and activity. It must be stressed that the use of orthotic devices is only part of a comprehensive intervention plan for persons with neurological conditions with UMNL manifestations.

In terms of research-based evidence, studies present conflicting recommendations, making the practice of orthotic provision to manage spasticity controversial. Systematic reviews such as those by Hellweg and Johannes,[34] Autti-Ramo and colleagues[3] and Mortenson and Eng[50] favor the use of orthoses to manage spasticity, whereas systematic reviews by Lannin and Herbert[42] and Katalinic and colleagues[38] provide counterevidence for the use of orthoses as a modality for spasticity management. Furthermore, a comprehensive review of theory and evidence indicates that "static splinting has not been able to demonstrably reduce either spasticity or contracture and since it was shown to do neither, a subsequent effect on activity was also not detected."[43] This statement should, however, not be construed as a call to abandon the practice of orthotic provision altogether. To reiterate, orthoses should not be regarded as the sole modality to manage spasticity but rather an important component of a multidimensional and multidisciplinary approach. Hardy and colleagues[33] studied the collaboration of use of an orthotic and electrical stimulation, which were shown to reduce spasticity as measured by the Modified Ashworth Scale and to improve overall function over time, specifically in the fingers.[33] An in-depth understanding of the pathophysiological process of spasticity, knowledge of current evidence to manage spasticity, and sound clinical judgment are keys to a successful orthotic intervention program.

ORTHOTIC DESIGNS FOR THE NEUROLOGICALLY IMPAIRED HAND

Applying orthotics to the neurologically impaired upper extremity is a widespread and long-held practice in physical rehabilitation. However, there remains a lack of consensus among practitioners and researchers on which approach is best. Two surveys of practitioners, conducted 30 years apart, illustrate this lack of consensus in terms of when orthotics is indicated and which design and theoretical rationale is preferred.[1,52] Scholars have criticized the continued use of orthoses for persons with neurological impairment in the clinic for its lack of "effect in reducing spasticity... or in preventing contracture."[43] Katalinic and colleagues[38] further concluded that stretch (as often accomplished through orthotic provision for the hand) "does not produce clinically important changes in joint mobility, pain, spasticity or activity limitation."[33] Others have found no significance in improvement of spasticity, range of motion, or function.[4] Alternatives such as adhesive taping have also proved to be more effective than manual stretching and passive splinting after botulinum toxin type A injections.[60] Although these evidence-based statements may be bothersome to adherents of clinical traditions, they should not be construed as a call to abandon orthotic provision altogether. As comparison, Charlton[16] highlights that because of muscle imbalance the potential exists for

TABLE 15.1 Evidence-Based Practice of Orthotic Intervention to Manage Spasticity

Author Citation	Design	Number of Participants	Description	Results	Limitations
Garbellini, S., Robert, Y., Randall, M., et al. (2018). Rationale for prescription, and effectiveness of upper limb orthotic intervention for children with cerebral palsy: A systematic review. *Disability & Rehabilitation, 40*(12), 1361–1371.	Systematic review	Sixteen studies met selection criteria. Two studies described a specific reason for orthosis prescription, six prescribed orthoses to manage a clinical symptom, and eight did not describe a reason. Eight studies were analyzed for effect according to intended outcome with no clear connection found among reasons for prescription, outcome measures used, and effect reported.	The study explored (1) reasons for upper limb orthosis prescription for children with cerebral palsy (CP), (2) the link between reason and effect according to intended outcome and outcome measure used, and (3) classifying the prescribed orthoses using standard terminology. A systematic review searched for experimental and observational studies investigating thermoplastic upper extremity orthotic intervention for children 0 to 18 years of age with CP. The Cochrane central register, MEDLINE, CINAHL, Embase, Scopus, and Web of Science databases were searched. Included studies were assessed for risk of bias.	Sixteen studies met the selection criteria. <ul><li>Two studies described a specific reason for orthosis prescription.</li><li>Six studies prescribed orthoses to manage a clinical symptom.</li><li>Eight studies did not describe a reason.</li><li>Eight studies were analyzed for effect according to intended outcome with no clear connection found between reasons for prescription, outcome measures used, and effect reported.</li></ul>	Limitations among studies were the lack of connection between the reason for orthosis prescription, intended outcome, outcome measure used, and observed effect. A lack of consistent orthotic terminology was also noted by the researchers.
Thibaut, A., Deltombe, T., Wannez, S., et al. (2015). Impact of soft splints on upper limb spasticity in chronic patients with disorders of consciousness: A randomized, single-blind, controlled trial. *Brain Injury, 29*(7/8), 830–836.	Randomized, single-blind, controlled trial	Seventeen patients with chronic (>3 months) disorders of consciousness were included (five VS/UWS; seven women; mean age = 42 ± 12 years; time since insult = 35 ± 31 months).	In this prospective single-blind controlled trial, a blind evaluator assessed spasticity (Modified Ashworth Scale and Modified Tardieu Scale), range of motion at the metacarpophalangeal, wrist, and elbow joints and the patients' hand opening before and after soft splinting, manual stretching, and a control condition (i.e., no treatment), as well as 60 minutes later.	Thirty minutes of soft splinting or 30 minutes of manual stretching both improved spasticity of the finger flexors. An increase of hand opening ability was observed after 30 minutes of soft splinting. Conclusion: 30 minutes of soft orthotic application reduced spasticity and improved hand opening of patients with chronic disorders of consciousness. Soft splinting was well tolerated and did not require supervision.	Small sample size

VS/UWS, Vegetative state/unresponsive wakefulness syndrome.
Contributed by Whitney Henderson.

contracture development due to loss of range of motion, which can lead to pain, impaired function, and hygiene and skin breakdown issues. Applying an orthotic can be used as prevention or work toward remediation of motion range. Thibaut and colleagues[68] found that using a soft design has advantages for clients with disorders of consciousness. This design allows for client contraction and reflexes while maintaining positioning specifically in the hand.[68] Therefore clinicians should undergo deep critical reflection on how orthoses should be used in practice. It should be noted that results of systematic reviews and meta-analyses are aggregates of select information to answer a broad clinical question. Nuances of original studies are lost. In an attempt to generate homogeneity, many smaller studies including "N = 1" or single-case designs and case series studies are routinely excluded from systematic reviews, even though they are considered acceptable alternatives to large randomized experiments. Given that clients are unique not only in their clinical manifestations but also in how they respond to rehabilitative interventions, it may be argued that managing spasticity is an "N = 1" practice. Evidence-based reasoning requires that clinicians not only critically appraise the evidence but also reflect on the individual client's needs and how they match with the evidence.

Client-centered practice indicates that the client's needs and concerns are the main consideration. To that end, therapists need to consider the individualization of the intervention plan based on the client's presentation. Not all clients with neurological impairment present with the same muscle tone, not all clients with spasticity benefit from the same orthotic type and prescription, and not all clients require an **orthosis.** One important consideration is whether the use of an orthosis for the neurologically impaired hand can, in some cases, contribute to disuse or learned nonuse.[66] If the impaired hand is further obstructed by the orthotic device during task performance, the potential benefit of the orthosis is outweighed by the negative consequence on function. Therapists must reflect on the clinical rationale for orthotic provision, including inhibition of tone, management or prevention of contractures, or active facilitation of neuromotor recovery. It stands to reason that depending on the goal or indications of the orthosis and the clinical presentation of the client, clinicians vary in their designs and prescriptions for use. Ways in which designs vary may be categorized based on theoretical orientation, biomechanics, and overall practical considerations. However, key to a successful management is constant monitoring of the client's response and ongoing problem solving with the client to attain therapeutic goals.

Design Based on Theory

There are two prevailing theoretical orientations that inform the use of orthoses for spasticity: neurophysiological and biomechanical. From a **neurophysiological** perspective, orthoses may be used to influence muscle tone by either inhibition or facilitation. From a **biomechanical** perspective, orthoses may be used to provide stretch to muscles to minimize the onset of contractures brought on by spasticity. The biomechanical orientation is discussed in later sections.

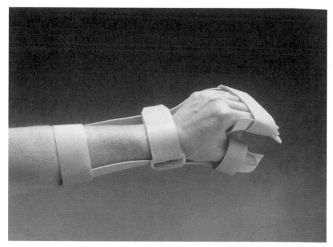

Fig. 15.1 Prefabricated resting hand orthosis. (Courtesy North Coast Medical, Gilroy, CA.)

In general, design incorporating the neurophysiological perspective varies according to (1) location of the hand-wrist-forearm platform and (2) the configuration of the hand component (including the position of the digits). Rehabilitation science literature contains proponents for volar platforms[10,54,74] and dorsal platforms.[13,15,37,63] Dorsal platform adherents argue that cutaneous stimulation of the volar surface of the hand and forearm triggers greater spasticity.[19,35,47] Volar platform adherents argue that sustained pressure on flexor tendon insertions results in muscle relaxation.[24,64] Both assertions have yet to be proven through well-designed empirical methods because other authors see no greater advantage for one platform design over the other.[42,49,59] Both volar- and dorsal-based forearm platforms may be custom fabricated (refer to Chapter 13) or prefabricated, which can be accessed through vendors and catalogs. Fig. 15.1 is an example of a prefabricated orthosis.

In terms of the configuration of the hand component, one design approach based on neurophysiological theory relies on the positioning of the thumb and fingers. As with the platform location, the positioning of the digits in either flexion over a rigid cylinder[24,25,58] or extension and abduction using a "finger spreader"[8,18,74] is purported to reduce spasticity. In addition to reducing spasticity, other factors such as improved mobility and functional ambulation have been connected to use of a reflex inhibitory design. This design involves the wrist at 20 to 25 degrees extension, thumb positioned in opposition, and fingers spread with a dorsal cover to provide complete volar contact to reduce stimulation potential for reflex.[65] Earlier designs incorporating positioning of the thumb and fingers did not incorporate a forearm platform to provide support to the wrist and take advantage of biomechanical leverage to maintain the position of the orthosis on the hand. Over the years, commercial providers of orthoses and expert clinicians (through textbooks) have incorporated the forearm platform as an important design feature (Fig. 15.2). Examples of the cone configuration are the Rolyan Deluxe Spasticity Hand Splint and the Comfy Adjustable Cone Hand Orthosis. An example of the finger spreader configuration is the Rolyan Deluxe Spasticity Hand Splint (Fig. 15.3). Adding a forearm

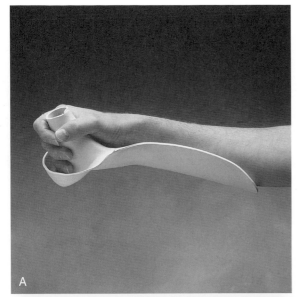

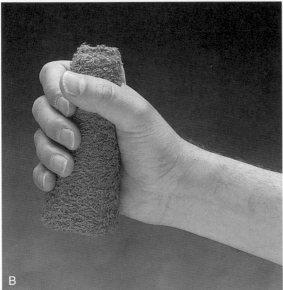

Fig. 15.2 A, Prefabricated cone orthosis with forearm trough. B, Prefabricated cone orthosis without forearm trough.

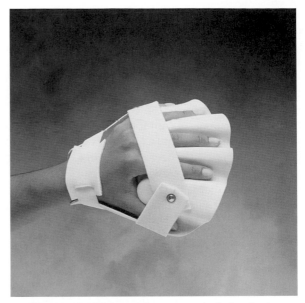

Fig. 15.3 Prefabricated finger spreader/ball orthosis.

component not only improves the leverage of the orthosis but also prevents the spastic long flexors from acting on the wrist.

There are two types of cylindrical orthotic designs for the hand component found in the literature: cone orthoses and dowel orthoses. Cone orthoses are constructed of rigid thermoplastic material with the smaller end placed radially and the larger end placed ulnarly to provide maximum palmar contact. The optimal contact is designed to provide deep tendon pressure on the wrist and finger flexor insertions at the base of the palm. Farber[24] observed that the total contact from the hard cone provides maintained pressure over the flexor surface of the palm, thus assisting in the desensitization of hypersensitive skin. MacKinnon and colleagues[45] adapted the standard hard cone to a solid wood dowel that exerts pressure on the palmar aspect of the metacarpal heads and exposes a larger surface area of the palm for sensory input compared to a cone. Although the shape of the hand may appear similar,

the authors' rationale could not be any more different from each other. Pressure on tendon insertion created by the cone orthosis was intended to inhibit spasticity,[25] whereas the pressure applied on the palmar surface around the metacarpal head region by the hard dowel was purported to provide facilitation of the deep hand intrinsics.[23,45] The efficacy of these orthotic designs has yet to be evaluated through studies with a larger sample and more rigorous methods.

In contrast to keeping the fingers in a flexed position, there are proponents of orthoses that require maintaining finger and thumb abduction and extension. Largely based on neurodevelopmental treatment,[8,18] the position of digital extension and abduction is considered a reflex-inhibiting pattern (RIP) that inhibits flexor spasticity of the hand. From Bobath's original foam block design that spreads the fingers apart, clinicians developed versions with more rigid and custom-molded thermoplastic materials that also incorporate the wrist and forearm.[21,41] The abducted thumb component is key to the RIP effect (relaxation of spasticity) and for proper fit and comfort.[21] The elements of the RIP pattern described earlier are to be contrasted with those of Pizzi and colleagues,[55] where the RIP pattern for the hand is described as the "…wrist in 30 degrees of extension, normal transverse arch, thumb in abduction and opposition with the pads of the 4 fingers, and metacarpal and proximal interphalangeal (PIP) joints in 45 degrees of flexion."[55]

Design Based on Biomechanics

Orthoses may be designed to address the biomechanical properties of muscles. Muscles are made of contractile and elastic components.[26] The contractile components are composed of the myofilaments that respond to neural excitation. These myofilaments are serially arranged into myofibrils, which are bundled to form muscle fibers. The elastic components of a muscle are part of connective tissue, along with collagen, that wraps around and runs parallel with the muscle fibers and muscle tissues.

The maintenance of the number of the contractile myo-filament units, or sarcomeres, and the size of the muscle are use dependent. Therefore, lack of use or disuse leads to muscle atrophy via reduction in the size or number of sarcomeres, especially when the muscle is in a shortened state.[30] Muscle disuse in persons with CNS conditions is brought on by lack of motor control, muscle weakness, decreased movement or immobilization, and spasticity. Confounding the loss of muscle mass is the onset of contractures, which causes a decrease in range of motion.

Contractures or shortening of soft tissues may occur to the joint capsule that is immobilized and to the connective tissue surrounding the inactive or disused contractile muscle tissues. The onset of contractures is time dependent; that is, with prolonged immobility or lack of use, there is loss of elasticity to the soft tissues, which makes for increased resistance to passive or active stretch. In spastic muscles the presence of contractures may accentuate the stretch reflex sensitivity[32,48] further, causing the muscles to shorten at rest and become more resistant to movement in the antagonist direction. The stretch reflex can be triggered at any point of the range of motion arc, thus limiting free range of motion. This phenomenon makes clinical measurement of spasticity challenging because it may be masked by the presence of contractures.

Given the biomechanical properties of muscles, an intervention program for spasticity incorporates promoting muscle activity to address disuse atrophy and maintain the elasticity of tissues through stretch to address the onset of contractures. Stretch for the hand, wrist, and/or elbow may be best achieved through prolonged orthotic use or casting. Orthoses may be preferred if the intervention plan requires active use since they are removable. Casts are preferred if prolonged and sustained stretch is needed, especially when the spasticity is severe and the soft tissue contractures significantly limit range of motion. At times a bivalve configuration allows for both prolonged stretch and removal for intervention. The bivalve cast can be removed to allow for additional techniques such as weight bearing and functional reaching to be incorporated into spasticity management. For the lower extremity, full weight bearing may suffice to maintain the requisite stretch.[72]

Controversies exist regarding the amount of time needed to sustain the stretch to maintain soft tissue length. In a meta-analysis conducted by Katalinic and colleagues[38] there is a wide variation in the frequency and duration in the application of stretch to address contractures in persons with neurological conditions. The pooled outcomes neither favor the control nor the intervention (stretch). Study results varied in relationship to the immediate, short-term, and long-term effects of the intervention. Despite the variations in intervention protocol and outcomes, the authors concluded the following: "Regular stretch does not produce clinically important changes in joint mobility, pain, spasticity or activity limitation in people with neurological conditions."[38] It must be noted that studies included in the meta-analysis are exclusively randomized control or

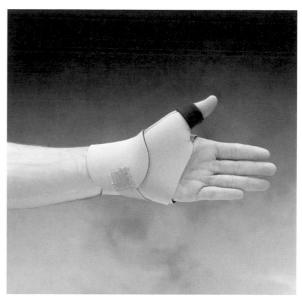

Fig. 15.4 Prefabricated Neoprene thumb orthosis.

controlled clinical trials. Thus, studies that do not have a control or comparison group were excluded.

Adding to the confusion is the debate on how much stretch is applied. Lannin and Ada[43] criticized the use of submaximal orthotic positioning (5 to 10 degrees below maximum passive range), citing the "functional" position described in textbooks is not supported by evidence and contradictory to findings about the benefits of maximal stretch. Many authors recommended positioning the spastic muscles in optimal stretch to achieve an inhibitory effect.[25,32,63,70] On the other hand, some authors recommended orthotic positioning with the wrist and hand in extension but with substantial consideration to the point when the stretch reflex is triggered.[48,54,59,69] Scherling and Johnson[61] suggested that wrist extension of 10 to 15 degrees and metacarpophalangeal (MCP) joint extension of −45 degrees offers a good starting position that is less likely to trigger the stretch reflex while gradually introducing passive stretch to the spastic muscles.

Given the dynamic nature of spasticity, the optimal position may not be the same for all clients. Even with the same client, spasticity can fluctuate at any given time. Anecdotal reports from clients indicate that the time of day, type of activity, fatigue/energy levels, emotional status, and weather may influence tone. In consideration of this issue, therapists should adopt a concept of spasticity management as a 24-hours-a-day regimen. With regards to the use of orthoses, there are alternatives that are flexible or conformable to the fluctuations in a client's tone. Examples of softer, more dynamic materials found to be effective in managing the spastic arm and hand include Lycra[7,22,31] and **Neoprene.**[14,67] Neoprene-based thumb orthoses such as the TheraKool Breathable Neoprene Thumb Spica and the Benik Pediatric Neoprene Glove are commercially available (Fig. 15.4). Another design that combines both flexible and rigid components is the SaeboStretch (Saebo Inc., Charlotte, NC), where the forearm volar platform is made of thin rigid

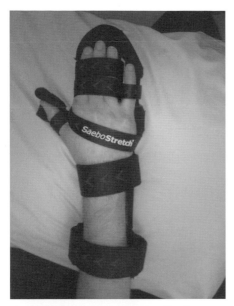

Fig. 15.5 SaeboStretch orthosis.

metal and the flexible metal-based volar hand component is interchangeable (Fig. 15.5). The metal components are padded adequately with Neoprene-based material, and the straps vary in widths according to the body part and are made of rigid silicone material. While case reports have been described,[9] the orthosis requires further examination through rigorous empirical studies. The dynamic hand wrist orthosis with Ultraflex hinge serves as an alternative, incorporating a low-load prolonged-stretch approach, which reduces spasticity and reduces pain caused from static stretch in chronic stroke clients.[2]

With various conflicting evidence to draw from, the best recommendation is always to be judicious in the interpretation of the studies and consider the client's unique clinical presentation. Because a client's neuromuscular presentation varies, a successful intervention plan is one that is consistently monitored and adjusted as needed in response to the client's changing status.

MANAGING THE NEUROLOGICALLY IMPAIRED HAND USING A PROBLEM-SOLVING APPROACH

When a client sustains an UMNL, a clinical syndrome consisting of impaired reflex function (hyperreflexia), muscle weakness, and impaired motor control is expected. As described earlier, spasticity, though associated with UMNL, may not be clinically manifested. In a longitudinal study of clients with stroke conducted by Wissel and colleagues,[73] nearly 25% developed spasticity in the first 2 weeks of onset. Some of the clients with initial spastic manifestation have a decrease in spasticity to levels that are not clinically detectable, whereas others have a worsening condition, especially if early intervention is not provided. There are clients who develop spasticity at a much later time, yet many will not develop any spasticity. With or without spasticity, the focus of intervention is on regaining active function and preventing secondary impairments (i.e., disuse, atrophy, and contractures).

Many clients who develop spasticity are preceded with a flaccid/hypotonic and a reflexive/hyporeflexive presentation. When muscles are flaccid, the hand rests in a dependent position, such as a "wrist drop" with an "ape hand" posture. The dropped wrist position is due to lack of extensor muscle control, whereas the ape hand position of hyperextended MCP joints with partial interphalangeal flexion is due to the passive tension of the extensor digitorum caused by the flexed wrist. To preserve the normal length-tension balance between the flexors and the extensors of the wrist and hand, an orthosis that positions the wrist in slight extension and the digits in **composite extension** is recommended. (*Note: Composite* means that the entire kinematic chain of a digit involving MCP, PIP, and distal interphalangeal joints is positioned as a unit.) The resting position of the hand places the digits in partial flexion (due to passive tension of the elastic components of the flexors). This position keeps the joints in extension, which provides gentle, static stretch to the flexors to preserve the length of the muscle fibers. A volar forearm hand immobilization orthosis is appropriate as a resting and positioning device, especially when muscle tone is considered flaccid. With a greater than neutral extension of the wrist, the orthosis may facilitate edema reduction to the hand.

In clients with acute UMNL, there is a propensity for flexor contractures. Early anticipation of the contracture and subsequent preventive orthotics in extension is good practice. Over time the elastic properties of the muscle adapt to the position of static stretch. Depending on the extent to which the extensors of the digits needed to approximate the requisite aperture size for the hand during pregrasp and release, the orthosis can be adjusted to increase the stretch on the flexors. For example, to actively grasp a water bottle, the wrist is stabilized in slight extension, and the fingers and the thumb must compositely extend to an aperture slightly greater than the diameter of the bottle. Therefore the clinician must assess whether the client can be passively stretched pain-free in composite wrist, hand, and elbow extension that approximates the desired hand-wrist position during reach-to-grasp. The therapist trains the client to tolerate this position through an orthosis. The elbow is included in the assessment of composite extension because the wrist and finger flexors are attached proximal to and can influence kinematics at the elbow joint. However, orthotic provision including the elbow is not necessary. Positioning the elbow in extension and encouraging motion in elbow extension assists with providing stretch to proximal and distal attachments of the hand and wrist flexors.

Using a **minimalist design**,[71] a dorsal forearm-based orthosis with a volar hand immobilization component and dorsal thumb extension is recommended to achieve passive stretch to the flexors. Unlike an entirely volar forearm and hand configuration, this "crowbar" design offers better leverage by pulling the "dropping" hand rather than pushing it into extension. As the client's hand evolves with spasticity, the orthosis is adjusted with increased wrist extension while maintaining the digits extended to provide constant stretch

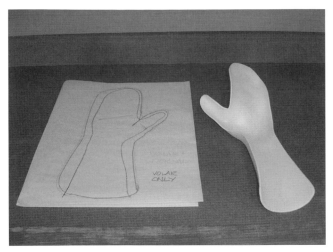

Fig. 15.6 Volar forearm hand immobilization orthosis (pattern and orthosis).

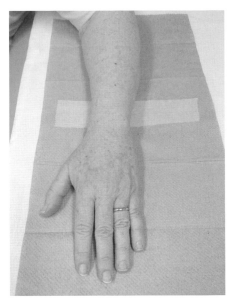

Fig. 15.7 Positioning the hand to trace the pattern.

to the finger and thumb flexors. Even with significant muscle stiffness, the orthotic design is mechanically more advantageous in dispersing pressure over a large surface area, unlike in volar designs, where significant flexor spasticity pulls the wrist and the MCP joints into greater flexion and away from orthosis contact. This design creates a three-point friction and concentrated pressure areas. The following are instructions on how to fabricate a dorsal forearm volar hand immobilization orthosis with a dorsal thumb extension component (Fig. 15.6).

Dorsal Forearm Volar Hand Immobilization Orthosis Construction

Material

The ideal thermoplastic material for this orthosis has moderate drape and resistance to stretch, moderate to excellent rigidity and memory, and low flexibility. The recommended dimensions are nonperforated to 1% perforated (for rigidity) and $3/32$- to $1/8$-inch thickness, depending on the severity of tone. Rolyan Ezeform, Kay-Splint III Basic, TailorSplint, and PolyFlex II meet these criteria.

Pattern Making

1. Place the hand and wrist in a neutral position over a tracing paper (Fig. 15.7). If the client has significant spasticity, the therapist may trace the less involved hand and then invert the pattern on the thermoplastic material before cutting.
   a. Trace the forearm (Fig. 15.8) and hand (Fig. 15.9), and mark the following anatomical locations: posterior one-third of the forearm, radial and ulnar styloids, and the middle of the second and fifth proximal phalanges.
   b. Exclude the thumb by not terminating at the first web space distally and at the base of the first metacarpal proximally. Connect the two thumb points to create a straight edge.
   c. Draw an arc that connects the phalangeal points (Fig. 15.10). Cut a slit along this arc.
   d. Trace the thumb on a separate piece of paper (Fig. 15.11). For the thumb, create $1/4$-inch margins on the medial and lateral sides and a 1-inch margin proximally.

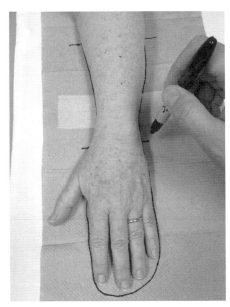

Fig. 15.8 Tracing the forearm.

2. Mark $3/4$-inch margins on the radial and ulnar side of the forearm and $1/2$-inch margins on the radial and ulnar side of the wrist shown in Fig. 15.12. Complete the pattern by drawing trim lines along the margins. The distal and proximal ends may not require additional margin because most thermoplastic materials appropriate for this type of orthosis tend to elongate when heated and draped on the body. The position of wrist extension may also create excess thermoplastic material during fabrication.

3. Transfer the hand-forearm and thumb patterns on the thermoplastic material. Mark the phalangeal arc using the slit on the pattern (refer to step 1c).
   a. Using a box cutter, cut the thermoplastic material in a rectangular configuration that contains the pattern before trimming the pattern to shape.
   b. Punch holes at the ends of the phalangeal arc using a leather puncher (Fig. 15.13).

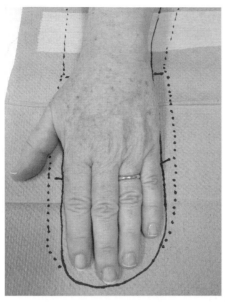

Fig. 15.9 Tracing the hand.

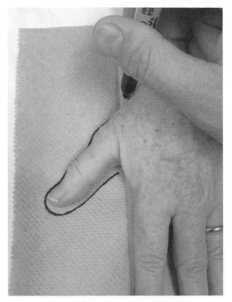

Fig. 15.11 Tracing the thumb.

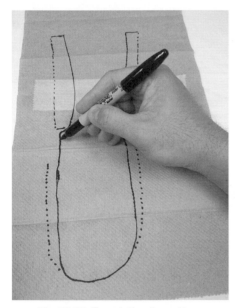

Fig. 15.10 Completing the pattern.

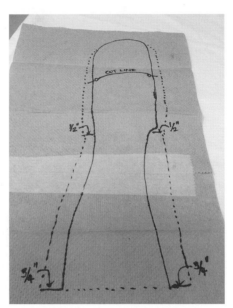

Fig. 15.12 Marking the margins.

c. Heat the material slightly and trim the thermoplastic material by the pattern. Cut a slit along the phalangeal arc as shown in Fig. 15.14. Do not heat the material to its maximum heating point to maintain its optimal integrity before molding.

Fabrication

4. Before molding, establish the optimal wrist position by performing the following:
   a. Place the forearm on a table surface with the elbow flexed at 80 to 90 degrees, the wrist flexed, and the hand resting freely over the edge of the table.
   b. Stabilize the forearm against the elbow and support the hand by the distal palm and fingers while maintaining the fingers in composite extension.

c. Slowly extend the wrist passively to minimize the stretch reflex response (spastic tone). Feel for a palpable stretch until the PIP and distal interphalangeal joints begin to passively or reflexively flex. Use this as a reference angle for optimal wrist extension. A goniometric measurement may be useful to have an estimate of the optimal position. Note, however, that this angle may change during fabrication because some clients will respond to the heat and/or pressure of the thermoplastic material with either relaxation or excitation of spasticity. Ideally, the greater the composite wrist and finger extension is, the more the stretch can be optimized.

5. Apply foam padding to the ulnar head and radial styloid (Fig. 15.15).

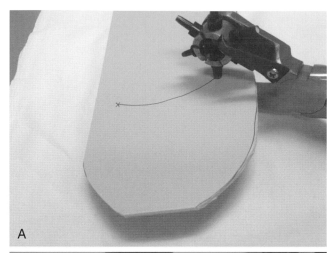

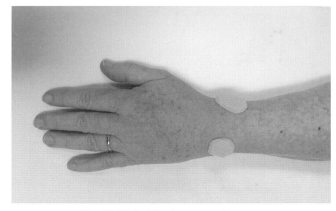

Fig. 15.15 Padding bony prominences.

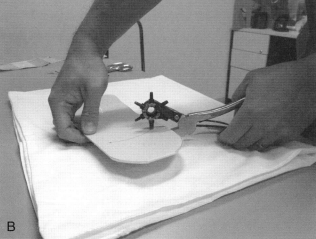

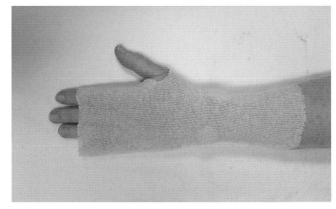

Fig. 15.16 Applying stockinette to protect the skin.

Fig. 15.13 A and B, Punching holes for the phalangeal arc.

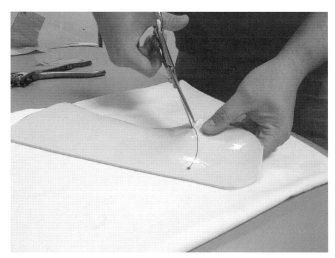

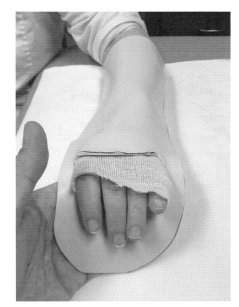

Fig. 15.14 Trimming the thermoplastic for the thumb piece.

Fig. 15.17 Draping the thermoplastic.

6. Apply a stockinette cover to the hand and forearm (Fig. 15.16).
7. Heat the thermoplastic material to the recommended time and optimum temperature per the manufacturer's instructions.

8. Begin the molding process by inserting the fingers through the phalangeal slit so that the fingers are supported to the proximal phalanx. Drape the rest of the material over the dorsum of the hand and the dorsal wrist and forearm (Fig. 15.17).

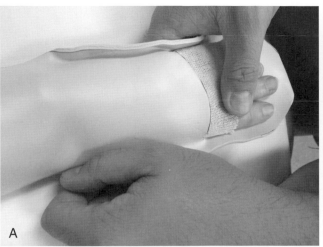

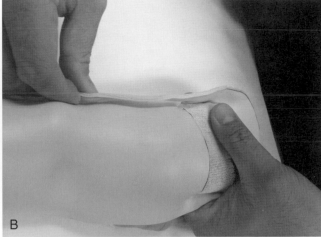

Fig. 15.18 A and B, Stabilizing the hand with digits in extension (A) and Folding the radial and ulnar sides for stability (B).

9. Stabilize the hand by maintaining the digits in extension. Fold the ulnar and radial margins dorsally from the digits to the wrist (Fig. 15.18).

10. While the material remains warm, contour the dorsal platform on the wrist and forearm to maintain the wrist and fingers in optimal composite extension (Fig. 15.19).

11. Heat the lateral and medial folds, and seal them against the body of the orthosis to reinforce the radial and ulnar folds (Fig. 15.20).

12. Smooth the edges and fit the orthosis to the client (Fig. 15.21).

13. Apply a 1½- to 2-inch rough adhesive-backed Velcro on the proximal forearm aspect of the dorsal platform. Secure the orthosis on the client using a 2-inch-wide Neoprene strap (Fig. 15.22).

14. Apply thin foam padding on the corresponding contours created by the ulnar head and radial styloid pads (Fig. 15.23).

15. Reapply the orthosis on the client, and check for comfort (Fig. 15.24). Ensure that the edges of the hand opening do not touch or cause pressure on the metacarpal heads.

16. Heat the thumb component, and drape thermoplastic material on the dorsal aspect of the thumb while the orthosis is on (Fig. 15.25A). Maintain the thumb in optimal extension and abduction (see Fig. 15.25B). Take caution when positioning the thumb by observing its color. Too much pressure or stretch causes the thumb to blanch and/or turn dark red to bluish purple.

17. Spot heat the proximal end of the thumb platform, and smooth it against the orthosis to keep it adhered. For materials that have a coating that prevents bonding, sand or scrape the surface coating or apply an adhesive agent before finishing (Fig. 15.26).

18. Apply adhesive-back rough-side Velcro to the dorsal aspect of the hand and the thumb (Fig. 15.27).

19. Secure the hand and the thumb with a 1½- and 1-inch wide Neoprene strap, respectively (Fig. 15.28).

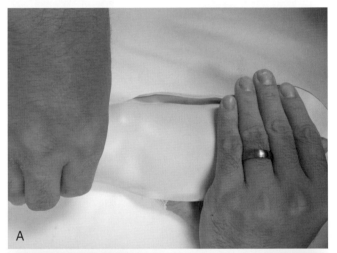

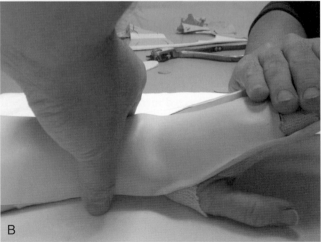

Fig. 15.19 A and B, Molding the wrist and forearm.

20. Optional step: The purpose of the hand strap is to prevent the hand (palm) and wrist from lagging volarly and the fingers from migrating proximally. This strap maintains the MCP joints in neutral. In rare occasions during wear, the MCP joints may become hyperextended and the PIP joints

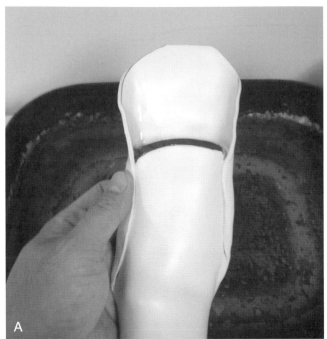

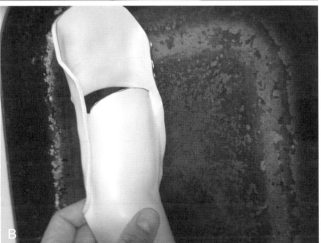

Fig. 15.20 A and B, Finishing and reinforcing the radial and ulnar folds.

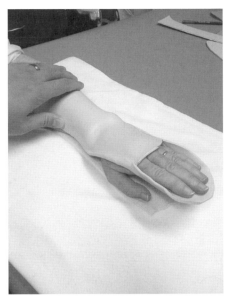

Fig. 15.21 Smoothing the edges of the orthosis.

flexed due to unexpected increase in long flexor tone. To prevent this "buckling" of the fingers, an extra strap over the proximal phalanx may be applied. The strap should not go over the PIP joint so as not to cause PIP hyperextension.

Orthotic Provision and Task-Oriented Intervention

At the earliest sign of volitional control of a mass movement pattern, the orthotic program is complemented with intensive task-oriented practice with or without therapeutic modalities that facilitate active control of the extensors to gain in passive motion that translates into daily functioning. The practice of positioning the hand and wrist to maintain the required alignment for arm and hand use in various daily living activities is deemed an effective method to prepare a client for intensive task training.[66]

The need to constantly monitor the success of the orthotic program in relation to the client goals cannot be overemphasized. As suggested in the study conducted by Wissel and

colleagues,[73] many clients may not develop spasticity, and of those who do, a few have diminished to full resolution of spasticity over time. Therefore, orthoses to manage the secondary effects of spasticity may outlast their usefulness. However, clients with diminished motor control, especially in hand opening for pregrasp and release and in achieving precision grip (e.g., picking up a pen or finger food), regardless of the presence and severity of spasticity, may require a different orthosis. This orthosis constrains select joints or positions for certain digits to enable more active and functional use of the hand. For example, for a client with a cortical thumb or thumb-in-hand resting posture (i.e., the thumb is flexed and adducted into the palm), a short opponens or C-bar orthosis may accomplish two purposes:

1. The orthosis preserves the soft tissue integrity of the structures around the thumb, including the first web space.
2. The orthosis positions the thumb in opposition and palmar abduction to facilitate precision or cylindrical grip during task practice (Fig. 15.29).

An alternative orthosis is a Neoprene- or Lycra-based thumb extension design.[14,22,67]

As discussed in the beginning of the chapter, there are two predominant theoretical orientations that guide the use of orthotic provision for the neurologically impaired hand—neurophysiological and biomechanical. With neurorehabilitation shifting toward more contemporary models of task-oriented and repetitive task training, therapists consider **task-oriented approaches** when it comes to the use of orthoses. Two additional examples of orthoses that promote intensive active practice of the hand are the SaeboFlex and the SaeboGlove (Saebo Inc., Charlotte, NC). The SaeboFlex orthosis is a dynamic forearm-based orthosis that positions the wrist in slight extension and the digits in composite extension through spring-loaded traction (Fig. 15.30) and is typically indicated for clients with significant to moderate spasticity. A client wearing

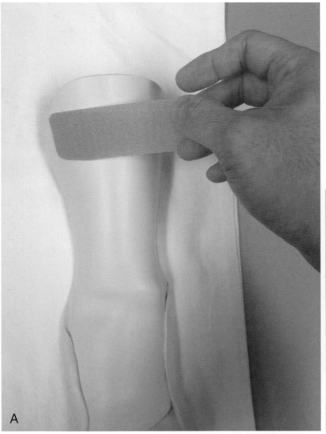

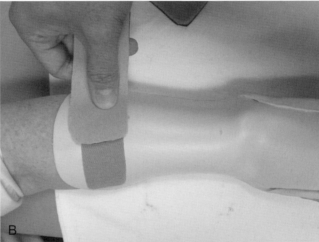

Fig.15.22 A and B, Applying straps to the forearm.

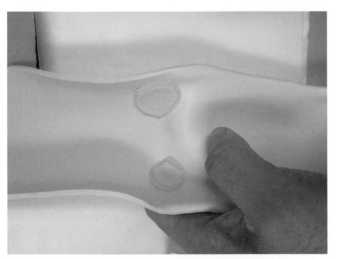

Fig. 15.23 Padding contours for bony prominences.

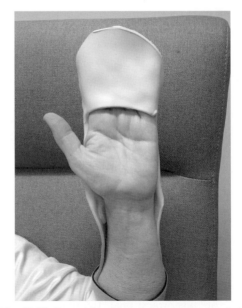

Fig. 15.24 Reapplying the splint to assess comfort.

the orthosis is trained to actively flex the fingers in limited excursion by grasping large-diameter balls against the resistance of the spring-loaded mechanisms followed by active relaxation of the finger flexors (Fig. 15.31A). The SaeboGlove has a similar purpose as the SaeboFlex but is low profile, made of semirigid parts, and best indicated for those with mild spasticity. The digits are positioned similarly in extension using silicone rubber traction anchored by a rigid plastic base (see Fig. 15.31B). As demonstrated in several studies,[11,27,36] the device when used in intensive repetitive task training facilitates gains in hand and arm function for persons with strokes.

Serial Casting to Manage Spasticity

In clients with significant joint and muscle stiffness due to severe spasticity and prolonged immobilization, **serial casting** presents an evidence-based solution that translates into

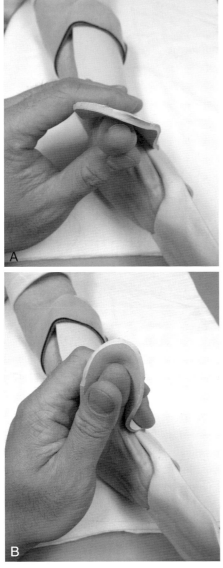

Fig. 15.25 A and B, Molding the thumb component.

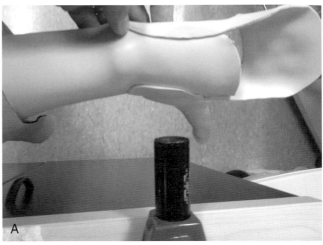

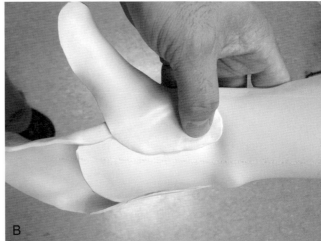

Fig. 15.26 A and B, Spot heating and bonding the thumb component to the rest of the orthosis.

increases in active and passive range of motion.[17,51,56,57,69] In addition to providing sustained passive stretch, the circumferential nature of the cast creates a warming effect on the soft tissue for increased relaxation.[39] Although effective, serial casting is known for various complications, such as pressure sores, pain, and swelling.[56] Therefore it is highly recommended that a therapist who is a novice in casting receive on-the-job or postprofessional training and appropriate supervision from an experienced practitioner before attempting the procedure.

Circumferential casting techniques involve specialized fabrication skills and orthopedic casting materials. Solid serial casting is designed to increase range of motion and decrease contractures caused by spasticity through a series of periodic cast changes. Typically, the affected joint is casted in **submaximal range** (5 to 10 degrees below maximum passive range). Cast change schedules range from every other day for recent contractures to every

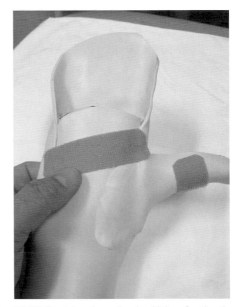

Fig. 15.27 Applying the adhesive Velcro for the thumb.

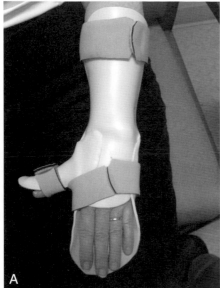

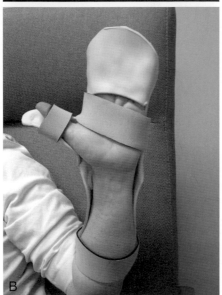

Fig. 15.28 A and B, Reapplying/applying the straps for the forearm and thumb.

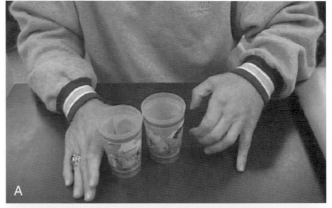

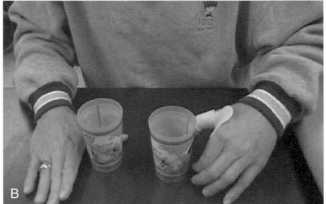

Fig. 15.29 A, Client with thumb extensor weakness is unable to grasp a cup. B, Client with thumb short opponens orthosis is more able to grasp a cup.

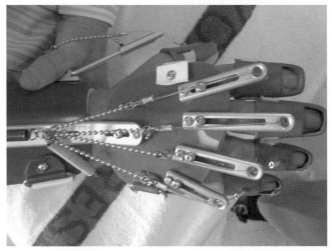

Fig. 15.30 SaeboFlex dynamic orthosis.

5 to 7 days for chronic contractures. Blood circulation, edema, skin condition, sensation, and range of motion are closely monitored during the casting process. The serial progression of the cast is discontinued when range-of-motion gains are no longer noted between a couple of cast changes. When no range-of-motion gains are noted, a final cast with bivalve configuration is applied daily to maintain range of motion.[28]

Therapists use plaster or synthetic resin materials such as fiberglass or stretch bandage with polyurethane resin for casting. Plaster is a cost-effective choice if the practitioner desires to gradually increase passive range of motion by using a series of static orthoses in brief intervals. A **plaster bandage** is easy to handle, and it conforms/drapes easily to body parts. However, the disadvantages of using plaster casts include porousness (non–water resistant), difficulty with maintenance, potential for allergic reactions, and heaviness compared to lighter weight alternatives. Fiberglass and bandage orthopedic resin materials

are more costly and require specialized training. These are lighter in weight, more durable, and ideal for long-term use. A review of studies[51,56] on serial casting reveals preference for synthetic materials for reasons not clearly specified. Both materials require six to eight layers of thickness for adequate strength. They harden in 3 to 8 minutes (depending on water temperature). A special type of synthetic material made of bandage impregnated with polyurethane resin (Delta-Cast Conformable, Depuy Orthopedics, Warsaw, IN) is layered to

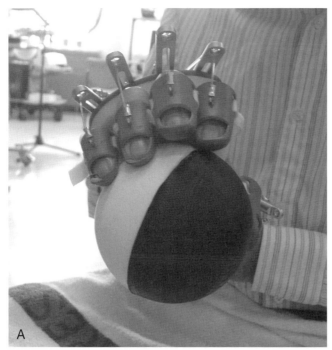

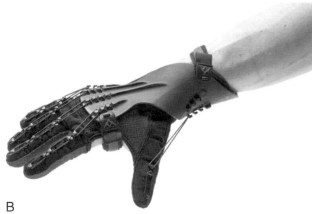

Fig. 15.31 A, Using the SaeboFlex to assist with hand extension after grasping ball. B, A SaeboGlove is best to use with mild spasticity. (B, Courtesy of Saebo, Inc.)

focus the rigidity on certain regions, thereby decreasing the need for multiple layers. Both plaster and synthetic bandages emit heat as a by-product in the curing process. (Refer to Chapter 19 for additional casting information.)

Materials, Tools, and Equipment

Specialized casting tools include the following:
- Electric cast saw
- Hand cast spreader
- Bandage scissors
  Casting program materials include the following:
- Plaster or fiberglass casting tape (2, 3, 4, 5 inch)
- Nylon or cotton stockinette (2, 3, 4, 5 inch)
- Rubber gloves (specialized casting gloves for fiberglass)
- Plastic water bucket
- Drop sheet to protect client
- Cast padding

Plaster Casting Procedures[28]

1. Measure and record joint range of motion.
2. The client should be sitting or lying comfortably and should be draped with sheets or towels to protect clothing and skin. Explain the procedure to the client clearly and reassure as needed. Some clients with brain injuries may be agitated during the casting procedure. In such cases the therapist must discuss the use of sedative agents with the referring physician to accomplish the task.
3. Tubular stockinette is placed over the extremity to be casted, extending it at either end 4 to 6 inches beyond where the cast ends.
4. Determine the targeted position of the extremity. Direct another person (therapist or aide) how and where to hold the extremity.
5. Strips of stick-on foam can be placed on either side of an area that may be susceptible to skin breakdown.
6. Apply cast padding in a taut fashion around the extremity, ending after three or four layers are applied. Extra padding or felt may be added if needed over bony prominences. Padding is applied 1 to 2 inches above the end of the stockinette.
7. Dip the plaster roll five to six times in warm water. Squeeze excess moisture from the roll.
8. Apply plaster to the extremity in a spiral fashion, moving proximally to distally.
9. Direct the person assisting to stretch the joint minimally as the plaster is being applied. The casting assistant should not apply direct pressure to the plaster as it is setting (breakdown or ischemia inside the cast can occur from this loading point effect). Rather, the assistant should stretch the joint above and below the cast or apply pressure with the entire surface of the hand to evenly distribute pressure.
10. Apply four to five layers of plaster. Smooth the plaster surface in a circular fashion as the plaster sets. Pay special attention to smoothing proximal and distal edges to prevent skin breakdown.
11. Before applying the last layer, turn back the ends of stockinette onto the cast. This gives a smooth finished surface to cast edges. Apply the last layer of plaster below this edge.
12. Instruct the casting assistant to maintain stretch on the joint until the plaster has set (3 to 8 minutes).
13. The plaster completely dries in 24 hours. Weight bearing on the casted extremity should be avoided until then.
14. Clean any dripped plaster from the client's skin, elevate the extremity comfortably, and check both ends of the cast for tightness. Check the client's circulation regularly. Some authors[17] recommend a post-casting management program of bivalve casting to maintain increased range of motion and tone reduction.

Fiberglass Casting Procedures[28]

1. Plastic gloves must be worn by anyone touching the fiberglass material during fabrication. Initially and throughout the procedure the plastic gloves are coated with petroleum

jelly or lotion. Fiberglass adheres to the skin or unlubricated gloves and is difficult to remove. Prepare the limb with padding and stockinette. Practice with the casting assistant to position the joint correctly.

2. Submerge the fiberglass roll in cool water, and gently squeeze it six to eight times. Remove the roll from the water, and apply it dripping wet to the extremity to facilitate handling of the material.

3. Fiberglass roll packages should be opened one at a time and applied within minutes. Fiberglass hardens and does not bond to itself when left exposed to air.

4. Fiberglass must overlap itself by half a tape width.

5. Blot the exterior of the cast with an open palm in a circular fashion after all layers are applied. This facilitates maximum bonding of all layers. Rubbing in a longitudinal fashion disrupts the fiberglass bond.

6. If one layer of the cast is allowed to cure (harden), subsequent layers will not bond well. All three to four layers are applied in efficient succession.

7. During the first 2 minutes after immersion, the fiberglass is molded while the extremity is maintained in the desired position. The extremity is held stationary during the last few minutes of the 5- to 7-minute setting time.

8. The cast is completely set in 7 to 10 minutes. Thereafter, the cast may be removed using a cast saw. Cast saws should be operated only by those individuals with training and experience.

The fiberglass cast can be made into a working bivalve in the following manner[28]:

1. Using the cast saw, cut the cast into anterior and posterior sections. Remove the cast with the cast spreader.

2. Remove the padding and stockinette from the extremity with the cast scissors and discard.

3. Inspect both fiberglass shells for protrusions and rough edges. Trim the edges of each shell and file smooth.

4. For soiled cast padding, use cotton padding to reline the shells, taking care to rip padding edges off to provide a smooth inner surface with no ripples. Reline with the same amount of padding used to fabricate the original cast. Extend the padding over all edges and sides of the shells.

5. Fold the padding over the edges of the shells, and secure with adhesive tape.

6. Cut a length of the stockinette approximately 4 to 6 inches longer than the length of the shell. Line each shell with stockinette. Secure both ends with adhesive tape.

7. Fashion straps using wide webbing and buckles. These straps can be taped or sewn onto stockinette covering the shell. Bivalves can also be secured with Ace wraps.

8. Carefully wean the client into the bivalve, modifying and adjusting as needed.

REVIEW QUESTIONS

1. How do the biochemical and neurophysiological approaches to hand orthotic provision differ?

2. Why would an orthosis that positions in submaximal range be less beneficial and potentially harmful to a client with evolving muscle tone?

3. What are the strengths and weaknesses of orthotic dorsal versus volar forearm platforms?

4. What is an appropriate rationale for orthotic design based on a biomechanical rationale?

5. What is the difference between the elastic and contractile properties of muscles, and what are the implications for orthotic provision?

6. What are the material options for casting?

7. What are two major characteristics for each of the materials below?
   - Plaster bandage
   - Fiberglass bandage
   - Neoprene or Lycra

REFERENCES

1. Adrienne C, Manigandan C: Inpatient occupational therapists hand-splinting practice for clients with stroke: a cross-sectional survey from Ireland, *J Neurosci Rural Pract* 2(2):141–149, 2011.

2. Andringa A, van de Port IGL, Meijer JWG: Tolerance and effectiveness of a new dynamic hand-wrist orthosis in chronic stroke patients, *Neuro Rehabil* 33:225–231, 2013.

3. Autti-Ramo I, Suoranta J, Anttila H, et al.: Effectiveness of upper and lower limb casting and orthoses in children with cerebral palsy: an overview of review articles, *Am J Phys Med Rehabil* 85:89–103, 2006.

4. Basaran A, Emre U, Karadavut KI, Balbaloglu O, Bulmus N: Hand splinting for poststroke spasticity: a randomized controlled trial, *Top Stroke Rehabil* 19(4):329–337, 2012.

5. Basmajian J, Burke M, Burnett G, et al.: *Illustrated Stedman's medical dictionary*, ed 24, London, 1982, Williams & Wilkins.

6. Bethoux F: Spasticity management after stroke, *Phys Med Rehabil Clin N Am* 26:625–639, 2015.

7. Betts L: Dynamic movement lycra orthosis in multiple sclerosis, *Br Neuro Nurs* 11(2):60–64, 2015.

8. Bobath B: *Adult hemiplegia: evaluation and treatment*, London, 1987, William Heinemann, Medical Books.

9. Bondoc S: *Management of the neurologic upper extremity with focus on the hand: an evidence base approach and practical solutions*, Chicago, IL, 2012. Seminar presented at the Rehabilitation Institute of Chicago.

10. Brennan J: Response to stretch of hypertonic muscle groups in hemiplegia, *Br Med J* 1:1504–1507, 1959.

11. Butler AJ, Blanton S, Rowe VT, et al.: Attempting to improve function and quality of life using the FTM protocol: a case report, *J Neurol Phys Ther* 30(3):148–156, 2006.

12. Burridge JH, McLellan DL: Relation between abnormal patterns of muscle activation and response to common peroneal nerve stimulation in hemiplegia, *J Neur* (69)353–361.

13. Carmick J: Case report: use of neuromuscular electrical stimulation and a dorsal wrist splint to improve the hand function of a child with spastic hemiparesis, *Phys Ther* 77(6):661–671, 1997.

14. Casey CA, Kratz EJ: Soft splinting with neoprene: the thumb abduction supinator splint, *Am J Occup Ther* 42(6):395–398, 1988.

15. Charait S: A comparison of volar and dorsal splinting of the hemiplegic hand, *Am J Occup Ther* 22:319–321, 1968.

16. Charlton PT: The use of orthoses in stroke rehabilitation, *Br J Neurosci Nurs* 10(Suppl 6):20–26, 2014.

17. Copley J, Watson-Will A, Dent K: Upper limb casting for clients with cerebral palsy: a clinical report, *Aust Occup Ther J* 43:39–50, 1996.

18. Davies P: *Steps to follow: a guide to the treatment of hemiplegia*, New York, 1985, Springer-Verlag.

19. Dayhoff N: Re-thinking stroke soft or hard devices to position hands, *Am J Nurs* 75(7):1142–1144, 1975.

20. Dietz V, Ketelsen UP, Berger W, et al.: Motor unit involvement in spastic paresis. Relationship between leg muscle activation and histochemistry, *J Neurol Sci* (75)86–103.

21. Doubilet L, Polkow L: Theory and design of a finger abduction splint for the spastic hand, *Am J Occup Ther* 32:320–322, 1977.

22. Elliott CM, Reid SL, Alderson JA, et al.: Lycra arm orthoses in conjunction with goal-directed training can improve movement in children with cerebral palsy, *Neuro Rehabil* 28(1):47–54, 2011.

23. Exner C, Bonder B: Comparative effects of three hand splints on bilateral hand use, grasp, and arm-hand posture in hemiplegic children: a pilot study, *Occup Ther J Res* 3:75–92, 1983.

24. Farber SD: *Neurorehabilitation: a multidisciplinary approach*, Toronto, 1982, WB Saunders.

25. Farber SD, Huss AJ: *Sensorimotor evaluation and treatment procedures for allied health personnel*, Indianapolis, 1974, Indiana University Foundation.

26. Farmer SE, James M: Contractures in orthopaedic and neurological conditions: a review of causes and treatment, *Disabil Rehabil* 23(13):549–558, 2001.

27. Farrell JF, Hoffman HB, Snyder JL, et al.: Orthotic aided training of the paretic upper limb in chronic stroke: results of a phase 1 trial, *Neurorehabilitation* 22:99–103, 2007.

28. Feldman PA: Upper extremity casting and splinting. In Glenn MD, Whyte J, editors: *The practical management of spasticity in children and adults*, Malvern, PA, 1990, Lea & Febiger.

29. Gelber DA, Jozefcyk PB: Therapeutics in the management of spasticity, *Neurorehabil Neural Repair* 13:5–14, 1999.

30. Goldspink G, Williams P: Muscle fibre and connective tissue changes associated with use and disuse. In Ada L, Canning C, editors: *Key issues in neurological physiotherapy*, Oxford, 1990, Butterworth Heinmann.

31. Gracies JM, Marosszeky JE, Renton R, et al.: Short-term effects of dynamic lycra splints on upper limb in hemiplegic patients, *Arch Phys Med Rehabil* 81(12):1547–1555, 2000.

32. Gracies JM: Pathophysiology of impairment in patients with spasticity and use of stretch as a treatment of spastic hypertonia, *Phys Med Rehabil Clin N Am* 12:747–768, 2001.

33. Hardy K, Suever K, Sprague A, Hermann V, Levine P, Page SJ: Combined bracing, electrical stimulation, and functional practice for chronic, upper-extremity spasticity, *Am Journal of Occ Ther* 64:720–726, 2010.

34. Hellweg S, Johannes S: Physiotherapy after traumatic brain injury: a systematic review of the literature, *Brain Inj* 22:365–373, 2008.

35. Jamison S, Dayhoff N: A hard hand-positioning device to decrease wrist and finger hypertonicity: a sensorimotor approach for the client with non-progressive brain damage, *Nurs Res* 29:285–289, 1980.

36. Jeon HS, Woo YK, Yi CH, et al.: Effect of intensive training with a spring-assisted hand orthosis on movement smoothness in upper extremity following stroke: a pilot clinical trial, *Top Stroke Rehabil* 19(4):320–328, 2012.

37. Kaplan N: Effect of splinting on reflex inhibition and sensorimotor stimulation in treatment of spasticity, *Arch Phys Med Rehabil* 43:565–569, 1962.

38. Katalinic OM, Harvey LA, Herbert RD: Effectiveness of stretch for the treatment and prevention of contractures in people with neurological conditions: a systematic review, *Phys Ther* 91(1):11–24, 2011.

39. King T: Plaster splinting as a means of reducing elbow flexor spasticity: a case study, *Am J Occup Ther* 36:671–673, 1982.

40. Knutson E, Martensen A: Posture and gait in Parkinsonian patients. In Bles Brandt, editor: *Disorders of posture and gait*, Amsterdam, 1986, Elsevier.

41. Langlois S, Pederson L, MacKinnon JR: The effects of splinting on the spastic hemiplegic hand: report of a feasibility study, *Can J Occup Ther* 58(1):17–25, 1991.

42. Lannin NA, Herbert RD: Is hand splinting effective for adults following stroke? A systematic review and methodological critique of published research, *Clin Rehabil* 17:807–816, 2003.

43. Lannin N, Ada L: Neurorehabilitation splinting: theory and principles of clinical use, *Neuro Rehabil* 28:21–28, 2011.

44. Little JW, Massagli TL: Spasticity and associated abnormalities of muscle tone. In DeLisa JA, Gans BM, editors: *Rehabilitation medicine: principles and practice*, ed 3, Philadelphia, 1998, Lippincott-Raven, pp 997–999.

45. MacKinnon J, Sanderson E, Buchanan D: The MacKinnon splint: a functional hand splint, *Can J Occup Ther* 42:157–158, 1975.

46. Mayer NH: Spasticity and the stretch reflex, *Muscle and Nerve* 6(Suppl 6):51–513, 1997.

47. Mathiowetz V, Bolding D, Trombly CA: Immediate effects of positioning devices on the normal and spastic hand measured by electromyography, *Am J Occup Ther* 37(4):247–254, 1983.

48. McPherson J, Becker A, Franszczak N: Dynamic splint to reduce the passive component of hypertonicity, *Arch Phys Med Rehabil* 66:249–252, 1985.

49. McPherson J, Kreimer D, Aalderks M, et al.: A comparison of dorsal and volar resting hand splints in the reduction of hypertonus, *Am J Occup Ther* 36(10):664–670, 1982.

50. Mortenson PA, Eng JJ: The use of casts in the management of joint mobility and hypertonia following brain injury in adults: a systematic review, *Phys Ther* 83:648–658, 2003.

51. Moseley AM, Hassett LM, Leung J, et al.: Serial casting versus positioning for the treatment of elbow contractures in adults with traumatic brain injury: a randomized controlled trial, *Clin Rehabil* 22:406–417, 2008.

52. Neuhaus B, Ascher E, Coullon B, et al.: A survey of rationales for and against hand splinting in hemiplegia, *Am J Occup Ther* 35:83–90, 1981.

53. O'Dwyer NJ, Ada L, Neilson PD: Spasticity and muscle contracture following stroke, *Brain* 119(Pt 5):1737–1749, 1996.

54. Peterson LT: *Neurological considerations in splinting spastic extremities*, Menomonee Fall, WI, 1980, Rolyan Orthotics Lab.

55. Pizzi A, Carlucci G, Falsini C, et al.: Application of a volar static splint in poststroke spasticity of the upper limb, *Arch Phys Med Rehabil* 86:1855–1859, 2005.

56. Pohl M, Mehrholz J, Ruckriem S: The influence of illness duration and level of consciousness on the treatment effect and complication rate of serial casting in patients with severe cerebral spasticity, *Clin Rehabil* 17(4):373–379, 2003.

57. Pohl M, Ruckriem S, Mehrholz J, et al.: Effectiveness of serial casting in patients with severe cerebral spasticity: a comparison study, *Arch Phys Med Rehabil* 83(6):784–790, 2002.

58. Rood M: Neurophysiological reactions as a basis for physical therapy, *Phys Ther Rev* 34(9):444–449, 1954.

59. Rose V, Shah S: A comparative study on the immediate effects of hand orthoses on reduction of hypertonus, *Aust Occup Ther J* 34(2):59–64, 1987.

60. Santamato A, Micello MF, Panza F, et al.: Adhesive taping vs. daily manual muscle stretching and splinting after botulinum tonix type A injection for wrist and fingers spastic overactivity in stroke patients: a randomized controlled trial, *Clin Rehabil* 29(1):50–58, 2014.

61. Scherling E, Johnson H: A tone-reducing wrist-hand orthosis, *Am J Occup Ther* 43(9):609–611, 1989.

62. Sinkjaer T, Taft E, Larsen K, Andreassen S, Hansen H: Non-reflex and reflex mediated ankle joint stiffness in multiple sclerosis patients with spasticity, *Muscle Nerve* 16:69–79, 1993.

63. Snook JH: Spasticity reduction splint, *Am J Occup Ther* 33:648–651, 1979.

64. Stockmeyer SA: An interpretation of the approach of Rood to the treatment of neuromuscular dysfunction, *Am J Phys Med* 46(1):900–961, 1967.

65. Suat E, Engin SI, Nilgun B, Yavuz Y, Fatma U: Short- and long-term effects of an inhibitor hand splint in poststroke patients: a randomized controlled trial, *Top Stroke Rehabil* 18(3):231–237, 2011.

66. Taub E, Uswatte G, Bowman MH, et al.: Constraint-induced movement therapy combined with conventional neurorehabilitation techniques in chronic stroke patients with plegic hands: a case series, *Arch Phys Med Rehabil* 94(1):86–94, 2013.

67. Ten Berge SR, Boonstra AM, Dijkstra PU, et al.: A systematic evaluation of the effect of thumb opponens splints on hand function in children with unilateral spastic cerebral palsy, *Clin Rehabil* 26(4):362–371, 2012.

68. Thibaut A, Deltombe T, Wannez S, et al.: Impact of soft splints on upper limb spasticity in chronic patients with disorders of consciousness: a randomized, single-blind, controlled trial, *Brain Inj* 29(7-8):830–836, 2015.

69. Tona JL, Schneck CM: The efficacy of upper extremity inhibitive casting: a single subject pilot study, *Am J Occup Ther* 47(10):901–910, 1993.

70. Ushiba J, Masakado Y, Komune Y, et al.: Changes of reflex size in upper limbs using wrist splint in hemiplegic patients, *Electromyogr Clin Neurophysiol* 44(3):175–182, 2004.

71. Van Lede P: Minimalistic splint design: a rationale told in a personal style, *J Hand Ther* 15(2):192–201, 2002.

72. Watanabe T: The role of therapy in spasticity management, *Am J Phys Rehab* 83(Suppl):45–49, 2004.

73. Wissel J, Schelosky LD, Faiss JH, Mueller J: Early development of spasticity following stroke: a prospective, observational trial, *J Neurology* 257(7):1067–1072, 2010.

74. Zislis JM: Splinting of hand in a spastic hemiplegic patient, *Arch Phys Med Rehabil* 45:41–43, 1964.

APPENDIX 15.1 CASE STUDIES

Case Study 15.1[a]

Read the following scenario, and answer the questions based on information in this chapter.

Rose is a 78-year-old client who is a resident of a long-term care facility, and she experienced an ischemic cerebrovascular accident (CVA) 2 months ago. She was admitted to the hospital for 12 days and returned to the facility for short-term rehabilitation. Before the CVA, Rose was independent in dressing and toileting, ambulatory using a walker, and able to participate in recreational activities. After a 2-week period of flaccidity, wrist and finger flexion spasticity emerged. Outside of the therapy schedule, the hand rests in wrist flexion most of the day. The dorsum of the hand is significantly edematous, causing the fingers to assume the position of deformity with the metacarpophalangeal (MCP) joints in slight hyperextension and the interphalangeal joints partially flexed. Pain-free range of motion is limited to 10 degrees of wrist extension. Composite finger extension can only be accomplished pain-free with the wrist in 5 degrees of extension. No active wrist motion is present, but reflexive digit flexion is emerging. From a position of maximum wrist flexion, the stretch reflex is elicited at −15 degrees of wrist extension until slightly past neutral. The family is concerned about Rose's hand becoming deformed. The nursing plan of care has been to position the hand elevated on a pillow resting on Rose's lap. The palm and the web spaces are moist, and a faint odor is detected along with slightly macerated skin. Additionally, the thumb is tightly flexed across the palm, thus causing skin irritation to the thumb web space.

1. Which of the following orthotic designs is most appropriate for Rose? Explain your rationale.
   a. A dorsal-based forearm platform with a volar hand component that positions the wrist and fingers in tolerable composite extension
   b. A volar finger spreader that positions the wrist and fingers statically in maximum extension
   c. A volar-based forearm platform and hard cone that positions the wrist in submaximal extension and fingers in partial flexion
   d. A volar forearm-based hand immobilization orthosis that stretches and positions the wrist and the fingers in composite extension
   e. A plaster cast that places the wrist in maximum extension and the fingers in a current resting position
2. The nursing staff reports that the orthosis is not applied regularly because Rose's edema worsens with wear. Meanwhile, Rose's hand at rest continues to be in the position of deformity of MCP joint hyperextension and proximal interphalangeal and distal interphalangeal joint flexion. How would you modify the intervention approach?

   Four weeks have passed, and Rose's hand and arm function as well as occupational performance are being assessed. Rose has been wearing the orthosis consistently for several

hours daily. The edema has reduced significantly, the joints remain passively mobile, but the spasticity is causing more muscle tightness. Rose is also getting more active mass grasp and partial release of 20 degrees of composite finger extension with effort—adequate to grasp and release a dish towel. There is evidence that the wrist stabilizers are activating as grip on an object can be sustained for a few seconds' duration before the hand fatigues. The thumb rests in an adducted and flexed position and is not able to engage in gross grasp tasks. The first web space and the thumb flexors are tight, but they can be passively positioned in extension and palmar abduction.

3. Which of the following orthotic designs should be considered for Rose at this time? Explain your answer.
   a. A finger spreader that positions the thumb in radial abduction and does not incorporate the wrist
   b. A hard cone that positions the thumb in opposition and does not incorporate the wrist
   c. A short (hand-based) opponens orthosis positioning the thumb in abduction with partial extension/opposition
   d. An orally inflatable orthosis that positions the wrist, fingers, and thumb in extension
   e. A Neoprene thumb abduction and extension orthosis that extends to the forearm radially
4. What specific suggestions would you offer the health care team and the family to encourage increased functional hand skills while Rose is wearing the orthosis?

Case Study 15.2[a]

Brian is a 25-year-old who was recently admitted to an inpatient rehabilitation unit after experiencing a traumatic brain injury following a motor vehicle accident. He was admitted to the emergency department, underwent a craniectomy, and was in the intensive care unit for 10 days. He was then transferred to the acute care floor for 2 weeks and was recently moved to inpatient rehabilitation. Brian is emerging from his coma and is in a minimally conscious state as evidenced by some automatic motor responses and object localization when being assessed using the JFK Coma Recovery Scale. Before the accident Brian was independent and working as an analyst at a hedge fund. Brian is displaying spasticity throughout his left upper limb, most specifically in the biceps, supinators, and wrist and finger flexors. The therapist can passively range Brian's arm. However, pain-free range of motion is limited in elbow extension by less than 10 degrees and wrist extension by 30 degrees, and composite finger extension can only be accomplished pain-free with the wrist in 10 degrees of flexion. He has no active movement. The Modified Ashworth Scale score is a 2 in his biceps and 3 in wrist and finger flexors. Hand hygiene is becoming a concern. Positioning, modalities, stretching, and weight bearing are proving beneficial during intervention sessions. The rehabilitation team wants orthosis for night use. Due to spasticity throughout his lower limb, serial bivalve casts have been provided.

[a] See Appendix A for the answer key.

1. Which of the following orthotic designs is most appropriate for Brian? Explain your rationale.
   a. A dorsal-based forearm platform with a volar hand component that positions the wrist and fingers in tolerable composite extension
   b. A volar finger spreader that positions the wrist and fingers statically in maximum extension
   c. A volar-based forearm platform and hard cone that positions the wrist in submaximal extension and fingers in partial flexion
   d. A volar forearm-based hand immobilization orthosis that stretches and positions the wrist and the fingers in composite extension
   e. A plaster cast that places the wrist in maximum extension and the fingers in a current resting position

   Three weeks have passed, and Brian has become more aware and engaging in therapy. He has 1 of 4 scores on shoulder movements against gravity. He is initiating reach-to-grasp with his left arm; however, his wrist and hand function is limited by spasticity. He can use his tone to perform gross grasp but is unable to perform release without passively moving his wrist into flexion. Modifications were made to his existing orthosis for nighttime to meet his needs.

2. What is an appropriate approach to augment Brian's therapy for spasticity management? Explain your rationale.
   a. A dynamic orthosis such as the SaeboFlex during active reach to grasp
   b. A static orthosis such as SaeboStretch during weight bearing
   c. A dorsal-based forearm platform with a volar hand component that positions the wrist and fingers in tolerable composite extension for pregrasp during simulated reaching

APPENDIX 15.2 LABORATORY EXERCISE

Laboratory Exercise 15.1

1. Practice fabricating a dorsal forearm based with volar hand immobilization orthosis on a partner. Use a goniometer and an acrylic cone to position the hand and wrist correctly.
2. After fitting the cone, use Form 15.1. This is a check-off sheet for self-evaluation of the hard-cone wrist and hand orthosis. Use Grading Sheet 15.1 as a classroom grading sheet.

APPENDIX 15.3 FORM AND GRADING SHEET

Form 15.1 Dorsal Forearm Based With Volar Hand Immobilization Orthosis

Name: _____	
Date: _____	
Answer the following questions after the orthosis has been worn for 30 minutes.	
(Mark NA for nonapplicable situations.)	

Evaluation Areas				Comments
Design				
1. The wrist position is at the correct angle.	Yes ○	No ○	NA ○	
2. The digits are in composite extension.	Yes ○	No ○	NA ○	
3. The thumb is positioned in palmar abduction and extension.	Yes ○	No ○	NA ○	
4. The hand platform extends slightly beyond the fingers.	Yes ○	No ○	NA ○	
5. The orthosis is two-thirds the length of the forearm.	Yes ○	No ○	NA ○	
6. The orthosis is half the width of the forearm.	Yes ○	No ○	NA ○	
Function				
1. The wrist is positioned in the target range.	Yes ○	No ○	NA ○	
2. The fingers are positioned to provide gentle stretch to the flexors.	Yes ○	No ○	NA ○	
3. The thumb position preserves the first web space.	Yes ○	No ○	NA ○	
Straps				
1. The straps avoid bony prominences.	Yes ○	No ○	NA ○	
2. The straps are secure and rounded.	Yes ○	No ○	NA ○	
Comfort				
1. The edges are smooth with rounded corners.	Yes ○	No ○	NA ○	
2. The proximal end is flared.	Yes ○	No ○	NA ○	
3. Impingements or pressure areas are not present. (The ulnar styloid is relieved.)	Yes ○	No ○	NA ○	
Cosmetic Appearance				
1. The orthosis is free of fingerprints, dirt, or ink marks.	Yes ○	No ○	NA ○	
2. The orthotic material is not buckled.	Yes ○	No ○	NA ○	
Therapeutic Regimen				
1. The person/caregiver has been instructed in a wearing schedule.	Yes ○	No ○	NA ○	
2. The person/caregiver has been provided with orthotic precautions.	Yes ○	No ○	NA ○	
3. The person/caregiver demonstrates understanding of the education.	Yes ○	No ○	NA ○	
4. Person/caregiver knows how to clean the orthosis.	Yes ○	No ○	NA ○	

Discuss adjustments or changes you would make based on the self-evaluation. What would you do differently next time?

_____

_____

_____

_____

Discuss possible areas to improve clinical safety when fabricating the orthosis.

_____

_____

_____

_____

Grading Sheet 15.1 Dorsal Forearm Based With Volar Hand Immobilization Orthosis

Name: _____
Date: _____
Grade: _____
1 = Beyond improvement, not acceptable
2 = Requires maximal improvement
3 = Requires moderate improvement
4 = Requires minimal improvement
5 = Requires no improvement

Evaluation Areas						Comments
Design						
1. The wrist position is at the correct angle.	1	2	3	4	5	
2. The digits are in composite extension.	1	2	3	4	5	
3. The thumb is positioned in palmar abduction and extension.	1	2	3	4	5	
4. The hand platform extends slightly beyond the fingers.	1	2	3	4	5	
5. The orthosis is two-thirds the length of the forearm.	1	2	3	4	5	
6. The orthosis is half the width of the forearm.	1	2	3	4	5	
Function						
1. The wrist is positioned in the target range.	1	2	3	4	5	
2. The fingers are positioned to provide gentle stretch to the flexors.	1	2	3	4	5	
3. The thumb position preserves the first web space.	1	2	3	4	5	
Straps						
1. The straps avoid bony prominences.	1	2	3	4	5	
2. The straps are secure and rounded.	1	2	3	4	5	
Comfort						
1. The edges are smooth with rounded corners.	1	2	3	4	5	
2. The proximal end is flared.	1	2	3	4	5	
3. Impingements or pressure areas are not present. (The ulnar styloid is relieved.)	1	2	3	4	5	
Cosmetic Appearance						
1. The orthosis is free of fingerprints, dirt, or ink marks.	1	2	3	4	5	
2. The orthotic material is not buckled.	1	2	3	4	5	

Therapeutic Regimen						
1. The person/caregiver has been instructed in a wearing schedule.	1	2	3	4	5	
2. The person/caregiver has been provided with orthotic precautions.	1	2	3	4	5	
3. The person/caregiver demonstrates understanding of the education.	1	2	3	4	5	
4. Person/caregiver knows how to clean the orthosis.	1	2	3	4	5	

Orthotic Intervention for Older Adults

Marlene A. Riley
Helene L. Lohman

CHAPTER OBJECTIVES

1. Describe special considerations for orthotic intervention with older adults in different environments.
2. Identify the complexity of age-related changes, medical conditions, and medication side effects that may impact orthotic provision.
3. Recognize how an older adult's performance in occupations and activities may influence orthotic use and design based on the Occupational Therapy Practice Framework.[2,55]
4. Select appropriate prefabricated off-the-shelf (OTS) orthoses.
5. Select appropriate materials to fabricate custom orthoses.
6. Describe factors that influence methods of instruction about safe use and care of an orthosis for an older adult and/or care partner.

KEY TERMS

anticoagulants	ecchymosis	soft orthosis
arteriovenous (AV) fistula	integumentary system	working memory

Donald is a 75-year-old man who plays basketball at a county senior center. He does not consider himself to be "old" and would not think of going to a senior center except that his friend invited him to join the indoor basketball team. He plays three times per week despite pain in his thumbs. The senior center director referred him to a county health department occupational therapist to explore options to minimize his pain and enable him to continue participation with the team. During the initial assessment, Donald said he had "his father's hands" and was interested in learning how to decrease his pain. The therapist recommended bilateral prefabricated thumb carpometacarpal (CMC) Push MetaGrip orthoses[39] because they would be appropriate for someone with osteoarthritis who is active and requires small, yet durable hand orthoses (Fig. 16.1).

Bonnie is a 78-year-old widow who lives alone. She just completed 5 months of chemotherapy for cancer and complains of weakness, numbness, and cold intolerance in her hands. Her history is also significant for flexor tenosynovitis in her dominant hand ring finger. She is pleased that her cancer seems to be in remission, yet she feels very de-

spondent that she is not able to drive or prepare meals due to the difficulty that she is experiencing with her hands. Her son accompanies Bonnie to an outpatient rehabilitation setting. Part of the therapy intervention for Bonnie includes an orthosis to restrict metacarpophalangeal (MCP) flexion for trigger finger.[18] There are a variety of trigger finger designs to choose from, including a lightweight thermoplastic custom-fabricated type (Fig. 16.2A), a silver ring that resembles jewelry[43] (see Fig. 16.2B), a soft prefabricated Neoprene orthosis (see Fig. 16.2C), and a prefabricated off-the-shelf (OTS) molded plastic orthosis (see Fig. 16.2D). Clinical reasoning to decide the most appropriate orthotic includes consideration of the availability of materials, payment source, and client input. In addition to the trigger finger orthosis, Bonnie may benefit from wearing a lightweight Showa Atlas nitrile-coated garden glove[41] to reduce cold intolerance and aid more secure grasping (Fig. 16.3).

Donald and Bonnie are both older adults who benefit from orthoses to improve their ability to participate in daily activities. Although close in age, their stories illustrate the broad range of knowledge and skills necessary when making decisions about orthotic provision for older adults. Donald is an active, independent older adult whose primary goal is to decrease thumb pain from osteoarthritis. Bonnie has a complicated medical history and requires ongoing therapy to address her decline in function.

Note: This chapter includes content from previous contributions from Serena M. Berger, MA, OTR; Maureen T. Cavanaugh, MS, OTR; and Brenda M. Coppard, PhD, OTR/L, FAOTA.

Late adulthood spans from age 65 until the end of life.[13] According to the U.S. Department of Health and Human Services Administration for Community Living, almost 1 in every 7, or 14.9%; of the population is an older American.[15] By 2040 the older adult population is projected to represent 21.7% of the total population.[15] Only 3.1% of the age 65 and older population in 2015 lived in institutional settings, such as long-term care settings. However, the percentage increases dramatically with age to 9% for persons 85 and older. The age 85+ population is projected to triple from 6.3 million in 2015 to 14.6 million in 2040.[15] The growth of the older adult population is a significant reason that the Bureau of Labor Statistics

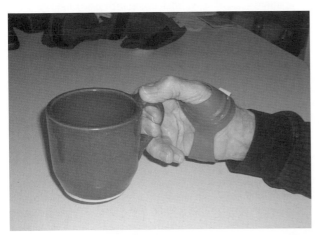

Fig. 16.1 Thumb carpometacarpal Push MetaGrip orthosis designed in consultation with Judy Colditz, Hand Lab.

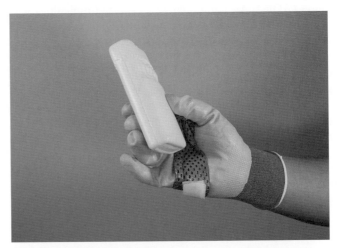

Fig. 16.3 Showa Atlas lightweight nitrile-coated garden gloves worn under an orthosis to reduce cold intolerance and assist with grasping.

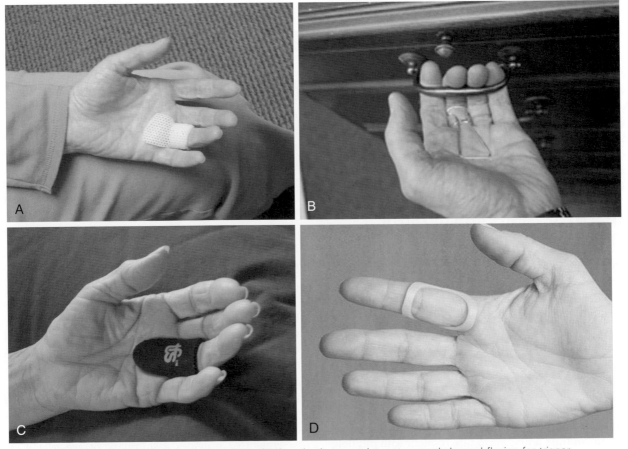

Fig. 16.2 A, Custom lightweight thermoplastic orthosis to restrict metacarpophalangeal flexion for trigger finger. B, Siris Silver Ring Trigger Finger Splint for chronic recurring flexor tenosynovitis. C, Neoprene Trigger Finger Solution (TFS). D, Oval-8 for trigger finger. (B Courtesy Silver Ring Splint Company, Charlottesville, Virginia. D Courtesy 3-Point Products,[53] Stevensville, Maryland.)

projects employment to grow by 21% for occupational therapists and 25% for physical therapists between 2016 and 2026.[7]

According to the U.S. Census Bureau's *American Community Survey,*[15] in 2013 over 30% of community-resident Medicare beneficiaries ages 65 and up reported some limitation in function that prevented them from being fully independent in performing one or more activities of daily living (ADLs). An additional 12% reported difficulties with instrumental activities of daily living (IADLs).[15]

Hands are one of the most common locations for musculoskeletal pain from osteoarthritis (OA).[14] The development of hand problems in older adults significantly impacts global physical functioning.[52] According to McKee and Rivard,[27] an orthosis that includes the needs of the client in the design process improves the ability to function by "relieving pain, providing protection and joint stabilization and enabling valued occupations."[27] Therapists who work with the older adult population need to have a strong foundation of interventions, including orthotic provision, to improve functional abilities in ADLs and IADLs.

Fundamental principles of clinical examination, design, and fabrication of orthoses do not change as people age. Therapists do, however, need to be aware of special considerations necessary to accommodate the unique needs of older adults. When designing an orthosis for an older adult, the therapist considers the specific needs of the individual, the goals of the orthosis, and the orthotic materials available. Clinical reasoning to determine the most effective orthosis for an older adult should consider:

- Age-related changes in body functions
- Medical history, including current medications
- Least restrictive designs
- Choice of lightweight but supportive materials
- Choice of materials for maintenance of skin integrity
- Simple designs for donning and doffing
- Awareness of payer source and cost effectiveness (e.g., prefabricated versus custom)
- The environment

TREATMENT SETTINGS AND ORTHOTIC DESIGNS

The older adult's environment is an important consideration for clinical decision making. Therapists provide interventions to older adults in multiple settings. Table 16.1 presents considerations and goals specific to different settings. The older adult's living situation (e.g., living at home, a long-term care setting, or an assisted living center) is important when the therapist determines the most appropriate orthosis. For example, an 80-year-old woman with OA who performs self-care independently and requires the use of her hands throughout the day may benefit from a thumb carpometacarpal (CMC) immobilization orthosis to improve her daily function. In contrast, a long-term care resident with multiple cerebrovascular accidents (CVAs) may require an orthosis to maintain sufficient range of motion (ROM) for assisted dressing and bathing. Hand ROM is necessary to prevent skin

TABLE 16.1	**Considerations for Orthotic Design in Different Settings**
Treatment Setting	**Special Considerations and Goals**

Short-term
  Acute hospital/ICU
  Subacute/SNF
  Comprehensive inpatient rehabilitation
	• Goals are to prevent secondary complications, such as loss of ROM and compromised skin integrity, while monitoring recovery
	• Positioning orthoses, such as a resting hand orthosis and neutral ankle-foot orthosis
	• Forward information related to the orthosis to the discharge setting

Long-term
  Assisted living
  Long-term care
  Geropsychiatry
	• Choose materials that are safe for clients who may have cognitive impairments or restricted mobility
	• Train staff members to monitor skin integrity when orthoses are used long-term (e.g., after discharge from skilled rehabilitation)

Community based
  Home health
  Outpatient
  Wellness center
	• Provide pictures and written instructions for use and care of orthoses and phone contact information in case questions arise
	• Orthoses are typically used to enable functional participation in ADLs and IADLs; orthoses must be versatile and durable

ADL, Activity of daily living; *IADL,* instrumental activity of daily living; *ICU,* intensive care unit; *ROM,* range of motion; *SNF,* skilled nursing facility.

maceration in the palm caused by sustained full-finger flexion. A prefabricated resting orthosis that is easily adjusted, such as the Comfy Hand Wrist Finger Orthosis (Fig. 16.4A) or a custom thermoplastic cylindrically shaped orthosis (see Fig. 16.4B), can prevent secondary contractures that impede skin care. Therapists who treat older adults during the acute stage of an illness must be aware of risk factors to prevent secondary complications, such as loss of passive range of motion (PROM), edema, and skin breakdown.

AGE-RELATED CHANGES AND MEDICAL CONDITIONS IMPACTING ORTHOTIC INTERVENTION

In addition to typical age-related changes, older adults' body systems are vulnerable to chronic diseases. For instance, someone referred for a hand orthosis following a CVA may have other health conditions more prevalent with aging, such as type 2 diabetes and OA. Besides obtaining a thorough medical history to determine the appropriate goals of an orthosis, the therapist needs to be familiar with how different medical conditions concurrently impact hand function.

Table 16.2 provides a summary of age-related changes and health conditions that affect the design and approach to orthotic intervention. The following client factors[2] are based on selected classifications from the World Health

Organization International Classification of Functioning, Disability and Health[55] as related to considerations for orthotic intervention.

Mental Functions

Therapists assess cognitive status to determine the older adult's ability to understand the orthosis' purpose, wearing schedule, and precautions. **Working memory** impairment may prevent the older adult from recalling the orthosis' storage location or application procedure. Sometimes a therapist can ascertain memory problems by noting how an older adult follows directions during orthotic fabrication. If memory is a problem, the therapist establishes a routine schedule for wear and care, fabricates a simple design, and labels the orthosis for easy application.

If the older adult has significant cognitive impairments, the therapist educates the care partner(s) about the orthosis' purpose, wearing schedule, care, correct application, and precautions. Individuals with later-stage dementias often posture in flexed positions and thus may require interventions to maintain skin integrity. If there are cognitive impairments, the risks versus the benefits of an orthosis must be carefully weighed against alternative positioning, such as the use of pillows or dense foam wedges. In addition, the therapist may consider using D-ring

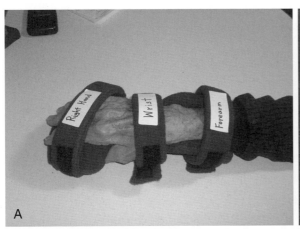 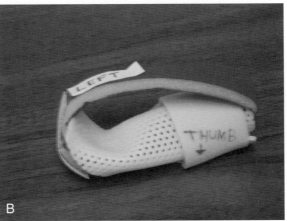

Fig. 16.4 A, Comfy Hand Wrist Finger Orthosis is an example of an adjustable prefabricated orthosis. B, A custom lightweight cylindrically shaped orthosis assists with keeping fingers out of the palm.

TABLE 16.2	**Summary of Age-Related Changes and Medical Conditions Impacting Orthotic Interventions**	
Body Functions	**Typical Age-Related Changes and Associated Conditions**	**Common Orthoses and General Hints**
Mental function: Cognition	Memory impairment Dementia	Assess individual's ability to understand the orthosis' purpose, schedule, and precautions. Establish routine schedule. Develop habit of keeping orthosis in same location when not in use. Provide thorough training to caregivers.
Sensory functions: Vision Hearing Touch Pain Temperature and pressure	Acuity loss (presbyopia) Cataracts Glaucoma Diabetic retinopathy Age-related macular degeneration (ARMD) Hearing loss (presbycusis) Diminished sensibility Joint pain Decreased ability to regulate body temperature to diffuse heat Hypersensitivity to cold	Written instructions should be simple. Use large font and provide high contrast. Use contrasting colors for orthosis and straps. Use tactile labels to mark reference points on orthosis (see Fig. 16.5). Use compensatory techniques, such as visual scanning. Use guidelines for talking to the hearing impaired (see Box 16.2). Share guidelines with family and caregivers. Perform visual skin checks; if vision is also impaired, instruct a caregiver how to do it. Consider if a soft orthosis or padding is an appropriate alternative to a rigid orthosis. Use neutral or resting positions for pain relief. Use an adjustable orthosis or adjustable straps to modify according to comfort level. Use an orthosis that can be easily removed. Use a stockinette on the extremity. Choose lightweight multiperforated materials. Provide a textured glove to wear under or over the orthosis (see Fig. 16.3).

Continued

TABLE 16.2   Summary of Age-Related Changes and Medical Conditions Impacting Orthotic Interventions—cont'd

Body Functions	Typical Age-Related Changes and Associated Conditions	Common Orthoses and General Hints
Neuromusculoskeletal and movement-related functions: Neurological Skeletal	Cerebrovascular accident (CVA) Peripheral neuropathies • Chemotherapy • Carpal tunnel • Cubital tunnel Parkinson disease/ tremorsldiopathic essential tremors	Use inhibition techniques to assist with application of antispasticity orthoses (refer to Chapter 15). Use resting hand and footdrop orthoses for flaccid extremities. Assess both sensory and motor function. Use a wrist orthosis in neutral. Position the elbow joint in 30 to 45 degrees of flexion. Provide elbow padding. Provide instruction in positioning and ergonomics (refer to Chapter 14). Use orthotic material to fabricate a base to hold assistive devices.
	Osteoporosis • Wrist fractures (Colles) Osteoarthritis (OA) • Heberden (DIPs) and Bouchard (PIPs) nodes • Thumb trapeziometacarpal involvement Loss of mobility	Choose a thermoplastic material with memory and moderate resistance to stretch if serial adjustments are indicated. Choose a prefabricated tubular design with D-rings for ease of application if fracture is healed. Immobilize PIPs/DIPs to rest joints or provide digit compression sleeves (see Fig. 16.8A–B). Use lightweight thermoplastic material. Ensure orthosis is easily donned and doffed. Use a hand-based thumb CMC custom or prefabricated design. Keep the orthosis within reach or easy walking distance. Maintain a consistent storage location. Keep the orthosis simple for easy application and removal. Permanently attach one end of each strap to the orthosis. Use D-ring straps.
Cardiovascular and hematological functions	Peripheral vascular disease (PVD)	Consider a footdrop orthotic design to float the heels and avoid pressure. Use padded volar knee extension orthosis for below-knee amputations. Choose a thermoplastic material with maximum resistance to stretch. Monitor skin carefully due to impaired sensation.
Digestive, metabolic, and endocrine functions	Diabetes related • Peripheral neuropathies • Trigger finger • de Quervain disease	Assess sensory and motor function. Educate to perform visual inspections. Keep fingertips and toes visible. Restrict MCP flexion. Immobilize thumb/wrist.
Genitourinary functions	End-stage renal disease (ESRD) Bladder conditions	In the presence of forearm AV fistulas, straps must be loose and easily adjusted to avoid constriction with fluctuations in edema. Orthoses may be contraindicated for insensate hands. For incontinence or frequent nocturnal urination, provide instructions on quick and safe removal of orthoses.
Skin functions	Fragile skin: • Corticosteroid adverse effect • Skin tears • Delayed wound healing • Flexion contractures of digits	Use stockinette or arm sleeves. Use gel orthotic pads or molded padding. Use lightweight thermoplastic materials or soft prefabricated orthoses. Inspect skin frequently. Modify wearing schedule to prevent skin maceration.

AV, Arteriovenous; *CMC,* carpometacarpal; *DIP,* distal interphalangeal; *MCP,* metacarpophalangeal; *PIP,* proximal interphalangeal.

straps for more secure positioning. Refer to Box 16.1 for a summary of general hints for orthotic instructions with older adults.

Sensory Functions

Vision

Older adults are particularly vulnerable to conditions that affect the visual system. Cataracts, glaucoma, age-related macular degeneration, and diabetic neuropathy are the primary conditions of visual impairment in older adults. According to a population-based study,[6] 81% of people with visual impairment are older than 50 years of age. Decreased vision may

impact a client's ability to adhere to orthotic instructions. For example, some older adults may be unable to apply their orthoses because of poor figure ground discrimination. Older adults may have difficulty seeing how the straps attach and may be unable to visually inspect their skin. Using thermoplastic material with contrasting color straps may assist the older adult who has poor visual discrimination. Bright colors may prevent the orthosis from being easily lost in bed linens or mistakenly sent to the laundry in an in-patient setting.

Older adults who have correctable vision should wear their glasses when they are instructed in orthotic use. The therapist needs to ask older adults to demonstrate proper orthotic application and removal. Simple, large-print instructions are best for this population. High contrast of ink and paper is helpful. The use of direct lighting and magnification devices helps with reading instructions and with performing skin inspections.

For older adults who have macular degeneration, glaucoma, cataracts, or poor visual acuity, the therapist encourages the use of compensatory techniques during application and removal of the orthosis and skin inspections. Compensatory techniques include eye scanning, head turning, and use of tactile labels to mark reference points on the orthoses (Fig. 16.5).

Auditory System

According to the American Federation for Aging Research, approximately 30% of older adults between 65 and 74 years of age and 50% of adults age 75 or older have hearing loss.[1] Hearing impairment impedes health literacy. Sometimes hearing problems can be detected during the initial interview or during orthotic fabrication. Therapists should not rely solely on printed information to relay instructions, because some older adults may be unable to read or have visual impairments that also limit reading capabilities. The therapist needs to use more tactile cues when positioning the person for orthotic intervention. When talking to an older adult who is hearing impaired, the therapist should use the guidelines outlined in Box 16.2.

Touch

A population-based study with community dwelling adults 57 to 85 years of age examined a potential common prevalence for global sensory loss of the five senses (visual, smell, hearing, touch, and taste).[12] Impaired touch was identified in 70% of the subjects. Two-thirds of the subjects had impairments in two or more senses.[12] Individuals with one identified sensory impairment should be evaluated for additional sensory deficits that may impact orthotic provision. Somatosensory function of two-point discrimination declines with age.[12] Because decline in somatosensory function is gradual over the life cycle, older adults may not be aware of their diminished sensibility. Vision is the primary sense used to compensate for decreased tactile sensation. When both vision and touch sensory functions decline, the older adult is at a greater risk for compromised skin integrity.

BOX 16.1 General Hints for Orthotic Instructions

- Keep the orthotic design simple for easy donning and doffing. Observe the client's/care partner's ability to don and doff the orthosis.
- Label the orthosis with individual's name, right or left extremity, hand or foot, and additional landmarks to identify how to properly position the orthosis.
- Provide written and oral instructions that include application, wearing schedule, and precautions for discharge.
- Identify a consistent location to store the orthosis within easy reach.
- Keep straps attached to the orthosis.
- Provide a picture of the orthosis on the extremity. Observe privacy regulations, and avoid public posting of information related to client's care.
- A dark-colored orthosis provides better contrast with light-colored bed linens.

BOX 16-2 Guidelines for Talking to the Hearing Impaired

- Seat or position the hearing-impaired person to see the face of the person speaking.
- Whenever possible, face the person with impaired hearing on the same level during verbal communication.
- Before talking, gain the older adult's attention by using touch, gesture, and eye contact.
- Use visual aids when possible. Take a photograph or draw a diagram that shows correct orthotic application.
- Use demonstration as part of the instructions.
- Keep hands away from face while talking.
- If the person misses statements, rephrase the statements rather than repeat the same words.
- Reduce background noises during verbal communication. When possible, work with the person one-on-one in a quiet room.
- Do not shout because doing so distorts voices. Talk in a normal voice but at close range.
- Avoid chewing gum during verbal communication, because this makes speech more difficult to understand.
- Be aware that people hear better if they are vertical rather than horizontal. If a person is standing or sitting, sound waves are directed into the ears. If a person is lying on a bed, sound waves are dispersed over the head.
- Recognize that persons with hearing impairments may not hear as well if they are tired or ill.
- If hearing is better in one ear, direct speech toward that ear. Never shout directly into the ear.
- Ask client to repeat the instructions back to you.

Data from Lewis SC: *Older adult care in occupational therapy*, Thorofare, NJ, 1989, Slack; Barlowe E, Siegal DL, Edwards F, et al: Vision, hearing, and other sensory loss associated with aging. In Doress PB, Siegal DL, editors: *Ourselves, growing older*, New York, 1987, Simon & Schuster, pp. 365-379; Hills GA: The changing realm of the senses. In Lewis BB, editor: *Aging: the health care challenge*, ed 4, Philadelphia, 2002, FA Davis.

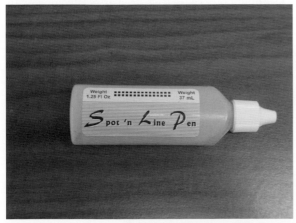

Fig. 16.5 Tactile label markers, such as the Spot 'n Line Pen, can be used to mark reference points on an orthosis for an older adult with impaired vision.

Tactile sensation may become impaired secondary to poor positioning of older adults with limited mobility. Decreased sensation may contribute to compression neuropathies of the median or ulnar nerves. Cubital tunnel syndrome, a compression of the ulnar nerve at the elbow level, may result from constant pressure on flexed elbows while sitting in a wheelchair or from prolonged bed confinement. A padded elbow protector (Fig. 16.6) or a padded elbow orthosis to restrict elbow flexion greater than 30 to 45 degrees (see Chapter 14) prevents further pressure on the nerve.[37]

Compression of the median nerve at the wrist or carpal tunnel syndrome may be due to prolonged wrist flexion posturing or secondary to an associated medical condition, such as rheumatoid arthritis (RA) or diabetes. A prefabricated wrist orthosis in neutral with D-ring straps is easier to don and can be used to prevent nerve compression (Fig. 16.7; see Chapter 7).

Pain

Perception of pain is subjective and variable among individuals regardless of age. A careful history, including documentation of location and particular activities that cause pain using a valid and reliable assessment such as the Patient-Rated Wrist Hand Evaluation (PRWHE), is an important part of the initial assessment.[26,51] The PRWHE is an example of an instrument that can be used for the self-care G-code set to convert scores for a G-code modifier to document percentage of impairment as required for Medicare B beneficiaries.[11] Once a baseline of pain and functional impairment is established, reassessments with the same instrument can determine if goals are met. It is important to assist the client in finding a balance between resting joints in the orthosis and actively using his or her hand.

Neuromusculoskeletal and Movement-Related Functions
Skeletal System

Several neurological and orthopedic problems are more common in older adults.[25] The skeletal system is most affected by aging. Osteoporosis and OA are common diagnoses that often require orthotic intervention. The National Osteoporosis Foundation reports that half of all women over 50 will break a bone due to osteoporosis because the loss of bone density accelerates after menopause.[31] Some older adults may sustain multiple fractures resulting from a fall (e.g., hip and distal radius fracture). Therapists may encounter such patients in a variety of settings, inpatient or outpatient, depending on the severity and healing progression.

The distal radius is especially vulnerable to fractures. A common fracture of the distal radius, a Colles fracture, typically occurs after falling on an outstretched arm.[32] Sustaining a Colles fracture can be associated with functional declines in physical performance in hand strength and walking speed.[32] A volar wrist orthosis is generally indicated for immobilization after removal of an arm cast or external fixator. As the fracture heals, the goal may change to one of mobilization, which can be achieved by serial adjustments to a thermoplastic orthosis to improve wrist extension (see Chapter 7). When treating a Colles fracture or any upper extremity condition, it is important to determine if there are other causes of upper extremity impairments. For example, a thorough assessment of a client referred with a wrist injury may reveal preexisting sensory loss in the dermatome distribution of C6-C7 due to compression of cervical nerve roots caused by OA. The sensory loss might otherwise have been associated only with the

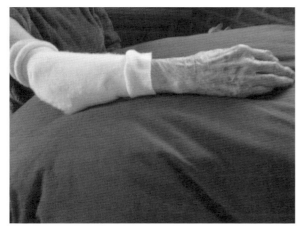

Fig. 16.6 Heelbo padded soft elbow sleeve protector to decrease pressure on the ulnar nerve.

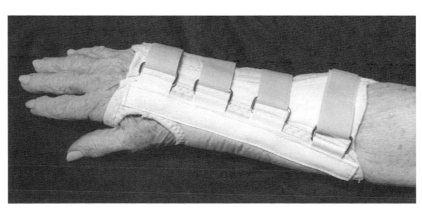

Fig. 16.7 This D-ring orthosis has a circumferential design that holds the orthosis in place during application.

wrist fracture. In older adults who have multiple medical conditions, the source of decreased sensorimotor function in the hand requires a careful differential diagnosis.

In addition to OA of the cervical spine, hand joints are frequently affected. OA typically becomes symptomatic in the 40s and 50s.[24] Primary OA is idiopathic or from known causes. Secondary OA results from conditions that impact joint cartilage such as trauma, congenital joint abnormalities, and endocrine and neuropathic diseases.[24] Most older adults have evidence of some cartilage damage.[36] Hand OA is characterized by enlarged nodules at the distal interphalangeal (DIP) joints (Heberden nodes) and/or enlarged proximal interphalangeal (PIP) joints (Bouchard nodes).[47] The nodules typically cause more impairment in the index finger because of the demands placed on the joint during pinch activities. An immobilization orthosis (Fig. 16.8A) or compression sleeves (see Fig. 16.8B) for DIP joints are conservative options to decrease pain. Surgical fusion may be warranted for more advanced degeneration if pain persists.

OA of the thumb at the CMC joint is another common reason for an orthotic referral. Initial conservative management usually requires a hand-based thumb immobilization orthosis (see Chapter 8). Individuals with CMC OA benefit from education on joint protection techniques to break the pain cycle. As discussed in Chapter 8, there are different approaches to orthotic intervention for arthritic hands. An effective conservative approach includes fabrication of a removable hand-based orthosis to immobilize only the CMC joint.[4]

Chronic flexion of the thumb MCP joint or an adduction contracture leads to a hyperextended interphalangeal (IP) joint. The hyperextended joint can be conservatively treated with a figure-eight orthosis to improve stability and function of the thumb (Fig. 16.9).

Neurological System

Central nervous system disorders are some of the most common causes of disability in older adults.[3] Progression of cardiovascular disorders may lead to CVAs resulting in abnormal tone on one side of the body. When making an orthosis for an older adult with abnormal tone, it is important to consider principles involved with orthotic design related to a coexisting condition, such as OA of the thumb CMC joint. Orthokinetic properties of materials should be cautiously selected because they may adversely affect tone (see Chapter 15).

Some neurological conditions cause tremors, which are particularly problematic for older adults. Tremors may be associated with Parkinson's disease, idiopathic essential tremors, or secondary to side effects from medications. An orthotic may be used to construct a base to hold assistive devices to improve self-care function in the presence of tremors, or thermoplastic material may be used to adapt self-care utensils, such as a spoon (Fig. 16.10A) or an electric razor (see Fig. 16.10B).

Peripheral neuropathies may be due to adverse effects of chemotherapy.[45] One study found that approximately 64% of patients treated with chemotherapy develop

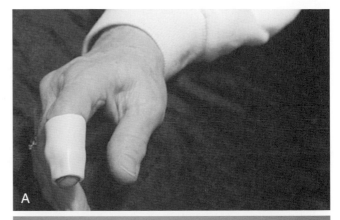

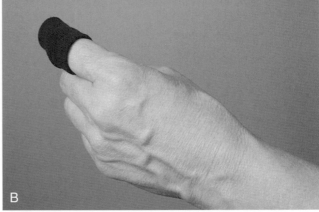

Fig. 16.8 Enlarged distal interphalangeal joints from osteoarthritis may become painful and benefit from (A) immobilization or (B) a compression sleeve to decrease pain.

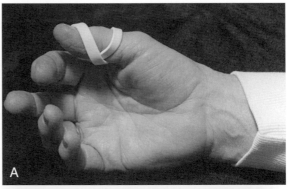

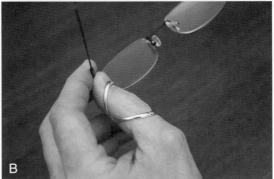

Fig. 16.9 A, A tripoint figure-eight design stabilizes the thumb interphalangeal (IP) joint to prevent hyperextension during pinch. B, Siris Swan Neck splint on the IP joint of the thumb to prevent hyperextension. (B Courtesy Silver Ring Splint Company.)

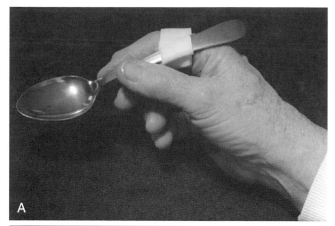

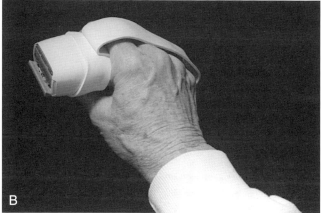

Fig. 16.10 Examples of adapted activity of daily living devices using thermoplastic materials. A, Eating utensils. B, Electric razor.

chemotherapy-induced peripheral neuropathy (CIPN).[45] Most cancer diagnoses occur in older adults, many of whom also have age-associated conditions.[29,42] Protocols for orthotic intervention of the particular nerve involved are followed. The skin must be routinely monitored due to loss of sensation.

Cardiovascular and Hematological Functions

Many older adults have cardiovascular disease, which may be the primary or secondary reason for referral. Older adults with cardiovascular disease may have limited energy. The therapist educates the older adult to store the orthosis in close proximity to conserve energy.

Peripheral vascular disease is a common accompanying condition for those who have cardiovascular disease. When fitting someone with a lower extremity orthosis like a volar knee extension orthosis to prevent flexion contractures post below-knee amputation (BKA), precautions for peripheral vascular disease are observed. The temperature of the thermoplastic material is carefully checked, and a double layer of stockinette should be considered instead of applying warm material directly to the skin. Older adults who have less ability to dissipate heat are vulnerable to burns and skin tears. Older adults with decreased cognition and thin skin may not be aware of the potential for burns. Furthermore, poor circulation results in delayed wound healing after skin breakdown. Footdrop orthoses should float the heel to avoid pressure.

Digestive, Metabolic, and Endocrine Functions
Digestive System

Dehydration, substance abuse, chronic disease, or poor diet in older adults may cause nutritional deficiencies.[56] Sensory testing is carefully completed with individuals who have digestive disorders and nutritional deficiencies because they may also present with impaired nerve function. Poor wound healing may be the result of a poor nutritional status. The condition of the skin and nails is observed to determine appropriate materials and orthotic care. Review of laboratory values gives therapists insight into nutritional status.

Endocrine System

Diabetes mellitus (DM), a disorder of the endocrine system, is a common condition reported by the Centers for Disease Control and Prevention,[8] which affects up to 25% of older adults. A chronic disease such as type 2 diabetes, which is more prevalent in the older adult population, is a source of hand impairment and activity limitations.[35] Individuals with long-standing DM have an increased incidence of other conditions that must be considered before an orthosis is made.

A careful sensory evaluation determines whether there are peripheral neuropathies in the hands or feet.[34] In the presence of diminished sensation, pressure caused by an orthosis may not be perceived by the older adult and may lead to skin breakdown. Straps must never cause constriction, especially if there is associated peripheral vascular disease. These considerations are particularly important when someone with diabetes is referred for a footdrop orthosis, a knee extension orthosis after a BKA, or a finger flexion contracture secondary to a CVA.

Individuals with DM are at greater risk for associated conditions that may require orthotic intervention for the upper extremity, such as carpal tunnel syndrome, flexor tendon nodules, and flexion contractures of the palmar fascia, which resemble Dupuytren disease.[21] Idiopathic Dupuytren disease (see Chapter 9) is most common in men age 45 and older.[46] These individuals develop flexion contractures of their fingers or thumbs with nodules at the palmar base of the involved digits. An orthosis is contraindicated preoperatively because the contracted palmar fibromatosis is caused by fascia tissue, which does not respond to low-load prolonged stress. Therefore, surgical intervention is necessary if the contracture is limiting function.[22] Orthotic intervention with a hand immobilization orthosis to regain extension of the digits[17] is appropriate only after a surgical release of the fascia or injection of clostridial collagenase.

When stenosing tenosynovitis occurs at the first dorsal extensor compartment on the radial aspect of the wrist, it is referred to as de Quervain disease. Conservative management includes a thumb spica orthosis (refer to Chapter 8). Orficast, a light, textile-like thermoformable taping material,[33] makes a comfortable thumb spica for an older adult with de Quervain disease (Fig. 16.11).

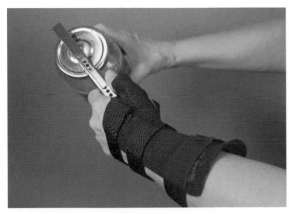

Fig. 16.11 Orficast thin and breathable thermoplastic fabric orthosis for de Quervain tenosynovitis.

Genitourinary Functions

Kidneys are part of the urinary system and have an endocrine function. When treating individuals with end-stage renal disease (ESRD), it is important to identify the subcutaneous **arteriovenous (AV) fistula.** Surgically created AV fistulas are typically located on the forearm and used for vascular access for hemodialysis. Because of the radial artery anastomoses with an adjacent vein, vascularity distal to the AV fistula is compromised[20] and can result in edema and peripheral neuropathies that affect sensorimotor hand function. Orthoses should be used selectively because any source of pressure could cause skin breakdown in an insensate hand with compromised vascularity.

Nocturnal urination is a common cause of sleep disturbances in older adults for a variety of reasons. The presence of comorbidities, medication usage, and several factors more prevalent in older persons influence the sleep-wake cycle.[5.] If an older adult needs to wear an orthosis during sleep periods, the history includes urinary function and a review of possible sleep-related disorders. With orthotic wear during sleep, it is especially important that the orthosis is easily donned and doffed for safe functional mobility and toileting.

Skin Functions

Aging of the **integumentary system** includes thinning of the epidermis and dermis.[19] Older adults with little subcutaneous fat are more susceptible to pressure sores. Fragile older adults are more likely to have skin tears. A **soft orthosis,** padding to line the orthosis, or a protective skin sleeve should be considered.

MEDICATIONS AND SIDE EFFECTS

Many older adults take medications that cause side effects[9] that may affect orthotic provision. More than 76% of older adults use two or more prescribed medications, and 37% use five or more.[9] A list of medications should be included in the history before an orthotic decision is made.[23] Corticosteroids are commonly prescribed for chronic conditions, such as rheumatic conditions and chronic obstructive pulmonary disease (COPD). Long-term steroid use can lead to **ecchymosis** (bruising), osteoporosis, and fragile skin that is vulnerable

to skin tears. Long-term steroid use can also lead to delayed wound healing. Anticoagulants, such as heparin, are prescribed for collagen vascular disorders. Side effects of **anticoagulants** include increased risk of ecchymosis and edema from minor soft-tissue trauma.[44.]

Antihistamines for respiratory conditions and psychotropic medications for mental health conditions can cause tremors. When designing orthoses for older adults who take these medications, the additional risks of fragile skin, osteoporosis, bruising, edema, or tremors are factored into the orthotic design. In older adults, sleep medications may affect orthotic wear. For example, the person may not notice problems if the orthosis becomes uncomfortable during the night, thus increasing the possibility of skin breakdown. In addition, the older adult may not be compliant with the wearing schedule and not routinely perform skin checks.

PURPOSES OF ORTHOSES FOR OLDER ADULTS

With the plethora of conditions that may affect older adults, the purpose of orthotic intervention may include, but is not limited to, the following:
- Prevent ROM loss
- Reduce pain
- Improve occupational performance
- Manage contractures
- Decrease edema
- Protect skin integrity
- Substitute for loss of sensorimotor function

Range of Motion

The design of an orthosis should always allow full ROM of noninvolved joints. Serial mobilization orthotic intervention is generally the preferred method to improve ROM for an older adult. An orthosis that is serially adjusted to improve ROM is easier to manage because the therapist has better control over the amount of force applied. For example, a volar wrist extension immobilization orthosis after a distal radius fracture may require several progressive adjustments to improve wrist extension (see Chapter 7).[28]

Pain Reduction

With acute and chronic conditions, one goal of orthotic intervention is to reduce pain by providing support and resting the involved joints. In addition to the design of the orthosis to rest specific joints, the wearing schedule should provide the appropriate balance between rest and activity. The hand-based thumb immobilization orthosis worn for CMC OA is an example of an orthosis removed periodically for ROM and reapplied during activities that otherwise cause pain and stress to the joint.

Improvement of Occupational Performance

An orthosis may improve or maintain an older adult's function. When possible, it is preferable to use compensatory strategies rather than restrict ROM in an orthosis. For example, rather than having an older adult wear a wrist orthosis for use during shaving, the therapist makes adaptations from thermoplastic material on an electric razor to allow the older adult to remain independent (see Fig. 16.10B). If adapting the task is not effective, then an orthosis may be indicated.

Contracture Management

Loss of mobility and neurological conditions place an older adult at increased risk of developing contractures.[38] Changes in the older adult's connective tissue and cartilage increase the risk for contractures, especially during inactivity.[38] Appropriate goals may be to prevent further contracture, decrease pain, or enable better skin care. Therapists determine whether to provide an orthosis by weighing the risks of additional complications that may arise from orthotic wear, such as contributing to skin breakdown.

If the orthosis is applied while PROM is still within normal limits, it may be possible to prevent a contracture. If the loss of PROM is recent, orthotic intervention may improve ROM and correct the contracture. An example is a footdrop orthosis to gradually position the ankle at 90 degrees after loss of active ankle dorsiflexion. Therapists also commonly use hand immobilization orthoses to prevent further deformity when there is a loss of active hand or wrist ROM.

Edema Management

With loss of active range of motion (AROM) combined with diminished circulation, edema can lead to secondary shortening of soft tissue. It is important to prevent edema through techniques such as elevation and AROM. The edematous hand is positioned in an orthosis to counteract adaptive tissue shortening and residual contractures. The position of deformity caused by edema in the hand results in thumb adduction, MCP extension, and IP flexion.[48] To prevent deformity the wrist is positioned in an intrinsic plus position. The intrinsic plus position consists of approximately 20 to 30 degrees of wrist extension, the thumb in palmar abduction to a level of comfort, and the fingers in MCP flexion with the PIP and DIP joints in extension (see Chapter 9). Adjunctive techniques may be necessary to treat edema when there is limited AROM. Wearing a compression glove concurrently with the orthosis may help control edema. If the noninvolved side of an older adult also appears edematous, a systemic cause, such as congestive heart failure (CHF), may be present.

Protection of Skin Integrity

The combination of impaired cardiovascular function and changes associated with aging, such as diminished sensation and thinning of the dermis and epidermis, creates the risk for loss of skin integrity. The heel is the most vulnerable area for skin breakdown in the lower extremity. Use of a densely padded positioning orthosis or footdrop orthosis with the heel elevated from the orthotic surface may prevent pressure sores from developing. Older adults who hold their hands in a fisted position or continually flex their elbows, knees, and hips create an environment conducive to skin breakdown.

The accumulation of perspiration within the skin folds allows bacteria to grow.[40] This constant posturing and the resulting bacteria growth may cause joint contractures, skin maceration, and possible infection. A thermoplastic orthosis, a hand roll, or a palm protector positions the involved joints in submaximum extension, allowing adequate hygiene of the hand. To accomplish goals, consider the following guidelines:

- An orthosis should not impede function unnecessarily. For example, the orthosis should not prevent an older adult from safely grasping an ambulation device or interfere with wheelchair propulsion.
- An orthosis should not exacerbate a preexisting condition. For example, an older adult who demonstrates a flexor-synergy pattern may wear a functional position orthosis at night for pain and contracture management. If the older adult also has OA in the thumb with joint deformities, consideration must be made not to aggravate the thumb CMC, MCP, and IP joints.
- An orthosis should not limit the use of uninvolved joints.

Substitution for Loss of Sensorimotor Function

When there is a nerve compression severe enough to cause loss of motor function, an orthosis may substitute for the lost function. In the case of median nerve compression, an orthosis can position the thumb in opposition to the index finger. If the ulnar nerve is affected, the fourth and fifth MCP joints are blocked in slight flexion to prevent a claw deformity with MCP hyperextension and IP flexion of the fourth and fifth digits. See Chapter 14 for more information on orthotic intervention for nerve conditions.[18] In the case of damage to the peroneal nerve, an ankle-foot orthosis can substitute for loss of ankle dorsiflexion (see Chapter 18).

ORTHOTIC INTERVENTION PROCESS FOR AN OLDER ADULT

Assessment

During an initial assessment the therapist completes a comprehensive rehabilitative evaluation to determine whether orthotic intervention is indicated. It is important to recognize that interactions with older adults require considerations such as those outlined by the National Institute on Aging in *Understanding Older Patients*[30] (Box 16.3).

All components of a therapy evaluation are essential for determining effective intervention strategies. (See Chapter 5 for a discussion of a hand examination.) The therapist pays special attention to the cognitive, sensory, physical, and ADL status of the older adult to determine the usefulness of orthotic intervention as part of the plan of care. The results of the assessment are used to develop a list of problems to be addressed. Typical goals include those listed in the section "Purposes of Orthoses for Older Adults." The therapist also documents functional goals based on orthotic usage.

During the initial assessment the therapist notes any current use of adaptive devices and techniques. For example, an older adult may already have an orthosis for a chronic condition, such as OA. The therapist evaluates the orthosis for its functional purpose, proper fit, and wearing schedule.

Observation during the assessment is vital to determining the purpose and orthotic design. It is important to observe and assess movement of the extremities in relation to the trunk. For example, an older adult who has hemiplegia with a spastic upper extremity may rest the hand on the chest, and provision of an orthosis may cause pressure.

Material Selection, Instruction, and Follow-Up Care

The choice of thermoplastic material, straps, and padding varies and is based on the older adult's needs.

Material Selection

Depending on client considerations and the goal(s) of the orthosis, the optimal material may be rigid, lightweight, multiperforated, less rigid thermoplastic material, or soft fabrics and dense foams. Selection of a low-temperature thermoplastic material is determined by the following:

- Extent to which an older adult's joint can assume and maintain a gravity-assisted position
- Size of the orthosis
- Performance requirements of the orthosis
- The padding requirements
- Weight of the orthotic material
- Therapist's skill level
- Environment

If the older adult is physically and cognitively able to hold the limb in the desired position, the therapist uses a material with high drapability and conformability to ensure an intimate fit. The therapist positions the extremity to ensure that gravity assists the material to more easily drape. Material with a high degree of conformability allows for a precise fit, thus increasing comfort and decreasing the risk of migration and friction over bony prominences.

Some older adults cannot assume positions that allow gravity to assist during molding. Clients may be anxious and respond to the stretch applied during orthotic fabrication by exhibiting increased tone. In such situations, or during the fabrication of large orthoses, materials with resistance to stretch are helpful. A material that lightly sticks to the stockinette placed on the older adult facilitates antigravity orthotic intervention (see Chapter 3). Preshaping techniques are helpful when fabricating an orthosis for an older adult with diminished cognition or abnormal tone.

Thinner thermoplastic materials (e.g., $3/32$ or $1/16$ inch) are less rigid. The therapist selects the thinnest material that can perform effectively. Minimizing the weight of an orthosis increases comfort and enhances adherence. Strength increases with more contouring to the underlying body part. Older adults usually appreciate lightweight orthoses because they are more comfortable. Orficast is a textile-like thermoformable taping material that is an alternative to traditional low-temperature plastics. It is a very lightweight knitted hybrid fabric and well suited for finger and/or thumb orthoses.[33]

Strapping material. Wide, soft, foam-like strapping material distributes pressure over more surface area than thin, firm straps. Soft strapping accommodates slight fluctuations of edema and can be fringed to decrease pressure against the skin. To prolong the durability of soft strapping material, it is beneficial to cut the material to the width of skin contact and weave a standard 1-inch loop strap through slits to keep the longer-lasting standard loop in contact with the adhesive hook on the thermoplastic material (see Fig. 16.12B). The loop strap should completely cover the hook portion on the orthosis' surface. This prevents skin abrasion or catching the orthosis on clothing and blankets. The use of presewn, self-adhesive straps can be an alternative to reduce the chance of losing straps.

There are advantages and disadvantages of using D-ring straps. An advantage is that D-ring straps provide mechanical leverage to effectively adjust the strap. Similarly, D-ring straps are useful for clients with dementia who may tend to spontaneously remove the orthosis. To minimize difficulty threading straps through D-rings, double over the ends to keep them loosely in position.

Padding selection. The two basic types of padding are open-cell foam (absorbent) and closed-cell foam (nonabsorbent). Open-cell padding absorbs moisture, is more difficult to keep clean, and can become a breeding ground for bacteria. Padding should be bonded with the thermoplastic material before molding to ensure a proper fit to accommodate the thickness of the padding. A composite thermoplastic material (i.e., with attached padding) can be placed in a resealable plastic bag before being immersed in heated water to keep it dry during fabrication (Fig. 16.12A). An alternative method is to first mold a removable padded liner. Plastazote,[57] a closed-cell foam available in a variety of thicknesses, is heated in a hot air oven at 285°F for 10 seconds for each 1 mm of thickness. The selected thickness of foam is softened to a pliable state and can then be molded directly on the extremity or over stockinette. The thinner widths can be used to mold a liner for an orthosis (see Fig. 16.12B), and the thicker widths can be used to fabricate an entire soft orthosis. Padding may also be molded on the

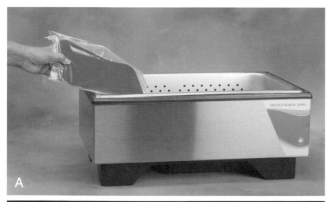

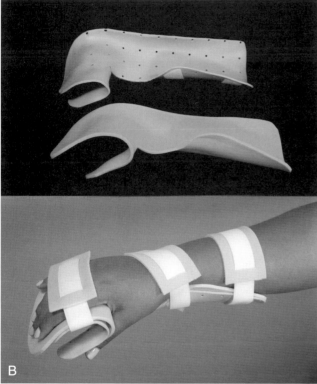

Fig. 16.12 A, A composite thermoplastic material put in a resealable plastic bag before placement in heated water keeps the padding dry. B, Foam, such as Plastazote, may be custom molded to line an orthotic if skin integrity is a concern. (A Courtesy North Coast Medical.)

outside of an orthosis if cushioning is needed when an orthosis rests against another body part. For example, an older adult who has hemiplegia and a flexed upper extremity may rest the orthosis against the rib cage, or a right ankle orthosis may press against the left leg when the older adult is side lying.

Choosing the correct strapping, padding, and thermoplastic materials is important. Clinical judgment and the ability to make adaptations is beneficial for older adult clients because they are most prone to contractures and pressure sores with illness.[49] Orthoses should fit well, achieve their goal(s), and be acceptable to the older adults and their care partners.

Technical tips. Therapists acquire technical skills through practice. With orthotic provision to older adults, one or more of the following technical tips may be helpful:

- Choose materials that have a slightly longer working time. For example, when fabricating a hand immobilization

orthosis (see Chapter 9), partially preshape the hand portion of the resting pan for a similar-size hand before applying it to the older adult.
- During the molding process, use latex-free resistance bands or an elastic bandage to temporarily secure the forearm trough. This technique permits more attention to contouring of the hand and wrist.
- Prepad bony prominences using circular pieces of adhesive-backed foam or gel padding over stockinette. Mold the orthosis over the padding, then reverse the adhesive side to position inside the orthosis and ensure congruous contact.
- Apply a stockinette to the extremity.
- Use uncoated and self-bonding material for orthoses if darts or tucks are necessary. Therapists often use this type of design for ankle, knee, and elbow orthoses.
- Use a coated material for thumb immobilization orthoses. Often the thumb IP joint is enlarged or deformed, thus making application and removal of a closed circumferential orthosis difficult. Use of a coated material allows circumferential wrapping around the thumb. After cooling the overlapping material pops open to allow for easier removal. If self-bonding materials are preferred, use a wet paper towel or tissue paper between the overlapping surfaces to prevent bonding.
- For serial repositioning, select a material that has a high resistance to stretch and memory.
- For a painful or deformed extremity, make the pattern on the opposite extremity, cut it out of the thermoplastic and then reverse it during fitting.
- To ease the fabrication process when working among multiple settings, create orthotic boxes or travel kits containing all necessary supplies.[50]

Older Adult and Care Partner Instructions for Follow-Through

Clear client and care partner instructions and consistent follow-through are important for successful orthotic intervention. Many factors influence adherence to an orthotic wearing schedule. The person responsible for the orthotic wearing schedule and care is the older adult or care partner(s). See Box 16.4 for information on adherence issues.

Instructions With Care Partners

Older adults unable to care for themselves will need assistance. Care partners are often family members or staff members from an agency or facility. When fitting an orthosis to an older adult, the therapist must provide thorough instructions. Instructions include information regarding (1) the orthosis' purpose, (2) wearing schedule, (3) orthotic care, and (4) precautions or safety factors. The therapist informs care partners about who and when to contact if a problem occurs. For example, for a client who has fluctuating edema, tone, and PROM, the responsible individuals are instructed in how to adjust the straps.

BOX 16.4 Factors That Influence Adherence to Orthotic Care and Wear Schedule

Older Adult Who Is Capable of Self-Management or Care Partner (Family and/or Staff)

- Explain the purpose and goals of the orthosis to the older adult and caregiver.
- Provide simple written and oral instructions with pictures.
- Use positive reinforcement for correct follow-through.
- Listen to the adult's complaints, and make adjustments as necessary.
- Use repetition with instructions as needed.
- Consider using analogies for instructions (e.g., "This is just like cleaning your dentures.")
- Ensure older adults wear their glasses and hearing aids.
- Label the orthosis for easy application when necessary.
- Ask if the patient/care partner has any questions about the orthotic wearing schedule and care instructions.
- Demonstrate proper orthotic application and removal.
- Encourage the patient or care partner to demonstrate the correct procedure several times.
- In an institutional setting, ensure that the orthotic-wearing schedule and hand hygiene are part of the older adult's care plan.
- Educate about precautions and safety. Provide contact information to report problems if they arise.

SELF-QUIZ 16.1ᵃ

For the following questions, circle either true (T) or false (F).

1. T F Observing the older adult's skin condition is important when the therapist is making orthotic intervention decisions.
2. T F The therapist should apply closed-cell foam only after the formation of an orthosis.
3. T F For an older adult who has spasticity, to ensure intimate contour, the therapist should use a material with high drapability.
4. T F The therapist should use wide straps on an orthosis for an older adult who has fragile skin.
5. T F A functional position orthosis is always appropriate to position the arthritic hand.
6. T F Older adults are more prone to joint contractures than younger persons who have similar diagnoses.
7. T F After orthotic completion for an older adult in a long-term care facility, there is little follow-up needed by the therapist.
8. T F Orthotic materials may be used to adapt ADL devices.
9. T F Medication use does not affect orthotic design.
10. T F It is always important to initially evaluate the entire upper extremity for an older adult with any injury.
11. T F Older adults with diabetes are at greater risk of associated conditions that may require orthotic intervention.
12. T F Poor positioning of older adults with limited mobility may contribute to neuropathies of the median and ulnar nerves.
13. T F When fitting an orthosis on an older adult with cardiovascular disease, the therapist should consider precautions for peripheral vascular disease.

ᵃSee Appendix A for the answer key.

The therapist provides oral and written instructions, demonstrates application of the orthosis, and observes for correct repeat of the demonstration until it is mastered.

The therapist labels parts of the orthosis for easier application (e.g., right/left, thumb/wrist/forearm). When possible, the therapist provides photographs of proper orthotic position in addition to a written wearing schedule. The therapist should include a list of precautions, safety factors, and maintenance information.

The therapist includes instructions in the medical record to ensure staff follow-through. All staff members involved with an older adult's care must receive instructions about the wearing schedule, precautions, and safety factors, particularly for those older adults who wear orthoses for only a portion of the day or evening. The wearing schedule may require modification to fit the staff schedule.

When appropriate, the therapist instructs care partners about the use of inhibition techniques to facilitate proper orthotic application. The therapist also provides instruction about the importance of intermittent PROM and active-assisted ROM to immobilized joints when appropriate.[16]

Skin care. Maintenance of skin integrity is important for older adults who need long-term orthotic intervention. The orthosis must be clean for application. A good cleaning method involves the use of isopropyl alcohol. Chlorine is appropriate for removal of stains. After removal of the orthosis, instruct to thoroughly wash and dry the hand. To manage moisture, have the older adult wear a stockinette under the orthosis.

Wearing schedule. To determine the wearing schedule, the therapist considers the goals of the orthosis. The goals establish whether a daytime, nighttime, or an intermittent wearing schedule is the most beneficial. For example, an intermittent wearing schedule allows air to reach the skin. A nighttime wearing schedule may be more appropriate if the older adult is able to use the extremity for functional assistance during the day.

COST AND PAYMENT ISSUES

Medicare is the primary insurance payer for older adults. Medicare Part A covers in-patient hospitalization, skilled nursing, and home health episodes of care. Medicare Part A services are typically paid under a bundled payment structure. Medicare Part B covers a percentage of outpatient rehabilitation and durable medical equipment (DME). The outpatient facility must be a DME supplier with Medicare to submit a bill with an L code for reimbursement for prefabricated off-the-shelf (OTS) or custom-fitted orthotics.[10] OTS orthotics are defined by the Centers for Medicare and Medicaid Services (CMS) as orthotics that require "minimal self-adjustment for appropriate use and do not require expertise in trimming, bending, molding, assembling, or customizing to fit to the individual."[10] When the orthotic does require

SELF-QUIZ 16.2ᵃ

Critical Thinking Case Scenarios

1. You are fabricating a volar hand immobilization orthosis for an older adult who is unable to actively supinate the forearm. Should you choose a material that has high drapability? Is this the best choice? Why?
2. You are treating an 86-year-old woman one year after a CVA. Since that time, she has held her left hand in a fisted position. Gentle passive extension is painful. The palm is macerated from perspiration. She does not have active motion in the left hand and does not use the hand for functional assistance during ADLs. Which type(s) of positioning device(s) would be appropriate?
3. An older adult who has RA complains of pain in the wrists and metacarpophalangeal joints. What problems would you anticipate if the therapist provides hand immobilization orthoses to rest all of the joints of the wrist and hands at night?
4. You fabricate a functional position hand immobilization orthosis for an older adult who has spasticity and hemiplegia and is in a flexor-synergy pattern. The older adult wears the orthosis at night for pain relief and contracture management. When the older adult is in bed, the orthosis is positioned against the rib cage. What can you do to relieve the pressure?
5. You fabricated a hand immobilization orthosis for an older adult with hemiplegia and congestive heart failure (CHF). You are concerned about the fluctuating edema noted in the hemiplegic hand. How would you modify the orthosis and straps?

ᵃSee Appendix A for the answer key.

SELF-QUIZ 16.3ᵃ

Matching

Match the intervention option with the problem that it would address.
1. _____ Silver ring orthotic
2. _____ Orficast custom orthotic
3. _____ Plastazote molded splint padding
4. _____ Nitrile-coated gloves under orthotic
5. _____ Soft, foam straps with fringed edges
a. Cold intolerance such as side effect from chemotherapy
b. Finger joint with chronic instability
c. Fragile skin or peripheral vascular disease
d. Need for lightweight breathable material
e. Edema

ᵃSee Appendix A for the answer key.

specialized fitting, the custom-fitting L code should be applied. The L-code payment structure covers the expertise required to provide an evaluation that is relative to provision of the orthotic. Follow up orthotic checks or training with an orthotic does not require the therapist to be a DME supplier. Medicare requires the use of timed Current Procedural Terminology (CPT) codes to bill for orthotic training and management during initial encounters and a separate code for subsequent encounters. Transmittals regarding codes, payment caps, and procedures frequently change. Therapists are encouraged to follow up-to-date information from their national and state level professional practice organizations as well as the CMS website. For additional details on cost and payment issues, see Chapter 6.

REVIEW QUESTIONS

1. What are the accommodations that a therapist can make for each of the following problems: edema, ecchymosis, fragile skin, contracture, diminished cognition, sensory loss, and motivation?
2. What are four possible goals of orthotic intervention with older adults?
3. Why are older adults prone to developing contractures?
4. What are five medical conditions more prevalent in older adults? What are the implications for orthotic intervention?
5. What are three common medication side effects that older adults typically experience? How might the side effects impact orthotic intervention?
6. How do instructions and selection of orthotic materials vary with an individual living independently in the community versus an individual in an inpatient setting?
7. What are three specific orthotic adaptations for older adults who have impaired cognition, sensory function, and poor adherence?

REFERENCES

1. American Federation for Aging Research (AFAR): https://www.afar.org/infoaging/healthy-aging/hearing/, 2018.
2. American Occupational Therapy Association: Occupational therapy practice framework: domain and process, ed 3, *Am J Occup Ther* 68(Suppl):S1–S48, 2014.
3. Bello-Haas VD, MacIntyre NJ, Seng-lad S: Neuromusculo-skeletal and movement function: muscle, bone, and joints. In Bonder BR, Bello-Haas VD, editors: *Functional performance in older adults*, ed 4, Philadelphia, 2018, FA Davis, pp 145–161.
4. Bertozzi L, Valdes K, Vanti C, Negrini S, Pillastrini P, Villafañe JH: Investigation of the effect of conservative interventions in thumb carpometacarpal osteoarthritis: systematic review and meta-analysis, *Disab Rehabil* 37(22):2025–2043, 2015.
5. Bliwise DL, Foley DJ, Vitiello MV, et al.: Nocturia and disturbed sleep in the elderly, *Sleep Medicine* 10(5):540–548, 2009.
6. Bourne RRA, Flaxman SR, Braithwaite T, et al.: Magnitude, temporal trends, and projections of the global prevalence of blindness and distance and near vision impairment: a systematic review and meta-analysis, *Lancet Glob Health* 5(9):e888–e897, 2017.

7. Bureau of Labor Statistics: Occupational outlook handbook. https://www.bls.gov/ooh/, 2018.

8. Centers for Disease Control and Prevention: *National Diabetes Statistics Report, 2017*, Atlanta, GA, 2017, Centers for Disease Control and Prevention, US Department of Health and Human Services.

9. Centers for Disease Control and Prevention: *Prescription drug use continues to increase: U.S. prescription drug data for 2007-2008, NCH Data Brief No. 42*. https://www.cdc.gov/nchs/data/databriefs/db42.htm, Sept 2010.

10. Centers for Medicare and Medicaid Services: Durable medical equipment, prosthetics/ orthotics, and supplies fee schedule. https://www.cms.gov/Medicare/Medicare-Fee-for-Service-Payment/DMEPOSFeeSched/OTS_Orthotics.html, 2018.

11. Centers for Medicare and Medicaid Services: Functional reporting. https://www.cms.gov/Medicare/Billing/TherapyServices/Functional-Reporting.html, 2018.

12. Correia C, Lopez KJ, Wroblewski KE, et al.: Global sensory impairment in older adults in the United States, *J Am Geriatr Soc* 64(2):306–313, 2016.

13. Crandell T, Crandell C, Zanden JV: *Human development*, ed 10, New York, 2012, McGraw-Hill.

14. Dahaghin S, Bierma-Zeinstra SM, Reijman M, Pols HA, Hazes JM, Koes BW: Prevalence and determinants of one-month hand pain and hand related disability in the elderly (Rotterdam study), *Ann Rheum Dis* 64(1):99–104, 2005.

15. Department of Health and Human Services: A profile of older Americans: 2016, Administration for Community Living. https://www.acl.gov/sites/default/files/Aging%20and%20Disability%20in%20America/2016-Profile.pdf, 2018.

16. Dittmer DK, MacArthur-Turner DE, Jones IC: Orthotics in stroke, *Phys Med Rehabil State Art Rev* 7(1):171, 1993.

17. Evans RB: Therapeutic management of Dupuytren's contracture. In Skirven TM, Osterman AL, Fedorczyk J, Amadio PC, editors: *Rehabilitation of the hand and upper extremity*, ed 6, St. Louis, 2011, Mosby, pp 281–288.

18. Fess EE, Gettle K, Philips CA, Janson JR: *Hand and upper extremity: principles and methods*, ed 3, St. Louis, 2005, Elsevier/Mosby.

19. Gregory CJ, Sandmire DA: The physiology and pathology of aging. In Robnett RH, Chop WC, editors: *Gerontology for the health care professional*, ed 3, Boston, 2015, Jones and Bartlett, pp 51–102.

20. Hechanova LC: Hemodialysis: Merck Manual professional version. http://www.merckmanuals.com/professional/index.html, 2018.

21. Hordon L: Limited joint mobility and other musculoskeletal problems in diabetes, *Diabetes Prim Care* 19(1):29–34, 2017.

22. Hurst L: Dupuytren's disease: surgical management. In Skirven TM, Osterman AL, Fedorczyk J, Amadio PC, editors: *Rehabilitation of the hand and upper extremity*, ed 6, St. Louis, 2011, Mosby, pp 266–280.

23. Knauf JJ: Drugs commonly encountered in hand therapy. In Weiss S, Falkenstein N, editors: *Hand rehabilitation: a quick reference guide and review*, ed 2, St. Louis, 2005, Elsevier, pp 441–446.

24. Kontzias A: Osteoarthritis: Merck Manual professional version. http://www.merckmanuals.com/professional/index.html, 2018.

25. Lewis CB, Bottomley JM: *Geriatric rehabilitation: a clinical approach*, ed 3, Upper Saddle River, NJ, 2008, Pearson Education, Inc.

26. MacDermid JC: Development of a scale for patient rating of wrist pain and disability, *J Hand Ther* 9(2):178–183, 1996.

27. McKee P, Rivard A: Orthoses as enablers of occupation: client-centered splinting for better outcomes, *Can J Occup Ther* 71(5):306–314, 2004.

28. Michlovitz S, Festa L: Therapist's management of distal radius fractures. In Skirven TM, Osterman AL, Fedorczyk J, Amadio PC, editors: *Rehabilitation of the hand and upper extremity*, ed 6, St. Louis, 2011, Mosby, pp 949–962.

29. Mohile SG, Fan L, Reeve E, et al.: Association of cancer with geriatric syndromes in older Medicare beneficiaries, *J Clin Oncol* 29(11):1458–1464, 2011.

30. National Institute on Aging: Understanding older patients. https://www.nia.nih.gov/health/understanding-older-patients#address, 2018.

31. National Osteoporosis Foundation: https://www.nof.org.

32. Nordell E, Jarnlo G, Thorngren K: Decrease in physical function after fall-related distal forearm fracture in elderly women, *Adv Physiother* 5(4):146–154, 2003.

33. Orfit. www.orfit.com.

34. Ponirakis G, Odriozola MN, Odriozola S, et al.: Nerve-Check for the detection of sensory loss and neuropathic pain in diabetes, *Diabetes Technol Therap* 18(12):800–805, 2016.

35. Poole JL, Santhanam DD, Latham AL: Hand impairment and activity limitations in four chronic diseases, *J Hand Ther* 26:232–237, 2013.

36. Poole JL, Siegel P, Tencza M: *Adults with arthritis and other rheumatic conditions*, Bethesda, MD, 2017, AOTA Press.

37. Porretto-Loehrke A, Soika E: Therapist's management of other nerve compressions about the elbow and wrist. In Skirven TM, Osterman AL, Fedorczyk J, Amadio PC, editors: *Rehabilitation of the hand and upper extremity*, ed 6, St. Louis, 2011, Mosby, pp 695–709.

38. Portnoi V, Ramzel P: Contractures. In Capezuti E, Malone M, Katz P, Mezey M, editors: *The encyclopedia of elder care: The comprehensive resource on geriatric health and social care*, ed 3, New York, 2013, Springer, pp 167–169.

39. Push Braces. http://pushmetagrip.com/.

40. Redford JB: Orthotics and orthotic devices: general principles, *Phys Med Rehabil: State Art Rev* 14(3):381–394, 2000.

41. Showa: Showa atlas gloves products. https://www.showagloves.com/.

42. Siegel RL, Miller KD, Jemal A: Cancer statistics, *CA Cancer J Clin* 65(1):5–29, 2015.

43. Silver Ring Splints. http://www.silverringsplint.com/, 2018.

44. Skidmore-Roth L: *Mosby's nursing drug reference*, ed 31, St. Louis, 2017, Elsevier Health Science.

45. Smith EML, Haupt R, Kelly JP, et al.: The content validity of a chemotherapy-induced peripheral neuropathy patient-reported outcome measure, *Oncol Nurs Forum* 44(5):580–588, September 2017.

46. Steinberg DR: Dupuytren contracture: Merck Manual professional version. http://www.merckmanuals.com/professional/index.html, 2018.

47. Steinberg DR: Osteoarthritis of the hand: Merck Manual professional version. http://www.merckmanuals.com/professional/index.html, 2018.

48. Strickland JW: Biologic basis for hand and upper extremity splinting. In Fess EE, Gettle K, Philips CA, et al.: *Hand and upper extremity: principles and methods*, ed 3, St. Louis, 2005, Elsevier/Mosby, pp 87–103.

49. Struck BD: Pressure ulcers. In Fillit HM, Rockwood K, Young JB, editors: *Brocklehurst's textbook of geriatric medicine and gerontology*, 8th ed, London, England, 2017, Elsevier, pp 939–942.

50. Swedberg L: Splinting the difficult hand, *WFOT-Bulletin* 35:15–20, 1997.

51. Taylor J, Kersten P: The patient-rated wrist and hand evaluation: a systematic review of its validity and reliability, NZ *J Physiother* 42(3):141–147, 2014.

52. Thomas E, Croft PR, Dziedzic KS: Hand problems in community-dwelling older adults: onset and effect on global physical function over a 3-year period, *Rheumatology* 48:183–187, 2009.

53. 3-Point Products. https://www.3pointproducts.com/, 2018.

54. University of California San Francisco Medical Center: Communicating with people with hearing loss. https://www.ucsfhealth.org/education/communicating_with_people_with_hearing_loss/, 2018.

55. World Health Organization: *International classification of functioning, disability, and health (ICF)*, Geneva, Switzerland, 2001, World Health Organization.

56. Youdim A, Geffen D: Nutrition in clinical medicine: Merck Manual professional version. http://www.merckmanuals.com/professional/index.html, 2018.

57. Zotefoams: http://www.zotefoams.com/product/azote/plastazote/, 2018.

APPENDIX 16.1 CASE STUDIES

Case Study 16.1[a]

Ruby is a 90-year-old right-hand–dominant woman who lives in an assisted living center. She was referred to occupational therapy to be evaluated and treated for an orthosis and activity of daily living (ADL) interventions. She underwent a trigger finger release of the right middle finger 2 years ago and has right thumb carpometacarpal (CMC) osteoarthritis (OA). Ruby no longer experiences triggering of the middle finger. However, she does have some loss of active metacarpophalangeal (MCP) extension. Ruby reports enjoying crocheting, but she finds that she has progressively crocheted less due to pain in her thumb. Upon observation of self-care performance, due to loss of active MCP extension of the middle finger, Ruby is noted to use only index-to-thumb opposition for activities that require pinch.

1. The therapist needs to consider which of the following to determine the most appropriate orthosis?
   a. Postoperative trigger finger protocols
   b. Grip strength
   c. Advantages and disadvantages of prefabricated and custom-fitted orthoses
   d. Prefabricated orthoses for trigger finger
2. The orthotic design should incorporate a combination of which of the following? Circle all that apply.
   a. Thumb CMC immobilization
   b. Thumb CMC mobilization
   c. Middle finger extension assist
   d. Middle finger MCP flexion block
3. Goals for the orthosis should include which of the following? Circle all that apply.
   a. Thumb mobilization
   b. Improved occupational performance
   c. Pain reduction
   d. Substitute for loss of motor function
4. To promote occupational performance, which of the following is least significant?
   a. Self-care function
   b. Leisure interest
   c. Location and degree of pain
   d. Age

Case Study 16.2[a]

Edward is a 74-year-old man who lives with his wife on a farm in a rural setting. He was recently discharged from an inpatient rehabilitation facility to his home. Edward receives home care services that include physical therapy, occupational therapy, and nursing. His referring diagnosis is left cerebrovascular accident (CVA) with right hemiparesis. Medical history is significant for congestive heart failure (CHF) and chronic obstructive pulmonary disorder. Edward's chief complaints are limited endurance and decreased use of his right upper extremity.

Upon evaluation, Edward presents with bilateral upper extremity (UE) tremors, good return of right UE function at the shoulder and elbow, minimal active wrist extension, finger and right-hand (dorsum) edema, and enlarged distal interphalangeal (DIP) finger joints. Although he is referred for orthotic intervention at this time, he was not fitted with an orthosis during his inpatient stay, because he was showing signs of motor return and was receiving daily treatment to prevent loss of motion.

1. Goals for the orthosis should include which of the following? Circle all that apply.
   a. Prevent loss of range of motion (ROM)
   b. Substitute for loss of sensorimotor function
   c. Decrease pain
   d. Decrease edema
2. What orthosis do you recommend?
   a. Wrist immobilization orthosis with D-ring straps
   b. Thumb immobilization orthosis
   c. Soft Neoprene prefabricated orthosis
   d. Prefabricated adjustable wrist-hand-finger orthosis
3. What type of straps would you choose?
   a. Long, soft, wide straps
   b. Thin loop straps
   c. D-ring straps cut to the exact size
   d. Wide hook straps
4. What wearing schedule would you suggest?
   a. Wear orthosis at all times
   b. Remove orthosis only for hygiene
   c. Wear orthosis only during the day
   d. Wear orthosis at night and periodically during the day when resting
5. What is the most likely cause of the enlarged DIP joints?
   a. Rheumatoid arthritis (RA)
   b. Osteoporosis
   c. Osteoarthritis
   d. Peripheral vascular disease

[a]See Appendix A for the answer key.

[a]See Appendix A for the answer key.

APPENDIX 16.2 LABORATORY EXERCISE

Laboratory Exercise 16.1ᵃ

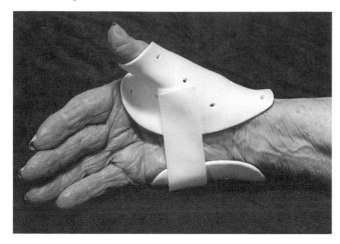

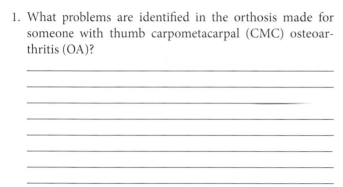

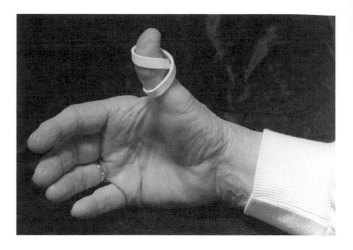

1. What problems are identified in the orthosis made for someone with thumb carpometacarpal (CMC) osteoarthritis (OA)?

   _____

   _____

   _____

   _____

   _____

   _____

   _____

   _____

2. How would the orthosis shown in the figure be modified for someone with hyperextension of the thumb interphalangeal (IP) joint?

   _____

   _____

   _____

   _____

   _____

   _____

   _____

   _____

   _____

   _____

ᵃSee Appendix A for the answer key.

Orthoses for the Pediatric Population

Yvette A. Elias

CHAPTER OBJECTIVES

1. Identify common diagnoses affecting the pediatric upper extremity.
2. Examine the impact of upper extremity orthoses on child development.
3. Describe common surgical procedures for select diagnoses and the postsurgical orthoses.
4. Describe orthoses fabricated specifically for the pediatric upper extremity.
5. Identify when thermoplastic versus soft orthotics are appropriate.
6. Describe challenges of orthotic fabrication for the pediatric population.
7. Describe wearing schedules and precautions for pediatric orthoses.
8. Discuss the importance and role of family members and other caregivers in orthotic intervention for children.
9. Assess and critique correct orthotic fitting.
10. Identify safety issues of orthotic intervention for children.
11. Identify resources for the purchase of prefabricated pediatric soft orthoses.
12. Examine current evidence for pediatric orthotic intervention.
13. Apply knowledge of pediatric orthotic intervention to a case study.

KEY TERMS

arthrogryposis	clinodactyly	radial longitudinal deficiency
brachial plexus palsy	congenital hand anomalies	spasticity
camptodactyly	Erb palsy	syndactyly
centralization	hypoplasia	tone
cerebral palsy (CP)	pediatric trigger thumb	ulnarization
clasped thumb	radialization	

Johnny is an 18-month-old boy who presents with right hemiparesis resulting from an intrauterine stroke. He has full passive range of motion in his right upper extremity and mild flexor tone, causing him to posture his elbow in slight flexion, forearm in pronation, wrist in flexion, thumb flexed into palm, and digits fisted. Active motion is limited at the end ranges of shoulder flexion/ abduction, elbow extension, forearm supination, and wrist extension. Although Johnny can actively extend his right-hand digits, he has difficulty grasping objects in his right hand because he approaches objects with his wrist flexed and has trouble abducting his thumb out of his palm most of the time. When his therapist stabilizes his wrist in extension, he can use a modified radial digital grasp on objects with more success but then has difficulty releasing objects from his hand and requires increased time for release tasks. Johnny's flexor tone causes him to have difficulty coordinating active wrist and digital extension simultaneously during grasping tasks (Fig. 17.1).

The therapist considers the following questions: In what ways might orthoses assist Johnny's function or prevent loss of function? Which orthoses are appropriate interventions for Johnny? What other interventions might enhance Johnny's volitional grasp and release, and how might orthoses be required with concurrent interventions?

This chapter introduces the most common conditions that affect the pediatric population and may require upper extremity orthotic intervention. A short description of each diagnosis is offered only as an overview. It is beyond the scope of this chapter to describe every pediatric hand condition. More detailed information is found in the cited references and in texts and journals. Orthotic fabrication is a therapeutic intervention used for children with orthopedic conditions and/or with developmental disabilities.[24] Surgical interventions for congenital hand anomalies are described with the postsurgical orthoses commonly required. General orthotic fabrication principles discussed in previous chapters apply to the pediatric population, but

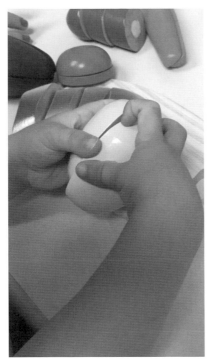

Fig. 17.1 Child with cerebral palsy (CP).

there are differences inherent in fabrication. This chapter addresses proper selection of orthotic materials, orthotic design, steps of orthotic fabrication, and tips for working with children and their caregivers. Typical orthoses fabricated for the pediatric population include elbow, forearm rotation, resting hand, wrist, and thumb orthoses. Children may benefit from commercially available orthoses. The measurements for and recommendations of a variety of commercial orthoses are described. The purpose of this chapter is to guide the novice therapist in applying knowledge of orthotic fabrication to the special needs of children with injuries, congenital hand anomalies, and/or developmental disabilities.

PURPOSE OF ORTHOSES FOR PEDIATRICS

The intents of pediatric orthoses are protective, preventive, or enhancement to the child's upper extremity function and skill development. Similar to orthotic provision for adults, pediatric orthoses may address issues at single or multiple joints. Orthoses may be applied in a variety of locations (e.g., shoulder to the distal interphalangeal [DIP] joints).

The different orthoses presented in this chapter are one small part of a comprehensive intervention program. A comprehensive intervention plan is developed beginning with an assessment of the child and incorporating all elements of the Occupational Therapy Practice Framework.[3] Using the Practice Framework as a guide ensures that the delivery of occupational therapy services is client centered and focused on occupations of importance to the child, the role within the family, and the performance of

play and learning, especially within the contexts of home and school environments. One quick method to apply the Practice Framework is to incorporate the following areas during evaluation:

- Areas of occupation: Make clinical observations of the child participating in activities. Does the use of an orthosis limit or improve function? What skill(s) does the child need to develop that might be enhanced with an orthosis?
- Client factors: Assess the child's muscle tone, range of motion (ROM), strength, and contractures. Will an orthosis improve or prevent further loss of any of these components?
- Performance skills: Evaluate the child's ability to reach, grasp, bear weight on the affected limb(s), and stabilize and manipulate objects. What are the child's sensory status, visual capabilities, and cognitive level? Will the use of an orthosis affect such systems?
- Context: Note the child's home and school environments. How does the use of an orthosis affect performance in these settings?

GOALS

The goals of orthotic intervention for children are similar to those for adults. Goals may include:

- Support the upper extremity
- Protect during healing
- Position for improved function
- Assist weaker muscle groups to improve function
- Facilitate or maintain tissue length and joint alignment
- Prevent deformity

However, orthotic fabrication for children involves more than simply making smaller-size orthoses.

Previous chapters discussed mechanical principles and orthotic fabrication techniques that apply to children. Orthotic fabrication for a child is different from orthotic fabrication for an adult in several key areas, including the following:

1. Different proportions between the palm and length of fingers in the growing hand versus the adult hand exist.[25]
2. Children are constantly growing and therefore require more frequent orthotic adjustments and/or new orthoses to accommodate for growth.
3. In many cases the parents or teachers are responsible for applying and removing the orthosis. They must understand the importance of the orthosis, wear and care schedule, and precautions.
4. Foundational movement patterns are set during the first 2 to 3 years of life. Interventions with orthoses assist the child with developing more typical movement patterns.
5. Children may be fearful about getting an orthosis and will typically not remain still while a custom orthosis is fabricated on their hand.
6. Children may remove their orthosis, and compliance with orthosis wear may be challenging.

DEVELOPMENT

Working with children requires a thorough understanding of normal and abnormal child development, knowledge of the specific pediatric conditions, and current evidence-based intervention practices, including orthoses. The parent or caregiver must be included in the orthotic process from the beginning to ensure adherence to the intervention plan. The parent should have a good understanding as to the purpose of each orthosis so that adherence to the wear schedule is optimal. The therapist should also consider the parent's specific goals and expectations for his or her child.

Normal Hand Development

Understanding normal hand development is required before orthotic fabrication. The upper extremity begins as a small outgrowth of tissue on the lateral body wall of the fetus, beginning on day 26 of gestation, even before growth of the lower extremity.[28] This small area contains all of the necessary information to form the limb. Development of the upper extremity proceeds proximally to distally. By the 31st day, the area of the hand is present. Fingers are evident by days 36 to 41. Bone, joint, muscle, and vascular development follows. Formation of the upper extremity is completed by the eighth week of fetal development.[28]

Abnormal Hand Development

Abnormal hand development may be affected by intrinsic factors (e.g., chromosomal abnormalities or mutant genes), extrinsic (i.e., environmental) factors, or a combination of the two. These factors contribute to the arrest of development of the forming limb or to the destruction of structures already formed.

Fine Motor Skill Development

A detailed description of hand and fine motor skill development is beyond the scope of this chapter. However, the therapist fabricating an orthosis considers the infant or child's current level of fine motor skills and thinks about how the orthotic intervention impacts future hand skill development. Through sensory exploration and play, children learn about their environments. Wearing an orthosis interferes to some degree with the ability to explore and play. The therapist provides appropriate scheduling of orthotic wear to ensure ample opportunities for play and development of grasp and release patterns. Table 17.1 is a guide to the development of gross and fine motor skills during the first year. Children develop these skills in a predictable manner. Proper orthotic selection takes this progression into account.

Atypical Upper Extremity Motor Development

Atypical upper extremity development occurs when the infant or child develops patterns of movement that compensate for weakness, spasticity, contractures, deformity, tightness, and/or sensory abnormalities. For example, if a child has an adducted thumb, grasp may result in using the ulnar fingers. Ulnar deviation and wrist flexion are reinforced with this pattern, whereas radial musculature may be overstretched and weakened through nonuse. This topic is discussed later in this chapter in the Cerebral Palsy section.

TABLE 17.1 Gross and Fine Motor Skill Development	
Approximate Age	**Gross and Fine Motor Skill**
Birth to 2 months	Physiological flexion
2 months	Grasp reflex
3 months	Hands together in supine
4 months	Objects held in midline, bears weight on forearm
5 months	Two-handed approach to objects, extended-arm weight bearing, displays some supination of forearm
6 months	Weight shifts on extended arms in prone, sits with straight back, elbows fully extend
7 months	Purposeful release, may pull to stand
8 months	Creeps on hands and knees
9 months	Reaches with active supination
10 months	Pokes with index finger
12 months	One hand stabilizes while one hand manipulates
15 months	Develops release with precision

Modified from Hogan, L., Uditsky, T. (1998). *Pediatric splinting: Selection, fabrication, and clinical application of upper extremity splints.* San Antonio, TX: Therapy Skill Builders.

COMMON PEDIATRIC UPPER EXTREMITY CONDITIONS

Children born with **congenital hand anomalies** require special consideration and a team approach. Intervention involves family members, therapists, surgeons, and teachers. The most common congenital anomalies include:

1. Common congenital hand anomalies
   a. Radial longitudinal deficiency/radial clubhand
   b. Hypoplastic thumb
   c. Pediatric trigger thumb
   d. Syndactyly
   e. Camptodactyly
   f. Clinodactyly
   g. Clasped thumb
2. Brachial plexus palsy
3. Arthrogryposis
4. Juvenile idiopathic arthritis
5. Cerebral palsy

Common Congenital Hand Anomalies
Radial Longitudinal Deficiency/Radial Clubhand

Radial longitudinal deficiency, also referred to as radial clubhand (Fig. 17.2), is the most common congenital longitudinal deficiency in the upper extremity.[15] The term describes congenital hand anomalies that present as a result of absent or abnormally developed or underdeveloped tissue on the radial

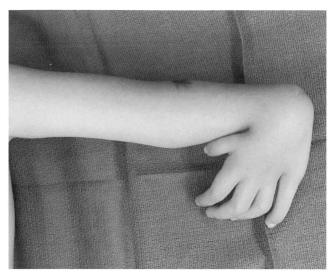

Fig. 17.2 Radial clubhand.

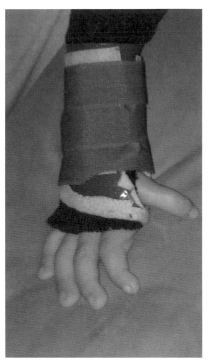

Fig. 17.3 Radial clubhand with orthosis.

aspect of the upper limb.[28] There is typically an absent or hypoplastic thumb with abnormalities seen in the other digits. The radial digits are usually stiff, while the more ulnar digits are more mobile.[43] There is no bony support on the radial side with carpal and musculotendinous abnormalities.[43] The combination of a stiff elbow, short forearm, radially deviated hand, and underdeveloped or absent thumb significantly impairs hand function.[43] The degree of severity determines the need for surgical intervention.

Radial deficiency conditions may occur in isolation but commonly occur to some degree in association with each other and in the presence of other syndromes.[1]

Passive stretching to all affected joints and fabrication of appropriate orthotics should be initiated soon after birth to distract and lengthen the tight radial structures at the wrist.[44] The implementation of passive stretching and use of orthotics is essential to preventing progressive contractures and to providing a supportive base for hand use. These approaches facilitate the best functional outcome postoperatively should they require a centralization procedure in the future, as is the case with more severe deficiencies. (**Centralization** is a surgical procedure to move the carpus to a central position on the ulnar to correct radial deviation and wrist subluxation.) Initially the radial gutter type of wrist orthosis (Fig. 17.3) (see Chapter 7) is molded on the radial border of the forearm and places the hand in a central position relative to the forearm, or as close to the center as passively possible. The orthosis is worn full-time and should allow the digits to be free for play and for hand to mouth exploration. Padding over bony prominences and lining the orthosis with moleskin is important for protecting the skin and promoting maximal comfort. Soft straps are better tolerated on the skin. If there is stiffness in the elbow, a posterior long arm orthosis can be fabricated for overnight use in the child's submaximal available passive flexion for prolonged stretching (see Chapter 10). This posterior long arm orthosis is serially modified into increased flexion as ROM improves. Full arm casting may be used to correct the positioning of the hand, wrist, and elbow.[36]

There are new surgical approaches being implemented to manage radial longitudinal deficiencies, but the most common procedure performed currently is soft tissue distraction followed by a wrist realignment procedure such as a centralization, radialization, or ulnarization.[32] (**Radialization** is a surgical procedure to move the hand closer to the radial border of the forearm. **Ulnarization** is a surgical procedure to move the hand closer to the ulnar border of the forearm.) A large retrospective review of 446 patients, including 137 patients managed nonsurgically and 309 patients managed with either a centralization or radialization procedure, found that those managed surgically had improvement in appearance and function, including improved alignment, ROM, and strength.[32]

Banskota and colleagues[5] recommend surgery for the wrist before 2 years of age because children quickly acquire adaptive functional skills. A delayed surgery may interfere with normal hand skill development. During the first phase of the surgery an external fixator is applied for soft tissue distraction. During this time the therapist may need to fabricate a protective orthosis over the external fixator to protect the pins and prevent injury to the child. This orthosis may need to be circumferential and may need to include the elbow for improved stability, especially if there is no thumb for anchoring the distal portion of the orthosis. Applying straps strategically can help prevent the orthosis from migrating. When strapping a short arm radial gutter orthosis, one strap can be used in a figure-eight pattern to best secure the orthosis, or one long strap can be applied to secure orthosis. A figure-eight pattern can also be applied to a long arm orthosis with wide straps crossing over the anterior elbow. A benefit to orthotic use is that, unlike casts, orthoses can easily be removed by

TABLE 17.2 Hypoplasia/Aplasia of the Thumb

Type	Findings	Treatment
I	Minor generalized hypoplasia	Augmentation
II	Absence of intrinsic thenar muscles	Opponensplasty
	First web space narrowing	First web release
	UCL insufficiency	UCL reconstruction
III	Similar findings as type II plus:	A: Reconstruction
	Extrinsic muscle and tendon abnormalities	B: Pollicization
	Skeletal deficiency	
	A: Stable CMC joint	
	B: Unstable CMC joint	
IV	Pouce flottant or floating thumb	Pollicization
V	Absence	Pollicization

CMC, Carpometacarpal; *UCL,* ulnar collateral ligament.

the surgeon to perform weekly distractions. The therapist must then modify the orthosis as needed to accommodate to the increased alignment of the wrist. The next phase is a formal centralization procedure, requiring the use of a forearm orthosis (see Chapter 7) throughout the 12-week postoperative period; which is removed for hygiene only. Again, if there is an absent thumb and there is difficulty in maintaining the orthosis in place, a long arm orthosis may be a better option to lessen chances of the orthosis being easily removed. This long arm orthosis is weaned to overnight use at around 12 weeks post surgery and is typically worn overnight until skeletal maturity.[28] Children with mild deformities are advised to follow the same overnight wearing schedule, with daytime use as needed.

Serial-static and static-progressive mobilization orthoses stabilize and position the wrist. These orthoses (and passive motion) align the wrist in a more neutral position and maximize function. Alternatively, children may benefit from nighttime resting hand orthoses (see Chapter 9) once full passive motion is achieved. Resting hand orthoses maintain digital alignment and prevent flexion contractures of the digits. A wrist support often improves functional grasp of the digits. With growth, children may require multiple surgeries and need frequent orthotic adjustments.

A number of challenges exist when fabricating an orthosis for a child with radial deficiency. These include:
- The child may easily remove the orthosis.
- Lack of a thumb to hook the thermoplastic material around during fabrication and wear.
- Tendency of the orthosis to migrate proximally and/or distally.
- Frequent serial adjustments of the orthosis are necessary with gains in passive ROM (PROM).
- The elbow may need to be included in the orthosis for leverage and mechanical length.

Hypoplastic Thumb

A thumb with some degree of deficiency in any of its anatomical parts—osseous, musculotendinous, or ectodermal—is referred to as a hypoplastic thumb.[28] The popular Blauth system classifies hypoplastic thumbs into five types (Table 17.2).[28]

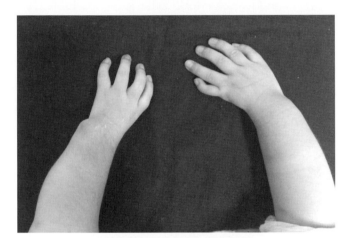

Fig. 17.4 Hypoplastic thumb.

Children with congenital thumb aplasia (total absence of the thumb) or hypoplasia (Fig. 17.4) are severely impaired with function.[28] These children lack an active thumb, which plays a key component in hand function. Surgical procedures vary from thumb reconstructions, including tendon transfers to enhance thumb function (for mild cases of thumb hypoplasia), to pollicization, creating a thumb from the index finger when the thumb is absent.[14]

Box 17.1 lists the indications for thumb hypoplasia orthotic intervention. Thumb orthoses (Fig. 17.5) for children with thumb hypoplasia include the carpometacarpal (CMC), metacarpal (MP), and interphalangeal (IP) joints, as needed. Such orthoses maintain an adequate first web space, hold the thumb in a functional position, and correct or prevent deformity. The appropriate thickness of thermoplastic material is based on the size of the child's hand. For small children and infants, even ¹⁄₁₆-inch thick thermoplastic material may be too heavy. A commercially available soft thumb orthosis, a ribbon, or a thin Neoprene strap in the web space may work best.

Pediatric Trigger Thumb

Pediatric trigger thumb generally presents early in childhood, but not at birth.[8] Most commonly the thumb is locked in flexion at the IP joint. There is a palpable nodule at the volar aspect of the metacarpophalangeal joint flexion crease,

BOX 17.1   Indications for Orthotic Fabrication for Thumb Hypoplasia

Preoperatively	Postoperatively
Orthoses to preserve and/or increase the first web space	Orthoses to protect the tendon transfers during healing
	Orthoses to protect pollicization of the index finger (in its new position)

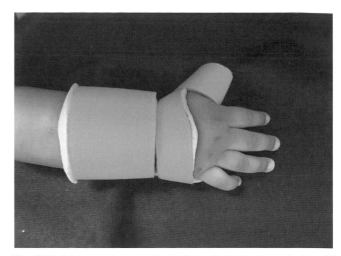

Fig. 17.6 A forearm-based orthosis is applied with the wrist in mild extension, thumb in radial abduction, and the IP joint in as much extension as passively available.

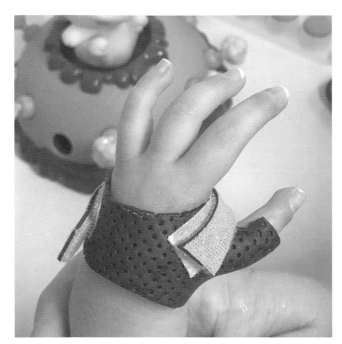

Fig. 17.5 Thumb orthosis.

known as a Notta nodule.[8] A recent ultrasound study of children with trigger thumbs demonstrated no abnormalities of the flexor pollicis longus (FPL) tendon or the A1 pulley. Rather, it is simply a size mismatch between the cross-sectional area of the tendon compared with that of the pulley.[8] There is some controversy as to whether pediatric trigger finger is an acquired deformity or a congenital anomaly.[8] In either case, orthotic intervention and stretching exercises can be successful. The evidence for the protocol includes full-time hyperextension orthotic intervention for 6 to 12 weeks followed by nighttime wear. Shiozawa and colleagues[42] recommended an immobilization orthosis at the first physician evaluation. A forearm-based orthosis is applied with the wrist in mild extension, the thumb in radial abduction, and the IP joint in as much IP extension as passively available (Fig. 17.6). A forearm orthosis is best suited for children, as small digitally based orthoses will typically slip off easily or will be removed by the child. These authors found that wearing an orthosis significantly reduced the need for further surgical intervention. Surgical release of the A1 pulley may be needed when there is no resolution after 1 year of conservative management.[31] Koh and colleagues[31] reported on the results of nonsurgical management of locked trigger

thumbs specifically. They found that 92% of those treated with nighttime use of an orthosis resolved completely at an average of 22 months after presentation, whereas 60% who were simply observed resolved completely at an average of 59 months.[31]

Trigger Finger

Pediatric trigger fingers often present in children with underlying conditions.[8] In contrast to trigger thumbs, trigger fingers more often present with classic triggering symptoms rather than fixed or locked in flexion posture.[8] Success has recently been reported in the nonsurgical management of idiopathic pediatric trigger finger. A recent comparative study of orthosis versus observation of pediatric trigger fingers found that 30% resolved in the observation group, whereas 67% resolved in the orthosis group.[8]

Syndactyly

Syndactyly (Fig. 17.7A) refers to the webbing of fingers. Syndactyly is classified as complete (full length of the fingers) or incomplete. Syndactyly may involve the skin only (simple syndactyly), or it may involve fusion of the bones (complex syndactyly).[27] Syndactyly is treated by surgical release for functional and cosmetic improvement. Surgery is typically performed before prehension patterns are established.[14]

For postsurgical syndactyly release, a web spacer or finger separator is formed from silicone or elastomer putty to maintain pressure on the surgically corrected interdigital web space. Highly conforming thermoplastic material is used. Web creep or the repeated fusion of the skin between the released digits may reoccur and is a significant complication that may require an additional surgical release.[27] The type of orthoses used in the treatment of syndactyly may include a resting hand orthosis (Fig. 17.8) with finger separators made from pellets of thermoplastic material or elastomer. A foam-padded dorsal piece of thermoplastic

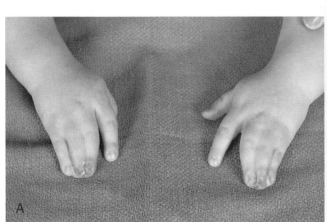

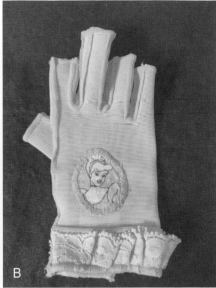

Fig. 17.7 A, Syndactyly. B, Compression glove to preserve webs after syndactyly release.

material can be clamshelled to the volar orthosis at the distal end to decrease existing PIP flexion contractures as well as to prevent the child from easily sliding fingers out of the orthosis. Coban can also be wrapped lightly around affected digits to aid in preserving webs and for scar remodeling purposes. Once the wounds are healed, some therapists measure the child's hand for compression gloves with slant inserts to preserve the web spaces and facilitate the development of a soft, flat, and mobile scar throughout the scar maturation period of 1 year (see Fig. 17.7B). It is recommended that the gloves be worn 23 hours a day for best outcome. The therapist has the option of lining a daytime glove with silicone within the webs and over the digital scars for 12-hour daytime wear and then alternating these with nighttime compression gloves without silicone lining for a total of 23-hour daily wear between both gloves. Parents should be instructed to perform scar massage frequently throughout the day and to monitor the child's skin for any signs of skin irritation or skin maceration. Those children with residual digital flexion contractures should continue to wear a static extension orthosis overnight.

Camptodactyly

Camptodactyly is a nontraumatic, flexion contracture of the proximal interphalangeal (PIP) joint that typically affects the little finger.[39] There are three basic types of camptodactyly:

- Type I appears in infancy and is present in both males and females. Type I affects the little fingers on both hands and may involve the ring and long fingers.
- Type II presents in adolescence and is more common among females. Type II worsens during growth spurts.
- Type III is a more severe form of camptodactyly and may involve multiple digits of both hands. Type III is associated with additional congenital anomalies.

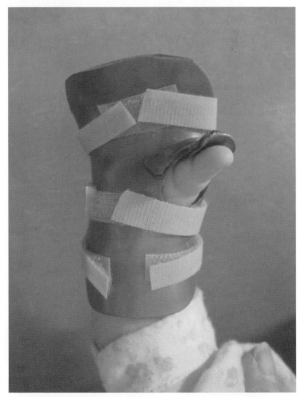

Fig. 17.8 Resting hand for infant. (Courtesy Orfit Industries.)

Intervention for camptodactyly, both operative and nonoperative, remains controversial and may depend on the severity of the deformity.[14] Nonoperative intervention with orthotics may sometimes be the only form of treatment needed for camptodactyly. Surgery is not the sole definitive treatment. Hand therapy plays a substantial role in achieving postoperative results and may also play a role in nonsurgical patients. Hand therapy must be individualized via clinical examination to decipher the best orthotic intervention to use.[39] Surgery is usually considered only when PIP skeletal changes are noted radiographically and the deformity is progressively worsening and interfering with function.[39] Types of orthoses for camptodactyly are PIP extension orthoses, including immobilization, mobilization, and/or static-progressive orthoses. Orthosis position is based on the clinical evaluation of the hand.[39] If the PIP joint remains flexed while the MP joint is flexed, the orthosis positions the hand in full MP joint and PIP joint extension.[39] If the PIP joint is flexed only when the MP joint is extended, the orthosis positions the hand in an intrinsic plus position with the MP joint flexed and the PIP joint extended (see Chapter 9 for a description of intrinsic plus position).[39] In young patients, excessive pressure to the skin and the joint may cause the DIP joint to be placed in excessive hyperextension, and this should be avoided.[39] It is preferable for young children to wear their orthoses during the night so that their hands are free to explore and develop appropriate developmental skills during the day. There is some evidence for the success of continuous orthotic wear to correct simple camptodactyly in young children.[28]

Orthoses are typically worn full-time at night until skeletal maturity is reached. Serial casting (see Chapter 19) and/or static-progressive orthoses may be more effective for rigid deformities.[12] Most if not all children require a forearm-based orthosis to prevent orthotic removal. Fabricating a circumferential orthosis or clamshelling the volar orthosis with a dorsal padded component distally helps prevent the child from sliding his or her fingers out of the orthosis and keeps the fingers as straight as possible. The fingertips should be visible for parents to monitor for any signs of discoloration.

Challenges providing orthoses for camptodactyly include difficulty keeping orthoses on the child's little finger only. Frequent orthotic adjustments are required during periods of growth. The best results occur when orthotic intervention is initiated early.

Clinodactyly

Clinodactyly refers to radioulnar deviation of the finger. Minor angulation, especially of the little finger, is so common that it is considered a normal variant. Pathological clinodactyly is usually described as greater than 10 or 15 degrees. Clinodactyly is usually present bilaterally and is caused by an abnormally shaped middle phalanx. For those whose function is impaired, an indication to operate can exist.[27]

Clasped Thumb

Clasped thumb refers to a classification of thumb anomalies that range from mild deficiencies of the thumb extensor mechanism to severe abnormalities of the thenar muscles, web space, and soft tissues.[33] A classification system was proposed by McCarroll and expanded by Mih.[33] A type I clasped thumb is supple, and the extensor mechanism is either absent or hypoplastic. Type II clasped thumbs are complex with additional findings of joint contracture, collateral ligament abnormality, first web space contracture, and thenar muscle abnormality. A type III clasped thumb is associated with arthrogryposis or its associated syndromes, in which case the extensor mechanism has minimal or no abnormality.[33] An extensor lag is usually observed at the MP joint as a result of a hypoplastic extensor pollicis brevis muscle tendon unit (Fig. 17.9A). A concomitant lag at the IP joint implies a deficiency of the extensor pollicis longus tendon as well. A thumb that postures in adduction may imply a deficiency of the abductor pollicis longus.[33]

Initial treatment of the type I clasped thumb is an orthosis for the affected joint in extension to prevent additional attenuation of the hypoplastic extensor mechanism and to allow hypertrophy over time.[33] A soft Neoprene thumb abduction orthosis is well tolerated by most infants (see Fig. 17.9B). In past studies, full-time orthotic wear for 2 to 6 months has

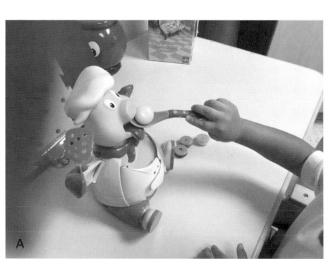
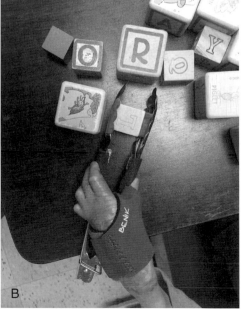

Fig. 17.9 A, Child with clasped thumb. B, A soft Neoprene thumb abduction orthosis is well tolerated by most infants with clasped thumbs.

been shown to be most effective when performed within 12 months of birth and less effective between the ages of 1 and 2 years.[33] Surgery is considered for children who have not responded to an orthotic regimen or who present after 2 years of age.[33] However, this all depends on the degree of impairment and its overall effect on hand function.[33] For example, a mild extensor lag at the MP joint usually does not affect hand function significantly.

Brachial Plexus Palsy at Birth

Brachial plexus palsy is an injury that occurs at birth. The typical posture of a child with brachial plexus palsy includes a shoulder that is adducted and internally rotated, an extended elbow, a pronated forearm, and a flexed wrist and digits. The thumb may be flexed in the palm. Most babies born with brachial plexus palsy recover spontaneously within the first 2 months. Those who do not recover the antigravity biceps by 5 to 6 months of age are considered for microsurgical reconstruction to facilitate a more functional outcome.[17] If recovery is not achieved by 3 months, there will be permanent ROM deficits, decreased strength, and a smaller upper extremity.[17]

Typically the injury affects the C5 and C6 roots of the brachial plexus **(Erb palsy)**. The palsy can affect the C7 root or even C8 and T1 (global brachial plexus palsy). Initial intervention is PROM to all joints. More recently a new Sup-ER orthosis has been used by some therapists early on after initial injury to position the shoulder in a functional position and prevent the shoulder from resting in an internally rotated posture, which positions the glenohumeral joint at risk for contractures, glenohumeral deformities, and posterior dislocations.[46] The Sup-ER orthosis protocol was implemented on 18 children with brachial plexus palsy during their study period. At a 2-year follow-up, those children who wore the orthosis performed better on the active movement scale than those who were treated without the orthosis.

The Sup-ER orthosis positions the shoulder in external rotation, the elbow in extension, and the forearm in supination (Fig. 17.10). The therapist fabricates a long arm elbow orthosis extending to the wrist. Two D-rings are riveted onto the upper medial aspect of the orthosis where two straps are applied. The long arm orthosis is kept in place circumferentially by a soft fabrifoam wrap. The therapist then manually rotates the shoulder into external rotation while keeping the arm fully adducted by the trunk. While this position is maintained, the two medial straps on the orthosis aspect are applied to the back side of a Neoprene diaper to maintain the position. The orthosis is worn 22 hours per day during the first month of its use. Then the orthotic wear is weaned to nighttime wear only. Full video instructions on the fabrication and application of the Sup-ER orthosis can be viewed online at https://bcchr.ca/brachial-plexus/treatment/splint. Further intervention depends on the severity of the paralysis. Children may have limitations in ROM at every joint and may develop contractures of the shoulder, elbow, forearm, and wrist. Orthoses (Fig. 17.11) are used for positioning, preventing elbow flexion contractures, and enhancing function.

Early intervention is the key to maximizing development of motor patterns. If an infant shows signs of muscle weakness or limited active range of movement, soft elastic orthoses are recommended. Signs of contracture development at the elbow, forearm, wrist, thumb, or digits indicate the need for immobilization or static-progressive orthoses.

Orthotic intervention for brachial plexus palsy includes immobilization orthoses (e.g., elbow positioning, wrist extension, forearm supination, thumb positioning, and nighttime resting orthoses). Static-progressive and/or mobilization orthoses may be used to lengthen tight structures and release joint contractures. Soft elastic orthoses that supinate the

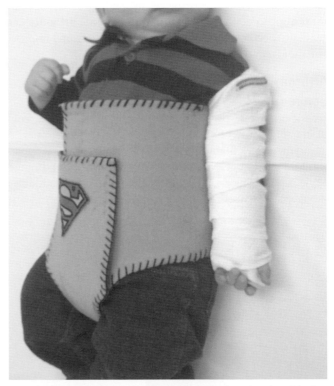

Fig. 17.10 Infant wearing Sup-ER orthosis for functional positioning.

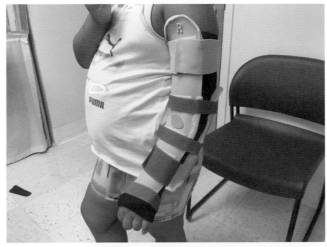

Fig. 17.11 Older child with brachial plexus injury wearing static elbow orthosis.

forearm and promote thumb opposition are used to improve functional skills (Fig. 17.10). A challenge in fabricating orthoses for brachial plexus palsy includes providing constant orthotic adjustments as the child grows. Adjustments ensure that the orthosis does not interfere with function.

Surgical Options for Brachial Plexus Palsy

There are multiple surgical procedures for children who do not spontaneously recover full upper extremity motion. Early surgery may include neurolysis, nerve grafts, or nerve transfers. Secondary surgeries typically occur between 2 and 10 years of age. These may include tendon transfers, free muscle transfers, arthrodesis, osteotomies, and others. Postoperative care requires protective orthoses, depending on the specific surgical procedure.[41] Creative use of dynamic orthotics can facilitate specific movements, enhance function, and improve bimanual play skills.

Arthrogryposis/Arthrogryposis Multiplex Congenita

Classic **arthrogryposis** or arthrogryposis multiplex congenita (Fig. 17.12) typically involves all four extremities. A pronounced lack of muscle mass and flexion creases is apparent. Joints have decreased ROM with an inelastic end range. Typical posturing includes internally rotated and adducted shoulders, extended elbows, pronated forearms, flexed and ulnarly deviated wrists, partially flexed fingers, and adducted thumbs.[47] Children who are born with *amyoplasia*, a form of arthrogryposis, also lack elbow flexor muscles and are born with elbow extension contractures.[35] These deficits significantly impact the child's ability to play and perform basic self-care tasks without assistance.[35] It is essential that physical and occupational therapy interventions begin at birth and include stretching, orthotics, positioning, and parent education on compensatory techniques to facilitate maximal independence with developmentally appropriate activities of daily living.[35] Orthotics are often needed to address contractures of the elbow, forearm, wrist, and hand. Often, bimanual patterns of upper extremity function are used due to lack of muscle strength. Children without passive elbow flexion are particularly compromised with an inability to self-feed. When passive elbow flexion is present, children can use mobilization elbow flexion orthoses or other strategies (e.g., tabletop propping or trunk swaying) to assist in self-feeding (see Chapter 10 and Fig. 17.13).

Multiple surgical procedures may be considered for children with arthrogryposis, including tendon transfers, posterior elbow capsulotomy, wrist arthrodesis or carpectomy, and thumb procedures. Orthotic intervention before surgery to increase passive joint ROM or to stretch tight contractures may be necessary. Postsurgical therapy and protective and positioning orthoses are an integral part of facilitating functional independence.

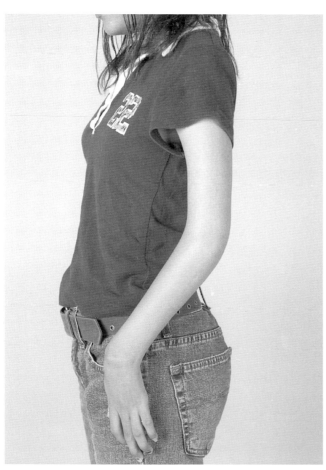

Fig 17.12 Child with arthrogryposis.

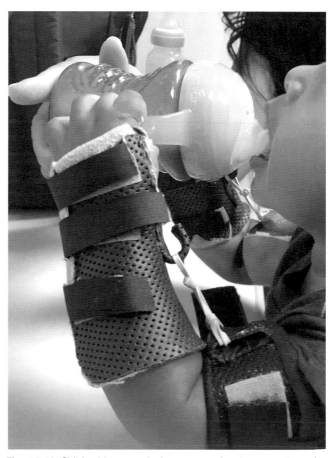

Fig. 17.13 Child with amyoplasia, a type of arthrogryposis, using dynamic elbow orthoses for feeding.

The intervention goal determines which type of orthotic intervention is appropriate for children with arthrogryposis. Soft elastic and/or thermoplastic immobilization orthoses for elbow, forearm, wrist, fingers, and thumb may be used to maintain or increase ROM. Orthotic intervention may improve the span of reach, quality and strength of grasp, and weight bearing. The orthoses protect the joint post surgery.

The challenges of fabricating orthoses for children with arthrogryposis include providing orthoses that allow maximal function while trying to preserve joint positioning. These children often require multiple surgeries and orthotic adjustments. Serial-static and static-progressive orthoses are fabricated for maximal passive stretching of tight joints and contractures. Bilateral use of immobilization orthoses may severely impair function; therefore consider wearing schedules carefully. Resting hand orthoses worn at night may be used to preserve and maintain joint motion and positioning.

Juvenile Idiopathic Arthritis

The term *juvenile idiopathic arthritis (JIA)* is the newer term for what used to be called *juvenile rheumatoid arthritis*. JIA encompasses different subsets of the disease.[40] Common to all subsets is the onset before 16 years of age and episodes lasting at least 6 weeks.[40] The disease is more prominent in females than males. JIA is a chronic, potentially lifelong disease causing joint inflammation. The goals of physical and occupational therapy are to enable children to participate in activities of everyday life. Goals of orthotic intervention are to preserve normal joint function and to prevent deformity and disability. Orthotic intervention should accompany joint protection techniques. Well-designed prefabricated orthoses are less expensive than custom-made orthoses and are typically better accepted by teens when long-term use is required. Usually orthoses are needed only during flare-ups.[34] Immobilizing orthoses are offered during periods of increased joint pain and inflammation to support and position joints. Mobilization orthoses are offered to enhance function in weak joints. Studies of adults with rheumatoid arthritis showed that patients using functional wrist orthoses reported decreased pain and improved function with orthotic use.[18,29]

Types of orthoses fabricated for children with JIA may include immobilization orthoses for the elbow, forearm, wrist (dorsal or volar based), fingers, and thumb. These orthoses:
• Protect the joints during flare-ups
• Prevent further deformity
• Support weak and inflamed joints
• Improve function of grasp and reach

Cerebral Palsy

Cerebral palsy (CP) (Fig. 17.14) is a lifelong disorder of sensory-motor development that originates from insult to the developing brain. CP is characterized by impaired ability to move and maintain posture and balance. Eighty-five percent of CP etiology is congenital, originating in utero or at the time of labor and delivery. The remaining 15% is acquired during early childhood from injury, poisoning, illness, and other causes.[13] CP ranges from mild to severe and can affect development of movement in one or all of the limbs, including the head and trunk. **Spasticity,** fluctuating muscle **tone,** muscle weakness, and/or reflex-dominated movement patterns are the hallmarks of impaired movement quality. These symptoms relate to where the initial brain damage occurred.[26] Co-occurring conditions (such as seizures, cognitive deficits, attention deficits, and visual, auditory, and other sensory disorders) are frequent and affect motor development.

Atypical Motor Development

A deep understanding of the development of movement is essential when providing intervention for CP and is beyond the chapter's scope. Key to appropriate and timely intervention is the notion that "Compensatory movement patterns develop and often become more extreme as the child ages because new functional sensorimotor patterns often are built on inefficient or inadequate foundations."[13]

At birth, spastic CP of the upper extremities usually presents as weakness with a prolonged period of fisting. Atypical and immature patterns of weight bearing, limited active movement, and weakness contribute to both excessive and diminished ROM in infants. For example, by 5 months typically developing infants push up into forearm prop. As infants tip from side to side, weight is transferred to the ulnar forearm and functionality moves from the ulnar to the radial side of the hand.[2] In a child with CP, if forearm prop is delayed (due to trunk and arm weakness), persistence of grasp typical of a 4-month-old is seen (i.e., adducted thumb and grasp attempts with the ulnar fingers only).[11] Infants with CP may attempt to grasp using atypical and immature patterns. Such patterns fail to serve as building blocks for more refined grasp development.[20] Likewise, limited experience in upper extremity weight bearing and unequal muscle strength between agonist and antagonist muscles leads to an inability to fully elongate shoulder flexors and elbow extensors. Inexperience in forearm prop leads to locking in pronation for

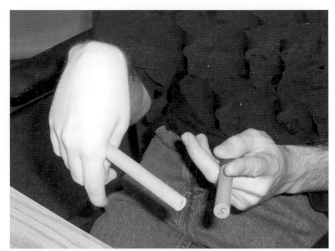

Fig. 17.14 Older child with cerebral palsy (CP). (From Burke, S. L., Higgins, J., McClinton, M. A., et al. (2006). *Hand and upper extremity rehabilitation: A practical guide* (3rd ed). St. Louis: Elsevier Churchill Livingstone.)

stability and nondevelopment or limited development of supination.[11] Full elongation of the wrist and finger flexors is present in typically developing children when they prop on extended arms, creep, and engage the thumb in grasp. With CP, children's inexperience with these milestones leads to underdeveloped range in wrist and finger extensors. Problems at the wrist are compounded if the child is allowed to creep while bearing weight on the dorsum of the hand. This destructive movement pattern overstretches and further weakens the already weak wrist extensors. Intervention of these movement patterns when first emerging improves the course of the child's motor development.

When evaluating for potential orthotic intervention for a child with CP, view the whole child and observe movement patterns during a typical day within the context of overall development. Therapists should:

- Observe the infant during supine, prone, and sitting positions for patterns of mobility, weight bearing, reach, and grasp.
- Watch toddlers play and note patterns of weight bearing, reach, and grasp, but also transitional patterns of movement (i.e., sitting to creeping or lying to standing). These observations give a clear understanding of whether the orthosis being considered will facilitate or inhibit function.
- Observe preschoolers and older children during play, school-related tasks, and self-care activities. If children are able to verbalize, ask them what they can do with their arms and hands. Note what types of activities they struggle to perform.

Specific upper extremity function observations should include:

- Any limitations or hypermobility in ROM at the shoulder, elbow, forearm rotators, wrist, thumb, and fingers
- Components of movement that appear to be diminished or absent during reach and weight bearing
- How the hand is incorporated into activities (e.g., hand used to stabilize a toy, hand neglect, sensation, volitional control of hand/digits, bilateral use, type of grasp pattern)

Orthotic Intervention for Children With Cerebral Palsy

Individuals with CP usually benefit from orthoses throughout their lives. Orthoses address issues of weakness and spasticity (Fig. 17.15), muscle fiber and connective tissue shortening, and maladaptive compensatory movement patterns. Orthoses address poorly aligned or subluxed joints and hygiene and skin integrity. All of these concerns are addressed through a comprehensive program of stretching, muscle strengthening, antispasticity medications, dynamic garments, and orthoses. Constraint-induced movement therapy, botulinum toxin type A (Botox), and electrical stimulation are emergent therapies used in conjunction with orthoses. Surgical interventions are used when less invasive techniques are inadequate. Orthoses are often an important component of presurgical and postsurgical intervention.

Types of Orthoses Used for Children With Cerebral Palsy

The intent of orthotic intervention determines the appropriate orthosis for children with CP. Orthoses may be fabricated for different purposes. Orthoses assist children with

developing more typical movement patterns (see Fig. 17.16). Elastic soft orthoses augment movement in weaker muscle groups.[10,37] These orthoses are made of Lycra, Neoprene, or similar elastic material and are worn during active play. Soft orthoses include shoulder-based rotation straps, flexible elbow extension orthoses (to assist with weight bearing and reach), forearm rotation straps, Neoprene thumb orthoses, and Neoprene wrist-hand orthoses. In a study that examined hand movements while performing functional tests, the children (who had CP) with the aid of a wrist extension and thumb abduction orthosis (Fig. 17.17 A & B) that was made of Neoprene and thermoplastic showed more improvement in overall hand function than those without the orthosis.[7]

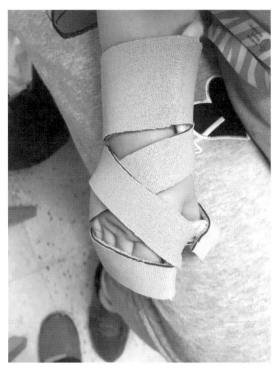

Fig. 17.15 Individuals with CP usually benefit from orthoses throughout their lives to address issues of weakness and spasticity.

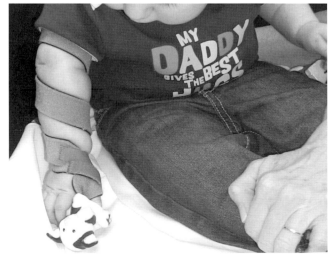

Fig. 17.16 Grasping with thumb orthosis with supinator strap.

Other orthoses block abnormal, nonproductive movement patterns, such as excessive wrist flexion, ulnar deviation, or thumb adduction. Rigid or semirigid stays may be added to soft elastic orthoses. Examples of these orthoses include Neoprene thumb orthosis with web stay, Neoprene wrist-hand orthosis with wrist stay and ulnar hand trough (see Fig. 17.17A), and Neoprene elbow band with an extension stay along the flexor surface of the elbow.

Functional thermoplastic orthoses block unwanted motion while allowing function. Examples include a dorsal wrist immobilization orthosis and a thumb abduction orthosis. These orthoses optimally position joints for function.

Orthoses reduce contractures, maintain ROM, and protect skin integrity. Orthoses that completely immobilize the joint and restrict function are best worn when the child is resting or napping. Immobilization orthoses include resting hand, elbow extension, thermoplastic thumb, and cone orthoses.

Orthoses assist in increasing ROM over time. Serial-static and static-progressive orthoses are fabricated for a stiff elbow, wrist, fingers, or thumb and may be used in combination with other interventions (see Chapter 13).

Postsurgical orthoses immobilize and protect joints, muscles, and soft tissues. Physicians typically determine the specifications for the orthosis and wearing schedule.

Finally, custom orthoses assist with specific skills to increase the child's functional repertoire, such as a pointer orthosis (Fig. 17.18). The bases for such custom orthoses are common orthotic patterns, such as a wrist immobilization orthosis that has a component added for the assist of function.

The challenges of orthotic fabrication for children with CP include the need to make adjustments as the child grows and develops. Implementing weight-bearing orthoses in a timely manner may be a difficult task. Therapists must be aware of the child's tone and how it affects function. Muscle tone may increase when a child is fearful, ill, cold, irritable, or when experiencing a growth spurt. In a small hand the weight and bulkiness of the orthotic material may present a barrier to movement. Therefore the therapist needs to use thin thermoplastic materials ($\frac{1}{16}$ inch to $\frac{1}{12}$ inch) or soft orthoses during function for the very young. In children with CP the wrist and long finger flexor muscles dominate over the extensor muscles. Over time the muscles may shorten in length if not positioned in a resting hand orthosis (see Fig. 17.8).

Because ulnar muscles dominate over radial muscles, wrist extension orthoses are designed to block excessive ulnar deviation. Due to the strength of the proximal muscles, there is a higher probability over time for hyperextension and subluxation at the thumb MCP joint.

When fabricating orthoses for children, it is always crucial that the parent and/or caregiver understand the reasons for the orthosis and be able to follow through with the wearing schedule. The child may need multiple orthoses. The therapist plans an appropriate wearing schedule to prioritize and accommodate the child's needs. For example, many children with CP need soft orthoses during the day to assist with function. But because soft orthoses do not maintain stretch on the wrist and long finger extensors, children also need resting hand orthoses at night to maintain ROM in the extensors.

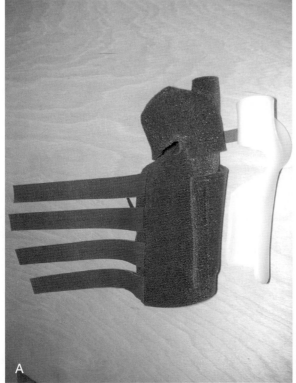
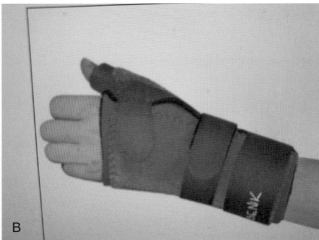

Fig. 17.17 A, Neoprene wrist hand orthosis with ulnar stay. B, Neoprene and thermoplastic wrist extension thumb abduction splint. (A, Courtesy Orfit Industries.)

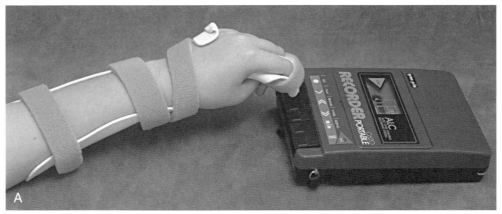

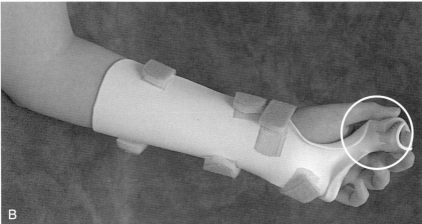

Fig. 17.18 A and B, Orthosis with pointer.

Hints for Orthotic Fabrication for Children With Increased Tone

Fabricating an orthosis on a child who has increased tone is challenging. With experience, therapists gain insight into methods that optimize the process. The following are hints for the novice therapist who is fabricating an orthosis for a child with increased tone:

- Choose a quiet location, and minimize other activity.
- Be conscious of lighting and room temperature.
- Invite parents/caregivers to assist if they can calmly help.
- Position the child in a comfortable position so that muscle tone is as close to normal as possible.
- Speak calmly and slowly, and handle the child's extremity gently.
- For a calming effect, use soft music, sing, or read a story.
- Do not use toys to distract the child because they can cause overexcitement, resulting in a crossover effect and increase tone.
- Prevent any sudden quick movements.
- Have parents assist in keeping the arm and specifically the elbow stable on the surface.
- Avoid touching the palm of the hand. First abduct the thumb out of the palm, and flex the wrist to normalize tone as much as possible. Then try extending the wrist while avoiding the palm as much as possible.

Cerebral Palsy and Botox Injections

Recent studies examined the benefits of a combined intervention strategy incorporating injections of Botox with orthotic fabrication for treatment of spastic muscles in the upper and lower extremities. This Botox injection causes a temporary weakening of the spastic muscles. One study demonstrated significant results following injections and the use of static nighttime upper extremity orthoses for children with spasticity.[30] Botox injections cause muscle relaxation, reductions in spasticity, and increased joint ROM. These results led to improved functional skills and fine motor function.

Cerebral Palsy and Surgery

Surgical procedures considered for children with CP include arthrodesis, contracture and joint release, tendon transfers, and muscle-lengthening procedures. Postoperative care requires a variety of protective orthoses depending on the specific surgical procedure.

GENERAL PRINCIPLES FOR ORTHOTIC FABRICATION

After a thorough initial evaluation and interview with the child and parents or caregivers, the key to successful orthotic fabrication is prioritizing the needs of the child.

- Create a list of the abilities and deficits.

BOX 17.2 Goals of Pediatric Orthoses

Orthoses for Positioning	Orthoses for Function	Orthoses for Hygiene	Orthoses for Protection
Mobilize joints, reduce contractures	Enable existing function to continue	Improve or prevent a hygiene problem	Keep the child safe
Provide stability	Improve existing function		Prevent undesired behaviors
Rest the extremity	Substitute for weak or absent muscles		
Provide proper alignment	Augment benefits of therapy		

- Prioritize the needs in accordance with age and ability to perform.
- Incorporate the family's stated outcomes and the child's stated outcomes.
- Fabricate an orthosis that first addresses one or two primary needs.
- Fabricate other orthoses to meet additional needs, and schedule alternate wear among the various orthoses.
- Reassess the fit of each orthosis and need for it frequently.

Consider the goal(s) for the orthosis (Box 17.2). Positioning orthoses mobilize joints, reduce contractures, provide stability, rest the extremity, and provide proper joint alignment. Functional orthoses enable continuation or improvement of existing function and can substitute for weak or absent muscles. Improvement or prevention of hygiene problems is assisted with orthotic intervention. Protective orthoses keep the child safe or prevent undesired behaviors.[25]

Always use a problem-based approach for orthotic intervention. Although a diagnosis helps predict probable outcomes with a given orthotic intervention, applying critical analysis allows for creative interventions.

Approaches to Pediatric Orthotic Fabrication

Several approaches are used for pediatric orthotic fabrication:
- To encourage motivation and acceptance of the orthosis, engage the child in design and color selections.
- Monitor the orthosis frequently due to growth. Consider not only the physical growth, but also psychomotor and mental growth.
- Children have unique hands that require custom designs and individualized intervention plans.
- It is essential that family/caregivers are invested.

Safety Tips and Precautions

When working with children, be mindful of safety. Consider the location of tools and equipment and the positioning of the child. The following safety guidelines are important:
- Place sharp tools and scissors out of reach.

- Do not leave scissors or other equipment unattended on the counter or table.
- When using hot water for orthotic fabrication, avoid splashing. Always cover the hydrocollator or fry pan when in use.
- Children's skin may be sensitive to heat and may react to thermoplastic materials. Allow the material to cool adequately before placing on the skin.
- Sharp edges on the orthosis' corners can scratch or cut skin. Smooth sharp edges and round corners on the orthosis and strapping materials. Securely attach straps and other small pieces to the orthosis so that they cannot be pulled off and swallowed.
- Verify that the thermoplastic material does not contain toxic ingredients.
- Use latex-free Neoprene.

Steps for Orthotic Fabrication

Once the goals are established, the orthotic fabrication process is initiated. The child and environment are prepared. The therapist designs the orthosis, selects the orthotic material, and makes the pattern. All three aspects are considered together. The orthotic design takes into account the child's unique hand shape and size, its purpose, intended wearing schedule, and the most effective material.

Prepare the Child

Position the child so that the effects of abnormal tone and postural reflexes on the arm and hand are at a minimum. This position depends on the assessment results of the child and may differ from how the child is typically positioned. It is important to provide external stability through equipment or handling for children who have not acquired internal stability of proximal joints. This stability may involve a seating system or other adaptive equipment. For the infant or young child, it may be possible for the parent to hold the child and provide external stability with the therapist's instructions.

It is important to reduce the child's fearfulness and maximize adherence. If the therapist does not already have a relationship with the child, spend time to allow the child to warm up. Even if the child knows the therapist, a brief time is provided to allow the child to acclimate to the equipment and setup for orthotic intervention. The therapist has toys, music, books, stickers, or other materials to establish a reciprocal interaction with the child before starting the fabrication process. With an infant the therapist talks in a soothing voice and touches the child in a playful manner before fabrication. With an older child the therapist shows the child what to expect by first fabricating an "orthosis" on a doll or stuffed animal or by making "thermoplastic jewelry" or other play objects.

When appropriate, the child is given the opportunity to touch and feel the material while it is warm and soft and again after it becomes cool and hard. The child's response to tactile stimuli is noted, and if signs of tactile defensiveness occur, the therapist follows sensory processing guidelines for improving sensory system modulation. If colored thermoplastic material is available, the child is encouraged to select a color. For some children, decorating the orthosis with stickers or leather stamps encourages acceptance.

Giving children a role to play in the fabrication process may increase adherence. The child's role may include keeping time by counting, holding the end of the Ace wrap, or any other task the therapist invents to keep the child involved. However, if associated reactions are present, it is best for the child to be involved without exerting effort because this may increase tone. Although preparing the child takes a few extra minutes at the beginning of a session, it can save hours of frustration in having to reschedule or remake an orthosis because of lack of adherence.

Prepare the Environment

Thoughtful preparation is especially important for orthotic intervention of children because of short attention spans. In addition to having orthotic and play materials close at hand, it is recommended that the therapist plan to have a second pair of adult hands to help with the fabrication.[4] This additional person might be a parent, teacher, paraprofessional, or another therapist. Extra help is especially important if the child has increased tone, is not able to follow verbal instructions, or is likely to be uncooperative. The therapist clearly explains the helper's role so that efforts assist the process and do not hinder it. This usually involves maintaining the child's overall position, calming or entertaining the child, holding the arm just proximal to the joint being positioned, or stabilizing the material once in place and while it is cooling.

Design

Orthoses can be fabricated on the volar, dorsal, ulnar, or radial borders, or circumferentially. Circumferential orthoses do not tend to migrate distally, especially when fabricated from a highly conforming material. Circumferential orthoses, which cover both the dorsal and volar surfaces, are more comfortable to take on and off than clamshell orthoses. Circumferential designs are strong and supportive. The number of joints included in the orthosis is considered. Although it is not usually recommended to include uninvolved joints in the typical adult orthosis, when working with the pediatric population, uninvolved joints might be included to maintain the position and keep the orthosis in place. When the therapist is creating a soft elastic orthosis, the elastic quality of the orthosis must cross the joint and pull in the same direction as the muscles do if the orthosis is intended to assist the weaker muscles.

Selection of Orthotic Materials

Pediatric orthoses are made of many different types of materials, depending on the purpose of the orthosis and the age and needs of the child. Thermoplastic materials are commonly used for the fabrication of static orthoses or those that require restricting motion at certain joints. Soft orthoses are commonly made of materials such as Neoprene. Soft orthoses may not totally immobilize a joint, but they provide support and allow greater freedom of movement. Children with athetosis or involuntary flailing movements should be protected from possible harm from the orthosis by selection of a soft material or by covering a thermoplastic material with a mitt or sock.

When working with Neoprene, take thickness into account. Although 3.0 mm is commonly used, consider 1.5-mm thickness because it is less bulky in a small hand. Check the stretch because the elastic quality is more prominent in one direction. It is possible to find Neoprene with one side smooth nylon and the other a Velcro-receptive material. Such material eliminates the need to sew on a Velcro loop where it is intended to adhere.

With Neoprene be alert to the possibility of skin irritation or rash. According to Stern and colleagues,[44] "skin contact with Neoprene poses two dermatological risks: allergic contact dermatitis (ACD) and miliaria rubra (i.e., prickly heat)." Although Neoprene hypersensitivity is rare, the authors recommend that therapists screen patients for a history of dermatological reactions; instruct clients to discontinue use and inform the therapist if a rash, itching, or skin eruptions occur. Cases of adverse skin reactions are reported to the manufacturer of the Neoprene material. The authors recommend that therapists limit their own exposure to Neoprene and Neoprene glue because exposure to thiourea compounds may contribute to allergic reactions.

Thermoplastic materials range in conformability, thickness, stretch, and rigidity. For an orthosis designed to stretch a tight web space, use a highly conforming material. Otherwise the skin may break down from the high resistance and unyielding shape. Generally, thermoplastic materials with a high plastic content have more conformability, whereas materials with high rubber content have less stretch but are less likely to be indented with fingerprints during fabrication. When making an orthosis that counteracts the forces of spasticity, it is especially important to select a thermoplastic material that resists stretch (i.e., one with high rubber content) because it is necessary to apply considerable pressure to obtain the desired position of the wrist, thumb, and fingers.[4] For children with spasticity or larger limbs, a ⅛-inch thick thermoplastic material might be the best selection. Smaller hands require thinner thermoplastic materials of ⅟₁₂ inch and ⅟₁₆ inch.

Some products combine the properties of plastic and rubber. Usually rubber-like (or combination) thermoplastic material is necessary when one is working against spasticity, even though it is less rigid than the plastic type. If necessary, a reinforcement component is added to the orthosis. Selecting a material with a high degree of memory is helpful when one is working with a child whose movements may be unpredictable and require the therapist to start over (sometimes more than once!). These plastics are elastic-like and self-adhere easily. Self-adherence can be problematic. One way to reduce the stickiness of the thermoplastic material is adding a tablespoon of liquid soap or shampoo to the hot water.[18] Ultimately with all these suggestions for thermoplastic materials, the therapist's experience and preferences affect the choice. (See Chapter 3 for a review of orthotic material.)

Pattern Making

Pattern making for a pediatric orthosis may be challenging, and intervention approaches are based on the child's developmental level. Older children can be encouraged to participate in the process by having them trace their own hands on the paper. Infants and toddlers might best be approached while napping or feeding. Younger children can be enticed to play a game where their hands are placed on the table. Making a photocopy of the child's hand may be helpful. A pattern drawn on a larger-size hand can be reduced by a photocopier to obtain the correct size.[25]

Using flexible material (such as paper towels or aluminum foil) to create the pattern allows the therapist to easily check the pattern on the child. Sometimes it is not possible to make an accurate pattern. Children with abnormal tone may be unable to lay their hands on a table surface for an accurate tracing. In this case the pattern must be held under the extremity in whatever position is least stressful. The therapist may consider using an uninvolved contralateral side to start a pattern, given that there is some symmetry of anatomy. Another approach is for the therapist to best estimate the design and sizing. It may be helpful to plan on extending the thermoplastic material beyond that of the finished product to give leverage to help hold joints in position. The extra thermoplastic material is cut away when the essential part of the orthosis is finished and hardened.[22] For patterns that tear, masking tape is used for repairs or to reinforce contours.

Heating the Thermoplastic Material

The therapist heats the water to the temperature range recommended by the manufacturer. After cutting out the orthosis, it may be necessary to reheat the plastic to obtain the desired degree of pliability before the molding process. Before placing the plastic on a child's extremity, the therapist dries off the hot water and makes sure the plastic is not too hot. Check the material's temperature by placing it against one's face or anterior portion of the forearm. Checking the material's temperature is especially important when spot heating with a heat gun because this method tends to result in higher surface temperatures.

Some children may be hypersensitive to temperature and react negatively, even though the temperature does not feel hot to the therapist. Because many children cannot communicate that the plastic feels too hot, the therapist watches the child's facial expressions and listens for vocalizations that indicate discomfort. The child's arm and hand can be moistened with cold water before molding. Another option is placing a wet piece of paper towel over the extremity, or waiting longer for the plastic to cool. Some therapists use a stockinette to protect the extremity. However, care must be taken that it does not wrinkle under the plastic during fabrication.

Hastening the Process

Time is of the essence when one is working with a moving target, a rebellious little one, or a difficult-to-position extremity. Rubber-based plastics, which are necessary to resist stretch, are somewhat slower to harden. Once the plastic is in place on the extremity, an ice pack can be rubbed on the orthosis to hasten the setting process. A rubber glove filled with ice chips can easily serve the purpose. After being partially hardened, the orthosis is carefully removed and put into a pan of ice water or placed under a faucet of cold running water. A TheraBand roll cooled in a freezer helps form the orthosis, which accelerates the cooling process.

A spray coolant may be used, but only with great care to spray after the orthosis is off the child. The spray is directed away from the child. The use of coolant spray is avoided with children who are unable to keep their heads turned away from the direction of the spray and those who have frequent respiratory problems.

An Ace wrap is useful to hold an orthosis in place while the therapist works on other portions of the orthosis—although this maintains heat and may increase setting time. The therapist should not apply the wrap or TheraBand too tightly and should flare the edges of the forearm trough away from the skin after formation of the orthosis.

Padding

Padding, or some form of pressure relief, may be necessary over bony areas to prevent skin problems. Padding does not compensate for pressure resulting from a poorly made orthosis. Padding takes up space, a factor the therapist considers before formation. Otherwise, the amount of pressure against the skin may increase. A variety of paddings exist, including closed- and open-cell foam and gel products. Pressure-relief padding with a gel insert is useful in protecting bony areas for children with little subcutaneous fat.

To ensure proper fit, the therapist lays the padding on the child's extremity before molding the plastic or places it on the thermoplastic material before molding the orthosis. When the therapist is molding with padding, the stretch of the thermoplastic material and the contourability may be compromised. Therefore the therapist adds padding only if necessary. In addition, padding becomes soiled and needs to be replaced. For more information on padding, see Chapter 3.

Another way to create pressure relief around a bony prominence without using padding is to cover the prominence with a small amount of firm therapy putty before forming the orthosis. The putty creates a built-in bubble and is removed from the orthosis after cooling.[25] Thin forms of padding are used to create friction and reduce migration or shifting of orthoses or for covering edges. Microfoam tape is useful for this purpose, especially on small orthoses.

Strapping

Many creative strapping solutions exist to keep orthoses on children (Fig. 17.19). The therapist considers strength, durability, elasticity, and texture when the strap is against the skin. Strapping with sharp edges is avoided with younger children and those with sensitive skin. The wider the strap, the more force is dispersed if the entire strap width is in full contact with the skin. Strap material may need to be cut narrower, especially around the wrist and fingers, to be proportionate to the size of the child's hand.

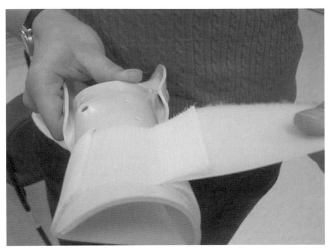

Fig. 17.19 Extra Velcro strap for closure. (Courtesy Orfit Industries.)

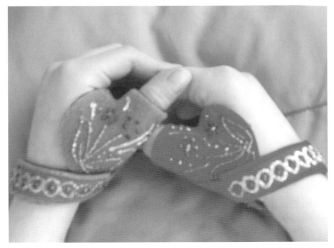

Fig. 17.20 Decorated Neoprene orthoses. (Courtesy Orfit Industries.)

D-ring straps are often used to increase the likelihood of nonremoval. Fasteners that require a two-handed release prevent easy removal. Swivel snaps, rings, and/or metal C-rings from hardware stores can be incorporated into strapping mechanisms.

Straps can be secured at each end with Velcro hook, which is attached to the orthosis. Velcro hook allows straps to be easily replaced when they become soiled, which is important if the child drools or mouths the orthosis. However, loose straps easily become lost and many times are not placed on the orthosis at the correct angle or location. An alternative is to secure the strap at one end with a rivet or strong contact adhesive. Another option is to create an extra attachment with Velcro hook that allows the child to open the orthosis. When soiled, straps are removed, and a new strap is attached. (See Chapter 3 for more detailed information about attaching straps.)

Increasing the likelihood that the child will not remove straps or the orthosis requires knowledge of child development and creativity. For infants and toddlers, consider the use of an Ace or Coban wrap to secure the orthosis. Children at certain ages (2- and 3-year-olds) are in the developmental stage of asserting their autonomy and may resist the parent's choice of clothing, food, or orthotic application. In this case, using principles of behavior analysis (such as shaping or rewarding successive approximations, finding times during the day when the child is most likely to be compliant, and contingent use of praise and attention) are helpful. Actively involving the child in choosing colors and decorations may increase the child's willingness to wear the orthosis (Fig. 17.20). Strap critter patterns are provided by Armstrong,[4] along with suggestions for using decorative ribbon, fabric paints, or shoelace charms. Armstrong suggests describing the orthosis as something cool to wear and providing the child with language to explain to peers, such as, "This is my shield or my princess glove."

If positive methods to prevent orthotic removal do not work, therapists use creativity to keep the little "Houdinis" in their orthoses, especially young children who do not

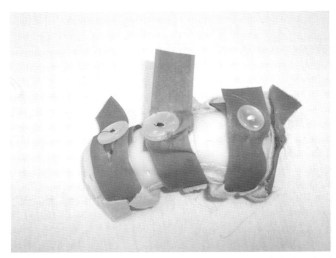

Fig. 17.21 Buttons on dorsum of orthosis. (Courtesy Orfit Industries.)

understand cause and effect. Some child-proof methods include using shoelaces, buttons (Fig. 17.21), buckles, or socks/stockinette/puppets. Lacing is done by punching holes along the lateral edges of the orthosis and lacing with wide decorative shoelaces. The therapist places padding under the laces and against the skin. To secure the laces, the therapist uses a "bow biter" (a plastic device available in children's shoe departments) to hold the laces in place.[16] Depending on the function of the orthosis, a sock puppet worn over the orthosis may be used as camouflage (see Fig. 17.8). Care must be taken not to provide any attachment that the child could bite off and swallow.

Providing Instruction for Orthotic Application

Those responsible for applying the child's orthosis (e.g., teachers, nursing staff, or parents) should be part of the assessment process and provide input on the orthotic design and agree with the need for the orthosis. They must understand the orthosis' purpose, rationale, precautions, and risks of incorrect usage. The correct application of the orthosis may not be obvious to those unfamiliar with orthotic intervention.

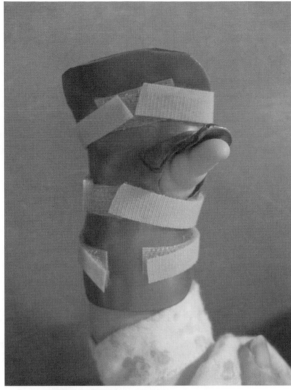

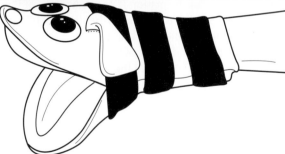

Fig. 17.22 Orthoses can be covered with a hand puppet.

The more complex the orthosis, the more detailed and explicit the instructions are. This is especially true when there are multiple care providers. The therapist provides written instructions along with a phone number and/or email address to contact for questions or concerns. A demonstration of the steps involved in donning the orthosis is provided, followed by an opportunity for the caretaker to practice applying the orthosis under supervision. A photograph of the child with the orthosis in the correct position is often an effective teaching tool if it does not conflict with policies regarding confidentiality.

Correct placement of straps is facilitated by writing a number or placing a small design on the strap end and a corresponding number or design on the orthosis. The therapist does everything possible to take the guesswork out of putting on the orthosis. Instruct caregivers to inspect the skin every time the orthosis is removed to assess for signs of excessive pressure.

Wearing Schedules

Wearing schedules vary according to the purpose of the orthosis, the child's tolerance, musculoskeletal status, occupations, and daily routines. Orthoses may be worn for long or short intervals during the day, at night, during functional activities, or a combination. It is necessary to gradually increase the wearing time initially to build up the child's tolerance for the orthosis and to make any modifications that become apparent with use.

When the purpose of the orthosis is to increase functional use, wearing the orthosis should occur during times when the child is engaged in occupations. If the purpose is tone reduction, the orthosis is worn before activities or occupations. When the purpose of the orthosis is to prevent a contracture, the orthosis is worn when the child is not engaged in occupations. Finally, if the orthosis is used to treat an existing contracture, it is necessary to wear it for prolonged periods of time.

The total time spent wearing the orthosis during a 24-hour period appears to be more important than whether it is worn continuously or intermittently.[25] The length of time an orthosis can be worn is affected by how much force is applied to achieve the desired position, which causes stress on the joints, muscles, and skin. Ultimately, wearing schedule decisions are based on developing and maintaining clinical competence, clinical reasoning, and collaborating with the child and/or family members or care providers.

The wearing schedule works only if the orthosis is placed on the child during the recommended times. Incorporating the orthotic schedule into the child's regular routine may increase adherence because it becomes less of a special chore for the parent, teacher, caregiver, or nursing staff. The therapist documents the agreed-upon wearing schedule and provides written copies to parents, caregivers, teachers, nurses, and child care providers. As the child's developmental or ROM status changes, the therapist evaluates the wearing schedule and possibly the orthotic design to make modifications.

Precautions

The skin is inspected frequently during the initial wearing phase. A distinct red area or generalized redness that does not disappear within 15 to 20 minutes after removal indicates excessive pressure and the need for revision.[23,25] During periods of monitoring the therapist should be aware of any problems associated with joint compression, pressure on nerves, compromised circulation, and dermatological reactions. Children's growth spurts often come without obvious signals, and during those times therapists and caregivers should be extra vigilant.

Evaluation of the Orthosis

A plan is made to reassess the orthosis on a regular basis to ensure proper fit and function. When possible, the therapist has the child don the orthosis 1 hour before the reassessment. This allows observation of how the orthosis is donned and whether the orthosis migrates. A poorly fitting orthosis can do more harm than good.

Special Pediatric Orthoses
Resting Hand Orthosis

The purpose of a resting hand orthosis is to prevent a contracture or deformity, to prevent an existing deformity from becoming worse, or to gradually improve or reduce a deformity (deformity-reduction orthosis). Children who are at the greatest risk of developing a contracture are those with moderately to severely increased tone or those with severely decreased tone who have no active movement. For children with severely increased muscle tone and tightly fisted hands, an additional purpose may be maintenance of skin hygiene.

Features. The components of a resting hand orthosis for a child are the same as those described in Chapter 9, except for the shape of the thumb trough and C bar. Components include a forearm trough, a pan for the fingers, a thumb trough, and a C bar. If spasticity is present in the thenar muscles, the thumb is positioned in partial radial abduction to elongate the opponens muscle. Sustained stretch of tight thenar muscles may inhibit tone in the hand.[39]

For children with moderately to severely increased tone, the ideal position of the wrist, fingers, and thumb may not be possible. Because its purpose is to prevent or reduce joint deformity, the orthosis provides as much elongation of the tight muscles as possible without causing excessive stress. The child should be able to tolerate wearing the orthosis for several hours to obtain the maximum benefit.

If the orthosis places the hand into the maximum range of passive motion, the forces generated may compromise circulation, cause skin breakdown, elicit pain, or reduce the length of time the child tolerates wearing the orthosis. Therefore the orthosis places the wrist joint in submaximal range,[21,23] which is a position especially important at the wrist to allow for finger extension. Low-load prolonged stretch provided by casts or orthoses is the best conservative way of increasing PROM.[19] When flexor spasticity is severe, using a serial-static orthosis may be necessary.[19,21]

The therapist determines the best orthotic position by handling the child's extremity and feeling the amount of passive resistance. After achieving the desired position manually, the therapist notes the angles of the joints involved and where pressure is applied to obtain this position. Handling the joints and feeling the resistance from muscles determines the most therapeutic position and the location of force application during orthotic fabrication and strap application.

Process to fabricate a resting hand orthosis

Thermoplastic material selection. When making an orthosis that counteracts the forces of spasticity, the therapist selects a low-temperature thermoplastic material that resists stretch. A considerable amount of pressure is applied on the material to obtain the desired position of the wrist, thumb, and fingers. This pressure can indent and inadvertently stretch materials that have conformability. Usually a thermoplastic material containing a high rubber content has the desired working characteristics (see the Steps for Orthotic Fabrication section).

Pattern. The pattern includes the measurements and markings of landmarks (see Chapter 9). Because the thumb position is different from the traditional resting hand orthosis, the thumb trough and C bar are shaped differently. After the pattern is drawn and cut out, it is fitted to the child for further modifications. While making the pattern and molding the orthosis, position the child to minimize the effects of abnormal tone and postural reflexes on the body and the extremities.

Padding. Before forming the orthosis the therapist considers the need for padding to allow the additional space necessary. Because padding places some restrictions on forming the orthosis and keeping it clean, it should not be used unless the assessment shows risk for skin problems. Creating bubbled-out areas over bony areas may be sufficient to avoid skin problems.

Forming the orthosis. Before placing the plastic on the child's extremity, the therapist prestretches the edge of the orthosis that forms the C bar. The therapist then places the soft plastic on the web space of the thumb. If available, an assistant stands beside the child and secures the forearm trough. The therapist forms the orthosis into the palmar arches and around the wrist and thumb. To obtain the desired contour and fit, the therapist needs to be aggressive when molding into the palm and around the thenar eminence—especially if working against spasticity.

The therapist forms the orthosis so that the bulk of pressure positioning the thumb is directed below the thumb metacarpophalangeal (MCP) joint and distributed along the thenar eminence. This formation is necessary to avoid hyperextension and possibly dislocation of the thumb MCP joint.[21] The thumb trough cradles the thumb and extends approximately ½ inch beyond the end of the thumb. The IP joint of the thumb is slightly flexed, and the C bar fits snugly into the web space and contours against the radial side of the index finger.

Forearm trough. After completing the wrist, palm, and thumb portion, the therapist completes the forearm trough. (See Chapter 9 for guidelines on securing the forearm in the trough and avoiding pressure points.) If the edges of the trough are too high, the straps bridge (i.e., the straps are raised from the skin's surface and do not follow the contour of the forearm, thus losing contact with the skin surface). To keep the forearm securely in place, the straps have maximum surface contact. If not secure, the forearm may rotate in the trough or the orthosis may shift distally, and the position of the wrist, fingers, and thumb are compromised.

Pan. Finally, the therapist forms the finger pan to position the fingers. The pan may require reheating because controlling all joints at the same time is difficult. (See Chapter 9 for the correct width and height of the pan.) In addition, the distal portion of the pan extends approximately ½ inch beyond the fingertips to allow for growth and for safety purposes. When forming the curve of the pan, contour into the proximal and distal transverse arches.

Straps. The correct placement of straps is as important as correct formation of the orthosis, especially when the orthosis is positioning joints against increased muscle tone. The straps and orthosis work together to create the necessary leverage and distribute pressure. If the forearm, palm, fingers, and thumb do not stay in the correct position, the benefit of the orthosis is greatly reduced. The optimum location and angle of each strap is determined in relation to the forces being applied by abnormal muscle tone.

The forearm trough requires two straps for an older child. However, for a smaller child or an infant, one wide strap across the forearm may be sufficient. Stability is provided at the proximal and distal areas of the forearm. If considerable wrist flexion is present, two straps are necessary to provide three points of pressure to secure the wrist.

One strap extends directly across the wrist distal to the ulnar styloid, and a second strap is angled from the thumb web space across the dorsum of the hand and secured proximal to the MCP joints on the ulnar side. Otherwise, one strap across the dorsum of the hand may be sufficient. If there is considerable finger flexion, straps may be needed across each of the three phalanges. Finally, the therapist adds a strap between the MP and IP joints of the thumb. When making a small orthosis for a young child, cut the straps narrower.

Adaptations. The resting hand orthosis provides a basic form for positioning the child in good alignment and serves as an inhibitor of hypertonicity. However, often the therapist deviates from the basic form to truly meet the needs of the child. One way the orthosis is adapted is the addition of finger separators (also described in Chapter 9) to abduct the fingers and assist in tone reduction. Separators are created by bubbling the material between digits or attaching a roll of thermoplastic material between the digits. Finger separators are also fabricated from thermoplastic pellets or elastomer.

Pellets are softened in hot water and kneaded together to the shape and size required. The pellets have 100% memory and are attached in the same way as any other thermoplastic material. Because of the putty-like consistency, pellets work well for individualized finger separators—such as for children who have arthrogryposis and different deformities in each finger.[25]

Elastomer is a silicone-based putty that is used in pediatric orthoses for thumb positioning or finger spacers. Pellets and elastomers are available from many product catalogs. The putty types of elastomers "with a gel catalyst or the 50/50 mix are probably the easiest to work with because they can be mixed in the hand and varied in stiffness by adding more or less catalyst."[4] Another option for modeling is Permagum, a silicone rubber dental-impression material.[6] Elastomers and pellets may also be used to maintain the palmer arches or as a base for a small hand orthosis.[16]

The therapist may choose to use a dorsal-based resting orthosis[4,45] as an alternative to the palmar-based orthosis already described. This design is illustrated in Chapter 9. The dorsal-based orthosis avoids sensory input to the forearm flexors, although it is somewhat more difficult to fabricate. For a child with very tight wrist flexors, donning the dorsal-based resting orthosis is easier than the palmar-based orthosis. The child's fingers are placed into the finger slot (with the fingers sufficiently positioned through the slot to support the MCP joints), pressure is placed across the wrist flexors, and slowly the forearm trough can be levered down onto the dorsum of the forearm. Armstrong[4] is a good source of information on fabricating this orthosis.

Infants with congenital finger contractures often need resting hand orthoses. However, when all digits are not affected, the orthosis is altered to free nonaffected digits to engage in movement and sensory experiences. Resting hand orthoses may be made with alternative materials, especially for infants. The therapist selects a semirigid pliable material for neonatal orthoses because it is less likely to cause abrasions. Bell and Graham[6] describe the use of Permagum, a silicone rubber dental-impression material, for neonatal orthoses. Several layers of adhesive cloth tape may also be an effective semirigid support.

Precautions. For orthotic provision against increased muscle tone, the therapist considers biomechanical principles of force distribution. The therapist monitors for any undesired lateral forces on the fingers or wrist that may result in poor anatomical alignment, dislocation, or deformity. The therapist is aware of any circulation compromise or pressure on nerves. The therapist's observations elicit important information from the child, parent, or caregiver—especially when assessing very young children or those with communication dysfunction.

Follow the same precautions for this orthosis as with any other orthosis. (See Chapter 6 for guidance in determining problems with skin, bone, or muscles.) For a child who has increased tone, the therapist shortens the initial wearing time to 15- to 20-minute intervals on the first day. The therapist carefully inspects the skin. A distinct red area or generalized redness on the skin that does not disappear within 15 to 20 minutes after orthotic removal indicates excessive pressure and the need for revision.[23,25] If no pressure areas are present, the therapist increases the wearing time to 30-minute intervals. The therapist then increases the wearing time by adding 15 to 30 minutes until the maximum wearing period is reached.

An additional precaution when making a resting hand orthosis for a child who has moderately to severely increased tone is maintaining the integrity of the MCP joint of the thumb. The therapist directs pressure below the MCP joint of the thumb. Exner[21] cautions that distal force to the spastic thumb can result in hyperextension and dislocation of the MCP joint.

Wearing schedule. The wearing schedule is determined on an individual basis, as are all other aspects of the intervention plan. In general, the more serious the threat of deformity, the longer the orthosis is worn over 24 hours. If tone continues to increase at night, extend the wearing schedule unless it interferes with the child's sleep or presses against another part of the body. During the day the orthosis is removed for periods of passive ranging, active movement, and opportunities for sensory experiences.

McClure and colleagues[38] provide a flow chart or algorithm for making clinical decisions regarding wearing schedules. They describe the biological basis for limitations in joint ROM and for increasing ROM. This information is especially applicable with existing contractures. According to the authors, "the primary basis for using [orthoses] to increase ROM is that by holding the joint at or near its end-range over time, therapeutic tensile stress is applied to the restricted periarticular connective tissues (PCTs) and muscles. This tensile stress induces remodeling of the tissues to a new, longer length, which allows increased ROM."[38] McClure and colleagues[38] defined remodeling as "a biological phenomenon that occurs over long periods of time rather than a mechanically induced change that occurs within minutes."

The child benefits from participating in occupations immediately after removal of the resting hand orthosis to capitalize on increased hand expansion and elongation of tight muscles. If developing or improving functional hand skills is a primary goal, the orthosis is removed more frequently or for longer periods of time.

Instructions for orthotic application. Applying the child's orthosis correctly is important. Caregivers should understand the purpose of the orthosis, precautions, risks of incorrect use, and how to reach the therapist with questions or concerns.

PROCEDURE FOR FABRICATION OF A DORSAL WRIST IMMOBILIZATION ORTHOSIS

When selecting thermoplastic material for the wrist immobilization orthosis, use highly conforming material. For children who have wrist flexor spasticity, use rigid material. For smaller children, use ½-inch thick thermoplastic material, whereas for larger children, use ⅛-inch thick material.

1. Position the child's hand palm down on a piece of paper. Make an outline of the child's hand from the fingertips to the forearm. The wrist is neutral with respect to radial and ulnar deviation. The fingers are in a natural resting position (not flat) and slightly abducted. Draw an outline of the fingers, hand, and forearm to the elbow.

2. While the child's hand is still on the paper, mark A at the MCP joint of the index finger, and mark B at the MCP joint of the little finger. Mark a C for the first web space. Mark a D for the ulnar border of the hand between the distal palmar crease and the wrist crease. Mark two-thirds the length of the forearm on each side with an X. Place another X on each side of the pattern approximately 1 inch outside and parallel to the two previous X markings for the approximate width of the orthosis. These markings are to accommodate for the side of the forearm trough.

3. Remove the child's hand from the pattern. Draw a line connecting the A and B markings of the MCP joints. Now, draw a new line 1 inch proximal to this line. This should match the child's distal palmar crease and marks the distal edge of the orthosis. Make sure that this line is angled toward the ulnar side of the hand.

4. Draw a kidney bean shape over the palmar area of the hand, leaving at least 1¼-inch border on each side and from the distal edge. This kidney bean shape matches with the first web space marked C on the radial side, and mark D on the ulnar side of the hand. This kidney bean–shaped area will be cut out. Redraw all borders of the orthosis pattern, and cut it out.

5. Trace the pattern onto the sheet of thermoplastic material.

6. Heat the thermoplastic material.

7. Cut the pattern out of the thermoplastic material. Carefully cut out the kidney bean–shaped opening in the palm. Reheat the thermoplastic material until fully activated.

8. Mold the orthosis onto the child's hand. To fit the orthosis on the child, have the child's elbow rest on a pad on the table with the forearm in a pronated position.

9. Slip the child's four fingers through the distal cut out, and pull the material over the dorsum of the hand and wrist. Make sure to stop midway over the back of the hand, halfway down the length of the MPs.

10. Fold over the dorsal material at the level of the wrist to provide extra support for extension.

11. Flare the material away from a prominent ulnar styloid and at the proximal edge of the forearm. Make other adjustments to the orthosis as needed.

12. Position the child's wrist in extension as the material cools and hardens. Use your thumb to mold the palmar arch. Make sure the wrist remains correctly positioned as the thermoplastic material hardens.

13. Cut the Velcro hook adhesive into two 2-inch oval-shaped pieces for the proximal edge of the orthosis. Heat the adhesive with a heat gun to encourage adherence before putting the Velcro pieces on the orthosis. If the material has a coating, use a solvent on the thermoplastic material or scratch the surface to remove some of the nonstick coating to increase adherence of the Velcro pieces.

14. The Velcro loop strap is placed at the proximal border of the orthosis. Depending on the child's size, it can be either a 1-inch or 2-inch wide strap. The strap should secure the orthosis snugly to the forearm.

15. Check the final fit of the orthosis. Make sure the orthosis is dorsally based and does not cover the volar surface of the forearm or wrist. Check the edges to ensure that they are not impinging on the skin or pressing on the bony prominences. Smooth all edges, and round all corners.

Evaluation of the orthosis. The self-evaluation described in Chapter 9 is used to evaluate the finished orthosis. The orthotic fit is reviewed at regular intervals. The orthosis' effectiveness in accomplishing stated goals and outcomes is reevaluated on an ongoing basis.

Dorsal Wrist Immobilization Orthosis

A dorsal-based wrist immobilization orthosis offers excellent wrist support while allowing the palmar surface of the hand to be free for sensory input and play. Remember that children gain information from the world through exploration with their hands and fingers. Even while the child is crawling, the dorsal-based wrist immobilization orthosis supports the wrist in extension for weight bearing. Using an appropriate thermoplastic material and slightly altering the pattern make weight bearing easier while wearing the orthosis. Blocking the entire palmar surface in a weight-bearing orthosis may not be appropriate for all children. During crawling and weight-bearing activities, ensure that the child's fingers are not hyperflexed, but rather extended.

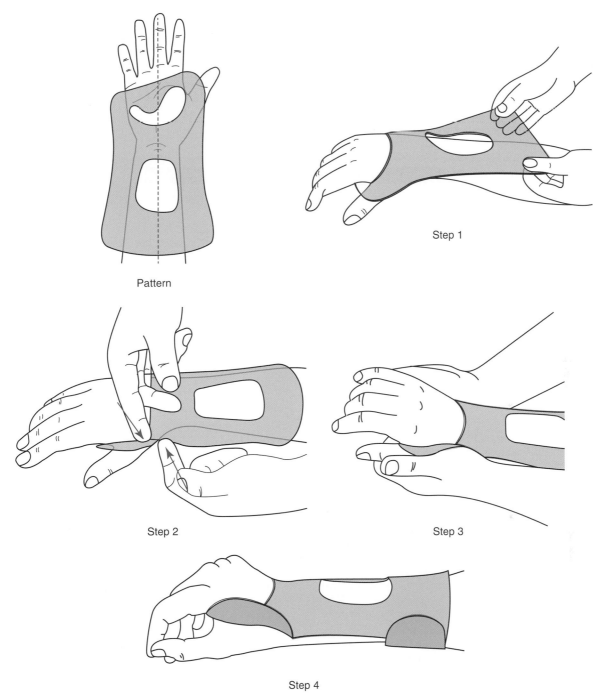

Pattern

Step 1

Step 2

Step 3

Step 4

Fig. 17.23 Instructions for dorsal wrist cock-up orthosis. (Courtesy Orfit Industries.)

Instructions for fabricating a dorsal wrist immobilization orthosis. The steps for fabricating a dorsal wrist immobilization orthosis can be found in the following procedure (Fig. 17.23).

Soft Thumb Orthosis

A soft thumb orthosis with a thumb loop is often used with children who have mild spasticity or increased tone. The orthosis positions the thumb out of the palm. The material used for the wrist band and thumb loop is made from Neoprene. The strap forming the thumb loop is wide enough to support the thumb but not so wide that it buckles or wrinkles in the thumb web space. The strap forming the wrist band is wide enough

to secure the thumb loop, remain in place on the wrist, and distribute pressure. The wrist band strap length is long enough to form an adequate overlap to secure the Velcro. Determine the specific dimensions by placing strap material on the child's arm and hand to measure lengths and widths to determine the desired angle of pull. Steps to fabricate a soft thumb orthosis can be found in the following procedure.

Rotation Strap

The rotation strap facilitates forearm supination or pronation, and it can be used to facilitate or augment shoulder rotation. The rotation strap is always coupled with a thumb or wrist orthosis. If used for shoulder motion, the strap must attach either to a therapeutic garment or strapping system at the trunk. A rotation strap is appropriate for children with flexor tone that pulls the forearm into pronation or shoulder internal rotation. The strap can also be used for positioning the forearm after surgeries.

To make the strap, use colorful soft Velfoam, Beta Pile, or Neoprene. To augment a weaker movement, use Neoprene because it is more elastic. Strap width varies from ¾ inch for infants to 1½ to 2 inches for older children and adolescents. Wider straps have greater elasticity than narrower straps. The length of the strap is approximately three to four times the length of the forearm (for forearm rotation) or three times the length of the arm for shoulder rotation (Fig. 17.24).

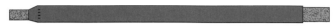

Fig. 17.24 Forearm rotation strap.

PROCEDURE FOR FABRICATION OF A SOFT THUMB ORTHOSIS

To make the pattern, the wrist band overlaps on the volar side of the wrist. The length of the thumb loop is the distance from the proximal edge of the wrist band, around the thumb, and back around to the point of origin.

The materials and tools needed for fabrication of the soft thumb orthosis include:

- Neoprene
- Hook-and-loop Velcro
- Needle and thread and/or Neoprene tape
- Tape measure
- Scissors or roller cutter
- Straightedge ruler

1. Measure the child's thumb IP circumference with accuracy to the 1/16 inch. This measurement is used to create the pattern. When measuring an infant or toddler, it may be simplest to knot one end of a piece thread, wrap the thread snugly—not tightly—around the child's IP, and mark where the thread and knot intersect. Then straighten the thread, and align it to a ruler's edge to obtain an accurate circumference measure.

2. Trace or photocopy the palm side of the child's hand with fingers and thumb outstretched. If tracing, mark points on the outline to indicate the four corners of the palm where the palm intersects the wrist and the index and little fingers. Mark the two points where the line of the thumb IP intersects the outline of the thumb. As accurately as possible, draw a line for the distal palmar crease on the hand tracing.

3. From the photocopy or tracing determine the following measurements:
   - Measurement A: From the web space, just below the distal palmar crease to the edge of the palm. Add 1 to 2 inches to this measurement.
   - Measurement B: Half the distance of the web space from the thumb IP to the index finger MCP.
   - Measurement C: Half of the thumb IP circumference. Add 1/16 inch if using 1.5-mm Neoprene. Add 1/8 inch is using 3.0-mm Neoprene.
   - Measurement D: Thumb IP to proximal edge of the thumb MCP joint.
   - Measurement E: Distance along the wrist crease from the ulnar to radial side of the wrist. Add 1 to 2 inches to this measurement.

4. Create the pattern using measurements A through E. Cut out the pattern, and trace it onto the Neoprene. Next cut the pattern from the Neoprene using either the scissors or

roller cutter. Trace and cut a second pattern from the Neoprene. (*Note:* If the Neoprene has back and front sides, cut out mirror images.)

5. To assemble the orthosis, abut the two pieces of Neoprene side D to side D. Sew this seam by machine using a wide zigzag stitch. You may alternatively apply Neoprene tape or sew these two pieces together by hand. If sewing by hand, follow the directions for sewing by hand in #6.

6. Tape or sew by hand side B to side B. Neoprene heat-sensitive tape can be used to bond the two pieces together because the thickness makes it difficult to sew together. If sewing by hand, use a single thread, and embed the knot in the foam rubber within the seam. Use a running stitch to sew fabric to the fabric on the outside of the orthosis. Turn the orthosis inside out, pierce the needle through, and use a running stitch to sew fabric to fabric. This method avoids compressing the Neoprene at the joint and thereby does not reduce the strength of the abutted joint. Using a single strand of thread reduces the possibility of creating irritation along the web of the child's hand.

7. Adjust volar and dorsal portions of the orthosis to achieve desired amount of thumb abduction, and cut excess accordingly (dorsal portion overlaps volar portion by 1 inch for hook-and-loop closure).

8. Sew hook-and-loop fastener onto thumb sleeve, loop side down on dorsal portion and hook side up on volar portion. The fit should be snug but not constricting.

9. Attach hook-and-loop Velcro to each end of the wrist band that is designed to overlap on the volar side of the forearm. To form the thumb loop, attach one end of the thumb loop to the dorsal portion of the wrist band. Then attach the loop Velcro to the free end of the thumb loop and hook Velcro to the dorsal portion of the wrist band (partially covering the origin of the thumb loop).

10. The thumb loop is directed up across the web space, around the thenar eminence, and pulled diagonally to attach to the dorsal portion of the wrist band. The amount of tension on the thumb loop and the attachment location of the free end to the wrist band influence the amount of radial and palmar abduction of the thumb. If the wrist band does not fit snugly, the orthosis shifts distally on the wrist, thus reducing the amount of tension on the thumb loop. The wrist band must avoid circulatory restrictions (see Fig. 17.25 A & B).

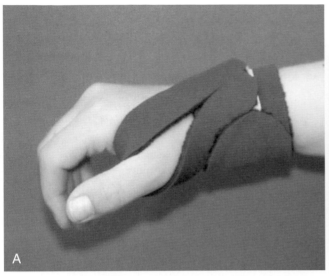

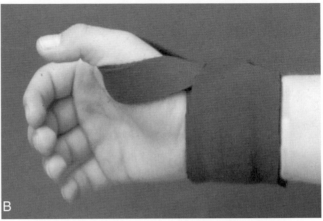

Fig. 17.25 A, Radial view soft thumb orthosis with loop. B, Volar view soft thumb orthosis with loop. (Courtesy Orfit Industries.)

Instructions for a rotation strap. Construction of a forearm rotation strap is simple. If cutting from a Neoprene bolt, use a roller cutter against a plastic ruler for accuracy. Before attaching the distal Velcro hook strip, trim the distal corners of the strap in a "V" to reduce bulk where the strap attaches to the hand or thumb orthosis. The proximal Velcro hook does not need to be sewn.

To apply the strap, attach to the hand thumb orthosis on the dorsal surface if promoting wrist extension. Likewise, attach to the palm side if promoting wrist flexion. Attaching the strap on the palm side and pulling through the web space may add unnecessary bulk to the orthosis and reduce hand function. Do not attach the strap ulnarly from the midline of the hand because it promotes ulnar deviation. The strap is always attached near the thumb. To fabricate the orthosis, position the child in a comfortable end range of desired rotation.

For a rotation strap that promotes supination, wrap the strap from the thumb side to ulnar side while spiraling up the forearm (Fig. 17.26). Likewise, for an orthosis that promotes pronation, wrap the strap from the thumb side to the radial side while spiraling up the forearm (Fig. 17.27).

Attach the strap to itself above the elbow with Velcro hook. You can assist in blocking elbow flexion if the strap is wrapped behind the elbow joint before securing it. This is a great addition to a thumb- or hand-based orthosis. The strap can sometimes provide enough assistance with wrist extension to promote weight bearing on the palm.

Anti–Swan Neck Orthosis

The goal of an anti–swan neck orthosis (Fig. 17.28) is to prevent hyperextension or swan neck deformity of the PIP joint of the finger.

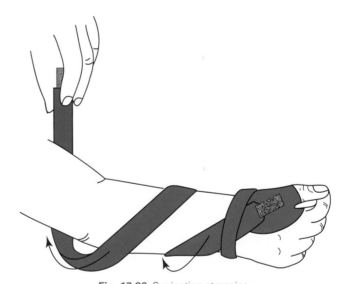

Fig. 17.26 Supination strapping.

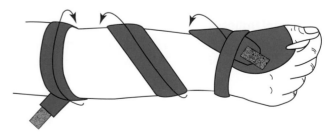

Fig. 17.27 Pronation strapping.

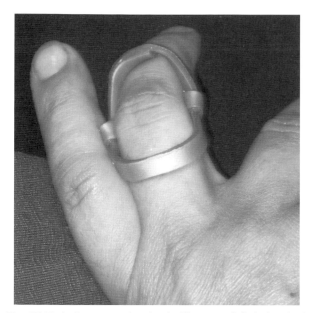

Fig. 17.28 Anti–swan neck orthosis. (Courtesy Orfit Industries.)

Fabrication of an anti–swan neck orthosis. The steps for fabricating an anti–swan neck orthosis can be found in the following procedure.

PROCEDURE FOR FABRICATION OF AN ANTI–SWAN NECK ORTHOSIS

The orthosis is fabricated from thin strips of 1/12-inch coated thermoplastic material.

1. Position the child's finger in PIP joint flexion. Construct a thermoplastic oval shape over the proximal phalanx and middle phalanx. Overlap the ends and let harden.
2. Place another strip of thermoplastic material directly under the PIP joint so that it overlaps onto the oval. Let harden. Carefully remove both strips and bond together with the use of a heat gun. Immediately dip into cold water to facilitate the bond and prevent overstretching of the material.
3. Ease the orthosis over the finger while it is flexed. The orthosis should allow for full finger flexion but prevent hyperextension or "swanning" of the PIP joint.

Commercial Orthoses

Sometimes the most cost-effective option for orthotic provision is a commercial orthosis. Therapists select a product and measure for correct sizing. The following companies specialize in prefabricated pediatric orthoses:

1. Bamboo Brace (elbow extension orthosis): The Bamboo Brace is a flexible pediatric arm brace (orthosis) placed around the elbow joint for children with CP and other developmental challenges. The Bamboo Brace assists children in maintaining a more extended elbow position to enable development of gross and fine motor skills.
2. Benik Orthoses (http://www.benik.com/): Benik sells custom Neoprene products, such as elbow, wrist, and thumb supports for adults and children. Measurement instructions are available online.
3. Comfy Splints (http://www.comfysplints.com/): These are prefabricated orthoses designed by occupational therapists and physicians. Their easy adjustability at multiple joints allows them to be used for many indications and deformities. They feature multilayers for softness and new drirelease with FreshGuard terry cloth covers. They are available in sizes for infants to large adults. The company sells a large selection of immobilization and mobilization orthoses.
4. The Joe Cool Company (http://www.joecoolco.com/): The Joe Cool thumb abduction orthosis maintains thumb abduction with minimal interference with grasp and sensation. Joe Cool thumb abduction orthoses are made of soft, flexible Neoprene and have an adjustable hook-and-loop closure system. They are latex-free and can be hand washed.
5. McKie Splints, LLC (www.mckiesplints.com): Dissatisfied with the bulkiness of commercially made thumb abduction orthoses for the 0 to 3-year-old population, Ann McKie, an occupational therapist, designed and patented the McKie thumb orthosis. Made from 1.5-mm Velcro-receptive Neoprene, the orthosis dynamically draws the thumb into opposition. The Velcro strap attaches at the head of the thumb MP to block hyperextension at the MCP joint. McKie Splints manufactures latex-free Neoprene thumb orthoses, supinator straps, and custom wrist-hand orthoses. All products are sized for premature infants, infants, children, teens, and adults and are available in a variety of colors. Low-temperature thermoplastic stays are available on custom orthoses.

EVIDENCE FOR ORTHOTIC INTERVENTION FOR CHILDREN

Table 17.3 summarizes evidence addressing the effectiveness of orthoses for children with a variety of diagnoses.

TABLE 17.3   Evidence-Based Practice About Orthotic Provision for the Pediatric Population

Author's Citation	Design	Number of Participants	Description	Results	Limitations
Cerebral Palsy					
Barroso, P. N., Vecchio, S. D., Xavier, Y. R., et al. (2011). Improvement in hand function in children with cerebral palsy via an orthosis that provides wrist extension and thumb abduction. *Clinical Biomechanics, 26,* 937–943.	Longitudinal study	Researchers investigated the hand movements of children with CP with and without an orthosis during functional tests. Thirty-two children with spastic hemiplegic CP participated in this study. Inclusion criteria: • Ages 5 to 12 years • Spastic hemiplegic CP • Cognition for simple commands to execute motor activities • Receiving OT or PT for at least 1 year • Manual Ability Classification System I and II • Limited wrist extension and abduction and TMC joint extension	Children wore a wrist extending/ thumb abduction (WETA) orthosis made of Neoprene and thermoplastic materials. The orthosis allows for freedom of movement of the fingers and IP of thumb. Researchers positioned the wrist at 20 degrees of extension. Researchers placed three passive reflexive markers on the hand and wrist and recorded movements with and without the orthosis.	Researchers measured ROM with digital image acquisition, grip strength with dynamometry, and hand function with Jebsen-Taylor Hand Function Test. When wearing the orthosis, the children demonstrated increased range of motion (flexion/extension and abduction/adduction); in the rest position, tripod pinches, and cylindrical grasp. The children demonstrated 50% greater muscle strength per dynamometry with the orthosis in place. Children demonstrated varied improvements on the four Jebsen-Taylor manual ability subtests with orthosis in place. Results indicate an orthosis has potential to improve ROM, strength, and manual ability with children with CP.	This research study did not consider the effect of rotations at the final phase of an opposition movement, which are crucial to provide stability for pinching and grasping. The sample size was small, and the study is of a lower level of evidence.
Elliott, C. M., Reid, S. L., Alderson, J. A., et al. (2011). Lycra arm splints in conjunction with goal-directed training can improve movement in children with cerebral palsy. *Neurorehabilitation, 21*(1), 47–54.	Randomized parallel group trial with wait list control	Researchers investigated the effectiveness of upper limb Lycra arm orthosis. Sixteen children with hypertonic CP participated in this study. One group of children wore the Lycra arm orthosis with goal-directed training for 3 months, whereas the other group completed goal-directed training (control). After the 3 months, group two wore the Lycra arm orthosis for 3 months with goal-directed training.	Participants wore the Lycra splint during school for 6 hours per day for 5 days per week. Goal-directed training included 25 minutes of active practice of task-specific activities that were related to each participant's individual goals.	Researchers collected data at baseline and upon orthotic application, after 3 months of splint wear, and immediately following removal of the orthosis. Researchers used the GAS and a motion analysis system to measure 3-D movement of upper limb. 94% of children in group 1 achieved goals on GAS over the 3-month orthotic wear period; whereas group 2 experienced little change during the control period. Children demonstrated improvement on joint kinematics with splint application and following 3 months of orthotic wear. Researchers observed a significant difference between baseline and 3 months of Lycra orthotic wear in the movement substructures (movement time, percentage of time, distance in primary movement, jerk index, normalized jerk, and percentage of jerk in primary and secondary movements).	This research study had a small sample size.

Continued

Author's Citation	Design	Number of Participants	Description	Results	Limitations
Jackman, M., Novak, I., Lannin, N. (2013). Effectiveness of hand splints in children with cerebral palsy: A systematic review with meta-analysis. *Developmental Medicine and Child Neurology, 56*, 138–147.	Systematic review and meta-analysis	Researchers reviewed studies to determine the efficacy of hand orthoses on hand function in children with CP. Sources of data included Cochrane Central Register of Controlled Trials *!* CENTRAL, MEDLINE, CINAHL, and PEDro.	Two reviewers selected articles for review based on specific inclusion criteria: • Study design was an RCT or a quasi-RCT. • All participants were 0–18 years of age. • All participants had a diagnosis of CP. • Intervention was a hand orthosis for the upper extremity. Studies that explored a hand orthosis in conjunction with another intervention were included in this review. Researchers excluded studies in which the orthosis was designed to restrain the upper limb or when the shoulder was the only area of orthotic application. Six articles with 224 participants were included in this analysis; 5 examined efficacy of nonfunctional hand orthoses; 1 investigated efficacy of a functional hand orthosis.	Researchers found a variety of splints and a variety of splint material used in these studies. Each study explored the use of hand splints in conjunction with therapy. Each of the six studies measured changes in body function and structure domain (e.g., ROM, 3-D motion analysis, Quality of Upper Extremity Skills Test), and three of the studies measured changes in the activity and participation domain (e.g., GAS, FIM, COPM) of the ICF. Results from these studies favored hand orthosis plus therapy over the sole use of a hand orthosis. Results also reported that benefits from orthosis plus therapy diminished 2 to 3 months after participants stopped wearing the orthosis (most frequent reported time was a 3-month follow-up).	None of the studies included in this review were free from bias and had a high level of heterogeneity. Researchers also included a small number of studies in this review due to lack of meeting inclusion criteria. In each of the studies it was impossible to blind the therapists to the hand orthosis due to inability to conceal. In five of the studies there was a lack of concealed group allocation. The assessors were not blinded to the treatment group in three of the studies. Data from these studies were reported in a way in which meta-analysis could not be conducted.
Louwers, A., Meesters-Delver, A., Folmer, K., et al. (2011). Immediate effect of a wrist and thumb brace on bimanual activities in children with hemiplegic cerebral palsy. *Developmental Medicine & Child Neurology, 53*, 321–326.	Pretest and posttest cohort study	Researchers investigated the immediate impact of a static wrist and thumb brace on the spontaneous use of an affected upper extremity during bimanual activities with children with hemiplegic CP. Inclusion criteria included: • Children between ages 4 and 12 years Diagnosis of spastic hemiplegic CP • Hand function classification of Zancolli I, IIA, or IIB25 children with CP participated in the study.	Researchers completed the AHA three times in which there was a 1-week intervention between each test. During AHA 1 the children did not wear the brace. During AHA 2 the children wore the brace, which was placed immediately before the assessment and removed immediately following the assessment. During AHA 3 the children did not wear the brace. Children did not receive any treatment between the assessments. Researchers used a static wrist and thumb brace (Ottobock).	In addition to the AHA, researchers also collected data before and during the first AHA using the following outcome measures: Gross Motor Function Classification System, Manual Ability Classification System, Zancolli classification, and House classification. When children with CP wore the brace, their performance of bimanual activities significantly improved. When wearing the brace, the children with CP increased by 3.2 points on the AHA.	This study used a small sample size, and researchers were unable to perform a subgroup analysis based on the Zancolli grade. Due to the study design, there is a lack of a comparison group and short follow-up times. The rater delivering the intervention was not blinded.

Author's Citation	Design	Number of Participants	Description	Results	Limitations
Sakzewski, L., Ziviani, J., Boyd, R. N. (2014). Efficacy of upper limb therapies for unilateral cerebral palsy: A meta-analysis. *Pediatrics*, e175–e204.	Meta-analysis	Researchers explored the efficacy of all nonsurgical upper limb therapies for children with unilateral CP. Sources of data included MEDLINE, CINAHL, Embase, PubMed, and Cochrane Central Register of Controlled Trials.	Researchers selected articles for review based on the following inclusion criteria: • RCT • Participants were children 0–18 years of age with diagnosis of unilateral CP • Study explored efficacy of nonsurgical upper limb therapy or adjunctive therapy with nonsurgical upper limb therapy • Outcomes from the study included upper limb unimanual or bimanual capacity or performance, achievement of individualized goals, or self-care skillsResearchers included 42 controlled trials in this review (13 different types of interventions).	Researchers reported that orthoses are often used as an adjunct to other upper limb treatment approaches. One study reported improved quality of movement 6 months after intervention when static night orthoses were used in conjunction with Botox and occupational therapy. Another study used a dynamic Lycra orthosis for 3 months with goal-directed training and demonstrated improved goal attainment when compared to a control group.	One study ncluded in this review related to orthotic wear and was a small study and had poor methodological quality.
Ten Berge, S. R., Boonstra, A. M., Dijkstra1, P. U., et al. (2012). A systematic evaluation of the effect of thumb opponens splints on hand function in children with unilateral spastic cerebral palsy. *Clinical Rehabilitation*, 26(4), 362–371.	Systematic evaluation of seven cases using a multiple baseline design	Researchers investigated the effects of a thumb opponens orthosis on hand function with children with unilateral CP. Inclusion criteria included: • Diagnosis of unilateral spastic CP • Thumb position of House 1, 2, or 4 • Between ages of 2 and 7 years 7 children participated in the study.	The children wore a Neoprene thumb opponens orthosis (McKie splints) at least 4 hours a day for 7 days a week. The parents donned the orthoses when the children were playing or participating in ADLs.	Researchers used the goal attainment scaling (bimanual ADLs) and VAS to assess hand function and task performance at baseline, during intervention, and follow-up. The time of these various data collection points varied from participant to participant. Researchers also completed a weekly semistructured interview with the parents. Parents reported good compliance with orthotic wear and that the children had more awareress of affected hand while wearing the orthosis. Of the seven children, four improved scores in GAS and/or visual analog scale after orthotic introduction, and the effects continued when the orthosis was not worn. Two of the seven children benefited from the orthosis only when it was worn.	This research study had a small sample size and had several areas of missing data. Researchers and parents were not blinded due to orthosis on, orthosis off conditions. There is potential for a co-intervention bias as all participants continued participation in physical and/or occupational therapy.

Continued

Author's Citation	Design	Number of Participants	Description	Results	Limitations
Trigger Finger Farr, S., Grill, F., Ganger, R., et al. (2014). Open surgery versus nonoperative treatment for pediatric trigger thumb: A systematic review. *Journal of Hand Surgery, 39*(7), 719–726.	Systematic review	Researchers explored the success rates of open surgery, orthotic intervention, and passive exercises with children with trigger thumb. Sources of data included PubMed, MEDLINE, Embase, Scopus, CINAHL, Cochrane Central Register of Controlled Trials, and Cochrane Database of Systematic Reviews.	Inclusion criteria included: • Children under the age of 10 with trigger thumb Minimum of 12-month follow-up Researchers included 18 articles in their systematic review: 12 with surgical intervention; 4 with orthotic intervention; 3 with exercise intervention; 1 with surgery and splinting	The four studies about orthotic intervention offered the orthotic intervention with or without passive exercise. The results are widely varied, ranging from 39% to 92% of participants experiencing full recovery of IP joint motion. The duration of orthotic wear varied, ranging from 2.9 to 22 months. In these studies, 5 of 115 participants experienced complications, and 11 of 138 participants had residual thumb triggering. In the study comparing surgery and orthotic intervention, 95% of participants with surgery achieved full IP motion, whereas only 67% of participants with orthotic intervention achieved this motion.	The majority of articles included in this review were of lower evidence (83% of articles at level IV evidence). One of the orthotic studies had a high dropout rate. The studies were not blinded due to nature of orthotic wear and lacked a control group.
Shiozawa, R., Uchiyama, S., Sugimoto, Y., et al. (2012). Comparison of splinting versus nonsplinting in the treatment of pediatric trigger finger. *Journal of Hand Surgery 37*(6), 1211–1216.	Retrospective study	Researchers compared orthotic provision and no orthotic provision in children with trigger finger. Researchers included 24 children with 47 affected fingers: 4 index, 28 middle, 11 ring, and 4 little.	One group included static orthotic provision, whereas the other group included observation. Researchers recommended static orthoses to all parents; however, 13 patients with 23 affected fingers elected not to receive orthotic intervention (observation group). 11 patients with 24 affected fingers were treated with a static orthosis. Researchers instructed parents to have children wear the orthosis one to two times per day during nap or for the first 2 to 3 hours of nighttime sleep for a minimum of 3 hours of wear time per day. Researchers fitted children with one of two types of orthoses depending on the number of affected digits. Children wore the orthosis for a mean time of 10 months.	Researchers collected data of active and passive range of motion and presence of triggering at various time points depending on the group. • Orthotic group—every 3 months for first 6 months; every 6 months for next year; once a year thereafter • Observation group—every 6 months for first 2 years; once a year thereafter Of the 24 fingers in the orthotic group, 67% resolved, 17% remain unchanged, 17% improved, and 29% required surgery. Of the 23 fingers in the observation group, 30% resolved without intervention, 4% improved, 65% remained unchanged, and 65% required surgery. The proportion of fingers requiring surgery in the orthotic-wearing group was significantly lower than in the observation group.	This study had a small sample size. There were also inconsistent data collection points between the two groups. The two groups were not randomly assigned. It does not appear researchers were blind to the group assignment. This study does not track orthotic adherence data.

Author's Citation	Design	Number of Participants	Description	Results	Limitations
Brachial Plexus Palsy					
Ho, E. S., Roy, T., Stephens, D., et al. (2010). Serial casting and splinting of elbow contractures in children with obstetric brachial plexus palsy. *Journal of Hand Surgery* 35(1), 84–91.	Retrospective review	Researchers investigated the effectiveness of serial casting and orthotic intervention with children with obstetrical brachial plexus palsy. Inclusion criteria included: • Diagnosis of obstetrical brachial plexus palsy • Referral for nonsurgical management of elbow flexion contracture • Minimum of two sessions for nonsurgical treatment Researchers included 27 patients in this retrospective review.	At this institution the treatment protocol included children with brachial plexus palsy who have an elbow contracture greater than 30 degrees with functional or cosmetic concerns. The traditional treatment protocol includes heat, range of motion and stretches, and serial casting or custom-made thermoplastic elbow extension orthosis. Orthoses are indicated when the contracture is reduced to 30 degrees or is initially between 20 and 40 degrees. The orthosis is worn at night and is placed anteriorly to maintain the elbow in maximum extension. The orthosis is modified with changes in elbow position.	An occupational therapist recorded the degree of passive elbow flexion contracture at each session. Researchers used the data from the initial treatment, best-achieved measurement, and final treatment. The type of orthosis, compliance, and complications were also recorded. Each participant experienced improvements in elbow range of motion. Researchers reported significant differences in passive range of motion from initial to best achieved and final time. 53% of patients reported noncompliance. Those patients who were more compliant demonstrated better results.	Researchers did not compare the two interventions. Due the nature of a retrospective review, there was not consistency in data collection. Researchers also had a small sample size, limiting the ability to complete statistical analysis. There was also a wide range of treatment duration.

ADL, Activity of daily living; *AHA*, Assisting Hand Assessment; *COPM*, Canadian Occupational Performance Measure; *CP*, cerebral palsy; *FIM*, Functional Independence Measure; *GAS*, Goal Attainment Scale; *ICF*, International Classification of Functioning, Disability and Health; *IP*, interphalangeal; *OT*, occupational therapy; *PT*, physical therapy; *RCT*, randomized controlled trial; *ROM*, range of motion; *TMC*, trapeziometacarpal; *VAS*, visual analog scale.
Contributed by Whitney Henderson.

SUMMARY

This chapter addressed the use of several types of orthoses for the management of children with a variety of conditions. Orthotic designs for a child differ from many of the adult designs. In addition to the dynamics of development, children differ from adults in the types of environments in which they live, learn, work, and play. Published case reports and research studies are needed to determine the effectiveness of pediatric orthotic designs and optimal wearing schedules. Such outcomes will allow therapists to make decisions based on clinical reasoning and evidence.

REVIEW QUESTIONS

1. How is orthotic intervention different with the pediatric population as compared to the adult population?
2. How would you prepare the room and the child to increase the probability of a successful orthotic fabrication session?
3. What factors should be considered when determining a wearing schedule for any pediatric orthosis?
4. What are the differences among the Bamboo Brace, Benik, Comfy Splints, Joe Cool, and McKie Splints commercial orthoses?
5. What are the pros and cons of using a soft orthosis versus thermoplastic material when providing an orthosis for a child?
6. What methods are appropriate for providing instructions to parents, teachers, and other caregivers to maximize correct application and use of an orthosis?

REFERENCES

1. Abzug JM, Kozin SH: Radial longitudinal deficiency, *J Hand Surg* 39(6):1180–1182, 2014.
2. Alexander R, Boehme R, Cupps B: *Normal development of functional motor skills: the first year of life*, ed 1, Tucson, AZ, 1993, Therapy Skill Builders, pp 71–157.
3. American Occupational Therapy Association: Occupational therapy practice framework: domain and process, ed 2, *Am J Occup Ther* 62:625–683, 2008.
4. Armstrong J: Splinting the pediatric patient. In Fess EE, Gettle K, Philips C, et al., editors: *Hand and upper extremity splinting: principles and methods*, ed 2, St. Louis, 2005, Mosby.
5. Banskota AK, Bijukachhe B, Rajbhandary T, et al.: Radial club hand deformity—the continuing challenges and controversies, *Kathmandu Univ Med J* 3(1):30–34, 2005.
6. Bell E, Graham HK: A new material for splinting neonatal limb deformities, *J Pediatr Orthop* 15(5): 613–616, 1995.
7. Barroso SD, Xavier Vecchio YR, Sesselmann M, et al.: Improvement in hand function in children with cerebral palsy via an orthosis that provides wrist extension and thumb abduction, *Clin Biomech* 26:937–943, 2011.
8. Bauer Andrea S, Bae Donald S: Pediatric trigger digits, *J Hand Surg* 40(11):2304–2309, 2015.
9. Deleted in review.
10. Ten Berge SR, Boonstra AM, Dijkstra PU, et al.: A systematic evaluation of the effect of thumb opponens splints on hand function in children with unilateral spastic cerebral palsy, *Clin Rehabil* 26(4):362–371, 2012.
11. Boehme R: *Improving upper body control: an approach to assessment and treatment of tonal dysfunction*, Tucson, AZ, 1988, Therapy Skill Builders, pp 86–118.
12. Bonhomme C, Trémoulet G, L'Kaissi M, et al.: Conservative treatment of camptodactyly by successive splinting, *Ann Phys Rehabil Med* 56(suppl 1):e173, 2013.
13. Colangelo C, Gorga D: *Occupational therapy practice guidelines for cerebral palsy*, ed 3, Bethesda, MD, 2004, American Occupational Therapy Association.
14. Comer GC, Ladd AL: Management of complications of congenital hand disorders, *Hand Clin* 31(2):361–375, 2015.
15. Colen David L, Lin IC, Levin SL, et al.: Radial longitudinal deficiency: recent developments, controversies and an evidence-based guide to treatment, *J Hand Surg* 42:546–563, 2017.
16. Collins LF: Splinting survey results, *OT Practice* 42–44, 1996.
17. Cornwall Roger, Waters PM: Pediatric brachial plexus palsy. In *Green's operative hand surgery*, ed 7, Philadelphia, 2017, Elsevier, pp 1391–1424.
18. de Boer IG, Peeters AJ, Rondays HK, et al.: The usage of functional wrist orthoses in patients with rheumatoid arthritis, *Disabil Rehabil* 30(4):286–295, 2008.
19. Duff SV, Charles J: Enhancing prehension in infants and children: fostering neuromotor strategies, *Phys and Occup Ther Ped* 24:129–172, 2004.
20. Erhardt R: *Developmental hand dysfunction theory: assessment and treatment*, Tucson, AZ, 1994, Therapy Skill Builders.
21. Exner CE: Development of hand skills. In Case-Smith J, editor: *Occupational therapy for children*, ed 5, St. Louis, 2005, Mosby.
22. Granhaug KB: Splinting the upper extremity of a child. In Henderson A, Pehoski C, editors: *Hand function in the child: foundations for remediation*, ed 2, St. Louis, 2006, Mosby, pp 401–432.
23. Hill SG: Current trends in upper extremity splinting. In Boehme R, editor: *Improving upper body control*, Tucson, 1988, Therapy Skill Builders, pp 131–164.
24. Ho Christine: Disorders of the upper extremity. In Herring JA, editor: *Tachdjian's pediatric orthopaedics*, ed 5, Philadelphia, Elsevier, pp 356–482
25. Hogan L, Uditsky T: *Pediatric splinting: selection, fabrication, and clinical application of upper extremity splints*, San Antonio, TX, 1998, Therapy Skill Builders.
26. Howle J: *Neuro-developmental treatment approach theoretical foundations and principals of clinical practice*, Laguna Beach, CA, 2002, Neuro-Developmental Treatment Association, pp 85–88.

27. Hovius Steven ER: *Congenital hand IV: disorders of differentiation and duplication: plastic surgery*, ed 3, Philadelphia, 2013, Elsevier, pp 603–633.

28. Jobe T, Mauck BM: Congenital anomalies of the hand. In Canale ST, Beaty JH, Azar FM, editors: *Campbell's operative orthopaedics*, ed 13, Philadelphia, 2017, Elsevier, pp 3826–3910.

29. Kahn P: Juvenile idiopathic arthritis—current and future therapies, *Bull NYU Hosp Jt Dis* 67(3):291–302, 2009.

30. Kanellopoulos AD, Mavrogenis AF, Mitdiokapa EA, et al.: Long lasting benefits following the combination of static night upper extremity splinting with botulinum toxin A injections in cerebral palsy children, *Eur E Rehabil Med* 49(4):501–506, 2009.

31. Koh S, Horii E, Hattori T, et al.: Pediatric trigger thumb with locked interphalangeal joint: can observation or splinting be a treatment option? *J Pediatr Orthop* 32:724–726, 2012.

32. Kotwal PP, Varshney MK, Soral A: Comparison of surgical treatment and nonoperative management for radial longitudinal deficiency, *J Hand Surg Eur* 37:161–169, 2012.

33. Kozin Scott H: Deformities of the thumb. In *Green's operative hand surgery*, ed 7, Philadelphia, 2017, Elsevier, pp 1289–1327.

34. Gay K, Davidson I: Occupational and physical therapy for children with rheumatic diseases. In *Textbook of pediatric rheumotology*, ed 7, Philadelphia, 2016, Elsevier 15, pp 176–187.

35. Lake Amy L, Oishi Scott N: Hand therapy following elbow release for passive elbow flexion and long head of the triceps transfer for active elbow flexion in children with amyoplasia, *J Hand Ther* 28:222–227, 2015.

36. Lutz CS, Kozin SH: Congenital differences in the hand and upper extremity. In Burke SL, Higgins J, McClinton MA, et al.: *Hand and upper extremity rehabilitation: a practical guide*, ed 3, St. Louis, 2006, Elsevier Churchill Livingstone, pp 659–688.

37. McKie A: *Effectiveness of a neoprene hand splint on grasp in young children with cerebral palsy*, Master's thesis, 1998, University of Wisconsin.

38. McClure PW, Blackburn LG, Dusold C: The use of splints in the treatment of joint stiffness: biological rationale and an algorithm for making clinical decisions, *Phys Ther* 74(12):1101–1110, 1994.

39. Netscher DT, Staines K, Hamilton KL: Severe camptodactyly: a systematic surgeon and therapist collaboration, *J Hand Ther* 28:167–175, 2015.

40. Petty RE, Laxer RM, Wedderburn LR: Juvenile idiopathic arthritis. In *Textbook of pediatric rheumotology*, ed 7, 15, Philadelphia, 2016, Elsevier, pp 188–204.

41. Ruchelsman DE, Pettrone S, Price AE, et al.: Brachial plexus birth palsy: an overview of early treatment considerations, *Bull NYU Hosp Jt Dis* 67(1):83–89, 2009.

42. Shiozawa R, Uchiyama S, Sugimoto Y, et al.: Comparison of splinting versus nonsplinting in the treatment of pediatric trigger finger, *J Hand Surg* 37(6):1211–1216, 2012.

43. Smith Paul J, Smith Gillian D: Radial club hand. In Guy Foucher, Raimondi Piero L, et al.: *The pediatric upper limb*, United Kingdom, 2002, Martin Dunitz Ltd, pp 153–182.

44. Stern EB, Callinan N, Hank M, et al.: Neoprene splinting: dermatological issues, *Am J of Occup Ther* 52(7):573–578, 1998.

45. Snook J: Spasticity reduction splint, *Am J of Occup Ther* 33(10), 1979.

46. Verchere C, Durlacher K, Bellows D, et al.: An early shoulder repositioning program in birth-related brachial plexus injury: a pilot study of the SUP-ER protocol, *Hand* 9:187–195, 2014.

47. Dan Zlotolow A: Arthrogryposis. In *Green's Operative Hand Surgery*, ed 7, Philadelphia, 2017, Elsevier, pp 1365–1390.

APPENDIX 17.1 CASE STUDIES

Case Study 17.1[a]

Read the following scenario, and use your clinical reasoning skills to answer the questions based on information in this chapter.

Matthew is an 8-month-old boy with arthrogryposis multiplex congenita. He lives with his mom and is cared for by a caretaker during the day, when his mom attends school. He has a supportive extended family. Matthew's shoulders rest in internal rotation, his elbows rest in extension, forearms rest in pronation, and wrists rest in flexion with thumbs adducted and digits partially flexed. Passive motion is limited and painful for end ranges of all shoulder motions, elbow flexion past 30 degrees, supination past 45 degrees, and wrist extension past 0 degrees. Active shoulder flexion is limited to 90 degrees. Matthew has only 30 degrees of active elbow flexion. There is no observable active wrist extension, and there is active finger flexion and extension. Matthew has difficulty grasping most toys. To compensate, he uses both hands during play and when attempting to grasp toys. He cannot hold a bottle or bring his hands to his mouth.

You have just completed Matthew's evaluation. Among the team goals are increasing his opportunities for play, increasing functional reaching and grasping skills, and increasing active participation in age-appropriate activities of daily living (ADLs). Specific objectives include increasing Matthew's ability to grasp and sustain hold on toys and improving functional reach and use of hands for play. You have selected the biomechanical frame of reference.

Orthotic intervention has never been used. You consider all of Matthew's limitations, and you are quite overwhelmed because you understand that it will be a challenge, but you are up for the task and decide to tackle it one step at a time. Which of the following treatment interventions would you select and why?

1. Option A: Educate his mom on passive range-of-motion exercises for both upper extremities, and inform his mom that once the child is able to tolerate passive motion without pain, you will implement the use of orthoses in your treatment plan.
2. Option B: Fabricate bilateral circumferential wrist orthoses in submaximal passive wrist extension for daytime wear. Fabricate bilateral posterior elbow orthoses for night use in submaximal passive elbow flexion.
3. Option C: Fabricate bilateral resting hand orthoses for daytime wear and bilateral posterior elbow orthoses for night wear in submaximal passive elbow flexion.
4. Option D: Fabricate bilateral circumferential wrist orthoses for daytime use, but remove orthoses during play activities. Fabricate bilateral resting hand orthoses for overnight wear.

Case Study 17.2[a]

Read the following scenario, and use your clinical reasoning skills to answer the question based on information in this chapter.

Luke is a 7-month-old boy who was referred to occupational therapy for indwelling thumb posture in his right hand. Mom is very concerned, explaining that Luke cannot bring his thumb out of his palm when attempting to grasp objects in his right hand. She reports that he keeps his thumb flexed in his palm when holding his bottle as well. You observe that Luke postures his right thumb metacarpal joint in flexion and that there is no active metacarpal extension during your evaluation. Luke has full active range of motion in bilateral upper extremities, with the exception of his right thumb. He has full passive right thumb metacarpal (MP) and interphalangeal (IP) flexion and extension, and this is interfering with the development of his fine motor skills. Which of the following orthotic interventions would you initiate now?

1. Option A: Fabricate a thermoplastic thumb spica for daytime use to facilitate improved functional positioning.
2. Option B: Fabricate resting hand orthoses for both hands and a thermoplastic material thumb orthosis for the right hand. Recommend wearing both resting hand orthoses at night and the left orthosis periodically during the day (depending on status of range of motion [ROM]). Recommend wearing the right thumb orthosis during functional grasp activities.
3. Option C: Fabricate resting hand orthoses for both upper extremities. Recommend that they be worn at night and during the day except during scheduled activities involving reach, grasp, and release.
4. Option D: Fabricate resting hand orthoses for both upper extremities. Because you are unsure if the orthoses would be put on correctly at home, recommend that they be worn only during the day at school. Both orthoses will be removed during scheduled activities involving reach, grasp, and release.

---

[a]See Appendix A for the answer key.

[a]See Appendix A for the answer key.

APPENDIX 17.2 LABORATORY EXERCISES

Laboratory Exercise 17.1[a] Recognizing Problems in Orthotic Fabrication No. 1

What problems in orthotic fabrication are present in the following picture?

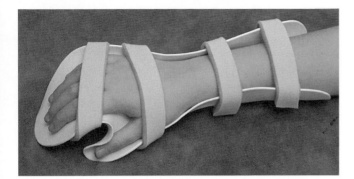

Laboratory Exercise 17.2[a] Recognizing Problems in Orthotic Fabrication No. 2

What problems in orthotic fabrication are present in the following picture?

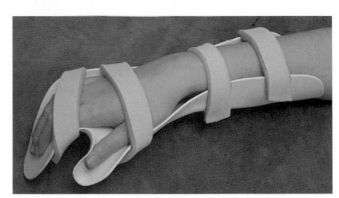

[a]See Appendix A for the answer key.

[a]See Appendix A for the answer key.

UNIT THREE

Topics Related to Orthosis

Lower Extremity Orthotics

Christopher Robinson
Stefania Fatone
Brittany Stryker

CHAPTER OBJECTIVES

1. Recognize the meaning of basic terminology used in lower extremity (LE) orthotic prescriptions.
2. Outline the role of the occupational therapist in the LE orthotic intervention program.
3. Recognize the importance of an interdisciplinary team approach to LE orthotic provision.
4. Describe the general purposes and basic functions of LE orthoses.
5. Describe the biomechanical principles of LE orthoses.
6. Describe the basic design principles of LE orthoses.
7. Describe various components and materials commonly used in the fabrication of LE orthoses.
8. Identify the basic components of normal and pathological gait.
9. Recognize commonly prescribed LE orthoses.

KEY TERMS

biomechanical principles
clinical considerations

normal gait
orthotic design principles

pathological gait

The International Organization for Standardization (ISO 8549-1:1989) defines an orthosis as an externally applied device used to modify the structural and functional characteristics of the neuromuscular and skeletal systems.[3,4] Orthoses are categorized based on the anatomical segments and joints encompassed (ISO 8549-3:1989)[4] with standard abbreviations for lower extremity (LE) orthoses listed in Table 18.1. Consistency in terminology ensures effective communication within the rehabilitation team.

Evidence of orthotic applications has been found as early as 2750 BC[2] in excavation sites where mummies have been uncovered with various orthoses still intact. Wars and battles have always dramatically increased the number of people in need of assistive devices. However, it was the polio epidemics of the 1950s and the introduction of thermoplastics in the 1970s that spurred increased interest and development in the field of orthotics in the United States.[6] Today, continued advancements in technology promote the development of new orthotic designs, materials, and components.

NOTE: This chapter includes content from previous contributions from Deanna Fish, MS, CPO; Michael Lohman, MEd, OTR/L, CO; Dulcey Lima, OTR/L, CO; and Karyn Kessler, OTR/L.

ROLE OF THE OCCUPATIONAL THERAPIST

In upper extremity orthotic practice, occupational therapists (OTs) typically provide comprehensive management, including the design, fabrication, fitting, and functional training of the client with the orthosis. With increased emphasis on interdisciplinary care, OTs are increasingly engaged in the care of clients who use LE orthoses. However, in these cases, certified orthotists (COs) are responsible for the design, fabrication, and fit of the LE orthoses, often working in concert with physical therapists in the provision of training in their use. OTs collaborate to ensure that LE orthoses are designed to facilitate successful occupational performance at each stage in the rehabilitation process. Common concerns addressed by OTs include acting as a client advocate, donning and doffing the orthosis, education regarding skin inspection for clients with insensate limbs, and integration of the orthosis into everyday use.

LE orthoses address specific biomechanical goals, such as providing knee stability during ambulation. In that case, it may require the OT to help the client learn how to perform mobility tasks with a locked knee. It is the OT's role to anticipate performance issues that may occur when wearing LE orthoses and collaborate with the orthotist to ensure that these issues are considered during the design and fabrication processes. The potential of a LE orthosis to address biomechanical and gait impairments is irrelevant if it is rejected because it is too difficult to don or doff or impedes activities of daily living (ADLs).

TABLE 18.1   Standard Abbreviations for Lower Limb Orthoses

Abbreviation	Name
FO	Foot orthosis
AFO	Ankle-foot orthosis
KO	Knee orthosis
KAFO	Knee-ankle-foot orthosis
HO	Hip orthosis
HKAFO	Hip-knee-ankle-foot orthosis

From Condie, D. (2008). International Organization for Standardization (ISO) terminology. In J. Hsu, J. Michael, & J. Fisk, *AAOS atlas of orthoses and assistive devices* (pp. 3–7). Philadelphia, PA: Mosby.

BOX 18.1   Clinical Objectives of Lower Extremity Orthotic Treatment

- Relieve pain
- Manage deformities
- Prevent excessive range of joint motion
- Increase the range of joint motion
- Compensate for abnormalities of segment length and shape
- Manage abnormal neuromuscular function (e.g., weakness or hyperactivity)
- Protect tissues
- Promote healing
- Provide other effects (e.g., placebo, warmth, postural feedback)

From Condie D. (2008). International Organization for Standardization (ISO) terminology. In J. Hsu, J. Michael, & J. Fisk, *AAOS atlas of orthoses and assistive devices* (pp. 3–7). Philadelphia, PA: Mosby.

With pediatric clients, LE orthoses affect occupational performance differently from adults. LE orthoses may focus, for example, on the development of balance and equilibrium as a foundation for skill development and motor milestone acquisition. LE orthosis designed to hold the hips in relatively extended and abducted position may provide a stable base of support to facilitate independent eating, playing, or writing skills but also impede crawling and transitional movements unless it is designed to avoid such problems.

An OT involved as part of the clinical team making decisions about LE orthotic management must have a working knowledge of terminology and basic biomechanical and **orthotic design principles** pertaining to LE orthoses. This chapter provides a basic understanding of LE orthotics but is not intended to be definitive or comprehensive in nature. Those with an interest in developing further expertise in this area should invest in additional training and reference texts, such as the *AAOS Atlas of Orthoses and Assistive Devices*.[17]

INTERDISCIPLINARY APPROACH

Although this chapter focuses primarily on the roles of the OT and the CO, all members of the interdisciplinary team contribute the expertise needed to facilitate a client's progression through a comprehensive rehabilitation program involving LE orthoses. The suggestion to provide a LE orthosis can come from any member of the interdisciplinary team with effective collaboration required to ensure the best possible clinical outcome. Consideration must be given to the client's sensory, motor, and occupational performance. Skin integrity and sensation influences the choice of material for interface components. The client's strength is considered in relation to the weight and forces required to use the orthosis. Fine motor strength and coordination also influence the design of the strapping system. ADLs are considered with regard to donning and doffing of the device. The client's physical and cognitive capabilities are also considered for successful use of the device.

Upper extremity orthoses made by OTs are typically fabricated from low-temperature thermoplastic materials and are intended for interim use with a typical life span of 3 to 6 months. The properties of low-temperature thermoplastic materials are described in Chapter 3 of this text. Limitations in material properties, such as lack of sufficient rigidity, preclude use of low-temperature thermoplastics in most LE orthotic applications. Orthotists must access a much wider variety of materials to successfully fabricate LE orthoses that may be worn for months or even years while being able to withstand forces such as weight-bearing activity. With the proper tools and skills, LE orthoses can be adapted to address the client's changing clinical presentation as the client progresses through rehabilitation.

ORTHOTIC DESIGN PRINCIPLES

General Concepts

When providing a client with LE orthoses, all involved must have a fundamental understanding of key biomechanical principles, clinical assessment, orthotic components, and material science to develop an orthotic intervention plan. Box 18.1 details the goals commonly addressed by LE orthoses. This intervention plan is created with input from the entire interdisciplinary team to ensure that it provides the client with the best possible outcome.

Biomechanical Principles

The orthotist's foundation for clinical decision making is based upon three fundamental **biomechanical principles**: three-point force systems, total contact, and kinaesthetic reminders. Although each of these principles may be used individually, they are often used in combination to achieve the best possible clinical outcome. These principles are summarized below in the context of LE applications.

Three-Point Force Systems

A three-point force system (Fig. 18.1) is used to change the alignment of a joint through the application of two forces working in opposition to a counterforce (or fulcrum). The counterforce is positioned on the convex side of the joint deviation, close to the joint requiring the angular change. The opposite two forces are positioned proximally and distally to the counterforce, on the side of the joint concavity. The greater the linear distance between opposing forces, the less force is required to achieve/maintain the angular correction.

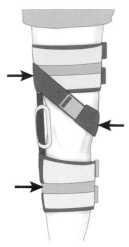

Fig. 18.1 Three-point force system to correct genu valgum. Pictured is a three-point force system applied in the coronal plane to effect an angular change at the knee joint (i.e., resistance to genu valgum).

Total Contact

Total contact is used to distribute forces from the orthosis more evenly over the client's body. The equation Pressure = Force/Area demonstrates that for the same force; an increasing area results in a relative decrease in pressure. It is important that pressures are kept at reasonable magnitudes; otherwise, the client is placed at risk for the development of skin breakdown. Breakdown could result in the inability to use the orthosis or infection if soft tissues are damaged and become a portal for bacteria. Some clinical presentations require relatively higher magnitudes of force from the orthosis to achieve biomechanical goals. The application of higher magnitudes of force requires increasing the surface area over which forces are applied, ensuring that tolerable and safe pressures are experienced by the soft tissues.

Kinaesthetic Reminder

A kinaesthetic reminder does not rely on the mechanical properties of an orthosis to achieve the intended function, but rather the sensation of wearing an orthosis. The sensation of being in physical contact with the orthosis may in some cases be sufficient to cue the client to alter movement patterns in a beneficial manner. For example, a child diagnosed with Down syndrome may present with excessive ankle dorsiflexion during the stance phase of gait (typically referred to as "crouch" gait) and can be provided a supramalleolar orthosis (SMO), which has elastic straps that circumferentially wrap just proximal to the malleoli. Although the elastic straps do not have the material properties required to mechanically limit excessive dorsiflexion and forward progression of the child's tibia during gait, the sensation of the strap across the tibial crest cues the child to volitionally limit movements of the ankle joint.

Clinical Assessment for Lower Extremity Orthotic Management

The ultimate design of any orthosis should explicitly address the intervention goals identified for each individual client.

BOX 18.2 Assessment for Lower Extremity Orthotic Intervention

- Personal history (e.g., initial presentation of disease, trauma, or problem; course of disease to date)
- Medical background (e.g., current medications, previous interventions)
- Comorbid conditions that affect orthotic management (e.g., diabetes, neurological impairment, hand dysfunction, and so on)
- Current and previous orthotic use
- Current exercise/therapy program
- Individual goals and expectations
- Daily activity level (current and anticipated)
- Sitting and standing posture and balance
- Description of body size and habitus (e.g., weight, height)
- Skin integrity
- Presence of edema
- Areas of pain/discomfort
- Neurological profile
- Sensation (e.g., light pressure, deep touch)
- Proprioception
- Range of available joint motion(s)
- Spasticity/tone
- Muscle strength
- Cognitive abilities (e.g., follow through with education and instructions regarding the orthosis)
- Static and dynamic alignment of joints
- Transfers and self-care tasks
- Observational gait assessment
- Functional testing to identify specific functional challenges (impact of condition on current functional status)

Data from Fish, D., Kosta, C., et al. (1997). *Functional walking: An EPIC approach. Oregon Orthotic System course manual*; Magee, D. (1987). *Orthopedic physical assessment*. Philadelphia, PA: WB Saunders; Uustal, H. (2008). The orthotic prescription. In J. Hsu, J. Michael, & J. Fisk. (2008). *AAOS atlas of orthoses and assistive devices* (pp. 9–14). Philadelphia, PA: Mosby.

Clinical objectives of orthotic treatment as identified by ISO 8551:2003 are listed in Box 18.1. Fabricating an orthosis without specific intervention goals identified will likely result in a less than optimal clinical outcome and decreased client acceptance of the orthosis. Making the client part of the clinical decision process is important because a single clinical presentation can be managed in many different ways. Defining appropriate orthotic intervention goals requires a thorough clinical assessment (Box 18.2). Physical examination includes both LEs to fully understand the client's current and potential function. LE orthoses may have intervention goals other than improving gait. Gait constitutes a large part of what LE orthoses address or compromise by their use. Hence it is important to understand gait when dealing with LE orthoses. An overview of both normal and pathological gait biomechanics is discussed.

Having a strong working knowledge of the major joints and structures that contribute to LE movement and how to assess them enables informed clinical decisions. The key joints and structures contributing to lower limb movement are the oblique midtarsal (Chopart), subtalar, ankle, knee, and

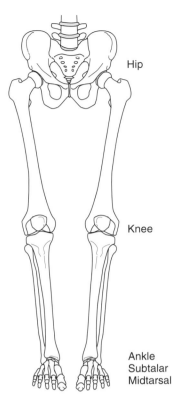

Fig. 18.2 Key joints and structures contributing to lower limb movement.

TABLE 18.2	**Control Options for Modification of Joint Motion by an Orthosis**
Terminology	**Description**
Free	Permit unencumbered motion in a plane or direction (e.g., free motion about the knee would allow flexion and extension of the knee through the full arc of motion).
Stop	To limit motion in a particular direction or plane (e.g., a plantar flexion stop mechanically blocks plantar flexion of the ankle but does not impede dorsiflexion).
Hold	To limit motion of a joint in both directions of a single plane of motion (e.g., a rigid orthosis preventing any motion at the ankle joint would be considered a hold).
Hold-variable	To limit motion of a joint in both directions of a single plane of motion without the joint being fixed (e.g., an orthosis made from a thin strut of flexible plastic posterior to the ankle can limit both plantar flexion and dorsiflexion without completely blocking all movement).
Assist	To encourage or facilitate motion in a specific direction for a plane of motion. Note assisting a motion will resist the opposing motion (e.g., a dorsiflexion-assist joint assists dorsiflexion movement while resisting plantar flexion movement).

hip joints (Fig. 18.2). When in contact with the ground, these joints work in concert to facilitate efficient movement patterns. When a single joint is deficient in strength or motion to perform a functional task, adjacent joint segments are often affected as well. For example, normal walking requires a person to have approximately 10 degrees of ankle dorsiflexion in order to allow the body to progress forward over the stance limb.[38] With a client who presents with a fixed plantar flexion contracture of 5 degrees at the ankle, tibial advancement is hindered. As a result, adjacent joints, including the oblique midtarsal joint and knee, may exhibit excessive motion so as to allow the tibia to continue to advance in the sagittal plane. The midtarsal joints may dorsiflex, and the knee may hyperextend, getting progressively worse over time as the client's body mass continues to progress forward with each step. This example describes movement in only a single plane. An orthosis aimed at addressing these impairments also accounts for coronal and transverse plane movements and the interplay that occurs between the joints, muscle groups, and motor control strategies needed to facilitate movement.

Once the orthotist has identified the specific joints, segments, and movements to address with the orthosis, the decision is made to control the joint directly or indirectly.[1] Direct control requires that the orthosis physically surrounds the segment or joint selected. Indirect control occurs when the orthosis attempts to modify the external forces acting on a joint beyond its physical boundaries. For example, an orthosis can address weak knee extensors using either direct or indirect control. The direct approach would involve fabricating an orthosis that physically surrounds the knee joint (e.g.,

a knee orthosis [KO] or knee-ankle-foot orthosis [KAFO]). Hinges that lock when the knee is fully extended act to stabilize the knee. An indirect approach would use an orthosis that encapsulates the foot, ankle, and calf musculature but terminates distal to the knee (i.e., an ankle-foot orthosis [AFO]). The AFO would rigidly hold the ankle joint in a fixed position, eliminating the ability of the tibia to advance over the foot during the stance phase of walking. Limiting ankle dorsiflexion in this way encourages the knee to remain extended during walking and standing without having an orthosis that physically surrounds the knee.

A helpful tool in the orthotic clinical decision-making process is the technical analysis form (TAF).[26] The TAF allows orthotists to identify specific motion constraints to impart at each joint and in each plane. Classifications for joint motion constraints are shown in Table 18.2.

Among other decisions the orthotist decides whether to provide a prefabricated or custom-fabricated orthosis. Prefabricated devices are also referred to as *custom-fit* because they still require a skilled orthotist to adjust and modify the device to ensure that it achieves the desired intervention goals. Custom-fit orthoses are beneficial in that they are potentially less costly than a custom-fabricated device, and they allow for immediate fitting so long as the desired orthosis is in inventory. The dilemma with custom-fit orthoses is that they are designed for a broad range of individuals and typically available in limited sizes that may not match the anatomy of the particular client. The severity of the pathology being treated may necessitate the use of a custom orthosis. For example, triplanar deformities often require a custom intervention because the affected segments lack the normal anatomical shape/alignment required to fit a prefabricated intervention. Custom-fabricated orthoses require additional time and skill, but they offer an intervention that is customized, allowing the orthotist to choose the most optimal combination of materials and components to address a particular client's needs. The criteria that is most important to the selection of a custom-fit versus a custom-fabricated intervention is the anatomical shape of the limb segments and the number of planes of motion.

Orthotic Components

Once the orthotist selects the motion controls to be incorporated into an orthosis, appropriate orthotic components are selected. Four categories of components are interface components, articulating components, structural components, and cosmetic components (ISO 13404:2005).[4]

- Interface components: Interface components are defined by ISO as those components that are in direct contact with the orthosis user, are responsible for transmitting the forces required for function, and help hold the orthosis in place on the body. Examples include shells, pads, straps and, when used with an orthosis that encompass the feet, shoes.
- Articulating components: Articulating components are defined by ISO as components used to allow or control the motion of anatomical joints. Articulating components are further defined by the joint that they are intended to control, the permissible motion of the joint in the final orthosis, the form of articulation (i.e., either by motion between parts, as in a hinge, or deformation of a part of the joint). These components control the axis of rotation (i.e., monocentric or polycentric) and the type of motion control, which is described in Table 18.2.
- Structural components: As defined by ISO, structural components are those that connect the interface and articulating components, acting to maintain the alignment of the orthosis (e.g., metal uprights and plastic shells).
- Cosmetic components: Cosmetic components are the means of providing shape, color, and texture to orthoses. Examples may include fillers, covers, sleeves, and patterns or pictures embedded into plastic shells.

When selecting orthotic components, the orthotist considers the client's height, weight, and activity level to ensure that the components are robust enough to function optimally and be durable without being excessively heavy or bulky. Articulating components are available in a variety of configurations and can influence joint motion in many ways. The simplest configuration is a single-axis joint that features a locking mechanism to create a hold in a specific plane. Orthoses may also feature relatively dynamic joints designed to impose an external torque across a joint. For example, a client who presents with a knee flexion contracture of 20 degrees may benefit from low-load, long-duration stretching if the interdisciplinary team feels that they have the

potential to improve muscle length and range of motion. The orthotist may fit a device that uses a spring-loaded articulation to apply an external extension torque at the knee, with the ultimate goal of increasing knee range of motion over time. This dynamic joint enables clients to continue to gain the benefits of stretching, while being able to remove the orthosis for skin hygiene and comfort in contrast to serial casts that must remain in place 24 hours per day.

Regardless of joint design, alignment of anatomical and mechanical joint axes is important. If the axes do not coincide, undesirable forces (both shear and compressive) and moments (i.e., torques) are generated as joints move through their range.[8] Appropriate alignment of joint axes has consequences not only for the soft tissue at the interface, but also the integrity of the joint. However, there are occasions for which joints are intentionally misaligned to create a desired outcome. For example, a posterior offset knee joint used in a KAFO places the mechanical knee axis posterior to the client's anatomical knee axis in the sagittal plane but parallel in all other planes. The objective of this alignment is to position the client's weight line anterior to the mechanical joint, thus creating an external extension moment (or torque) across the knee during stance phase. This facilitates knee stability without having to lock the mechanical knee joint entirely.

Materials Science

Once the orthotist chooses the specific components to be included in the orthosis, selection of the appropriate materials to create the structural components of the device occurs. Orthotists fabricate the vast majority of orthoses from thermoplastics, thermosets, metals/alloys, and foam interface materials. Within the realm of LE orthotics, metal or alloy systems were prominent until the 1970s when high-temperature thermoplastic materials and vacuum-forming techniques were introduced into clinical practice. Although metal orthoses are still used (often by long-time users), thermoplastic systems have become the standard so long as there are no contraindications to their use, such as an allergy to the thermoplastic, heat sensitivity from total contact, or uncontrolled fluctuating edema.

High-temperature thermoplastics are typically used in the fabrication of LE orthoses, because they have greater strength and fatigue resistance when compared with the low-temperature thermoplastic materials typically used in the fabrication of upper extremity orthoses. High-temperature thermoplastic materials become malleable at temperatures above 80°C (180°F) and must therefore be shaped over a heat-resistant model of the client's limb. Thermoplastic materials are relatively inexpensive and available in a wide variety of strengths and thicknesses. They are popular because they can be heated multiple times and remolded, allowing for alterations to the contours of an orthosis to accommodate any changes in limb shape and volume. The most common high-temperature thermoplastic materials used in LE orthoses are polypropylene, copolymer, and polyethylene. Polypropylene is a strong but notch-sensitive plastic that is typically used where rigidity is required, especially in clients who have higher weight or activity levels. Copolymer is also a relatively strong thermoplastic material but typically lacks the rigidity of polypropylene of the same thickness, often being used in instances where some flexibility is desired. Polyethylene is a flexible plastic that is well suited to applications where weight is not necessarily borne through the material. Polypropylene and copolymer offer adequate tensile and bending strength for LE applications in pediatric and adult clients so long as the resultant orthosis is fabricated with appropriate thickness.

Thermoset materials used in LE orthoses generally consist of fiber-reinforced, laminated resins with layers of natural or synthetic fibers. Thermosets are composed of three principal materials: resin, matrix, and promoter. The resin is in a liquid form until it is combined with a promoter. The promoter converts the liquid into a solid material. While in its liquid state, the resin is poured over the matrix and is allowed to set or cure until the material hardens. To manufacture a laminated orthosis, the orthotist relies on a positive model of the client's limb due to the exothermic reaction that occurs during curing. The material properties of the finished orthosis are more reliant on the type and orientation of the matrix materials than the chosen resin or hardener, which serves to bind the layers of matrix together. Common resins used in orthotic practice include polyester, acrylic, and epoxy, whereas common matrices include nylon, carbon, and glass fiber. Adding fibers and orienting them in an optimal manner increases the maximum strength and stiffness of the thermoset. Thermosets have the potential to provide relatively lightweight and stronger orthoses in contrast to thermoplastics but are potentially more costly. Once cured, thermosets cannot be reheated or reformed, although they can be sanded and trimmed; therefore they are best used with clients who are stable with regard to fluid volume.

Where durability is critical, orthoses can be fabricated primarily from metal and alloys. Metals and alloys are also used in thermoplastic or thermoset orthoses as many orthotic joints, rivets, screws, and chafes are manufactured from alloys. The most common metals/alloys used in the manufacture of LE orthoses are aluminum, stainless steel, and titanium. All of these materials can be treated and manufactured to create different properties. Aluminum and stainless steel are used more commonly in clinical practice as they are easier to work with from a fabrication standpoint and less expensive than titanium alloy.

Interface materials are the final consideration in the manufacture of orthoses. Orthotists use a wide array of natural and synthetic materials to create an interface between the client and the orthosis. The simplest interface is the application of a sock; a cotton or wool sock allows the skin to breathe while wicking sweat and oils from the LE. Interface components may also be lined with materials designed to increase wearing comfort. Nylon, Neoprene, and thermoplastic foams can be attached to the inner surface of the interface component during the manufacturing process or as needed at follow-up assessments. For example, clients with peripheral neuropathy are at high risk of ulceration on the plantar surface of their feet. The orthotist may elect to line the plantar interface component of an orthosis with a foam such as Plastazote, which is similar in durometer to soft tissue. With pressure, this material yields over areas of bony prominence and helps redistribute pressure over the plantar surface of the foot.

Gait Biomechanics

Observational gait analysis. As already mentioned, prescription criteria for LE orthoses are based on a thorough assessment of the client, including evaluation of gait where appropriate. Ideally, observational gait analysis (OGA) is performed with the client wearing minimal and/or snug-fitting clothing. This allows the observer to relate the function of the lower limbs to the stability of the upper torso. Walking is observed with the client barefoot and then while wearing any existing orthoses or ambulation aids. Observation of gait is facilitated by use of video recordings that can be replayed and/or played in slow motion.

Normal gait. **Normal gait** is characterized by smooth, rhythmic patterns of motion that require relatively little effort. Normal gait is often described in terms of a gait cycle, which is defined as initial contact of one foot to the next initial contact of the same foot (Fig. 18.3). The gait cycle is partitioned into

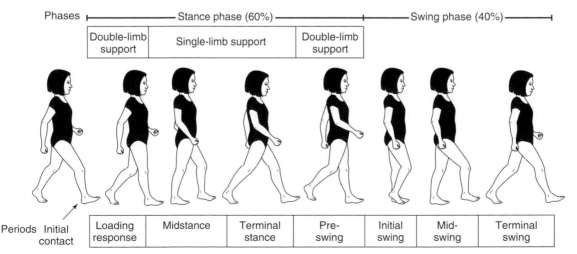

Fig. 18.3 The normal gait cycle consists of swing and stance phases with periods of double- and single-limb support. Swing and stance phases are further subdivided into seven functional subphases.

stance and swing phases, with stance phase including periods of double- and single-limb support. Stance phase is further divided into more specific functional subphases: loading response, midstance, terminal stance, and preswing; whereas swing phase can be divided into initial swing, midswing, and terminal swing.[38] Gard and Fatone[12] described the following important functions associated with normal walking: gait initiation and termination, balance and upright posture, stability of the stance leg, execution of the stepping motion, forward progression, shock absorption, and energy conservation. These functions are further detailed later.

Two-thirds of the body mass is carried above the hips when standing. Being top-heavy in this way challenges stability with active intervention required to maintain balance of the head, arms, and trunk over the legs and pelvis. Abdominal and pelvic muscular effort is reduced by holding the trunk vertical and positioned over the legs. During standing, static balance is achieved by positioning the body's center of gravity (weight line) within the base of support created by the perimeter of the feet. If the center of gravity moves outside the base of support, the person falls over. However, during walking the center of gravity does not need to be positioned directly over the base of support. The person walking maintains a dynamic equilibrium in which the motion of the body mass plays a role in maintaining an upright posture and balanced state. The dynamics associated with forward momentum of an able-bodied person enable body configurations to be assumed during gait for which static balance would not be possible.

Walking requires that a person successfully accelerate the body forward from a standing position and stop walking while maintaining an upright, balanced state.[12] In able-bodied people, steady-state walking speed is achieved within two to three steps. During standing and walking, the stance leg must have the ability to support the weight of the body, especially during single support, when the body progresses forward over the supporting leg while the contralateral leg is swinging forward. This requires a combination of adequate muscular strength and appropriate leg positioning. During walking the body appears to increase stability of the lower limb joints through careful control of the ground reaction force (GRF) vector, reducing joint moments (i.e., torques) and muscle forces. The GRF is the reaction to the force exerted by the body on the ground.

Weight transfer onto the leading leg during gait is rapid and fairly abrupt. Weight transfer creates the challenge of accepting fast-moving body weight in a manner that both absorbs the shock of floor contact and creates a stable limb over which the body can advance.[38] Normal ambulation is characterized by knee flexion during loading response, which serves to provide shock absorption by decreasing leg stiffness.[13]

Normal walking requires the ability to advance the leg from behind to in front of the body so as to execute the stepping motion in a smooth, efficient manner that does not disrupt forward progression. To accomplish this objective the leg must be sufficiently shortened so that it does not contact the ground during swing, and it must then be rapidly lengthened as it moves in front of the body in preparation for initial contact and stance phase.

Able-bodied walking is characterized by symmetry with the stance and swing phases of one leg nearly equal in duration to those of the other, providing an even, rhythmic pattern. Stance phase duration during freely selected able-bodied gait is approximately 62% of the gait cycle, with swing phase constituting approximately 38% and double-support phases lasting approximately 12%. Phase durations are modified with faster or slower walking speeds.[31] The stepping rate (i.e., cadence) is influenced significantly by the swing leg: walking speed is difficult to change without the ability to control swing phase duration.

Able-bodied adults generally adopt a freely selected walking speed of approximately 1.3 to 1.4 m/s and are able to comfortably walk across a range of speeds from approximately 0.8 to 1.8 m/s.[24] Walking speed is determined by both step length and step rate. As the limb prepares for initial contact, the swing leg hip is flexed and the knee extended so as to move the foot to a position in front of the body, allowing for an adequate step length. Inability to flex the hip or extend the knee sufficiently results in short step lengths and slows forward progression. Faster walking speeds tend to be accompanied by greater pelvic rotation,[35] which serves to further increase step length. Rate of stepping relies on the ability to transfer body weight to the leading leg and swing the trailing leg forward without hindering forward progression.

Knee flexion is the primary mechanism by which the leg is effectively shortened for swing phase ground clearance of the foot. Knee flexion during swing phase converts the leg into a double (i.e., compound) pendulum, enabling the leg to swing forward with less effort and energy. Effort required to rotate the leg is reduced by knee flexion as it brings the foot and shank masses closer to the hip joint's axis of rotation. This also enables the leg to swing forward in shorter time than if the leg were fully extended.[23]

Able-bodied people use mechanisms to conserve mechanical energy and preserve forward momentum of the body, enabling forward progression with only relatively small additions of metabolic energy from step to step. Perry and Burnfield[38] suggested that three rocker mechanisms (heel, ankle, and forefoot) serve to facilitate forward progression, whereas Gard and Childress[11] proposed that these three rocker mechanisms can be integrated during walking to create a single, smooth "roll-over shape." Regardless of how it is defined, an altered foot rocker mechanism disrupts forward momentum of the body and decreases walking speed.[9]

During double support, body weight is rapidly transferred to the leading leg so that the trailing leg can be lifted and advanced in front of the body. Weight transfer must occur quickly and efficiently so that the knee of the trailing leg can begin flexing in preparation for swing phase and the leg can begin accelerating forward. Knee flexion and ankle plantar flexion in the trailing leg during double-support phase serve to lengthen the leg. This allows the trailing leg to maintain contact with the ground and provide stability while facilitating transfer of load to the leading leg. Serving as a mobile link between the two legs, the pelvis facilitates smooth transmission of body weight from one leg to the other and provides shock absorption.[10] Rapid flexion of the hip in late stance accelerates the leg forward, and further knee flexion occurs passively. Inhibition of knee flexion at the end of stance phase or delay in knee flexion initiation reduces acceleration of the trailing leg, prolonging double-support phase and slowing forward progression of the body.

Cushioning of impact forces generated during normal walking are achieved through the physical properties of biological tissues, footwear, and walking surfaces[20] and through actions of the lower limb and pelvis, such as stance phase knee flexion and coronal plane pelvic motion (i.e., pelvic obliquity).[10,13,38,43] The motions that occur during loading response provide shock absorption. At initial contact, ankle plantar flexion and knee flexion serve to lessen the impact of floor contact.[32,37,41] Increasing knee flexion in early stance decreases the stiffness of the leg and diminishes transmission of mechanical shock to the head.[15,20,27]

Able-bodied walking is characterized by remarkable efficiency, which seems to be accomplished by two primary means: managing the GRFs in such a manner that the internal muscle moments (i.e., torques) about joints are reduced and by conserving mechanical energy associated with moving the segment masses of the body. Able-bodied people are able to capitalize on these energy-conserving mechanisms, reducing the amount of metabolic energy that must be added from step to step. Recordings of muscle activity during walking show that for much of stance phase muscles are largely silent, indicating that little effort is required to maintain stability and advance the body forward.[38] Muscles appear to be used primarily to accelerate and decelerate the head, arms, trunk, and lower limb segments, with significant reliance on momentum of the body masses that enable muscles to be turned off in midstance and midswing. Perry and Burnfield[38] suggested that sufficient gait velocity is required to preserve the advantages of momentum and reduce demand on muscles.

Pathological gait. A **pathological gait** pattern often develops secondary to neuromuscular deficits, joint instabilities, pain, disease processes, congenital impairments, and many other conditions. Excessive or insufficient joint motion can lead to exaggerated, inhibited, or compensatory movements of the body throughout the gait cycle.[38] As a result, the normal walking speed of the individual is often diminished. Clinical training in OGA ensures the identification of all pathological gait deviations in need of LE orthotic intervention. Gait deviations are considered as either primary and directly caused by the pathology, or secondary compensatory maneuvers. When a primary deviation is identified, the observer looks for secondary gait deviations. Where a secondary gait deviation is observed, the observer looks elsewhere for the primary problem. It is important to realize that correction of the primary deviation will resolve the secondary deviation, but not vice versa. Deviations can occur in combination with each other (e.g., stiff knee gait coupled with hip hiking), and the magnitude of deviations in any individual subject may vary with severity of the pathology. Commonly observed primary gait deviations include footdrop, tone-induced equinovarus, knee hyperextension, knee instability, genu varum, genu valgum,

and stiff knee gait. Commonly observed secondary or compensatory gait deviations include increased step width, vaulting, steppage gait, circumduction, hip hiking, and lateral, anterior, and posterior trunk lean. These gait deviations are described in more detail in the following sections.

Primary deviations. Primary gait deviations may be due to the impairment or may also be caused by orthotic interventions acting appropriately or inappropriately (e.g., due to worn-out orthotic components). Examples of primary gait deviations include footdrop (insufficient dorsiflexion during swing as a result of dorsiflexor muscle weakness) and tone-induced equinovarus (excessive plantar flexion during swing as a result of calf muscle spasticity or hypertonicity). A worn out plantar flexion stop or dorsiflexion assist spring on an AFO can also create problems with the ankle alignment needed for swing phase ground clearance of the limb. When dorsiflexion of the ankle is compromised in any of these ways, not only will the toes drag on the ground during swing phase, but initial contact with the ground during loading response will occur with the toes or forefoot rather than the heel. In response to these problems, clients will, if possible, adopt secondary gait deviations that provide ground clearance of the plantar flexed foot during swing phase, such as exaggerated hip and knee flexion (i.e., steppage gait) or hip circumduction. However, without the assistance of a LE orthosis, it is very difficult to compensate for the inappropriate initial contact. Disruption of the heel rocker in this manner compromises forward progression and slows walking.[34]

Secondary deviations. Secondary (compensatory) gait deviations are a functional response to an impairment or orthotic intervention that disrupts the ability to walk. However, although secondary deviations facilitate walking, they can often be in and of themselves inefficient and energy expensive. Examples of common secondary gait deviations include vaulting, circumduction, and hip hiking. Each of these deviations compensate for a limb that is functionally too long during swing phase or cannot be shortened at the appropriate time (e.g., where knee motion is reduced due to a locked KO or hypertonicity/spasticity of the knee extensors; where there is a limb length discrepancy; where the dorsiflexor muscles are weak and the toe drags during swing). Vaulting involves exaggerated plantar flexion of the contralateral (uninvolved) ankle during midstance. By rising up on the stance limb, extra ground clearance is created for the swing limb in which hip and knee flexion or ankle dorsiflexion are compromised. When circumducting, the impaired limb follows a laterally curved path during swing rather than swinging straight forward; less knee flexion is therefore needed for the foot to clear the ground during swing. Hip hiking involves elevation of the pelvis (and consequently the hip) on the impaired side in the coronal plane during swing. Hip hiking raises the leg more than it otherwise would be raised. Although these deviations help ensure that the swing limb clears the ground during swing phase, they require larger displacement of segment masses, which increases muscular effort and energy expenditure and diminishes conservation of mechanical energies.

These energetic issues are even worse when trunk deviations (such as lateral, anterior, or posterior trunk lean) are used to compensate for lower limb impairments, such as weak hip abductors, weak knee flexors, and weak hip extensors, respectively. Weakness of these muscles compromises stance phase stability at the respective joint. Shifting the trunk center of mass during stance on the impaired/weakened limb reduces the moments (or torques) that the weakened muscles must counteract to maintain upright stability. Moving the trunk laterally over the stance limb reduces the internal hip abductor moment needed from the muscle to maintain a level pelvis during single-limb stance. Similarly, moving the trunk anteriorly over the stance limb increases the external knee extensor moment acting to stabilize the knee during single-limb stance.

Some pathological motions are more difficult to compensate for in a functional manner. Knee hyperextension is such a condition (Fig. 18.4). This occurs as the knee moves in a backward direction during midstance (i.e., opposite to the direction of walking), often secondary to weakness of the quadriceps and/or calf muscle groups. Without hyperextension the person experiences uncontrolled knee flexion and collapse. Unfortunately, ongoing knee hyperextension results in increasing knee deformity and pain and disrupting the efficiency of gait because the LE is forced backward as the body mass is attempting to move forward over the stance limb.

FOOT ORTHOSES

General Description

The most common LE orthoses are foot orthoses (FOs), not only because they form the basis of many of the more proximal LE orthoses, but also because they are prescribed for an extremely broad range of pathologies from mild to severe. FOs are those devices that encompass all or part of the foot but terminate distal to the ankle joint.[4] A variety of FO designs are shown in Fig. 18.5. They may extend the length of the foot or terminate at the toe sulcus or proximal to the metatarsal heads. FOs benefit the foot primarily in stance and are held in position against the foot by shoes.[30] FOs may be used to treat foot instability or deformity caused by muscle weakness and/or imbalance, structural malalignment, and loss of structural integrity due to ligamentous laxity or rupture. FOs may also address more proximal disorders because the foot is the base of support for the entire body during standing and walking. Alignment of the foot can affect plantar pressure distribution, center of pressure progression, and moments occurring at proximal joints by altering the orientation of the GRF vector with respect to joint axes.

Shoes are an integral part of LE orthosis function because they form the base upon which almost all LE orthoses must work. Footwear must be spacious enough to accommodate the orthosis (e.g., they may be a half-size larger or have removable inserts). To appropriately support the orthosis, it is helpful for the shoe to be of stable construction, including a heel counter and a nonskid sole. For dysvascular feet at high risk of pressure ulcers, shoes should be made of soft materials, constructed without seams and provide extra depth to ensure the toe box does not place pressure on the dorsum of the foot. Velcro closures with longer openings can facilitate donning.

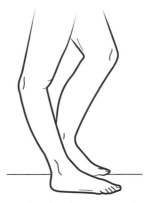

Fig. 18.4 Knee hyperextension (genu recurvatum) is a progressive stance phase deformity. The knee moves posteriorly upon weight bearing, serving to disrupt forward momentum and functionally shortening the limb during loading response.

Most FOs are biplanar by design, addressing joint deviations and providing support in the sagittal (e.g., midfoot depression) and coronal planes (e.g., hindfoot varus or valgus). More involved FO designs, such as the University of California Biomechanics Laboratory (UCBL), offer triplanar support with added control for transverse plane deviations (e.g., forefoot abduction or adduction).

Michael[29] identified three broad categories of FOs: accommodative or soft FOs, intermediate or semirigid FOs, and corrective or rigid FOs (see Fig. 18.5). Soft FOs are made from soft or flexible materials, such as closed and open cell foams. Soft FOs accommodate and protect rigidly deformed or dysvascular feet. These orthoses attempt to increase the weight-bearing surface area, redistribute the plantar pressures, and decrease the forces applied to the tissues at risk for ulceration and breakdown. Semirigid FOs are made by layering different density foam materials. The composition of the layers dictates the degree of support and biomechanical control. Semirigid FOs include many prefabricated, commercially available FOs. Accommodative and semirigid devices are fabricated by molding foam directly to the plantar surface of the foot or by using crush boxes (blocks of foam whereby an impression of the foot is made by crushing the foam beneath the foot and subsequently filling the indentation with plaster to create a positive model of the foot used to vacuum-form the FO). Rigid FOs correct flexible deformities, especially those that include hind-foot varus or valgus. The orthosis must be rigid to contour to the calcaneus (heel) and provide control of hind-foot alignment and motion, especially during weight-bearing activities. Rigid orthoses are generally made from high-temperature thermoplastic materials and require a heat-resistant positive model of the foot.

Clinical Considerations for the Occupational Therapist

When wearing FOs it is recommended that OTs educate clients with insensate feet about visual skin inspection. Education is important to ensure skin integrity and prevent skin breakdown. Handheld skin inspection mirrors are indicated for clients with reduced LE range of motion to ensure comprehensive

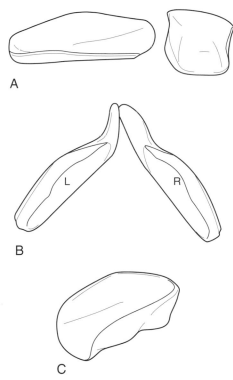

Fig. 18.5 Common foot orthosis (FO) designs. A, Accommodative or soft FO. B, Intermediate or semirigid FO. C, Corrective or rigid triplanar FO. (Courtesy University of California Biomechanics Laboratory.)

inspection of the plantar surface of the foot. Checking the skin's color and temperature is essential for clients with major vascular issues and neuropathy. The OT plays an important role in educating the client in regular skin inspection and implications to overall health. Communicating any concerns to the interdisciplinary team is helpful to developing a long-term care plan and to voice concerns to family members or caretakers.

ANKLE-FOOT ORTHOSES

General Description

AFOs are devices that encompass the ankle and the whole or part of the foot (Fig. 18.6).[4] AFOs primarily provide ankle motion control in the presence of various foot and ankle pathologies. AFOs may also provide some control of subtalar motion. Some AFOs and SMOs have trimlines that terminate immediately proximal to the ankle. The more common AFO design includes a proximal trimline that terminates 20 mm distal to the neck of fibula. The trimline provides the longest possible lever arm for ankle motion control, particularly with spasticity of the calf muscle. Depending on the lever arm, an AFO not only controls the ankle directly but also influences the knee (and perhaps the hip) indirectly by altering the moments acting about it.[4] AFOs are usually prescribed for clients who have muscle weakness controlling ankle-foot position, who have muscle hypertonicity or spasticity, or who have conditions resulting in pain or instability due to a loss of integrity of the structures of the lower leg, ankle, and foot.

AFOs may be made of metal, plastic, or a hybrid of metal and plastic. In most AFO designs, an anterior opening allows for donning and doffing. The anterior closure (calf strap) secures the orthosis to the limb. The closure mechanism varies depending on the manual dexterity of the client. Most AFO designs incorporate a foot plate to control the foot and ankle, an articulated or nonarticulated ankle (depending on the desired motion control), and a calf section to provide mechanical leverage for ankle and knee control. Metal AFO designs are attached externally to a shoe or incorporated into a foot plate that fits within the shoe. Thermoplastic material and thermoset AFO designs use a molded foot plate to improve midtarsal and subtalar joint control. This AFO improves aesthetics and allows different shoes to be worn. A common heel height when changing shoes is needed to maintain the desired anklefoot and tibia-to-vertical alignment. In a thermoplastic AFO the degree of ankle motion control is determined by material selection, trimline placement around the ankle, conformity, and articulation configuration. The function imparted by an AFO relies largely on the degree of resistance provided to rotation about the ankle.[42] One function common to many AFOs is the support of the foot at an appropriate angle for clearance of the ground during swing. Clearance is usually accomplished by limiting plantar flexion range.

AFOs are either articulated or nonarticulated. Nonarticulated AFOs are used to rigidly encase the ankle joint (usually leaving only an anterior opening for donning and doffing), limiting ankle motion in the coronal and sagittal planes. Nonarticulated AFOs are used when the ankle requires complete immobilization to reduce pain and/or ensure stability. However, a posterior leaf spring AFO is an example of a nonarticulated AFO that permits dorsiflexion motion but provides resistance to plantar flexion. By virtue of its trimlines around the ankle joint, the posterior leaf spring orthosis is more flexible in one direction than the other, permitting dorsiflexion through bending of the plastic. Articulated AFOs allow ankle motion in the desired plane and direction by incorporating orthotic ankle joints and motion control devices (mechanical stops). Orthotic ankle joint components are configured to provide motion within a specific range, limit motion in a particular direction (e.g., a plantar flexion stop), and/or assist motion in a particular direction (e.g., dorsiflexion assist joints) (see Table 18.2).

An AFO is designated as a floor-reaction AFO if it is designed specifically to act indirectly at the knee. Manipulating ankle-foot alignment alters moments at the knee. Any AFO that affects ankle-foot alignment has an indirect effect at the more proximal joints. Creating an external knee extension moment during stance provides knee stability when it is absent or compromised. This moment is achieved with or without articulation at the ankle joint. An external knee extension moment is created during the stance phase by either a rigid AFO set in slight plantar flexion or an articulated AFO with a dorsiflexion stop.

Clinical Considerations for the Occupational Therapist

Similar issues apply for AFOs as for FOs with people who have insensate feet. The need for education regarding visual skin

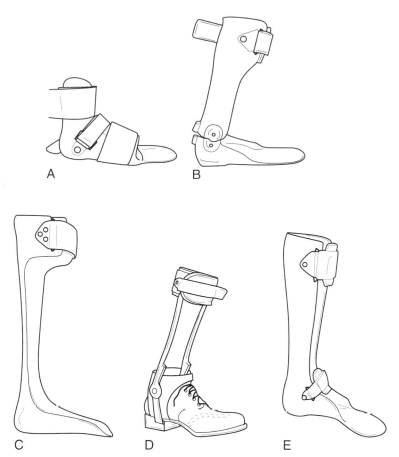

Fig. 18.6 Various ankle-foot orthosis (AFO) designs. A, Supramalleolar orthosis (SMO). B, Articulated AFO with posterior plantar flexion stop and full-length foot plate. C, Posterior leaf spring AFO. D, Double-upright design with medial T-strap and dorsiflexion-assist ankle joints. E, Solid ankle AFO with instep strap.

inspection exists. AFOs may be needed when the client is in a critical recovery or rehabilitation period, as in the case of cerebrovascular accident (CVA). OTs assist in making this process acceptable to the client by educating them on what to expect from the AFO. Educating clients on how the orthosis works, what muscles it may be assisting, and why it has to be constructed, is vital to acceptance of the orthosis, orthotic use, and recovery. Certain AFO design options positively or negatively influence occupational performance tasks. For example, a rigid ankle design provides appropriate biomechanical alignment and joint correction. The rigid design completely restricts ankle range of motion. The ankle movement restriction results in difficulty with activities, such as operating an automobile gas pedal, kneeling, bending at the waist, using stairs, or rising from a chair. Helping clients learn adaptive techniques to perform such activities while wearing the orthosis is important.

KNEE ORTHOSES

General Description

KOs are generally prefabricated or custom fit to encompass the knee, and they act in the coronal and sagittal planes (Fig. 18.7). As classified by the American Academy of Orthopaedic Surgeons (AAOS), the KO function falls into three categories: prophylactic, rehabilitative, and functional.[46] Prophylactic

KOs prevent or reduce the severity of injury for otherwise healthy able-bodied persons involved in high-impact or contact sports. In these circumstances, KOs act kinesthetically to remind the wearer of a recent injury. Rehabilitative KOs are prescribed after a surgical procedure to limit knee range of motion while soft-tissue structures (e.g., reconstructed ligaments) heal. Functional KOs provide ongoing mechanical stability to the chronically unstable or reconstructed knee joint or alter knee moments and unload knee joint compartments affected by osteoarthritis.

Fit, joint alignment, and suspension are critical factors in the effectiveness of KOs. Given the cylindrical shape of the limb, mitigating distal migration of the orthosis can be challenging. If the orthosis is not maintained in proper position, joint alignment is sacrificed. Often a discrepancy is created between the anatomical and mechanical joint axes. Single-axis and polycentric joint designs refer to the pivoting motion of mechanical knee joints. A single-axis joint functions as a single hinged action. Polycentric joints produce a shifting axis to mimic the functional motion of the anatomical knee. Size, weight, function, and durability are important factors in selection. Specially designed straps, supracondylar pads, or inner sleeves prevent distal slipping of the orthosis during ADLs. The client must properly don and do periodic checks of the alignment of the orthosis throughout the day.

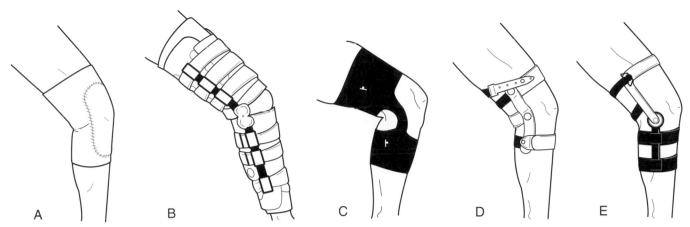

Fig. 18.7 Various knee orthosis (KO) designs. A, Soft Neoprene knee sleeve. B, Postoperative KO controls flexion and extension range of motion with adjustable joints. C, Prophylactic KO with lateral joint. D, Rehabilitative design to control knee hyperextension. E, Custom KO to stabilize injured knee.

Clinical Considerations for the Occupational Therapist

People receiving functional KOs to prevent further osteoarthritic knee deformity may also experience upper extremity degenerative changes that limit hand function. Although most KO designs use Velcro closure systems, deciding between medial and lateral placement of closures is critical to enhancing available functional dexterity. Closures that include a wider chafe opening allow the client with impaired hand function to feed Velcro straps through the opening with less difficulty.

Wherever possible, KOs are generally designed to provide total contact and are worn directly against the skin. Donning/doffing procedures are reviewed with the client to ensure that an effective dressing routine is established. For older adult clients the sequencing of how to cinch straps is important to prevent migration of the orthosis and skin breakdown.

KNEE-ANKLE-FOOT ORTHOSES

General Description

KAFOs encompass the knee, ankle, and whole or part of the foot.[4] KAFOs include an AFO component and therefore incorporate some of the same concepts described previously. Compared to AFOs, KAFOs extend proximally, bridging the knee and containing the thigh tissues. KAFOs allow for coronal and sagittal plane control of the knee. Transverse plane control is determined distally by the AFO foot plate design. Skeletal knee alignment is achieved by applying corrective forces through the soft-tissue structures of the thigh. Therefore a well-molded and fitted thigh shell is an important component of the orthotic design. Excessive gapping reduces the mechanical effect of the design and reduces potential stability and function. Most KAFOs are custom made from measurements or casts and are fabricated from metal and leather, thermoplastic, laminates, or combinations of these materials. Material selection is generally based on height, weight, activity level, and functional requirements (Fig. 18.8).

The most proximal component of the KAFO is the thigh section. Posterior shells with anterior straps, anterior shells with posterior straps, and full circumferential shells are common thigh designs. Thigh shells are fabricated of rigid or flexible material. The thigh shell may be designed to "unweight" or "unload" the lower limb by providing a shelf for the ischium to sit on in combination with soft-tissue containment of the thigh tissues (see Fig. 18.8B). The principal impairments addressed by KAFOs are weakness of the muscles controlling the knee (and perhaps the hip and ankle), upper motor neuron lesions resulting in LE hypertonicity (spasticity), or loss of structural integrity of the hip or knee. KAFOs improve stability and functional mobility for clients with significant genu valgum, genu varum, genu recurvatum, or knee flexion instability.[7]

Similar to KOs, orthotic knee joints may be single axis or polycentric. There are four basic knee control options available in KAFOs (Fig. 18.9):
1. Free motion joints
2. Posterior offset joints (see Fig. 18.9A)
3. Joints with a manual lock (see Fig. 18.9B–D)
4. Stance control joints

Free motion joints provide support in the coronal plane while allowing sagittal plane motion. A mechanical block limits movement of the knee into an abnormal extension range. A locked knee KAFO provides support in the sagittal and coronal planes. The lock may be manually disengaged for sitting. Common locking mechanisms include the drop lock and bail or lever lock designs.[5] Drop locks are designed to fall into place over the mechanical hinge when the client stands. These locks must be manually lifted before engaging in any activity that requires knee flexion (e.g., sitting). Bail or lever locks are designed to snap into place, locking the knee once it is extended. The joints must be unlocked before sitting and can sometimes be disengaged by bumping the posterior lever mechanism on the seat of a chair. Although a locked KAFO is able to reliably provide stability in stance, it does not allow for flexion of the knee in swing, resulting in a functionally longer

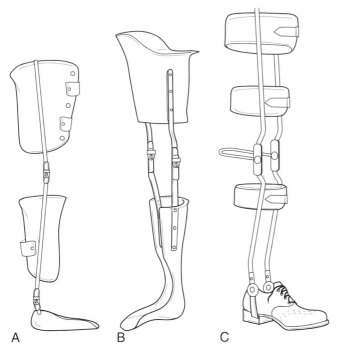

Fig. 18.8 Various knee-ankle-foot orthosis (KAFO) designs. A, Thermoplastic KAFO with molded foot plate, articulated ankle, long anterior tibial shell, drop locks, and circumferential thigh shell. B, Thermoplastic KAFO with molded foot plate, solid ankle, drop locks, and quadrilateral thigh shell for weight support. C, Double-upright KAFO attached to shoe with articulated ankle, posterior calf band, bail lock knee, and two posterior thigh bands.

limb. The longer limb leads to secondary gait maneuvers, such as vaulting, hip hiking, and circumduction, to ensure clearance of the ground by the foot during swing phase.[21,47] Walking with a locked knee results in a slower, more asymmetrical gait and increases the energy expenditure of walking.[16,18,25,39,44]

Posterior offset knee joints allow swing phase knee flexion and rely on geometric alignment to ensure stability of the knee in stance. The posterior offset knee joint assumes that in a normally aligned knee the vertical GRF vector is oriented through the knee joint during limb loading. The alignment ensures stability with little muscular effort. By positioning the mechanical knee joint axis posterior to the anatomical knee joint axis in the sagittal plane, the vertical GRF vector is positioned anterior to the mechanical joint during the first part of stance. This alignment creates an external extensor moment (torque) and ensures that the mechanical joint is stable during weight bearing. Consequently, stability of the anatomical knee joint is ensured. However, stability provided in this manner can be unreliable, especially over uneven terrain and slopes. Posterior offset knee joints should be used only when the client has:

- Adequate muscular control around the hip
- Proprioception at the knee
- Good balance

Such criteria ensure stumble recovery if geometric stability of the knee cannot be achieved.

Stance control knee joints employ various mechanisms to lock the knee in stance and automatically unlock in swing. Stance control knee joints include cable control, a position-dependent pendulum, and microprocessors.[7] Depending on the mechanism, these joints are used with KOs and KAFOs. Stance control joints allow for a more normal gait pattern because the knee is not required to be locked during stance and swing to prevent stance phase knee flexion. Some of these joints offer a triphasic mode of operation: automatic lock/unlock, always unlocked, and always locked. Different modes are selected for different activities (e.g., the automatic mode for walking, unlock for sitting, and lock for standing or added security when walking over uneven terrain). The ideal candidate for stance control knee joints presents with isolated unilateral quadriceps weakness, a relatively sound contralateral side, minimal contractures, minimal spasticity, and reasonable hip musculature.[36]

Genu recurvatum is a common condition for KAFO application. Specifically, knee joint laxity allows the anatomical knee center to move posteriorly during weight bearing. Genu recurvatum is usually an acquired deformity that develops secondary to weakness of the quadriceps or posterior calf muscles. The client compensates by maintaining the knee posteriorly and shifting the body weight anteriorly through hip flexion and anterior trunk lean. The compensations effectively place the body weight in front of the knee joint to prevent collapse and falling. Genu recurvatum may also develop secondary to a plantar flexion contracture at the ankle pulling the tibia backward, forcing the knee posteriorly during loading response and disrupting forward progression during stance. Load-bearing stresses cause permanent damage to the posterior capsule and soft-tissue structures. Such deformity continues to progress over time. The potential for the development of a severe deformity with permanent damage to the knee necessitates prompt attention.

The objective of a KAFO varies for clients with genu recurvatum (see Fig. 18.4). In some orthotic designs, complete sagittal plane correction is the goal as long as there is a mechanical means of providing stance stability to prevent collapse into knee flexion when weakness is noted. For other clients, partial correction reduces the deforming forces to the knee and limits progression of the deformity.

Clinical Considerations for the Occupational Therapist

Using a KAFO that locks the knee in extension is a significant issue with regard to occupational performance. Unfortunately, locking of the knee during walking was once unavoidable for clients who required knee stability and were at risk of falling because of quadriceps weakness. To some extent, locked knees are ameliorated with the availability of stance control orthotic knee joints. However, some clients still use locked knee KAFOs. Then the OT considers the manual dexterity required to engage and disengage the locking mechanism safely. Additionally, a locking knee interferes with activities, such as rising from a chair, toileting, getting in and out of a car or confined space, and so on. Helping clients learn

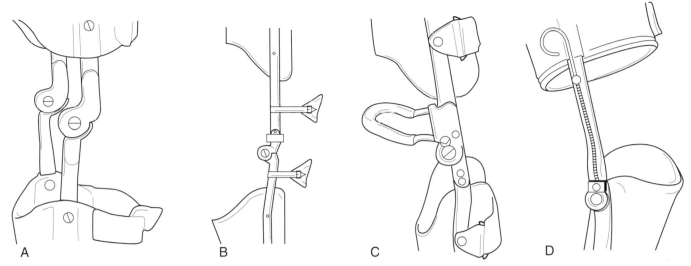

Fig. 18.9 Various knee joint locking mechanisms. A, Free posterior offset. B, Posterior offset with drop locks. C, Bail lock. D, Trigger lock.

adaptive techniques for how to perform these activities with an immobile knee plays a major role in the successful occupational performance while wearing the KAFO. KAFOs in general have a number of straps and can be awkward to don and doff. This likewise will deserve the attention of an OT.

HIP ORTHOSES
General Description

Hip orthoses (HOs) are devices that encompass either unilaterally or bilaterally the hip(s), consisting of a pelvic section, mechanical hip joint(s), and thigh cuff(s). Occasionally a shoulder strap is used to assist with suspension of the orthosis. HOs are primarily prescribed for problems associated with the femoral head or acetabulum where there is a need to control range of motion, alignment, and dislocation. However, the hip is a universal ball-and-socket joint with motion in all three planes. Although many orthoses control abduction/adduction and flexion/extension reasonably well, controlling internal/external rotation is difficult.

HOs are used to treat congenital, dysplastic, traumatic, or degenerative hip conditions (Fig. 18.10A–C) or after postoperative hip procedures (see Fig. 18.10D).[14] Pediatric and adult populations require different orthotic approaches. Pediatric HOs for congenital hip disorders are typically designed to maintain good joint alignment during bone growth. Dysplastic joints present with varying degrees of severity. In the beginning of the disease process, occlusion of blood supply to the head of the femur promotes necrosis. Although revascularization eventually occurs, the bony contouring of the femoral head does not develop normally. Continued weight-bearing stresses increase deformation of the hip joint and can result in permanent disability. Maintaining maximum joint congruency and controlling forces through the hip joints using a variety of HO designs (see Fig. 18.10) promotes normal development of the head of femur and acetabulum. As with most HOs, this type of orthotic treatment is temporary.

HOs for adults usually address the effects of joint deterioration. Clients with degenerative conditions are usually placed in HOs that limit range of motion to support and control compromised muscles, prevent dislocation following primary or revision surgery, and decrease pain. In adults who have had a hip replacement surgery, the HO is designed to provide different alignment options as the client progresses through the rehabilitation process. Usually the hip joint is aligned to maintain 10 to 20 degrees of abduction and allows 0 to 70 degrees of flexion when there is risk of posterior dislocation following surgery.[22] When there is risk of anterior dislocation postoperatively, hip motion is blocked at 40 degrees extension and 70 degrees flexion. Flexion and extension ranges are limited to prevent dislocation while allowing the client sufficient motion to sit and walk. Internal and external rotation control is limited to some degree by "grasping" the soft tissue of the thigh. Proper fitting, adjustment, and donning of the orthosis are critical to maximizing function and benefit. Postoperatively the HO is usually worn at all times for 3 to 6 months to allow the soft tissue to heal and to serve as a kinesthetic reminder to maintain proper positioning during ADLs. Although recurrent hip dislocation after surgical repair is rare, occasionally ongoing external support may be required for complicated procedures, revisions, or poor surgical outcomes.

Children with spasticity of the hip muscles may develop hip instability and pain, requiring surgical release of the hip adductors, flexors, and internal rotators or more complicated bony osteotomies of the pelvis or femur. HOs used postoperatively in these cases ensure that the hips are maintained in an appropriate position for healing while still allowing some small amount of motion to facilitate function. Additionally, HOs are usually equipped with two sets of liners that can be washed daily to eliminate odor and improve hygiene. When the HO is no longer used 24 hours a day to protect the surgical correction, it transitions to a functional orthosis during the day or a positioning orthosis at night.

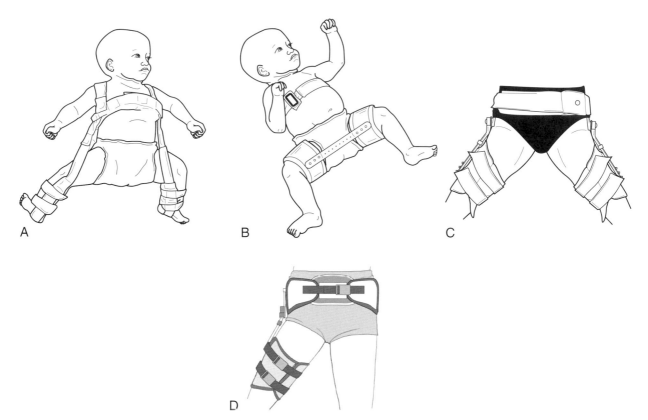

Fig. 18.10 Various hip orthosis (HO) designs. A, Pavlik harness used to manage congenital dysplasia of the hip. B, Ilfeld orthosis used to manage congenital dysplasia of the hip. C, Bilateral hip abduction orthoses with pelvic band. D, Postoperative hip abduction orthosis.

Clinical Considerations for the Occupational Therapist

After total hip surgery and while wearing an HO, both adult and pediatric clients require training in self-care activities, such as dressing, bathing, toileting, and hygiene. An OT is essential in assisting a client to maintain hip precautions while donning the orthosis. An OT educates the client in the use of adaptive equipment (e.g., a reacher, sock aid, long-handled bath sponge, long-handled shoe horn, and raised toilet seat) and may reduce excessive hip motion during hygiene and self-care.

HIP-KNEE-ANKLE-FOOT ORTHOSES

General Considerations

Hip-knee-ankle-foot orthoses (HKAFOs) encompass all three major lower limb joints and build upon the basic concepts already outlined for KAFOs. HKAFOs provide varying levels of mechanical control (Fig. 18.11). Most simply, a unilateral KAFO is attached to a pelvic band with a single-axis joint to control rotational alignment of the limb during swing (see Fig. 18.11B). This alignment allows proper positioning of the limb for stance. Bilateral mechanical hip joints and a pelvic/trunk section are used to provide additional control and stability for paraplegic standing and ambulation. HKAFOs may be used for neurological conditions resulting in severe muscle weakness (see Fig. 18.11A and C). The hip or pelvic section consists of a narrow band, or it may completely enclose the pelvis and trunk with a spinal orthosis attached to the LE orthoses. The amount of bracing of the trunk segment depends on the functional abilities, control, and upper body strength of the client. Hip and knee joints may be locked in extension during standing and walking, and the knees usually are locked.

Standing frames, such as the parapodium and swivel walker,[40] are bilateral HKAFOs mounted to a base plate. These devices are designed to provide support for hands-free standing or limited mobility by swiveling, wherein shifting weight laterally by rocking or rotating the trunk unweights one limb and causes the orthosis to swivel forward on the weight-bearing side. Swivel walkers are used effectively only on smooth, flat surfaces and provide extremely slow ambulation. Children are prescribed standing frames because standing is believed to provide a stimulus for normal development of bones and bowel and bladder function. In adults, standing is believed to reduce osteoporosis and improve peripheral circulation.

Ambulation with bilateral HKAFOs requires a "swing-through" gait pattern assisted by a walker or crutches. The HKAFO is used to lift the whole body from the ground and swing it forward. Variations in this pattern of ambulation are known as "swing-to" and "drag-to" gait. HKAFOs are used for daily activities and therapeutic intervention programs. High energy costs of these type of gaits may prohibit use of this orthosis for all ADLs, and wheelchair mobility may be a better option for some clients.[7,45]

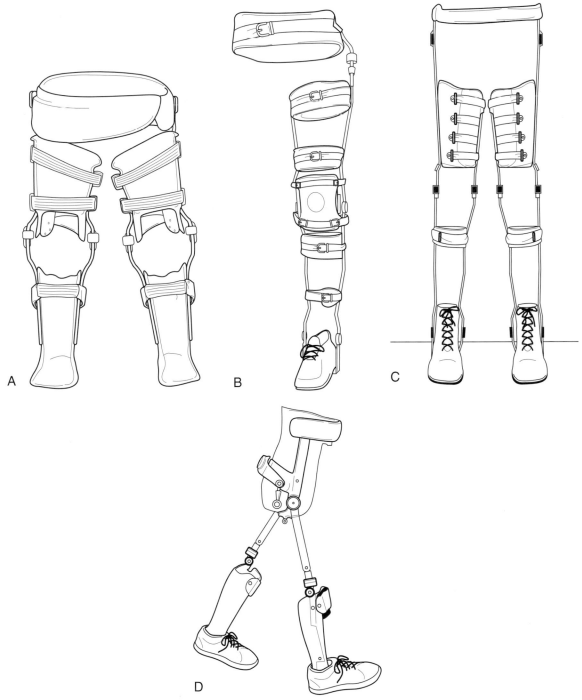

Fig. 18.11 Various hip-knee-ankle-foot orthosis (HKAFO) designs. A, Bilateral thermoplastic HKAFOs. B, Unilateral double-upright HKAFO. C, Bilateral double-upright HKAFOs. D, Reciprocating gait orthosis (RGO).

More complex HKAFO designs facilitate a reciprocal gait pattern so that extension of one limb promotes flexion of the contralateral limb and vice versa (see Fig. 18.11D). These reciprocating gait orthoses (RGOs) employ a linkage between the hip joints either by interlinked cables or a posterior, pivoting metal bar. RGOs are used in pediatric and adult populations, primarily for clients with flail bilateral lower limb involvement. Good upper extremity strength and adequate trunk control are prerequisites for RGOs because the main propulsive forces for this form of ambulation come from the arms via crutches or similar assistive devices. Reciprocal gait is more cosmetic and stable than swing-through gait. However, a greater level of training is required to ensure effective ambulation, and the complexity of orthotic design increases the need for maintenance. Although RGOs are used effectively by children with growth and body mass increases, it becomes more energy efficient to use a wheelchair than to ambulate with an RGO. Hence the use of RGOs is lower among adults.[7]

HKAFOs are commonly prescribed for clients with spina bifida or spinal cord injury or for any client presenting with a flail lower limb and limited hip control. Individual height, weight, strength, endurance, motivation, physical assistance requirements, donning abilities, and psychosocial situations are evaluated with regard to the potential success of the orthotic program. Upright weight bearing is believed to improve cardiopulmonary function, bowel and bladder function, circulation, and bone density.[19,28,33] Children benefit from the social interaction with their peers and can alternate with wheelchair mobility as needed. Almost all adult clients with traumatic spinal cord injury retain the desire to walk as a primary goal throughout their rehabilitation program.

Clinical Considerations for the Occupational Therapist

HKAFO systems require much higher levels of energy expenditure, upper extremity strength, and endurance than many clients are able to maintain on a regular basis. Although it may be apparent to members of the interdisciplinary rehabilitation team that the client achieves higher levels of functional independence when using a wheelchair for mobility, the client may prefer to focus on ambulation as a primary goal. Adding a pelvic component, hip joint, knee joint, or ankle control to an orthosis increases the difficulty of dressing and undressing. Difficulty with dressing tasks is magnified when the client is at work or school, and it will require loose-fitting clothing and adaptive strategies for donning and doffing clothing. In addition, the OT provides consultation for proper seating for toileting, desk work, and transportation.

SUMMARY

An interdisciplinary approach is important for all aspects of rehabilitation care, including LE orthotic management. The OT should confer with the CO in the development of the LE orthotic prescription to ensure that the orthosis addresses the client's occupational goals. Such goals include but are not limited to the ability to don/doff the orthosis successfully and integrate the LE orthosis into ADLs. LE orthoses address a large number of issues from pain management to mobility. Regardless of the goals it is important that the health care team have a working knowledge of the biomechanical principles necessary to achieve the intervention goals. LE orthotic management is unique when compared with the upper extremity in that it often requires more robust designs and materials due to the magnitude of the forces associated with weight-bearing activity and ambulation. Sound understanding of normal gait is important when assessing a client with mobility deficiencies. Knowing whether a gait deviation is primary or secondary (compensatory) is important to determine the ultimate design of the orthotic intervention. Once the specific biomechanical deficiencies are identified, the practitioner has a wide variety of orthotic designs available to address the client's specific needs from relatively simple FOs to the reciprocating gait orthosis, which spans all major joints associated with LE function.

REVIEW QUESTIONS

1. What health care professional provides custom orthotic services to persons with LE impairments?
2. What are four clinical objectives of a LE orthosis?
3. What are the major joints that contribute to lower limb function?
4. What are the three key biomechanical principles of LE orthotic management?
5. What are the basic differences between low-temperature and high-temperature thermoplastic materials?
6. What are the seven subphases of gait?
7. What is the main distinction between a primary and secondary gait deviation?
8. What is the role of the OT in the development of the orthotic intervention program?
9. What skin inspection techniques are taught to the person with insensate feet?
10. What are two control options for the ankle joint of an articulated AFO?
11. What are two design parameters that can be integrated into a KO to prevent migration and to ensure proper alignment of the anatomical and mechanical joint axes?
12. What are the four main types of knee joints used in KAFOs?
13. What type of training would a person wearing a postoperative HO require?
14. What clinical presentation would most benefit from a RGO?

REFERENCES

1. Bowker P: The biomechanics of orthoses. In Bowker P, Condie D, Bader D, et al.: *Biomechanical basis of orthotic management*, Oxford, 1993, Butterworth-Heinemann.
2. Bunch W, Keagy R: *Principles of orthotic treatment*, St. Louis, 1976, Mosby.
3. Condie D: International Organization for Standardization (ISO) terminology. In Hsu J, Michael J, Fisk J, editors: *AAOS Atlas of orthoses and assistive devices*, ed 4, Philadelphia, 2008, Mosby, pp 3–7.
4. Condie E, Campbell J, Martina J: *Report of a consensus conference on the orthotic management of stroke patients*, Copenhagen, Denmark, 2004, International Society for Prosthetics and Orthotics.

5. Dibello T, Kelley C, Vallbona C, et al.: Orthoses for persons with postpolio sequelae. In Hsu J, Michael J, Fisk J, editors: *AAOS Atlas of orthoses and assistive devices*, ed 4, Philadelphia, 2008, Mosby, pp 419–432.

6. Fatone S, Orthotics: In Akay M, editor: *Wiley encyclopedia of biomedical engineering*, Hoboken, NJ, 2006, John Wiley & Sons, Inc.

7. Fatone S: A review of the literature pertaining to KAFOs and HKAFOs for ambulation, *J Prosthet Orthot* 18(3):137–168, 2006.

8. Fatone S, Hansen AH: A model to predict the effect of ankle joint misalignment on calf band movement in ankle-foot orthoses, *Prosthet Orthot Int* 31(1):76–87, 2007.

9. Fish D, Kosta C: Walking impediments and gait inefficiencies in the CVA patient, *J Prosthet Orthot* 11(2):33–37, 1999.

10. Gard S, Childress D: The effect of pelvic list on the vertical displacement of the trunk during normal walking, *Gait Posture* 5(3):233–238, 1997.

11. Gard S, Childress D: What determines the vertical displacement of the body during normal walking? *J Prosthet Orthot* 13(3):64–67, 2001.

12. Gard S, Fatone S: Biomechanics of lower limb function and gait. In Condie E, Campbell J, Martina J, editors: *Report of a consensus conference on the orthotic management of stroke patients*, Copenhagen, Denmark, 2004, International Society for Prosthetics and Orthotics, pp 55–63.

13. Gard SA, Childress DS: The influence of stance-phase knee flexion on the vertical displacement of the trunk during normal walking, *Arch Phys Med Rehabil* 80(1):26–32, 1999.

14. Goldberg B, Hsu J: *Atlas of orthoses and assistive devices*, St. Louis, 1997, Mosby.

15. Greene P, McMahon T: Reflex stiffness of man's anti-gravity muscles during kneebends while carrying extra weights, *J Biomech* 12(12):881–891, 1979.

16. Hanada E, Kerrigan DC: Energy consumption during level walking with arm and knee immobilized, *Arch Phys Med Rehabil* 82(9):1251–1254, 2001.

17. Hsu J, Michael J, Fisk J: *AAOS Atlas of orthoses and assistive devices*, ed 4, Philadelphia, PA, 2008, Mosby Elsevier.

18. Kaufman KR, Irby SE, Mathewson B, et al.: Energy-efficient knee-ankle foot orthosis: a case study, *J Prosthet Orthot* 8(3):79, 1996.

19. Kraft G, Lehmann J: Orthotics, *Phys Med Rehabil Clin N Am* 3(1):1–241, 1992.

20. Lafortune M, Lake M: Human pendulum approach to simulate and quantify locomotor impact loading, *J Biomech* 28(9):1111–1114, 1995.

21. Lage KJ, White SC, Yack HJ: The effects of unilateral knee immobilization on lower extremity gait mechanics, *Med Sci Sports Exerc* 27(1):8–14, 1995.

22. Lima D: Orthoses in total hip replacement. In Hsu J, Michael J, Fisk J, editors: *AAOS Atlas of orthoses and assistive devices*, ed 4, Philadelphia, PA, 2008, Mosby Elsevier, pp 335–341.

23. Maillardet F: The swing phase of locomotion, *Imeche* 6(3):67–75, 1977.

24. Margaria R: Biomechanics of human locomotion. In Margaria R, editor: *Biomechanics and energetics of muscular exercise*, Oxford, 1976, Oxford University Press, pp 67–144.

25. Mattsson E, Brostrom LA: The increase in energy cost of walking with an immobilized knee or an unstable ankle, *Scand J Rehabil Med* 22(1):51–53, 1990.

26. McCollough NC 3rd, Fryer CM, Glancy J: A new approach to patient analysis for orthotic prescription—part I: the lower extremity, *Artif Limbs* 14(2):68–80, 1970.

27. McMahon TA, Valiant G, Frederick EC: Groucho running, *J Appl Physiol* 62(6):2326–2337, 1987.

28. Merritt JL, Yoshida MK: Knee-ankle-foot orthoses: indications and practical applications of long leg braces, *Phy Med Rehabil: Stat Art Rev* 14(3):239–422, 2000.

29. Michael J: Lower limb orthoses. In Goldberg B, Hsu J, editors: *AAOS Atlas of orthoses and assistive devices*, ed 4, St. Louis, 1997, Mosby.

30. Mojica M: Foot orthoses. In Hsu J, Michael J, Fisk J, editors: *AAOS Atlas of orthoses and assistive devices*, ed 4, Philadelphia, PA, 2008, Mosby Elsevier, pp 335–341.

31. Murray MP, Kory RC, Clarkson BH, et al.: Comparison of free and fast speed walking patterns of normal men, *Am J Phys Med* 45(1):8–24, 1966.

32. Nack J, Phillips R: Shock absorption, *Clin Podiatr Med Surg* 7(2):391–397, 1990.

33. Nene A, Hermens H, Zilvold G: Paraplegic locomotion: a review, *Spinal Cord* 34(9):507–524, 1996.

34. Nolan KJ, Yarossi M: Preservation of the first rocker is related to increases in gait speed in individuals with hemiplegia and AFO, *Clin Biomech (Bristol, Avon)* 26(6):655–660, 2011.

35. Wall J, Nottrodt J, Charteris J: The effects of speed on pelvic oscillations in the horizontal plane during level walking, *J Hum Mov Studies* 8(1):27–40, 1982.

36. Otto JP: The stance control orthosis: has its time finally come? The O&P Edge. http://www.oandp.com/articles/2008-03_02.asp.

37. Perry J: Kinesiology of lower extremity bracing, *Clin Orthop* 102:18–31, 1974.

38. Perry J, Burnfield J: *Gait analysis: normal and pathological function*, Thorofare, NJ, 2010, Slack Inc.

39. Ralston H: Effects of immobilization of various body segments on the energy cost of human locomotion, *Ergonomics* 8(Suppl):53–60, 1965.

40. Rose GK, Henshaw JT: A swivel walker for paraplegics: medical and technical considerations, *Biomed Eng* 7(9–2):420–425, 1972.

41. Snyder RD, Powers CM, Fontaine C, et al.: The effect of five prosthetic feet on the gait and loading of the sound limb in dysvascular below-knee amputees, *J Rehabil Res Devel* 32(4):309–315, 1995.

42. Stills ML: Thermoformed ankle-foot orthoses, *Orthot Prosthet* 29(4):41–51, 1975.

43. Sutherland D, Kaufman K, et al.: Kinematics of normal human walking. In Rose J, Gamble J, editors: *Human walking*, Baltimore, MD, 1994, Williams & Wilkins, pp 23–44.

44. Waters RL, Campbell J, Thomas L, et al.: Energy costs of walking in lower-extremity plaster casts, *J Bone Joint Surg Am* 64(6):896–899, 1982.

45. Waters RL, Mulroy S: The energy expenditure of normal and pathologic gait, *Gait Posture* 9(3):207–231, 1999.

46. Wolters B: Knee orthoses for sports-related disorders. In Hsu J, Michael J, Fisk J, editors: *AAOS Atlas of orthoses and assistive devices*, ed 4, Philadelphia, PA, 2008, Mosby Elsevier, pp 335–341.

47. Zissimopoulos A, Fatone S, Gard SA: Biomechanical and energetic effects of a stance-control orthotic knee joint, *J Rehabil Res Dev* 44(4):503–514, 2007.

APPENDIX 18.1 CASE STUDIES

Case Study 18.1[a]

Read the following scenario, and answer the questions based on information in this chapter.

A 67-year-old man sustained an acute cerebrovascular accident (CVA) to the right hemisphere of his brain and now presents with left-sided hemiparesis. The client complains of difficulty ambulating, standing for long periods of time, and performing his activities of daily living (ADLs). During ambulation the client's left lower extremity (LE) presents with paralytic equinus during swing phase, lateral forefoot initial contact, and asymmetrical step lengths.

1. What are some of the potential roles an occupational therapist (OT) may play in the intervention of this client?
2. What intervention goals can be addressed for this client using a LE orthosis?
3. What biomechanical principles might be implemented in the design of this client's LE orthosis?
4. What type of LE orthosis might this client benefit from?

Case Study 18.2[a]

A 62-year-old male client has a diagnosis of type 2 diabetes mellitus and associated peripheral neuropathy. The client complains of callousing on the plantar aspect of metatarsophalangeal (MTP) joints and tightness wearing the Oxford style shoes he typically wears. On clinical examination the client presents with clawed toes, atrophy of the intrinsic muscles of the foot, and depressed medial longitudinal arches during weight bearing. Results from a monofilament assessment of the plantar aspect of the foot confirmed peripheral neuropathy. LE strength and active range of motion are within normal limits at all major joints. The client receives bilateral, custom-fabricated, full-length accommodative foot orthoses (FOs) manufactured from multidurometer foams and extra-depth footwear to accommodate the claw toe deformity. The multidurometer foam construction allows for distribution of forces throughout the plantar aspect of the foot, which reduces peak plantar pressures and minimizes the risk of plantar ulceration. The extra-depth footwear allows for needed adjustments of volumetric changes of the foot and accommodates the thickness of multidurometer FOs.

1. How might neuropathy negatively impact this client?
2. What benefits do extra-depth footwear have?
3. Why was the client provided accommodative instead of corrective foot orthoses?

Case Study 18.3[a]

A 62-year-old male client is 2 weeks post right total knee arthroplasty. During the surgery he sustained an iatrogenic peroneal nerve lesion at the level of the fibular head. He complains of difficulty walking and is dragging his toe. The client is otherwise healthy and has no edema. On clinical examination the client presents within functional limits for bilateral passive range of motion at the midfoot, ankle, subtalar, hip,

and knee joints. A manual muscle test reveals he has 0/5 dorsiflexion and eversion. He has sensory loss over the dorsal aspect of the foot and lateral compartment of the leg. While ambulating the client exhibits secondary compensations with hip hiking during the swing phase on the affected limb and initial contact with the lateral forefoot. The client receives a custom thermoplastic ankle-foot orthosis (AFO) with a flexible ankle trimline fabricated from $\frac{5}{32}$-inch (4 mm) copolymer (similar to Fig. 18.5C). Resistance to plantar flexion from the AFO coupled with the full-length foot plate provides the client with improved swing phase clearance. The foot plate eliminates the need for compensatory hip hiking and encourages a normal heel strike at initial contact. A flexible ankle trimline allows the tibia to progress forward during stance, and the thermoplastic design allows for a lightweight orthosis that can be readily changed from shoe to shoe with equal heel heights.

1. Why does the client present with both dorsiflexion and eversion weakness?
2. How would the client's gait be affected if he were provided a solid ankle AFO instead of the orthosis described above?

Case Study 18.4[a]

A 54-year-old female client has right lateral compartment osteoarthritis with associated genu valgum. The client complains of knee pain during weight-bearing activity that increases proportionally with activity level. Clinical evaluation reveals bilateral genu valgum and palpable swelling over the lateral joint line of the right knee. The client receives a functional knee orthosis (KO) to unload the lateral joint compartment of the right knee. The KO's three-point force system (acting through straps in the coronal plane) applies medially directed forces at the proximal and distal aspects. The KO's laterally directed force at the medial femoral condyle results in unloading of the lateral compartment of the knee joint. Polycentric knee joints are used to match the natural movements of the knee. Composite construction of the articulating and structural components ensures that the orthosis is structurally sound yet lightweight.

1. Why are polycentric articulations most appropriate when providing a knee orthosis?
2. What is the primary biomechanical objective for the provided orthosis?

Case Study 18.5[a]

A 47-year-old client has paralytic postpolio syndrome. The client complains of severe left knee pain while walking. The client was diagnosed with acute polio at 3 years of age and has noted increased symptoms of weakness with age. Clinical examination reveals that the client has a 15-degree plantar flexion contracture and 30 degrees of knee hyperextension during loading response. There is laxity of the right knee in the sagittal plane and palpable swelling throughout the popliteal fossa. Sensation, vascular function, and proprioception are within normal limits. With ambulation the client exhibits secondary hip hiking during swing, initial contact with the forefoot, and severe hyperextension during stance. The client receives a thermoplastic knee-ankle-foot orthosis (KAFO) with posterior offset knee joints, solid ankle, and metatarsal-length foot plate. The thermoplastic KAFO design accommodates the client's plantar flexion and knee hyperextension. The design allows the weight line to pass anterior to the anatomical knee and posterior offset knee joints. The posterior offset knee joints create a knee extension moment at both joints throughout stance phase. The KAFO serves to limit additional knee hyperextension and increases stability. The three-quarter–length foot plate facilitates heel off in pre-swing, allowing the transition to swing phase.

1. How is the sensation and proprioception affected in a client with paralytic postpolio syndrome?
2. How would your recommendation change if the client presented with a 10-degree knee flexion contracture instead of knee hyperextension?

Case Study 18.6[a]

A 62-year-old client is seen in the postanesthesia recovery unit after a total hip arthroplasty revision. The client has a history of hip joint subluxation. The physician would like the hip to be maintained in a flexed and abducted position. The client has normal anatomy and a thin dressing placed at the incision anterior to the greater trochanter. The client receives a prefabricated hip orthosis (HO) with an adjustable range-of-motion joint. This articulation enables the orthotist to set the hip joint to a fixed abduction angle while allowing some flexion for ADLs. The orthotic alignment is intended to encourage proper healing of the soft tissues surrounding the hip prosthesis. Although the HO provides mechanical control of the hip joint, it is imperative that the OT reinforce hip joint precautions and facilitate the integration of the orthosis into ADLs.

1. Why would the physician request a flexed and abducted alignment?
2. What activities might the patient have difficulty achieving given the motion limitations the hip abduction orthosis is set to?

Case Study 18.7[a]

A 6-year-old child diagnosed with a low thoracic myelomeningocele lesion presents with absent sensation and motor function of bilateral LEs. The intervention goal is an orthosis that facilitates static standing and the ability to ambulate in as normal a manner as possible. The child has access to both pediatric physical therapists and OTs at school and has excellent upper limb strength and dexterity. The child is provided a custom reciprocating gait orthosis (RGO) because it facilitates static standing and step-over-step ambulation. To take advantage of this orthosis, it is imperative that the child have access to therapists to develop the skills needed to successfully integrate the orthosis into ADLs and have the requisite training to use crutches or other assistive devices necessary to successfully ambulate with the orthosis.

1. Why couldn't this client be provided ankle-foot orthoses instead of the relatively cumbersome RGO?
2. What advantage does the RGO have over a hip-knee-ankle-foot orthosis (HKAFO) with locked hips and knees and fixed ankles?

---

[a]See Appendix A for the answer key.

[a]See Appendix A for the answer key.

Casting

Audrey Yasukawa

CHAPTER OBJECTIVES

1. Identify the types of upper extremity casts and the criteria for use.
2. Describe casting interventions for common upper extremity range-of-motion limitations and alignment issues that affect function.
3. Describe the rationale for upper extremity casting.
4. Describe therapeutic methods to use in conjunction with and after implementation of a casting program.
5. List three criteria for a successful upper extremity casting program.

KEY TERMS

antagonist
contracture

myostatic
submaximal range

Troy is a 16-year-old varsity football player who sustained a Bennett fracture (an intra-articular fracture-dislocation of the thumb metacarpal at the carpometacarpal joint). Troy sustained the fracture during a football game, and he received a Neoprene thumb spica sleeve for stabilization for the remainder of the game. Once confirmed by computed tomography (CT) scan, Troy's fracture was reduced in a long thumb spica cast that extended beyond his wrist but allowed motion at the metacarpophalangeal (MCP) joints of the fingers. Troy was concerned about the limitations of motion and asked the physician if he could get a "game day" cast that allowed more motion. The physician referred him to occupational therapy.

Julie is a 5-year-old who experienced brachial plexus palsy at birth. Subsequently, she presents with an elbow flexion contracture associated with the palsy. Her elbow is contracted more than 30 degrees in a flexed position. The occupational therapist now seeing Julie is considering a serial casting intervention to increase Julie's elbow extension, which will benefit her performance in tasks such as putting on shirts and coats.

DIAGNOSTIC INDICATIONS FOR CASTING

Casting intervention may be considered for a variety of conditions (Box 19.1), including orthopedic and neurological conditions.

Orthopedic Conditions

As exemplified by the story of Troy, a fracture is an orthopedic condition requiring immobilization, which is often accomplished with casting. The traditional intervention for an upper extremity fracture is to apply an elbow cast, long arm cast, wrist cast, or hand cast. The physician and cast technician generally apply the cast to stabilize the fracture site. The physician continues to reevaluate the bone healing and assess the injury site and stability of the area during healing. Depending on the injury, the cast may be left in place from 3 to 8 weeks.[7]

Burns are another diagnostic group that may benefit from casting. With burns, contractures result from the damage to the soft tissue and muscles and scar formation.[3,11,47]

Neurological and Neuromuscular Conditions

Casting can also be appropriate for neurological conditions such as the case with Julie. Such clients clinically present with abnormal tone, muscle imbalance, and muscle weakness that may limit passive and active range of motion (ROM) of the upper extremity. Therefore casting is used as an adjunct to therapy for an individual with motor disorders, in which contracture or spasticity are often present.[46] Clients with abnormal tone often have stiffness, muscle imbalances, spasticity, or abnormal response to stretch. Muscles, soft tissue, or joints that remain in a shortened position for extended periods of time often present with decreased extensibility.[19,41,54] Once a contracture occurs, slow gradual stretch of the connective tissue and muscles can gradually improve ROM.[20,32,33,44]

BOX 19.1 Casting Indications and Contraindications

Indications to Cast	Contraindications to Cast
• Soft tissue contracture • Increased spasticity limiting function • Improve AROM or PROM (e.g., for hygiene) • Inability to tolerate an orthosis • Poor biomechanical alignment of the arm/hand inhibiting active motion • Improve motor training • Stabilize a joint • For CIMT	• Severe rigidity • Severe athetosis • Fluctuating tone • Unstable medical conditions • Long-standing contractures • Bilateral casts to patients with hypertension • Skin surface that is not intact • Joints with heterotopic ossification • For CP: Over time increased activity with the arm positioned in pronation and elbow flexion may cause posterior dislocation of the radial head • For CP: Torsion of the bone warrants consultation before casting

AROM, Active range of motion; *CIMT,* constraint-induced movement therapy; *CP,* cerebral palsy; *PROM,* passive range of motion.

Common neurological diagnoses that may require casting intervention include spinal cord injury, traumatic brain injury, stroke, and cerebral palsy.[5,15,18,29,39,49]

Brachial plexus birth palsy refers to the paralysis of the upper extremity due to a traction or compression injury sustained to the brachial plexus during birth. In children with brachial plexus injury, muscle imbalance, weakness in the antagonist muscle group, and habitual compensatory movement patterns often lead to the development of contractures, which may require casting.[12,21]

Traditional intervention techniques to address contractures include passive stretching to restore the normal ROM when the range is limited by muscle tightness and loss of soft tissue elasticity. However, muscle/soft tissue tightness is likely to recur with the client who is dependent on a caregiver for movement. For example, casting may be used to improve ROM for care and hygiene and to prevent skin breakdown in a tightly fisted hand or flexed elbow. Increasing joint ROM may be accomplished by providing the client with an orthosis. An increase in range may be difficult to maintain unless the extremity can be positioned using an orthotic device.[35,56–58]

Thus primary indications for casting are soft tissue contracture and increased spasticity that limits function. Further considerations for casting are decreased active and passive ROM, inability to tolerate an orthosis, and poor biomechanical alignment of the arm/hand inhibiting active movement. Casts can be used to improve motor training to stabilize a joint, (e.g., wrist stabilization to allow the client to learn finger extension). Further assessment helps determine if casting is an appropriate option.

Although casting is often provided for orthopedic and neurological/neuromuscular conditions, this chapter focuses on casting for clients with neurological and neuromuscular conditions. However, some of the discussed concepts can be applied with either type of condition.

CONTRAINDICATIONS TO CASTING

Casting is not always appropriate for all clients (see Box 19.1). In cases of severe skin redness, open wounds, shoulder subluxation, edema, heterotopic ossification, or rigidity, the application of a cast may be contraindicated. Other contraindications to casting include clients with severe rigidity, athetosis, fluctuating tone, unstable medical conditions, or long-standing contractures. For example, a teenager with cerebral palsy who has a long-standing contracture of the elbow may not benefit from a casting program if the goal is to gain full ROM. Increased activity with the arm postured in pronation and elbow flexion over long periods of time might cause posterior dislocation of the radial head.[43] This dislocation impairs achievement of elbow extension actively and passively.

For a developing child with cerebral palsy, as the bones grow, the muscles may maintain a shortened position. The bony modeling of the radius and ulna with a forearm in constant forearm pronation and elbow flexion suggests that bony deformities may result from the lack of full rotation into supination.[10] In a developing child presenting with movement restriction due to the long-standing contracture into elbow flexion and forearm pronation, torsion of the bone may occur. In this case a consultation with an orthopedic specialist is helpful before the casting procedure.

EVIDENCE FOR CASTING

Cast provision to address contractures and motor disorders associated with muscle imbalance and spasticity is well established in rehabilitation practice. Therapists have identified those patients who are most likely to benefit from cast intervention.[20,21,32,44,46] A lack of evidence to support the use of upper extremity casting with stroke exists.[14,40,48] Upper extremity casting is more successful for clients with traumatic brain injuries or cerebral palsy.[5,20,44,45] Regardless, the use of casting and the outcome for each individual varies due to the severity, tone, and functional status.

The influence of upper extremity casting continues to be speculative, with a low level of evidence to assist with the clinical decision making for developing protocols (Table 19.1). Randomized controlled trials are scarce, with little consistency in outcome measure, except for the measure of ROM.[27,28,38,50] The evidence base for lower extremity casts exists; however, it is limited.[4] It is difficult to conduct a randomized controlled group of human subjects with adequate sample size to detect the treatment effects for upper and lower extremity casting. Many subjects in rehabilitation settings receive medical and pharmaceutical

TABLE 19.1   Evidence-Based Practice for Casting

Author Citation	Design	Number of Participants	Description	Results	Limitations
Lannin, N. A., & Cusick, A. (2007). A systematic review of upper extremity casting for children and adults with central nervous system motor disorders. *Clinical Rehabilitation, 21,* 963–976.	Systematic review	23 studies were included within the review (including 3 RCTs and 4 systematic reviews) *Inclusion criteria:* human subjects; >50% of participants described as having BI, CP, or CVA.	Authors searched the Cochrane Database of Systematic Reviews, MEDLINE, Embase, CINAHL, PEDro, OTSeeker, Google Scholar, and reference lists of retrieved articles to gather studies that provided evidence on UE casting in adults and children with neurological conditions and met inclusion criteria. The PEDro scale was used to determine quality of RCTs.	Authors found mixed results. Two RCTs noted positive effects of casting on ROM or quality of motion; however, these improvements were of small magnitude or short-term duration. Only one study noted adverse events or safety issues caused by casting. Indications for casting were reported to be (1) presence of soft-tissue contracture; (2) presence of spasticity; (3) limitations in joint AROM; (4) pathological reflexes; (5) inability to fabricate a splint/orthosis; (6) prevention of contracture; (7) clinical decision to use casting to stabilize the wrist to promote motor learning of active finger extension. Contraindications for casting were listed as (1) rigid tone in the upper limb; (2) athetoid or fluctuating tone; (3) unstable medical condition; (4) absent sensation; (5) joint calcification; (6) open wounds/poor skin condition; (7) <5 years of age; (8) intellectual impairment; (9) hypertension and/or raised intracranial pressure; (10) long-standing contracture (>6 months). There was great variability among studies in terms of degrees of stretch (ranging from 5 to 10 degrees less than full ROM to neutral to end of available ROM), duration of stretch, cast change frequency, and presence of concurrent therapies. The following concurrent therapies were listed within some articles: (1) weight-bearing activities; (2) functional BUE tasks; (3) OT based on NDT approach; (4) PROM. Postcasting therapy regimens also varied greatly. Reported options included stretching through long-duration positioning or splinting, which varied in intensity, movement training, CIMT using a cast on the unaffected hand, weight-bearing activities, and PROM.	The review was inclusive of published studies in the English language. Studies could have been missed due to the search terms used. Additionally, with only 3 RCTs and high variability in study designs, methods, casting protocols, and outcomes, causation cannot be made. *Overall, there is insufficient high-level evidence to support or negate upper limb casting in individuals with CNS motor disorders. Evidence speaking to long-term benefits or adverse effects is nonexistent. There is a definitive need for additional sufficiently powered RCTs to make stronger conclusions.*

Author Citation	Design	Number of Participants	Description	Results	Limitations
Kuipers, K., Burger, L., & Copley, J. (2012). Casting for upper limb hypertonia: A retrospective study to determine the factors associated with intervention decisions. *NeuroRehabilitation, 31*, 409–420. https://doi.org/10.3233/NRE-2012-00811	Retrospective design that involved auditing records of children and adults with UE hypertonicity due to BI.	64 "primary intervention decisions" were gathered retrospectively from initial evaluation reports. *Inclusion criteria for records:* (1) involved children or adults with UE performance difficulties secondary to BI; (2) contained an initial assessment that was completed between 1999 and 2010; (3) recorded a primary intervention decision.	Before this study, Copley and Kuipers developed "the Protocol," which meant to structure therapists' clinical reasoning and decision making related to management of UE hypertonicity. Researchers explored whether OTs consistently used the UE characteristics described in the Protocol as being commonly associated with "moderate disability" to inform casting decisions to reduce contracture, which UE characteristics were the most powerful predictors for choosing casting, and the proportion of clinical decisions that resulted in casting (p. 411).	Of the records reviewed: • UE hypertonicity was present in 84.4% of the participants in the sample. • Of 5 possible clinical aims, *reduction of hypertonicity* (54.7%) and *enhancement of function* (46.9%) were the most commonly recorded aims. • Casting was listed as the most common primary intervention choice (n = 30, 47%), followed by resting splints (19%), and functional splints (17.5%). • Clinicians were less likely to use casting in individuals with mild or mild/moderate UE hypertonicity or rigidity. Individuals with moderate or severe hypertonicity were highly correlated with casting. • Adult clients were deemed more likely to receive casting than children. • Reasons as to why casting was indicated, yet not implemented, included older age (75–95 years), limited caregiver support, and a clinical aim of hygiene/comfort maintenance and/or pain reduction. • The decision to cast was highly associated with cases for which the clinical aims were to reduce hypertonicity, reduce contracture, or both.	This retrospective study contained a small sample size, which reduces the power of overall results and restricts the extent of statistical analysis that could be performed. Larger, prospective studies on this topic are warranted.

AROM, Active range of motion; *BI,* brain injury; *BUE,* bilateral upper extremities; *CIMT,* constraint-induced movement therapy; *CINAHL,* Cumulative Index to Nursing and Allied Health Literature; *CNS,* central nervous system; *CP,* cerebral palsy; *CVA,* cerebrovascular accident; *NDT,* neurodevelopmental therapy; *OT,* occupational therapy; *PROM,* passive range of motion; *ROM,* range of motion; *RCT,* randomized controlled trial; *ROM,* range of motion; *UE,* upper extremity.
Contributed by Andrea Coppola.

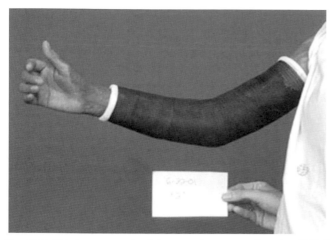

Fig. 19.1 This is an example of documenting range-of-motion (ROM) status during serial casting process. (Photo courtesy Serghiou, M., Cowan, A., & Whitehead, C. [2009]. Rehabilitation after a burn injury. *Clinics in Plastic Surgery, 36*[4], 675–686.)

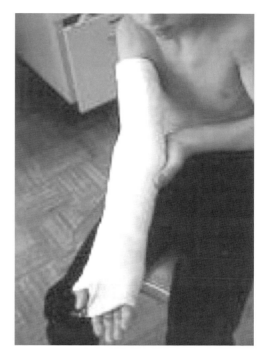

Fig. 19.2 Inhibitory cast—forearm supination cast.

treatment. Most studies are of single case reports, which describe the use of casting, case series, or chart review. Therefore therapists must rely on their clinical judgment to determine if casting is an appropriate intervention. Despite the inherent limitations associated with single case reports or case series, they do provide some guidance for treatment interventions. Moreover, they are an impetus for future research.

Casting Options

Three general casting options are available: serial casts, inhibitory casts, and drop-out casts.[15] A serial cast is applied and removed progressively as ROM increases (Fig. 19.1). Cast changes of 1 to 4 days are common.[15] Often with increased muscle tone, casting is most effective 2 to 3 weeks post botulinum toxins.[15]

An inhibitory cast places a joint in a position that reduces spasticity in a reflex-inhibiting position (Fig. 19.2). The reflex-inhibiting postures for the upper extremity include shoulder abduction, elbow extension, forearm supination, wrist extension, and finger and thumb extension and abduction.[15]

Drop-out casts for a spastic joint allow movement in a desired position while concurrently preventing the joint from returning to a contracted position (Fig. 19.3).[15] For example, an elbow with a flexion hypertonicity may be casted with the posterior portion of the upper cast cut away to allow the person to extend the elbow, while preventing the elbow from moving to a flexed position.[15]

UPPER EXTREMITY ASSESSMENT FOR CASTING

Selection of a casting program requires a comprehensive analysis of the involved upper extremity, including a baseline assessment before casting. Ongoing assessments are essential to determining the effectiveness of the casting program. Assessment is conducted between consecutive cast application(s) and upon completion of the casting program.

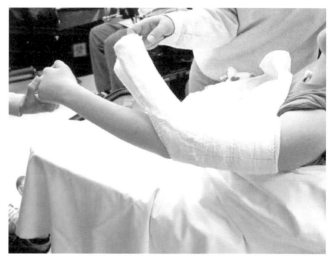

Fig. 19.3 Drop-out cast.

Assessment tools used for the casting program must be objective and reliable, and have valid outcome measures to determine the efficacy of the casting intervention. The following discussion includes considerations for assessment of neurological conditions for possible casting. Although casting for an orthopedic issue may require some of the same assessments, not all the following apply. For example, casting a fracture has no relationship to assessment of spasticity.

Range of Motion

ROM assessment is an essential component throughout the casting program, before and after casting, as well as between each cast application in the series. Goniometric assessment improves reliability of measurements when taken by the same examiner.[52] The therapist measures the specific joint being casted, and the joints proximal and distal. ROM improvements may be noted in the casted joint, but they may also occur in other joints. Both active and passive ROM are measured.

Manual Muscle Test

Motor function assessment of the involved arm or hand is important, especially in evaluating a short, tight muscle or weakness in an overlengthened muscle. It is important to examine the specific muscle or muscle group as compensatory movement patterns can compromise the function of the muscle. The therapist may need to use clinical observation of active muscle control if it is difficult to isolate specific muscles and assess selective motor control (e.g., ability to isolate wrist extension). Test the performance and strength of the muscle according to the guidelines of manual muscle testing.[26]

Grip Strength

To take the measurements of grip strength, the therapist uses a dynamometer for adult clients or a rubber bulb dynamometer for children. A change in wrist ROM into extension and the forearm into supination may assist with increased strength and dexterity.[13] To maintain consistency in measurements, document the position of forearm and wrist and any support given.

Modified Ashworth Scale

The Modified Ashworth Scale (MAS) is a numerical scale that grades the resistance felt by the therapist during a quick-stretch maneuver opposite to the pull of the muscle group being tested. The MAS measures the level of resistance to passive movement but does not evaluate the velocity of passive joint movement. The MAS is effective in clinical practice because of its ease of use, but it shows only moderate to good intrarater reliability and poor to moderate interrater reliability.[6,17,31] However, if it is consistently used by the same evaluator, the MAS assists with assessment of tone in the upper extremity and the joint to be casted. Table 19.2 describes scale of resistance to passive movement of the MAS.

Severity of hypertonicity (spasticity and muscle stiffness) is characterized as mild, moderate, or severe. The therapist documents the availability of active movement and the presence of soft tissue contracture. A client with mild hypertonicity may display a stretch reflex only at the end range of movement, or no hypertonicity at rest. A client with moderate hypertonicity may display a stretch reflex at midrange, and a client with severe hypertonicity may display a stretch reflex at the beginning of range.[51]

Sensibility

The identification of sensory deficits is an important consideration when establishing functional goals and predicting success of a casting program. Evaluation of sensory function requires the client to interact with the examiner to answer questions. If the client is unable to respond, the examiner uses clinical observation to note sensory neglect of the arm or hand during functional tasks. There are many possible ways of testing hand sensation, as described in previous chapters. These include touch, pain, two-point discrimination, stereognosis,

TABLE 19.2	Modified Ashworth Scale
0 =	No increase in muscle tone
1 =	Slightly increased muscle tone, manifested by a catch and release or minimal resistance at end ROM
1+ =	Slightly increased muscle tone, manifested by a catch and release or minimal resistance through remainder (less than half) of the ROM
2 =	More marked increase in muscle tone through most of range, but affected parts are easily moved
3 =	Considerable increase in muscle tone; passive movement difficult
4 =	Affected part(s) rigid in flexion or extension

ROM; Range of motion.

and position sense. Sensory impairment may be an important factor that limits functional outcome. Evaluation of deficient sensation of the hand or arm may have implications for training in activities of daily living and use of appliances in aspects of the client's management after the casting program.[9,36,58]

Skin Condition

The condition of the skin is important to consider before casting. Assessment of circulation and temperature of the hand to be casted is compared with the other hand. At times there may be a temperature difference in the more involved upper extremity when comparing it with the less involved arm. This temperature difference should be noted before placing the cast. After cast application the therapist always rechecks the extremity temperature, the pulse at the wrist (as able), fingers and thumb tips for blanching, and any tendency for edema.

Postural Control

Children and adults with neuromotor impairments may have poor postural control and demonstrate instability or insecurity when sitting or standing up against gravity. Casting may assist with reduction in spasticity, but as the client becomes upright in standing, it may also place more demands and stress on the arm. The therapist evaluates and documents the posture of the client's arm during ambulation, going up and down stairs, and when performing functional tasks. The client who has difficulty weight shifting onto the more involved leg/foot may demonstrate posturing of the arm due to a poor base of support. The client may use the arm for postural control when upright, limiting freedom of control during challenging motor tasks. An example of this is decreased reciprocal arm swing during ambulation. The therapist assesses postural alignment and the position of the arm at rest, in standing, and during movement.

Functional Use

Functional assessment is important and needs to include active placing and holding of the arm and active flexion and extension of the elbow during functional tasks. Functional assessment considers the ability to rotate the forearm to orient the hand for grasp and release of objects to use for activities of daily living.

TABLE 19.3   Functional Classification System

Class	Description	Activity Level
0	Does not use	Does not use
1	Poor active assist	Uses as stabilizing weight only
2	Fair passive assist	Can hold onto object placed in hand
3	Good passive assist	Can hold onto object and stabilize it for use by other hand
4	Poor active assist	Can actively grasp object and hold it weakly
5	Fair active assist	Can actively grasp object and stabilize it well
6	Good active assist	Can actively grasp object and then manipulate it against other hand
7	Spontaneous use, partial	Can perform bimanual activities easily and occasionally uses the hand spontaneously
8	Spontaneous use, complete	Uses hand completely independently without reference to the other hand

Data from House, J. H., Gwathmey, F. W., & Fidler, M. O. (1981). A dynamic approach to the thumb-in-palm deformity in cerebral palsy. *Journal of Bone and Joint Surgery, American Volume, 63*, 216–225.

House et al.[23] devised a nine-level functional classification system (House Classification [HC]) to describe the characteristics of hand function in children with cerebral palsy (Table 19.3). The scale was further modified. The Modified House Classification (MHC) can be used objectively in children with unilateral cerebral palsy and may be useful in measuring the functional capability of the affected hand.[16] A standard group of tasks that require a variety of upper extremity motions can be used, as well as tasks devised for a particular client.

ASSESSMENT BETWEEN CASTS

During application of a series of casts, ROM of the joint casted, spasticity, and active motor control are reassessed before each new cast is fabricated. The skin is checked to ensure there are no reddened or open areas resulting from the cast. If there is skin breakdown, the cast program may need to be placed on hold until the skin area heals. If edema and swelling are noted, a delay in the application of another cast is likely. This may require discussion with the physician before placing another cast.

CLIENT PARTICIPATION AND OTHER CLIENT FACTORS

After the assessment has determined the need for a cast, the ability of the client to participate in treatment is a key factor in a successful casting program. As the tight muscle/soft tissue

is lengthened, the opposing and overstretched weak muscle requires a strengthening program. Ultimately, the weak antagonist, the muscle that opposes the action of the tight muscle, can be activated and strengthened.[29,55] Improved muscle balance around the joint may result, decreasing the potential for recurrence of the myostatic contracture. Strengthening the muscle opposing a contracted muscle is an intervention approach that should be incorporated into the client's activities of daily living. The long-term effectiveness of maintaining a good outcome is dependent on the practice of the functional activities that are to be performed when the casting program is completed.

Clients with significant spasticity or stiffness may require oral medication such as baclofen to help relax the muscles to improve the ease of cast application. Botulinum toxin type A (BtA) injection is used to inhibit the release of acetylcholine, functionally denervating or decreasing neural input to the tight muscle. Return of the neural input occurs with regeneration and collateral sprouting of the nerve endings. The chemodenervation effect generally lasts for 3 to 5 months, depending on the size and function of the muscle injected. Changes in muscle tone, ROM, and functional activities have been reported.[14,22,34,42] BtA weakens the injected muscle, but it will not increase the muscle length. Casting is frequently used in conjunction with BtA management to elongate the injected muscle. BtA in conjunction with an occupational therapy program, including casting, has improved outcomes compared with BtA only.[14,24,34,40,53]

TYPES OF CASTS, RATIONALE FOR USE, INSTRUCTION FOR APPLICATION

After the initial assessment the therapist selects the type of cast that is deemed most effective to improve ROM and optimize function. The therapist uses clinical judgment and problem-solving skills to decide which cast is the most appropriate and determines the appropriate follow-up treatment during and after the casting program.

During casting, joints are positioned statically in submaximal range to avoid elicitation of the stretch reflex and to prevent microtearing and overstretch of the soft tissue, nerves, and blood vessels. Submaximal range is defined as 5 to 10 degrees less than the range available with maximal stretch. When casted at maximal stretch, there is a chance that the muscle will rebound when the cast is removed. Microtearing of the overstretched muscle may occur and cause pain, muscle spasm, or loss of ROM. The goal of gentle serial casting at submaximal range is to provide a low-load, prolonged stretch. An increase of at least 5 degrees in passive ROM is expected when the cast is removed. The casting program is discontinued when ROM has not increased or there is no improvement in volitional movement. If changes in spontaneous movement or ROM are noted later, the casting program may be reestablished.

Inhibitory casts are those used to reduce the effects of abnormal muscle tone. Casting one portion of the arm may have a relaxing effect on the other muscles in that extremity. For example, positioning the thumb into extension with input into the thenar eminence and palmar arch may relax the tightness in the fingers. Positioning the forearm in supination with elbow extension may have an inhibitory effect on the spasticity or stiffness in the elbow, wrist, or hand.

The tight muscle is maintained in a gradually lengthened range, while the antagonist is in a shortened range, to improve active and passive ROM.

Cast fabrication and application requires two therapists or the primary therapist casting and an aide or assistant instructed in the casting and holding techniques. It is extremely important that the assisting person who holds the arm and the person applying the cast work as a team. The holder is responsible for assisting with maintaining the alignment of the arm or hand during the casting procedure. The holder of a cast is crucial when applying a cast on a client who has significant spasticity or muscle weakness to ensure that the involved arm is in good alignment and position to optimize achievement of ROM during the casting process.

PROTOCOL

Casts are often applied in series, with each cast being left in place for 3 to 7 days, depending on the severity of tone or stiffness and the type of cast.[5,20,30,44] For a client with burns the cast may be left on for 2 to 3 days, depending on the skin integrity and precautions.[3,11] When one cast in the series is removed, the skin is cleansed and checked for pressure areas. The therapist assesses the ROM and muscle tone, and then another cast is immediately applied. The casting series is generally limited to five to seven casts to prevent stiffness and to incorporate gains made with the casting program into functional movement.

A bivalve cast or orthosis can be fabricated to maintain the ROM while other treatment methods are explored. When a cast is intended to be used as a bivalve splint or orthosis for maintenance, fiberglass casting materials are often used for durability. A bivalve cast is cut into two halves, with the edges finished and straps applied to hold both sections together.

After a cast is applied, the client or caregiver is provided with information on care of the cast and receives instructions on areas to be monitored. The client is instructed in warning signs and provided with written instructions (Table 19.4). For a cast that must be removed using a cast saw, it is helpful to provide a letter to present to the emergency department physician describing the purpose of the cast (Table 19.5).

It is further important to incorporate active movement and exercise upon removal of the cast to translate the gains from casting into functional movement.

CASTING MATERIALS

Therapists will likely develop preferences for casting materials as they become more familiar with the various properties. Local hospital and orthopedic supply vendors often present updates and training about casting products, such as stockinette, padding, fiberglass, and plaster. There are many choices of casting products in terms of the texture, feel, and setting

---

TABLE 19.4 Cast Care and Precautions

This cast will be removed on _____. Please read the following to learn about the cast and precautions for your cast.

Precautions

If your cast causes any of the following conditions, contact your therapist.
1. Swollen or puffy fingers
2. Differences in temperature or color between the casted and uncasted arm
3. Pain
4. Numbness or tingling
5. Blueness in fingernails
6. Bad odor

Do not get your cast wet since it will become soft and cause skin problems. Cover the casted arm with a plastic bag when taking a shower or bath. If the cast becomes wet, it must be removed as soon as possible to prevent skin breakdown.

If the cast is able to be taken off by unraveling, please remove immediately if there is a problem. If it is too tight, unravel some of the cast and monitor the skin to see if this will alleviate the problem.

Elevate your casted arm/hand periodically. Do not let it just hang at your side.

Initially check the cast every hour to monitor skin.

Therapist Telephone _____

TABLE 19.5 Sample Letter to Emergency Department Physician Describing Purpose of the Cast

Name:
DOB:
Type of cast:
Date:

Emergency Department Letter

To whom it may concern:

I have applied plaster/fiberglass cast(s) to the _____ of _____, who is an outpatient at _____ Hospital. The cast has been applied to gain range of motion and improve strength. There is NO fracture or joint instability to be concerned about if the cast is removed. The patient has been instructed to go to the nearest emergency department if problems arise when we are not available.

Please remove the cast(s) if there is any question of compromised circulation or if the patient is complaining of significant pain. There is a minimum of three (3) layers of cotton padding under the shell of the cast.

If there are problems with the cast, please call me at _____.

Thank you for your assistance. _____

---

characteristics. For example, a therapist may choose a type of padding because it is easy to tear, conforms easily, or is more durable. Plaster materials are available from fast setting to

TABLE 19.6 Casting Materials

	Size	Characteristic	Amount needed	Removal
Stockinette	3-inch width	Cotton	See specific	
	2-inch width	Polyester	measurements	
	1-inch width		for each cast	
Cast padding	3-inch width	Cotton	2–5 rolls	
	2-inch width	Polyester	depending on	
		Cotton and rayon blend	size of arm	
Plaster cast	3-inch width	Heavy	3–5 rolls adult	Cast saw
	2-inch width	Strong	1–2 pediatric	
Fiberglass	3-inch width	Strong-lightweight	3–5 rolls adult	Cast saw
	2-inch width	Fiberglass	1–2 pediatric	
Delta-Cast Conformable	3-inch width	Polyester cast tape—used for	2–3 rolls adult	Bandage scissors and cutting
	2-inch width	functional cast therapy (FCR)	1 roll pediatric	strip placement in cast
Semirigid soft cast				
Delta-Cast Soft	3-inch width	Lightweight, flexible, soft	3–5 rolls adult	Unravel
	2-inch width	Polyester fabric impregnated with	1–2 pediatric	
		low-tack polyurethane resin		
	1-inch width	Fiberglass, flexible, soft	3–5 rolls adult	Unravel
3M Scotchcast Soft Cast	2-inch width	Knitted fiberglass fabric impreg-	1–2 pediatric	
	3-inch width	nated with a water-activated		
		polyurethane resin		

Soft Cast Supplies
3M Scotchcast Soft Cast (fiberglass)
3M Health Care
3M Center Building 275-4E-0
Saint Paul, MN 55144-1000
1-800-228-3957

Delta-Cast Soft (polyester cast tape)
Delta-Cast Conformable—functional cast therapy (polyester cast tape)
BSN Medical, Inc.
5825 Carnegie Blvd.
Charlotte, NC 28209-4633
1-800-552-1157

Felt Strip—Regular Purchased Felt Material (See Illustrations in Instruction for Application)

Humerus	One 1½-inch width the circumference of the humerus below the axilla
Ulnar styloid	One 1½-inch width the circumference of the forearm over the ulnar styloid
Elbow	Two 1½-inch width by 6 inches—place on the elbow across the olecranon vertically along the ulna and up onto the humerus, and the other piece horizontally across both epicondyles
Thumb	One 1½-inch width by 5 inches, one 1-inch width by 3 inches
	Fold the wider strip (1½ × 5 inches) in half lengthwise, and cut a half circle one-third from the top. Place the smaller felt strip through the hole of the larger strip. Place the felt strip piece through the thumb covering the web space and the longer strip placed along the radial border.

Additional Materials
Paper tape, masking tape, or hospital tape for holding the felt strips on stockinette
Towels
Bucket/water: warm, not hot. Placing fiberglass or plaster cast with hot water may elevate the temperature beneath an applied cast with risk of thermal injury.[1,25]
Bandage scissors
Gloves—latex-free to use when applying casting materials

extrafast setting, with varying smoothness and conformability of the material (Table 19.6).

When unrolling the padding, place the roll facing up and unwrap gently, without pulling the material, as this may cause increased tightness and circumferential restriction. During application of the plaster or semirigid soft cast, hold the material at the end of the roll and dip into warm water. Gently squeeze the roll to get rid of excess water, and begin

TABLE 19.7 Rigid Circular Elbow Cast Using Plaster or Semirigid Materials

	Size	Amount	Removal
Stockinette	3 inch, adults 2 inch, smaller adults/pediatric 1 inch width for toddlers or infants		
Cast padding	3 inch, adults 2 inch, smaller adults/pediatric	1–5 rolls depending on size of arm	
Plaster cast	3 inch, adults 2 inch, smaller adults/pediatric	1–5 rolls depending on size of arm	Cast saw
Semirigid soft cast	3 inch, adults 2 inch, smaller adults/pediatric	1–5 rolls depending on size of arm	Unravel

Felt: 4 strips	Humerus—One 1½-inch width by circumference of
	    humerus below axilla
	Ulnar styloid—One 1½-inch width by circumference of
	    forearm over the ulnar styloid
	Elbow—Two 1½-inch width by 6 inches		

Additional supplies	Bucket for warm water, towel, bandage scissors, tape,
	    gloves **needed** for semirigid soft cast but may prefer
	    not to use gloves for plaster		

application on the arm. The plaster or the semirigid cast material sets quickly, so plan and practice the technique and position needed for the holder before application. Unroll the material similar to the padding method.

RIGID CIRCULAR ELBOW CAST

Rationale for Use

A loss of elbow extension with contracture results in serious impairment in performance of activities of daily living. A series of rigid circular elbow casts is applied to gradually increase elbow ROM. The elbow cast is effective for improving elbow extension in clients with central nervous system (CNS) dysfunction, muscle imbalance from peripheral nerve injury, or myostatic contracture. In clients with fluctuating tone the elbow cast assists with providing equalized pressure for gradual improvement in extensibility. If the client presents with severe rigidity or heterotopic ossification and immobility is contraindicated, the elbow cast should not be used.

When casting the elbow of clients with severe to moderate spasticity, it is important to apply equalized pressure throughout the humerus and forearm to prevent pressure directly on the olecranon. It is important to wrap around the olecranon in a figure-eight wrap, rather than a direct pull over the bony prominence. The figure-eight padding wrap distributes the pressure evenly over the olecranon.

The rigid circular elbow cast is left in place for 5 to 7 days to provide a slow, gradual stretch. After removal the arm is checked and cleaned, and ROM is documented. A new cast is applied to continue increasing ROM into further elbow extension. Materials for elbow casts are listed in Table 19.7.

Cast Application Instructions (Box 19.2)

Measure stockinette from the acromion to the posterior aspect of the olecranon to accommodate for the length of the material to the distal proximal interphalangeal (PIP) joint (Fig. 19.4).

1. For a severe to moderate elbow flexion contracture of 45 degrees or more, cut a slit on the stockinette at the anterior elbow crease horizontally from one epicondyle to the other. Overlap the stockinette. This is to keep the stockinette from bunching and wrinkling at the antecubital crease.

2. Apply the felt strips to the following: distal to the axilla circumferentially, over ulnar styloid circumferentially, across the olecranon vertically along the ulna and up on the humerus, and horizontally across both epicondyles (Fig. 19.5).

3. Apply padding beginning proximally or distally, and wrap circumferentially, overlapping each wrap by third. If the padding is bulking on one side, tear the opposite side to conform the material smoothly on the arm (Fig. 19.6A–B). The padding should cover the ulnar styloid distally and extend fully up onto the axilla.

   a. For plaster cast, apply five or six layers of padding at both distal and proximal ends and four or five layers covering the midsection of the arm.

   b. For semirigid soft cast less padding is required as the material can be unraveled and peeled off versus using a cast saw.

4. Apply a figure-eight padding wrap at the olecranon for the elbow flexed at 45 degrees or more. Padding should crisscross at the anterior elbow crease and overlap approximately 1 inch over the olecranon; wrap again to overlap by 1 inch over the olecranon. There are initially two layers of padding over the olecranon (Fig. 19.7A–B). Continue to figure-eight again around the olecranon to provide four layers, and continue down the arm. If going up the arm again, you can unroll the padding without doing the figure-eight wrap to complete.

5. Apply plaster cast ½ inch below the top of the padding at the axilla, down the humerus to ½ inch proximal to the ulnar styloid. If the plaster bulks or narrows, tuck it where it is bulking (Fig. 19.8).

A. OT staff will evaluate for and apply casts to patients' UEs on referral from physician.

B. Types of casts applied include rigid circular long arm, elbow, wrist, wrist with thumb enclosed, or MCP wrist cast.

C. Casts will be applied to improve passive range of motion for hygiene care/skin care, to reverse contracture, to manage abnormal tone in conjunction with botulinum toxin or oral baclofen, to assist with strengthening/rebalancing muscles, or to assist with application of orthoses for positioning or CIMT.

D. Application of casts is not recommended in the following:
Bilateral casts to patients with hypertension
Skin surface that is not intact
Joints with heterotopic ossification

E. Special consideration should be taken when casting patients with the following:
Heterotopic ossification
Decreased circulation/edema
Decreased sensation
Decreased orientation/alertness
Decreased stability of proximal joints

F. Qualified OT staff will assume responsibility for monitoring casts and documentation of process results and complications.

Procedure

1. A. Referrals may be made to OT by any referring physician who states: "Evaluate for cast and splints as needed."
   - Referrals may include area to be casted (elbow, wrist, digits), extremity to be casted, and type of cast
   - Or a qualified OT may recommend casting and request orders from the physician.

2. Qualifications of OT personnel assessing for and applying cast.
   A. OTRs may be qualified to assess for and apply casts.
   B. To be qualified, therapist must be able to review the following information to a qualified staff member:
      1. Indication for the cast to be used
      2. Contraindications
      3. Safety precautions/emergency removal procedures
      4. Casting application procedure
   C. To be qualified, therapist must demonstrate cast technique for qualified staff by applying and removing cast on another staff member.
   D. Cast applications, monitoring, and removal to be directly supervised by qualified therapist until technique skill is ensured.
   E. Before cast application, a qualified staff member must okay type of cast for QA monitor.
   F. OT students may be qualified but MUST continue to be directly supervised in all aspects of casting.

3. Application of casts
   A. Precast evaluation to include:
      1. Goniometric evaluation
      2. Notations of skin condition
      3. Goniometric measurement of point-of-stretch reflex
      4. Goniometric measurement of wrist position when hand is fully flexed and extended
      5. Recording sensory status over area to be casted
      6. Cognition
      7. Spontaneous functional use
      8. Functional arm placement/hand use
   B. Cleanse area to be casted
   C. Apply stockinette
   D. Apply felt over bony prominences and distal and proximal borders if needed

E. Apply material:
   1. Plaster—requires cast saw for removal, except for finger cast
   2. Fiberglass—requires cast saw for removal
   3. 3M Scotchcast soft cast—unravels off, but has fiberglass
   4. Delta-Cast soft—unravels off, made of polyester
   5. Delta-Cast Conformable—polyester, FCT. This material is used for fabricating a splint. No padding is needed; must use the special Terry-Net stockinette. The technique is to provide rigidity where the patient will need it and flexibility in areas not requiring rigid immobilization. This requires a cutting stick to be placed before application of the material for safe removal.

4. Monitoring
   A. Document date cast applied and date to be removed. If applying the soft cast, instruct caregiver on the removal process. The caregiver should remove cast at home if there are any problems with child's ability to tolerate the cast.
   B. After cast application, always monitor the following:
      1. Red areas
      2. Pulse at points distal to cast
      3. Temperature comparison both UEs
      4. Pain
      5. Edema
      6. Discoloration of hand/nail beds
   C. Qualified OT will monitor cast and notify nurse in charge for inpatients. For outpatients, discuss precautions and instruct in removal technique. Parents/caregivers should remove the cast if there are any difficulties at home. If the soft cast is too tight, let caregiver know that the cast can be gradually unwrapped to loosen the cast without having the cast totally removed.
   D. Use of the cast saw
      1. For plaster cast or fiberglass materials, the cast saw must be used for removal.
      2. OT staff must practice removal from a qualified OT before using the saw.
      3. Before removing the cast, explain the use of cast cutter.
         a. The sound may be loud and frightening, may use headphones for child.
         b. The cast blade runs back and forth and not around, so will not cut through padding.
         c. Hold the cast saw in the middle, and go up/down to cut; do not hold blade down in material for long periods or the blade will heat up. Do not run the blade across materials, only up/down.
         d. When a "give" is felt with the cast saw going down in the material, lift the cast saw back up. Do not leave the blade down in material, or that position will heat the blade.
         e. If the blade feels overheated, stop cutting; may require a new blade or need to cool off.
         f. After cutting the cast use the cast spreader to open the cast.
         g. Cut the padding first, running the cast scissors on the stockinette.
         h. Lift the stockinette off the skin, and cut the stockinette. Prevent running the scissors on the client's skin.

5. Documentation
   A. The OT will document in the medical chart the cast application and observations of how the client tolerated the casting procedure.
   B. The OT will document status before casting, changes and status on removal of cast, and goals.

CIMT, Constraint-induced movement therapy; *FCT,* functional cast therapy; *MCP,* metacarpophalangeal; *OT,* occupational therapist, occupational therapy; *OTR,* occupational therapist, registered; *QA,* quality assurance; *UE,* upper extremity.

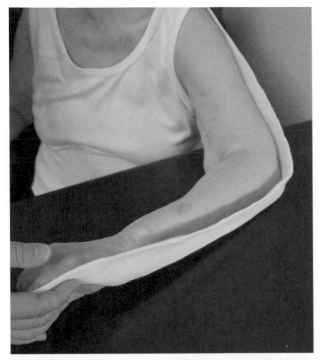

Fig. 19.4 Measure stockinette from the acromion to the posterior aspect of the olecranon to accommodate for the length of the material to the distal proximal interphalangeal (PIP) joint.

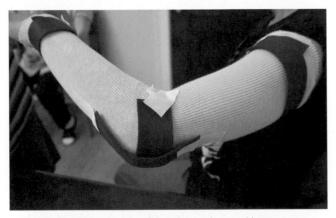

Fig. 19.5 Applying felt strips to the stockinette.

6. The holder can assist with pulling the stockinette over the edge of the plaster cast and secure the stockinette with the plaster cast material.
7. Rub the plaster cast well into the gauze, and allow it to set. Flare the proximal and distal edges with a circumferential motion combined with outward pull of the index finger. Do not apply counterpressure with thumb. The completed rigid circular elbow cast is shown in Fig. 19.9.

RIGID CIRCULAR WRIST CAST

Rationale for Use

The rigid circular wrist cast is indicated for the wrist that exhibits spasticity, muscle imbalance, or weakness, as well as contractures where wrist flexion is more dominant and may lead to myostatic contracture. The wrist cast may be positioned in flexion, extension, or deviation depending on the clinical problem and alignment concerns. As the wrist ROM improves, the hand can be properly fitted and maintained by a lightweight, low-temperature thermoplastic orthosis.

By improving the balance between wrist flexion and extension and stabilizing the wrist in a functional hand position, the wrist cast may promote fine motor control of the thumb and fingers. This cast stabilizes the wrist for the client to actively coordinate thumb and finger movement with the wrist in a better alignment. Poor wrist strength requires a wrist orthosis and active wrist strengthening to be incorporated after the casting program. Gradual improvement into wrist extension may occur over time as the client practices hand function and strengthening.

The wrist cast is generally left in place for 5 to 7 days unless contraindicated. The upper extremity should be reevaluated after each cast, according to the goal and aim of the casting program.

Wrist Cast Application Using Plaster Material (Table 19.8)

1. Measure stockinette from the olecranon to the PIP joint.
2. Cut a small ¼-inch slit approximating the placement of the thumb, and apply the stockinette (Fig. 19.10).
3. Apply the felt strips to the following: one over the ulnar styloid and the two smaller strips for the thumb piece.

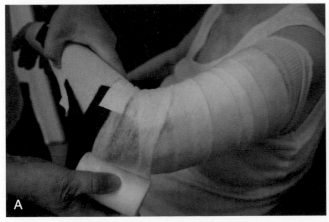

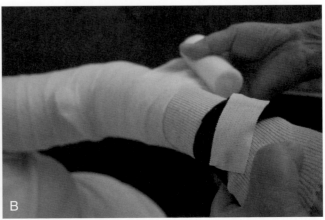

Fig. 19.6 A and B, Initially there are two layers of padding over the olecranon with the application of padding in a figure-of-eight manner.

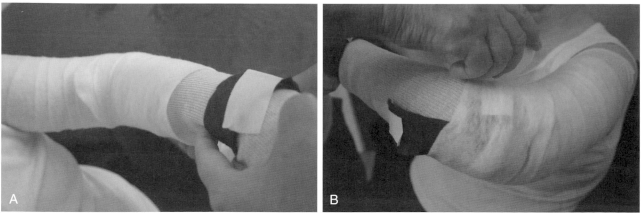

Fig. 19.7A-B Padding should crisscross at the anterior elbow crease and overlap approximately 1 inch over the olecranon; wrap again to overlap by 1 inch over the olecranon. There are initially two layers of padding over the olecranon.

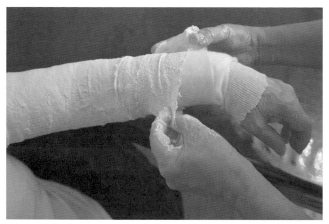

Fig. 19.8 Apply plaster from ½ inch below the top of the padding at the axilla, down the humerus to ½ inch proximal to the ulnar styloid.

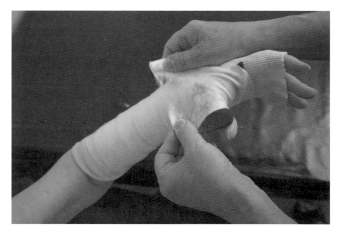

Fig. 19.10 Cut a small ¼-inch slit in the stockinette for the thumb.

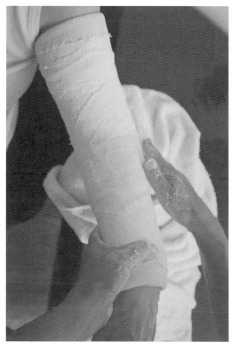

Fig. 19.9 Completed rigid circular elbow cast.

Fold the larger strip in half lengthwise, and cut a half circle one-third from the top. Place the smaller felt strip through the hole of the larger strip, and place the felt strip piece through the thumb slit, covering the web space. The longer piece is placed along the radial border of the forearm. Tape the felt pieces in place (Fig. 19.11A–B).

4. Apply padding proximally approximately 2 inches below the olecranon to wrap circumferentially, overlapping by one-third on each wrap. If bulking occurs on the narrow side of the forearm while wrapping the distal forearm, hold the padding and tear at the opposite end of the bulking to contour the forearm shape.

5. When wrapping around the thumb, pull the padding going radial to ulnar on the dorsum of the hand above the wrist, and then from ulnar to radial on the volar surface to reinforce wrist extension. Place the middle of the padding in the middle of web space (Fig. 19.12). Tear the padding horizontally at the third metacarpal on the dorsal surface. Wrap the lower half of the padding around the metacarpal joint of thumb. Wrap back around the carpometacarpal (CMC) and MCP joint of the thumb. Repeat as needed.

TABLE 19.8	Wrist Cast Materials Using Plaster or Semirigid Material		
	Size	**Amount**	**Removal**
Stockinette	3 inch, adults 2 inch, smaller adults/pediatric 1 inch width for toddlers or infants		
Cast padding	3 inch, adults 2 inch, smaller adults/pediatric	1–5 rolls depending on size of arm	
Plaster cast	3 inch, adults 2 inch, smaller adults/pediatric	1–5 rolls depending on size of arm	Cast saw
Semirigid soft cast	3 inch, adults 2 inch, smaller adults/pediatric	1–5 rolls depending on size of arm	Unravel
Felt: 3 strips	Ulnar styloid—one 1½-inch width by circumference of forearm over the ulnar styloid Thumb—one 1½-inch width by 5 inches, and one 1-inch width by 3 inches		
Additional supplies	Bucket for water, towel, bandage scissors, tape, gloves **needed** for semirigid soft cast material but may prefer not to use gloves for plaster		

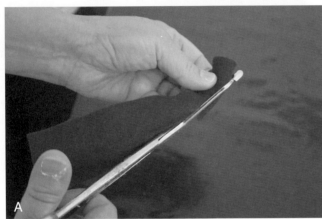
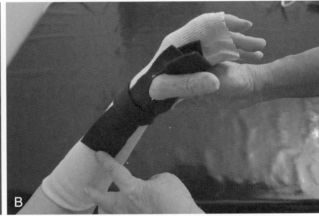

Fig. 19.11 A, Fold the larger strip in half lengthwise, and cut a half circle one-third from the top. Place the smaller felt strip through the hole of the larger strip, and place the felt strip through the thumb slit covering the web space. Apply the felt strips—the longer piece is placed along the radial border of the forearm. B, Apply the felt strips—the longer piece is placed along the radial border of the forearm.

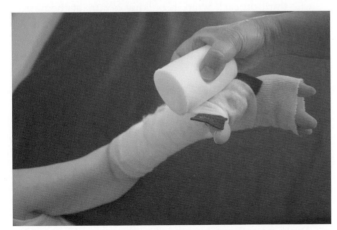

Fig. 19.12 Place the middle of the padding in the middle of the web space.

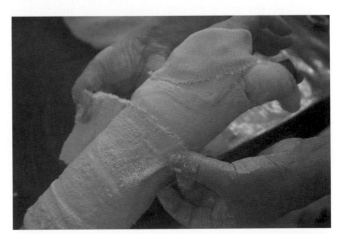

Fig. 19.13 Begin application by applying the plaster ½-inch below the proximal end of the forearm and unrolling, leaving ½ inch of padding at the distal and proximal ends.

6. Begin application by applying the plaster ½ inch below the proximal end of forearm and unrolling, leaving ½ inch of the padding at the distal and proximal ends. If bulking occurs with the plaster, take the extra piece of plaster and tuck (Fig. 19.13). Apply the plaster again, radial to ulnar, on the dorsal side and ulnar to radial on the volar side to reinforce the pull into extension.

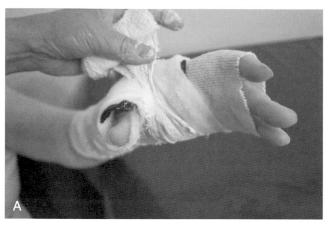

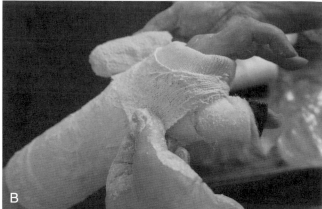

Fig. 19.14 A and B, Angle the plaster on the dorsum of the hand, and tuck to continue unrolling in a radial-to-ulnar direction.

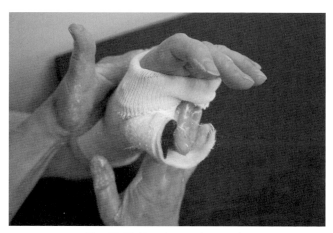

Fig. 19.15 Forming a palmar arch.

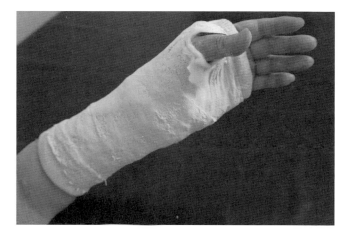

Fig. 19.16 Completed wrist cast.

7. To apply plaster through the web space, squeeze the plaster together so that it lays in the middle of the padding. Angle the plaster on the dorsum of the hand, and tuck to continue unrolling radial to ulnar (Fig. 19.14A–B). Come through the web space with the plaster only two to three times, or it may become too bulky and cause difficulty using the thumb for prehension.

8. After applying two to three rolls of plaster, form a palmar arch. (Fig. 19.15). Use only the palm, and not the thumb or fingertips, when applying counterpressure on the dorsum of the cast to prevent indentation into the cast material.

9. Turn the stockinette over the plaster edge distally and proximally, and secure with the plaster cast or plaster strips. The felt strip at the thumb can be folded over and secured with the stockinette for the web space.

10. Check for tightness at the distal and proximal end of the cast. The completed wrist cast is shown in Fig. 19.16.

Cast Application for Soft Wrist Cast Using Semirigid Soft Cast Material (Similar to the Wrist Cast Procedure)

1. Measure stockinette from the olecranon to the PIP joint.
2. Cut a small ¼-inch slit approximating the placement of the thumb, and apply the stockinette.

3. Apply the felt strip to the following: one over the ulnar styloid.

4. Apply padding proximally approximately 2 inches below the olecranon, and wrap circumferentially, overlapping by one-third on each wrap. If bulking occurs at the narrow end while wrapping the distal forearm, hold the padding and tear at the opposite end to contour the forearm shape.

5. When wrapping around the thumb, pull up on the padding going radial to ulnar on the dorsum of the hand above the wrist, and then from ulnar to radial on the volar surface to reinforce wrist extension. Place the middle of the padding in the middle of the web space. Tear the padding horizontally at the third metacarpal on the dorsal surface. Wrap the lower half of the padding around the metacarpal joint of the thumb. Wrap back around the CMC and MCP joint of the thumb. Repeat as needed. The padding around the thumb is required to keep the sticky casting material away from the skin.

6. Apply the soft cast ½ inch below the proximal end of the forearm, and unroll, leaving ½ inch of the padding at the distal and proximal ends. Apply the soft cast again radial to ulnar on the dorsal side and ulnar to radial on the volar side to reinforce the pull into extension.

7. Wrap through the web space by cutting a slit, starting at the third metacarpal on the volar surface of the soft

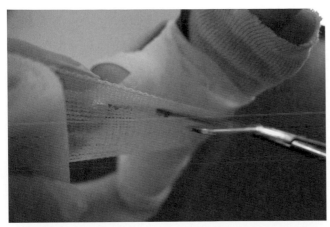

Fig. 19.17 Wrap through the web space by cutting a slit for the thumb to slide into.

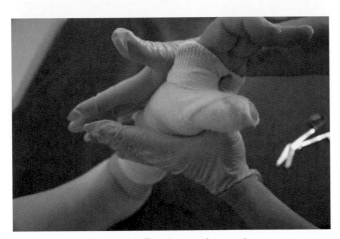

Fig. 19.18 Forming a palmar arch.

cast and moving toward the index finger on the dorsal side on the distal third portion of the wrist cast material. The smaller third portion of the cut cast material should lay on the web space as the thumb is placed through the opening of the cast (Fig. 19.17).

8. Apply the soft cast material through the web space, wrapping two to three times depending on the size of the hand. Turn the stockinette back over the edge on the distal and proximal end, and secure the cast.

9. Form a palmar arch (Fig. 19.18). Using the palm to avoid pressure from the thumb or fingertips, apply counterpressure on the dorsum of the cast.

10. Check for tightness at the distal and proximal ends of the cast. The completed wrist cast is shown in Fig. 19.19. Finish the thumb area by removing the padding so that the thumb can be incorporated into activities requiring prehension.

LONG ARM CAST

Rationale for Use

The long arm cast can be effectively used for clients with minimal to moderate involvement and spasticity of the arm. The long arm cast may reduce the dominance of spasticity

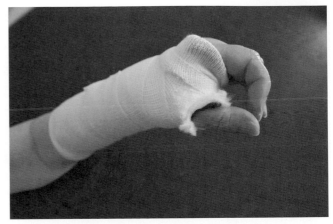

Fig. 19.19 Completed wrist cast.

and assist with rebalancing the antagonistic motor group. Furthermore, a common pattern of clients with poor postural alignment is the forward shoulder, with an abducted or downwardly rotated scapula. This position biomechanically places the humerus into internal rotation, and the upper extremity into elbow flexion, pronation of the forearm, and flexion or ulnar deviation of the wrist with flexion of the fingers and an adducted thumb or thumb-in-palm. The client often demonstrates difficulty with dissociation of the wrist and forearm during active grasp, decreased ability to extend the wrist using thumb-finger opposition for grasp, and difficulty supinating the forearm during lifting the object with the fingers. The malalignment of the joints and tightening of muscles often prevent activities that require thumb-finger opposition for fine prehension.

The long arm cast includes the elbow, forearm, and wrist. It is used to simultaneously manage problems with alignment of the humerus, elbow, forearm, and wrist. The long arm cast is the only cast effective in controlling alignment of forearm rotation by incorporating the wrist, as well as the elbow, into extension. This cast may be inappropriate in the presence of extreme tightness throughout the arm. Microtearing of the soft tissue may occur when tight muscles are stretched over multiple joints. It is also contraindicated for use with a client with a subluxed shoulder.

Clients can simultaneously work on proximal stability and improve scapular control as they increase the strength of their shoulder girdle.[55] As the forearm and elbow soft tissue is gradually lengthened, improvement may be seen in active forearm control and reach into extension.

The long arm cast has also been used for children with brachial plexus birth palsy, which affects the upper plexus involving the fifth and sixth cervical nerve root. The long arm cast assists with improving shoulder girdle alignment and strengthening shoulder girdle and scapula stabilizers from the muscle imbalance. Often children with brachial plexus injury posture the affected arm into humeral internal rotation and compensate by lifting the affected arm into humeral abduction, elbow flexion, and forearm pronation. The long arm cast may reduce the habitual dominance of the arm posture and assist with rebalancing the antagonistic motor group. Muscle reeducation is important

TABLE 19.9   Long Arm Cast Materials

	Size	Amount	Removal
Stockinette	3 inch, adults 2 inch, smaller adults/pediatric 1 inch width for toddlers or infants		
Cast padding	3 inch, adults 2 inch, smaller adults/pediatric	1–5 rolls depending on size of arm	
Semirigid soft cast	3 inch, adults 2 inch, smaller adults/pediatric	1–5 rolls depending on size of arm	Unravel
Felt: 3 strips	Ulnar styloid—One 1½-inch width by circumference of forearm over the ulnar styloid Thumb—One 1½-inch width by 5 inches, and one 1-inch width by 3 inches		
Additional supplies	Bucket for water, towel, bandage scissors, tape, gloves		

in facilitating isolated control, because muscle weakness is a common problem.

In cases with muscle paralysis, such as a client with spinal cord injury C5-6, the unopposed biceps may develop into a supination contracture as the forearm is pulled into supination during elbow flexion. Early positioning and long arm casting into pronation is critical for assisting the client to work on hand-to-mouth patterns and to eventually use an orthosis to facilitate a functional tenodesis for tabletop skills. The bicep relaxes in the cast as the arm is positioned into forearm pronation and the elbow is gradually extended.[18]

To position the arm before the cast the therapist gently holds the involved hand and positions the elbow into extension and forearm in the desired position. The therapist then feels for the decrease in the tension or pull of the arm. The therapist typically holds the arm at the submaximal range while applying the padding and casting material.

Cast Application for Long Arm Using Semirigid Soft Cast Material (Table 19.9)

1. Measure stockinette from the acromion, and on the posterior aspect of the olecranon to accommodate for the length of the material to the fingertips (Fig. 19.20), and approximate placement of the thumb. Apply the stockinette (Fig. 19.21). When the elbow is flexed 45 degrees or more, cut a slit in the stockinette at the anterior elbow crease to prevent wrinkling of the stockinette, similar to the elbow cast instruction.
2. Apply the felt strips to the following: one over the ulnar styloid, and the two smaller strips for the thumb piece, similar to the wrist cast.
3. *Note:* If the elbow is flexed 45 degrees or more, apply felt strips similar to the elbow cast vertically across the olecranon, up on the humerus, and down along the ulna. The horizontal strip is across the olecranon covering the medial and lateral epicondyles.
4. Apply padding as described for the elbow and wrist cast. If applying semirigid soft cast, fewer layers of padding can be used as the material can be unraveled and peeled off.

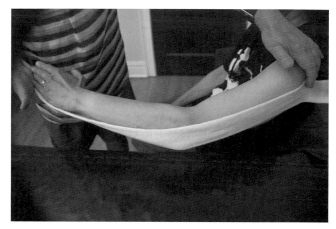

Fig. 19.20 Measure the stockinette from the acromion to the fingertips.

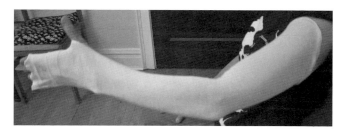

Fig. 19.21 Applying stockinette.

5. Apply the soft cast material ½ inch below the top of padding at the axilla, down the humerus to ½ inch of padding at the distal end.
6. Apply the soft cast material ½ inch below the proximal end of the forearm and unroll, leaving ½ inch of padding at the distal and proximal ends. Apply the soft cast again radial to ulnar on the dorsal side and ulnar to radial on the volar side to reinforce the pull into extension.
7. Wrap the soft cast through the web space similar to the wrist soft cast procedure. Cut a slit in the material so that the distal width (one-third portion) of the cast material lays in the web space as the thumb is placed through the opening of the cast. Cut a slit in the soft cast to place the thumb through the opening.

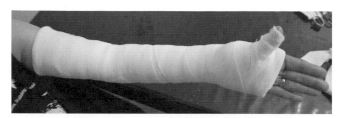

Fig. 19.22 Completed long arm cast.

8. Wrap the soft cast through the web space two to three times, depending on the size of the hand. Turn the stockinette back over the edge on the distal and proximal ends, and secure with soft cast.

9. Form a palmar arch. Use one's palm to avoid pressure from the thumb or fingertips, and apply counterpressure on the dorsum of the cast to prevent indentation.

10. Check for tightness at the distal and proximal end of the cast. Finish the thumb area by removing the padding or leave in place. The completed long arm cast is shown in Fig. 19.22.

WRIST CAST WITH THE THUMB INCLUDED

Rationale for Use

The alignment of the wrist and forearm influences the ability of the thumb to oppose the index and middle finger for prehension and manipulation of objects. When the wrist is pulled into flexion and ulnar deviation, the thumb is held in adduction and flexion, which eventually develops into a shortened and tight web space. Improving the muscle balance and joint alignment gained through a casting program may stretch the tightness of the thumb and lead to improved ability to use the thumb for functional activities.

A thumb-in-palm deformity is caused by abnormal muscle pull of the flexor pollicis longus or brevis, adductor pollicis, and/or the first dorsal interossei, which can lead to a fixed myostatic contracture. This deformity prevents the thumb from participating in grasp and pinch. The tightness and contracture of the thumb may cause shortening of the web space, an unstable MCP joint, or an overstretched extensor pollicis longus and brevis.

A wrist cast with the thumb included can improve the range into thumb abduction and extension and gradually improve palmar expansion. Opening the hand and bringing the thumb out of the palm assists with the development of the transverse or carpal arch, as well as the oblique arch, formed when the thumb moves toward the fingers for opposition.

It is important to contour the casting material at the thenar eminence, supporting the MCP and interphalangeal (IP) joint of the thumb. The thumb should be gradually stretched and the material molded in the web space to assist in providing palmar expansion and stability. Gradual positioning of the thumb in a stretched position is provided at submaximal range to elongate the thumb extensors and abductors, with the wrist in neutral or in 10 to 15 degrees of extension. A series of casts that provides a slow, gradual stretch prevents overstretching or pain in the thumb. This is key for rebalancing muscle forces and controlling the opposing muscle groups. Follow-up after casting may include a night orthosis to maintain the thumb in good alignment and strengthening to optimize functional use of the hand and thumb.

A wrist cast with the thumb enclosed may assist with stabilizing a dystonic thumb with hyperextension at the IP or MCP joint and tightness of the thenar eminence. The client practices grasp and release of objects with the wrist and thumb stabilized in the cast. The distal IP joint is stabilized with the enclosed cast, or the cast can be wrapped proximal to the IP joint or IP crease to allow the client to practice distal IP control.

Careful evaluation and palpation is needed to assess the best position of the thumb to promote a gentle stretch, or to provide stability, as indicated.

Casting Materials

A moldable material is needed for wrapping around the thumb, providing contour of the palmar arch, thenar eminence, and enclosing the thumb. Plaster cast material or polyester soft cast is recommended. Fiberglass material will not conform to the thumb or provide the needed molding of the hand (Table 19.10).

Cast Application for Thumb-Enclosed Wrist Cast Using Polyester Soft Cast

1. Apply the stockinette and felt strips as described for wrist cast.

2. Wrap the forearm as described for padding the wrist cast.

3. Another method for wrapping the thumb is to go up the center of the web space with the padding and tear horizontally to angle the padding toward the thumb. Wrap snuggly around the thumb beyond the IP joint two times. On the third time around come up through the web space; check that the CMC joint and thenar eminence are covered with the padding (Fig. 19.23). Continue to wrap around the thumb, covering the thenar eminence.

4. Apply this cast similar to the wrist cast, using the polyester soft cast material or plaster.

5. Wrap the material between the web space, angle slightly toward the MCP joint of the thumb, and wrap the material two to three times around the thumb, depending on the size of the hand (Fig. 19.24). Bring the material up through the web space on the dorsal side of the hand and around the volar surface and back up through the web space.

6. Turn the stockinette back over the soft cast, and secure the edges with the material.

7. Form the palmar arch, and contour the thenar eminence, supporting the MCP and IP joint of the thumb.

8. Allow the tip of the thumb to be seen, and trim the padding on the edges of the thumb for the skin to be monitored. The completed thumb-enclosed wrist cast is shown in Fig. 19.25.

TABLE 19.10	Thumb Enclosed Wrist Cast Using Plaster or Polyester Soft Cast Material		
	Size	**Amount**	**Removal**
Stockinette	3 inch, adults 2 inch, smaller adults/pediatric 1 inch width for toddlers or infants		
Cast padding	3 inch, adults 2 inch, smaller adults/pediatric	1–5 rolls depending on size of arm	
Plaster cast	3 inch, adults 2 inch, smaller adults/pediatric	1–5 rolls depending on size of arm	Cast saw
Semirigid soft cast	3 inch, adults 2 inch, smaller adults/pediatric	1–5 rolls depending on size of arm	Unravel
Felt: 3 strips	Ulnar styloid—One 1½-inch width by circumference of forearm over the ulnar styloid Thumb—One 1½-inch width by 5 inches, and one 1-inch width by 3 inches		
Additional supplies	Bucket for water, towel, bandage scissors, tape, gloves **needed** for semirigid soft cast material but may prefer not to use gloves for plaster		

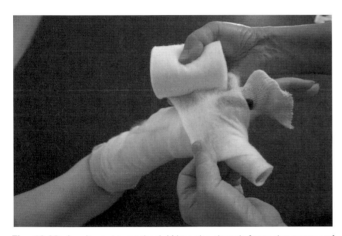

Fig. 19.23 An alternate method: Wrap the thumb from the center of the web space with the padding, and tear horizontally to angle the padding toward the thumb.

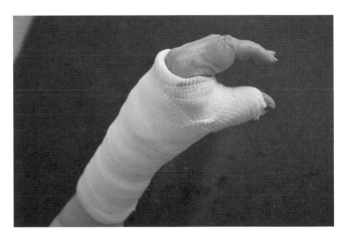

Fig. 19.25 Completed thumb-enclosed wrist cast.

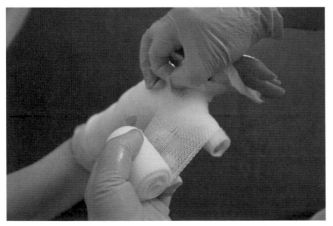

Fig. 19.24 Wrapping the material between the web space and angling slightly toward the metacarpophalangeal joint of the thumb.

METACARPOPHALANGEAL WRIST CAST

Rationale for Use

When weakness of the intrinsic muscle or spasticity of the lumbricals causes flexion contractures of the MCP joints, this inhibits the client from fully extending at the distal PIP and IP joints of the fingers. For a client with spasticity the pull of the intrinsics into flexion at the MCP joint can lead to an intrinsic plus hand and further lead to a myostatic contracture. The MCP cast can be applied just distal to the MCP or PIP joint to allow the client to actively work on end-range finger extension. This cast positions the wrist and finger MCP into extension and facilitates active finger extension. The support of the distal cast beyond the MCP joint or PIP joint assists with gradual elongation of the intrinsic musculature to facilitate active extension of the IP joints when the MCP joints are extended.

End the distal portion of the cast where the fingers require the support, to gradually assist with active end range of finger extension, or to lengthen the long finger flexors in the presence of intrinsic muscles tightness.

The MCP cast is used to gradually improve the tightness of the intrinsic muscles to improve finger extension, thus improving the ability of opening of the hand for grasp-and-release functional activities.

Casting Materials

Any casting materials can be used for the MCP cast (Table 19.11).

Refer to the wrist cast materials, and apply the cast according to the procedure.

Cast Application for Metacarpophalangeal Wrist Cast Using Semirigid Soft Cast

1. Apply the stockinette from the olecranon to the DIP joints and approximate placement of the thumb. Cut a straight slit for the thumb.
2. Apply the felt strips as described for the wrist cast, to the ulnar styloid and thumb.
3. Wrap the forearm as described for padding the wrist cast.
4. Wrap padding around the thumb to prevent the sticky material from adhering to the skin of thumb. Apply the padding proximally extending three-fourths the length of the forearm and distally beyond the MCP joint or PIP joint depending on your assessment.
5. Apply the soft cast similar to the wrist cast. Apply the cast material ½ inch below the padding proximal, and end the material ½ inch distal to the padding.
6. Apply the soft cast material radial to ulnar on the dorsal surface of hand, and ulnar to radial on the volar surface. Cover the thumb CMC joint wrap radial to ulnar on the dorsal surface. Lay the soft cast going up through the web space so it lies partially in the trough formed by the padding and past the MCP joints (Fig. 19.26). Continue the soft cast ½ inch to the distal padding
7. Turn the stockinette back over the soft cast, and secure the edges with the material.
8. Form the palmar arch.
9. Finish the thumb area by removing the padding or leave in place. The completed MCP wrist cast is shown in Fig. 19.27.

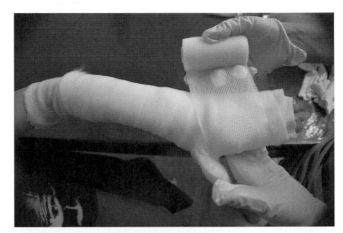

Fig. 19.26 Application of soft cast material in a radial-to-ulnar direction on the dorsal surface of the hand.

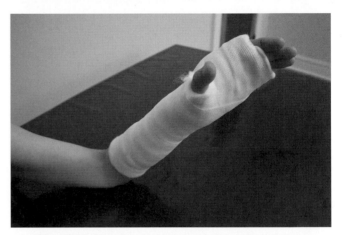

Fig. 19.27 Completed metacarpophalangeal wrist cast.

TABLE 19.11	Metacarpophalangeal Wrist Cast Using Plaster or Semirigid Soft Cast Material		
	Size	**Amount**	**Removal**
Stockinette	3 inch, adults 2 inch, smaller adults/pediatric 1 inch width for toddlers or infants		
Cast padding	3 inch, adults 2 inch, smaller adults/pediatric,	1–5 rolls depending on size of arm	
Plaster cast	3 inch, adults 2 inch, smaller adults/pediatric	1–5 rolls depending on size of arm	Cast saw
Semirigid soft cast	3 inch, adults 2 inch, smaller adults/pediatric	1–5 rolls depending on size of arm	Unravel
Felt: 3 strips	Ulnar styloid—One 1½-inch width by circumference of forearm over the ulnar styloid Thumb—One 1½-inch width by 5 inches, and one 1-inch width by 3 inches		
Additional supplies	Bucket for water, towel, bandage scissors, tape, gloves **needed** for semirigid soft cast material but may prefer not to use gloves for plaster		

METACARPOPHALANGEAL WRIST CAST TO INCREASE FLEXION OF THE METACARPOPHALANGEAL AND PROXIMAL INTERPHALANGEAL JOINTS

Rationale for Use

In an intrinsic minus hand there is hyperextension of the MCP joints and flexion of the PIP joints, referred to as a claw hand. The claw hand is caused by paralysis of the interossei and lumbrical muscles. The client can flex and extend the fingers with the MCP joints in hyperextension or extension but is unable to flex at the MCP for fine prehension. For example, a client with significant burns on the dorsum of the hand with scarring can pull the fingers into hyperextension at the MCP, which leads to an intrinsic minus hand with myostatic contractures.

The MCP wrist cast can be applied just distal to the MCP or PIP joint to work on increasing range into MCP and PIP flexion. When using the soft cast material, it is difficult to position the MCP into flexion, because of the flexibility and sponginess of the material. After applying the padding, a piece of Aquaplast is draped over the dorsum of the forearm and MCPs. The Aquaplast is pulled to hold the MCP joints in the position needed to improve flexion. The soft cast material is then applied, similar to the MCP wrist cast. The MCP cast for the intrinsic minus hand is used to gradually improve the tightness of the MCP for improved hand grasp and release and fine prehension.

Casting Materials
Semirigid Soft Cast Materials

This technique is used when working with a client when you want the client or caregiver to be able to remove the cast at home if issues arise (Table 19.12).

Cast Application for Metacarpophalangeal Wrist Cast Using Soft Cast

1. Apply the stockinette from the olecranon to the DIP joints and approximate placement of the thumb. Cut a straight slit for the thumb.
2. Apply the felt strips as described for the wrist cast.
3. Wrap the forearm as described for padding the wrist cast.
4. Wrap padding around the thumb to prevent the sticky material from adhering to the skin of the thumb. Apply the padding distally, extending three-fourths the length of the forearm and distally beyond the MCP joint or PIP joints, depending on needs per assessment.
5. Drape the Aquaplast on the dorsum of the hand over the padding, and pull the MCP and PIP joints into flexion while holding the splint material (Fig. 19.28).

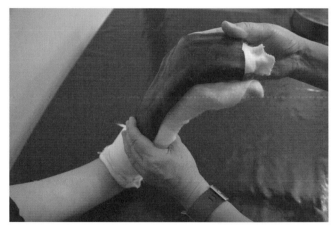

Fig. 19.28 Drape the Aquaplast on the dorsum of the hand over the padding, and pull the metacarpophalangeal and proximal interphalangeal joints into flexion.

TABLE 19.12	Metacarpophalangeal Wrist Cast Using Semirigid Soft Cast Material and Aquaplast		
Semirigid soft cast materials are used when working with a client and you want the client or caregiver to be able to remove the cast at home if issues arise.			
	Size	**Amount**	**Removal**
Stockinette	3 inch, adults 2 inch, smaller adults/pediatric 1 inch width for toddlers or infants		
Cast padding	3 inch, adults 2 inch, smaller adults/pediatric	1–5 rolls depending on size of arm	
Semirigid soft cast	3 inch, adults 2 inch, smaller adults/pediatric	1–5 rolls depending on size of arm	Unravel
Felt: 3 strips	Ulnar styloid—One 1½-inch width by circumference of forearm over the ulnar styloid Thumb—One 1½-inch width by 5 inches, and one 1-inch width by 3 inches		
Aquaplast	A sheet of 4 × 10 inch Aquaplast (adjust sheet according to size of hand)		
Additional supplies	Bucket for water, splint pan for Aquaplast material, towel, bandage scissors, tape, gloves		

6. Apply the cast similar to the MCP wrist cast over the Aquaplast to position in place. Apply the cast material ½ inch below the padding proximal and end the material ½ inch distal to the padding.
7. Turn stockinette back over the soft cast, and secure the edges with the material.
8. Form the palmar arch. The completed MCP wrist cast to increase MCP flexion is shown in Fig. 19.29.

FUNCTIONAL CAST THERAPY

Functional cast therapy (FCT) is a casting method using Delta-Cast Conformable Polyester Cast Tape to apply a form-fitting orthosis that is molded directly onto the client's hand. The knitted polyester material is easy to apply and molds similar to plaster or semirigid polyester soft cast. The material provides the rigidity needed to support specific joints and also offers the flexibility for areas where immobilization is not required. The material is easy to apply and is used for a variety of orthotic needs. Further information on the different types of functional cast therapy applications is described in the application manual using Delta-Cast Conformable by BSN Medical, Inc.

THUMB SPICA WITH FUNCTIONAL CAST THERAPY MATERIALS

Rationale for Use

The thumb spica orthosis is used to decrease movement and provide support and comfort through stability of an injury. It is often used for clients with de Quervain tenosynovitis, traumatic thumb injuries, or rheumatoid arthritis. Stabilizing the thumb and wrist can also be used to manage dystonia or hypertonicity, which positions the thumb in palmar flexion and adduction. By positioning the thumb in abduction and opposition of the index and middle fingers, motions for functional prehension are possible. The position of the thumb in a thumb spica orthosis varies depending on the client's diagnosis.

FUNCTIONAL CAST THERAPY MATERIALS (TABLE 19.13)

Cast Application for Thumb Spica Using Delta-Cast Conformable

1. Apply the thumb stockinette liner with the padded side on the client's skin.
2. Apply sticky-back foam over the ulnar styloid on the stockinette.
3. Insert the cutting strip under the stockinette on the dorsal side of the forearm and hand, covering the area to be casted (Fig. 19.30).
4. Before applying the FCT cast decide what part of the wrist splint requires stabilization to support the hand (three to four layers to provide stability) and what part of the splint can remain flexible.

TABLE 19.13	**Functional Cast Therapy Using Delta-Cast Conformable**		
	Size	**Amount**	**Removal**
Stockinette	Terry-Net Thumb Spica		
Delta-Cast Conformable	3 inch, adults 2 inch, smaller adults/pediatric	1–3 rolls depending on size of arm	Cutting strip and bandage scissors
Sticky-back foam padding	Over ulnar styloid		
Terry-Net adhesive hook and stretch loop	2 inch 1 inch		
Additional supplies	Bucket for water, towel, bandage scissors, tape, gloves, felt-tip pen		

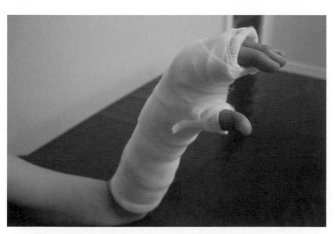

Fig. 19.29 Completed metacarpophalangeal wrist cast.

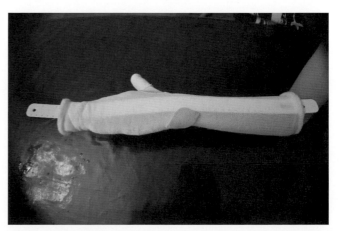

Fig. 19.30 Insert the cutting strip under the stockinette on the dorsal side.

a. Measure the desired length from palm to proximal third of the forearm. Place the three to four layers on the volar surface of the hand (Fig 19.31). The holder can assist with holding in place. *Note:* The layers do not need to be placed in the water.

5. Place the remaining roll in the water, and begin to unroll. Start at the proximal end unwrapping around the forearm with two layers. Overlap each layer by *half the width of the material,* unwrapping the cast down to the CMC joint. Remember overlapping by half, and continue in a radial-to-ulnar direction (Fig. 19.32). Continue up through the web space.

6. Wrap around the thumb to the IP joint two times while having the holder maintain the position of the thumb in abduction. Come back up around the dorsum of the hand over the MCP joint.

7. Form the palmar arch and thenar eminence, and rub the remaining cast (Fig. 19.33). Place gloves in the water before rubbing in the cast. Once the tackiness is gone, then the cast is ready to be cut off.

8. To remove the cast, place the scissors on top of the cutting strip. Gently squeeze the cast in the area you are cutting and work your way down the cast (Fig. 19.34).

9. Reposition the cast on the client's hand, and decide what area needs to be trimmed to improve the fit of the splint. Mark directly on the cast the areas on the dorsal and volar surface (e.g., palmar crease) that can be trimmed to provide MCP flexion to all of the fingers (Fig. 19.35). If some areas are too difficult to trim, use the special small tin snip–like scissors for the rigid areas.

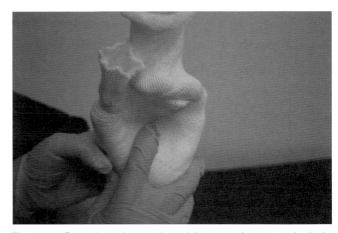

Fig. 19.33 Form the palmar arch and thenar eminence, and rub the remaining cast.

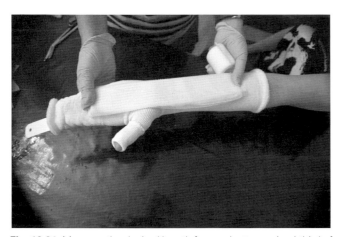

Fig. 19.31 Measure the desired length from palm to proximal third of the forearm, placing three to four layers on the volar surface.

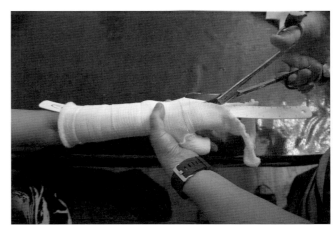

Fig. 19.34 Gently squeeze the cast in the area you are cutting, and work your way down the cast.

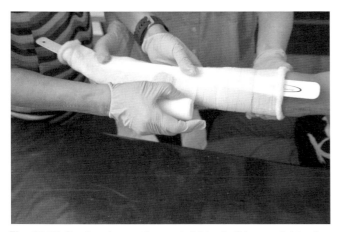

Fig. 19.32 Overlap the casting material by half in a radial-to-ulnar direction.

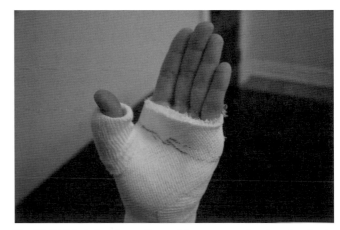

Fig. 19.35 Mark directly on the cast the areas on the dorsal and volar surfaces to trim to allow metacarpophalangeal flexion.

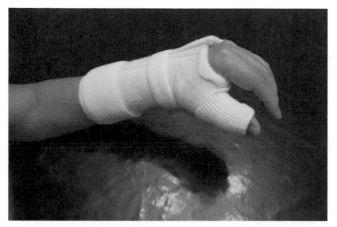

Fig. 19.36 Apply the Velcro stretch loop to complete the orthosis.

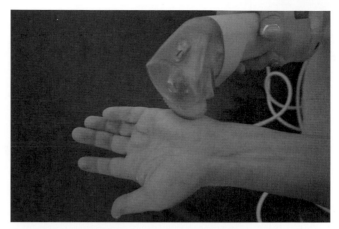

Fig. 19.37 Explain to the client how the cast saw works by demonstrating on your own hand.

10. Complete the orthosis by placing the adhesive fleece edger around the edges of the orthosis. Once the orthosis is totally dry, apply the adhesive hook. Use a heat gun to heat the sticky side of the adhesive hook before applying to the orthosis. Once the heated hook Velcro is applied to the orthosis, rub the Velcro with the blunt edge of the scissors to secure it to the material. Apply the 1-inch or 2-inch Velcro stretch loop to complete the orthosis. The completed thumb spica is shown in Fig. 19.36.

CAST REMOVAL

As discussed, some types of casting material require removal with a cast saw or cutter, and others constructed of materials, such as the FCT, that can be cut off with scissors. With respect to the cast saw, the therapist must (1) be knowledgeable about how to safely operate the cast saw, (2) be familiar with the cast removal techniques, and (3) be knowledgeable about use of the equipment. Staff must complete competency training by a qualified staff member who is experienced in the use of a cast saw. A system of checking for equipment maintenance must be established to ensure that the cast saw and blade are in proper working condition.

The most common cast saw is the electrically motorized cast cutter. Some of the cast cutters are attached to a cast dust vacuum that has a strong airflow, facilitating hygienic surroundings. Safety glasses are worn to protect the eyes of the client and therapist during the cutting procedure. The blade of the cast saw does not rotate but rather oscillates back and forth for an excursion of approximately ⅛ inch. The therapist should explain to the client by demonstrating how the blade oscillates and touch lightly on their own hand to show how the saw works (Fig. 19.37). The blade is designed to cut through plaster or fiberglass and is not intended to cut through padding or stockinette. When properly used, the cast saw should not cause damage or abrasion to the skin. The sound of the cast saw can be loud; therefore when working with children, headphones can be used to muffle the sound of the saw.

The technique for using the saw requires the therapist to grip the cast saw securely by the handle and hold it perpendicular to the cast using a down-and-up motion to cut. When cutting

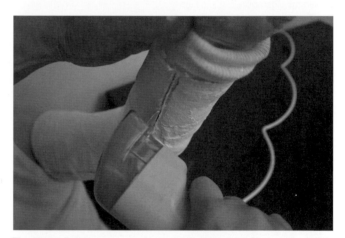

Fig. 19.38 Pull the saw up as soon as a "give" in the material is felt.

down into the cast material with the saw, the therapist will feel a "give." Pull the saw up as soon as a "give" in the material is felt (Fig. 19.38). Do not leave the saw in the casting material for an extended period as the blade becomes hot. If there is more than one cast saw, dedicate one cast saw for cutting fiberglass and one for removing plaster. The blade for cutting the fiberglass may require more frequent changes, and the use of a vacuum attachment assists with control of airborne fiberglass material.

When using the cast as a bivalve orthosis, determine and mark the cut line before cutting. Avoid cut lines over the antecubital fossa and olecranon (Fig. 19.39).

Use of a Cast Cutter

Hold the cast cutter securely by the handle in the middle of the saw.

1. Press down firmly until a "give" is felt in the material. When there is less resistance, the saw has cut through the plaster or fiberglass. Lift the saw up, then place the saw back down, going only up/down.
2. Do not leave the saw down in the cast for extended periods or use the saw to cut or run parallel across the cast. This overheats the blade and may cause a burn to the client. If the cast saw is hot, allow the motor to cool.
3. Insert a cast spreader between the cut area of the cast, and spread the edges apart (Fig. 19.40).

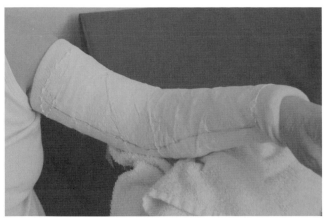

Fig. 19.39 When using the cast as a bivalve orthosis, determine and mark the cut line before cutting, and avoid lines over the antecubital fossa and olecranon.

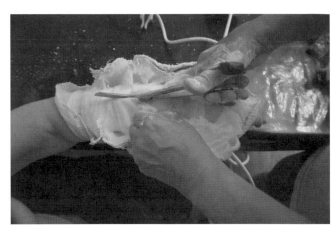

Fig. 19.41 Use a bandage scissors to cut the padding while gliding the scissors on the stockinette.

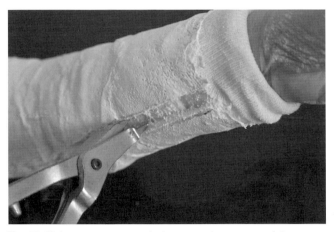

Fig. 19.40 Insert a cast spreader between the cut area of the cast to spread the edges apart.

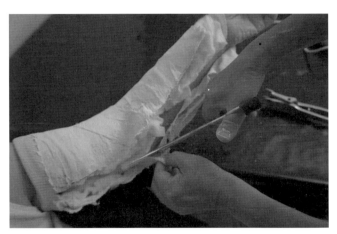

Fig. 19.42 Pull up the stockinette to avoid pressure on the skin from the bandage scissors.

4. Use bandage scissors to cut the padding, gliding the scissors on the stockinette (Fig. 19.41).
5. Pull up the stockinette so there is no pressure from the bandage scissors felt on the client's skin, and cut the stockinette (Fig. 19.42).

Removing Semirigid Soft Cast

The soft cast materials can be removed by unwrapping the layers or cutting off with bandage scissors (Fig. 19.43). The use of a cast saw is not recommended as this material is flexible and less padding is used. When the cast is completely dry, demonstrate how to unwrap the soft cast material by unraveling a small amount and then trimming the edge. If the cast feels too tight, inform the caregiver that a small amount of the casting material can be unwrapped instead of removing the entire cast.

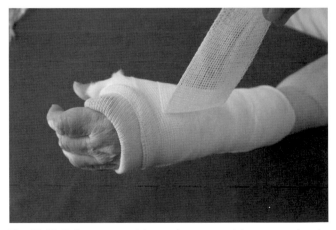

Fig. 19.43 Soft cast materials can be removed by unwrapping the layers or cutting with a bandage scissors.

SUMMARY

A thorough assessment of underlying tissue causing joint restrictions is critical to determine the effectiveness of any casting program. The evaluation assists clinicians with determining what type of cast to use. Furthermore, the assessment findings guide the therapist with sound clinical reasoning for cast implementation.

REFERENCES

1. Ahmed SS, Carmichael KD: Plaster and synthetic cast temperatures in a clinical setting: an in vivo study, *Orthop* 34(2):99, 2011.
2. Autti-Ramo SJ, Anttila H, Maimivaara A, et al.: Effectiveness of upper and lower limb casting and orthosis in children with cerebral palsy: an overview of review articles, *Am J Phys Med Rehabil* 85:89–103, 2006.
3. Bennett GB, Helm P, Purdue GF, et al.: Serial casting: a method for treating burn contractures, *J Burn Care Rehabil* 10(6):543–545, 1989.
4. Blackmore AM, Boettecher-Hunt E, Jordan M, et al.: A systematic review of the effects of casting on equinus in children with cerebral palsy: an evidence report of the AACPDM, *Dev Med Child Neurol* 49(10):781–790, 2007.
5. Booth BJ, Doyle M, Montgomery J: Serial casting for the management of spasticity in the head-injured adult, *Phys Ther* 63:1960–1966, 1983.
6. Brashear A, Zafonte R, Corcoran M, et al.: Inter-and intrarater reliability of the Ashworth scale and the disability assessment scale in patients with upper-limb poststroke spasticity, *Arch Phys Med Rehabil* 83:1349–1354, 2002.
7. Clinkscales C: Sports-specific commentary on Bennett's fractures in professional basketball players: Bennett fractures and metacarpal fractures, *Hand Clin* 28(3):391–392, 2012.
8. Copley J, Watson-Will A, Dent K: Upper limb casting for clients with cerebral palsy: a clinical report, *Aust Occup Ther J* 43:39–50, 1996.
9. Dannenbaum RM, Jones LA: The assessment and treatment of patients who have sensory loss following cortical lesions, *J Hand Ther* 6(2):130–138, 1993.
10. de Bruin M, van de Giessen Vroemen JC, et al.: Geometrical adaptation in ulna and radius of cerebral palsy patients: Measures and consequences, *Clin Biomechanics* 29:451–457, 2014.
11. Dewey WB, Richard RL, Parry IS: Postitioning, splinting, and contracture management, *Phys Med Rehabil Clin N Am* 22(2):229–247, 2011.
12. Duijnisveld BJ, Steenbeek D, Nelissen RG: Serial casting for elbow flexion contractures in neonatal brachial plexus palsy, *J Pediatr Rehabil Med* 9(3):207–214, 2016.
13. Eliasson AC, Ekholm C, Carlstedt T: Hand function in children with cerebral palsy after upper-limb tendon transfer and muscle release, *Dev Med Child Neurol* 40:612–621, 1998.
14. Fehlings D, Rang M, Glazier, et al.: An evaluation of botulinum-A toxin injections to improve upper extremity function in children with hemiplegic cerebral palsy, *J Pediatr* 137:331–337, 2000.
15. Flinn SR, Craven K: Upper limb casting in stroke rehabilitation: rationale, options and techniques, *Top Stroke Rehabil* 21(4):296–302, 2014.
16. Geerdink Y, Lindeboom R, de Wolf S, et al.: Assessment of upper limb capacity in children with unilateral cerebral palsy: construct validity of a Rasch-reduced modified house classification, *Dev Med Child Neurol* 56(6):580–586, 2014.
17. Ghotbi N, Nakhostin AN, Naghdi S, et al.: Measurement of lower-limb muscle spasticity: intrarater reliability of the modified Ashworth scale, *J Rehabil Res Dev* 48:83–88, 2011.
18. Goga-Eppenstein P, Hill J, Philip PA, et al.: *Casting protocols for the upper and lower extremities*, Gaithersburg, MD, 1999, Aspen Publishers.
19. Gracies JM: Pathophysiology of impairment in patients with spasticity and use of stretch as a treatment of spastic hypertonia, *Phys Med Rehabil Clin N Am* 12:747–768, 2001.
20. Hill J: The effects of casting on upper extremity motor disorders after brain injury, *Am J Occup Ther* 48:219–224, 1994.
21. Ho ES, Roy T, Stephens D, et al.: Serial casting and splinting of elbow contractures in children with obstetric brachial plexus palsy, *J Hand Surg Am* 35(1):84–91, 2010.
22. Hoare BJ, Imms C: Upper-limb injections of botulinum toxin-A in children with cerebral palsy: a critical review of the literature and clinical implications for occupational therapists, *Am J Occup Ther* 58(4):389–397, 2004.
23. House JH, Gwathmey FW, Fidler MO: A dynamic approach to the thumb-in-palm deformity in cerebral palsy, *J Bone Jt Surg Am* 63:216–225, 1981.
24. Hurvitz EA, Conti GE, Brown SH: Changes in movement characteristics of the spastic upper extremity after botulinum toxin injection, *Arch Phys Med Rehabil* 84:444–454, 2003.
25. Hutchinson MJ, Hutchinson MR: Factors contributing to the temperature beneath plaster or fiberglass cast material, *J Orthop Surg Res* 3(10), 2008.
26. Kendall FP, McCreary ER, Provance PG: *Muscles: testing and function with posture and pain*, ed 5, Baltimore, 2005, Lippincott Williams and Wilkins.
27. Kuipers K, Burger L, Copley J: Casting for upper limb hypertonia: a retrospective study to determine the factors associated with intervention decisions, *NeuroRehabil* 31:409–420, 2012.
28. Lannin NA, Novak I, Cusick A: A systematic review of upper extremity casting for children and adults with central nervous system motor disorders, *Clin Rehabil* 21(11):963–976, 2007.
29. Law M, Russell D, Pollock N, et al.: A comparison of intensive neurodevelopmental therapy plus casting and a regular occupational therapy program for children with cerebral palsy, *Dev Med Child Neurol* 39:664–670, 1997.
30. LeahyP: Precasting work sheet: an assessment tool, a clinical report, *Phys Ther* 68, 2002. 72–72.
31. Lee KC, Carson L, Kinnin E, et al.: The Ashworth scale: a reliable and reproducible method of measuring spasticity, *J Neurol Rehabil* 3:205–209, 1989.
32. Lehmkuhl LD, Thoi LL, Baize C, et al.: Multimodality treatment of joint contractures in patients with severe brain injury: cost, effectiveness, and integration of therapies in the application of serial/inhibitive casts, *J Head Trauma Rehabil* 5:23–42, 1990.
33. Leong B: Critical review of passive muscle stretch: implications for the treatment of children in vegetative and minimally conscious states, *Brain Inj* 16:169–183, 2002.
34. Lukban MB, Rosales RL, Dressler D: Effectiveness of botulinum toxin A for upper and lower limb spasticity in children with cerebral palsy: a summary of evidence, *J Neural Transm (Vienna)* 116:319–331, 2009.
35. MacKay-Lyons M: Low-load, prolonged stretch in treatment of elbow flexion contractures secondary to head trauma: a case report, *Phys Ther* 69(4):292–296, 1989.
36. Meyer S, Karttuen AH, Thijs V, et al.: How do somatosensory deficits in the arm and hand relate to upper limb impairment, activity, and participation problems after stoke? A systematic review, *Phys Ther* 94(9):1220–1231, 2014.
37. Meyerding HW, Krusen FH: The treatment of Volkmann's ischemic contracture, *Ann Surg* 110(3):417–426, 1939.
38. Mortenson PA, Eng J: The use of casts in the management of joint mobility and hypertonia following brain injury in adults: a systematic review, *Phys Ther* 83:648–658, 2003.

39. Moseley AM, Hassett LM, et al.: Serial casting versus positioning for the treatment of elbow contractures in adults with traumatic brain injury: a randomized controlled trial, *Clin Rehabil* 22:406–417, 2008.

40. Newman DJ, Kennedy A, Walsh M, et al.: A pilot study of delayed versus immediate serial casting after botulinum toxin injection for partially reducible spastic equinus, *J Pediatr Orthop* 27(8):882–885, 2007.

41. O'Dwyer NJ, Ada L, Neilson PD: Spasticity and muscle contracture following stroke, *Brain* 119:1737–1749, 1996.

42. Ozcakir S, Sivrioglu K: Botulinum toxin in poststroke spasticity, *Clin Med Res* 5(2):132–138, 2007.

43. Pletcher D, Hoffer M, Koffman D: Non-traumatic dislocation of the radial head in cerebral palsy, *J Bone Joint Surg Am* 58(1):104–105, 1976.

44. Pohl M, Ruckriem S, Mehrholz J, et al.: Effectiveness of serial casting in patients with severe cerebral spasticity: a comparison study, *Arch Phys Med Rehabil* 83:784–790, 2002.

45. Pohl M, Mehrholz J, Ruckriem S: The influence of illness duration and level of consciousness on the treatment effect and complication rate of serial casting in patients with severe cerebral spasticity, *Clin Rehabil* 17:373–379, 2003.

46. Preissner KS: The effects of serial casting on spasticity: a literature review, *Occup Ther Health Care* 13(2):99–105, 2002.

47. Serghiou M, Ott S, Whitehead C, et al.: Comprehensive rehabilitation of the burn patient. In Herndon DN, editor: *Total burn care*, cd 4, St. Louis, Elsevier Inc, 2012.

48. Stevanovic M, Sharpe F: Management of established Volkmann's contracture of the forearm in children, *Hand Clin* 22(1):99–111, 2006.

49. Stoeckmann T: Casting for the person with spasticity, *Top Stroke Rehabil* 8(1):27–35, 2001.

50. Thibaut A, Chatelle C, Ziegler E, et al.: Spasticity after stroke: physiology, assessment and treatment, *Brain Inj* 27(10):1093–1105, 2013.

51. Van de Pol RJ, van Trijffel E, Lucas C: Inter-rater reliability for measurements of passive physiological range of motion of upper extremity joints is better if instruments are used: a systematic review, *J Physiother* 56(1):7–17, 2010.

52. Yang TF, Fu CP, Kao NT, et al.: Effect of botulinum toxin type A on cerebral palsy with upper limb spasticity, *Am J Phys Med Rehabil* 82(4):284–289, 2003.

53. Yarkony GM, Sahgal V: Contractures. A major complication of craniocerebral trauma, *Clin Orthop Relat Res* 219:93–96, 1987.

54. Yasukawa A: Upper extremity casting: adjunct treatment for a child with cerebral palsy hemiplegia, *Am J Occup Ther* 44(9):840–846, 1990.

55. Yasukawa A, Malas BS, Gaebler-Spira DJ: Efficacy for maintenance of elbow range of motion of two types of orthotic devices: a case series, *J Prosthet Orthot* 15:72–77, 2003.

56. Yasukawa A, Lulinski J, Thornton L, et al.: Improving elbow and wrist range of motion using a dynamic and static combination orthosis, *J Prosthet Orthot* 20(2):41–48, 2008.

57. Yasukawa A, Cassar M: Children with elbow extension and forearm rotation limitation: functional outcomes using the forearm rotation elbow orthosis, *J Prosthet Orthot* 21(3):160–166, 2009.

58. Yekutiel M, Jariwala M, Stretch P: Sensory deficit in the hands of children with cerebral palsy: a new look at assessment and prevalence, *Dev Med Child Neurol* 36:619–624, 1994.

APPENDIX 19.1 CASE STUDIES

Case Study 19.1[a]

Read the following scenario, and answer the questions based on the information in this chapter.

Ella is a 10-year-old girl who has spastic cerebral palsy (CP) and is dependent on her parents to assist her with most of her daily care. Her family includes her parents and a younger brother. She has moderate to severely increased muscle tone in all four extremities with reduced tone in her trunk. She takes oral baclofen in the morning to assist with managing her tone. Ella's functional use of her upper extremities is limited because of limited active control and both hands present with increased tone. Mother reports that during the winter months it is extremely difficult to position her wrist through the sleeves of her coat because of the flexed and myostatic contracture of her wrist. Her range of motion at both wrists is 100 degrees flexion to 60 degrees wrist flexion. Modified Ashworth Scale of her wrist flexors is 3, with considerable increase in muscle tone, and passive movement is difficult. Ella displayed severe hypertonicity with a stretch reflex felt at the beginning of range, at 85 degrees of flexion. Functional classification is 0, she does not use. Ella has been unable to be positioned in a night orthosis because of her tightly fisted hands. Ella is scheduled to be seen by her physiatrist to receive a botulinum toxin type A (BtA) injection. The physician will place the BtA into her wrist to relax the flexors and long finger flexors and to decrease the pull into flexion.

You will be following up with Ella's intervention program to address the tightness in both of her hands.

1. What are three baseline evaluations that should be used?
2. What are two different types of cast that you may consider? What is the rationale for each?
3. In what position should the wrist be placed in the initial cast?
4. How long should each cast be applied in the series?
5. What follow-up should be provided after casting?
6. What is the primary goal for casting Ella?

Case Study 19.2[a]

Paul is a 25-year-old man who was injured in a motor vehicle accident. He was hospitalized for 6 weeks and in a coma for 4 of the 6 weeks. When he was admitted for rehabilitation, Paul showed only localized response to visual and auditory stimuli. He responded to simple yes/no questions inconsistently, and displayed a mass flexor response with imposed movement with his arms.

Paul's posture was markedly asymmetrical, with his head rotated and laterally flexed to the left. The left upper extremity exhibited a strong flexor pattern, and the right was moderately involved, with minimal active movement. Minimal passive motion could be achieved with relaxation and positioning techniques, but increased spasticity/stiffness and

myostatic upper extremities deformities were present bilaterally. No spontaneous motion in the upper extremities was present with the exception of the mass flexor synergy pattern of flexion at the elbow, wrist, and hand.

Treatment goals were to decrease the spasticity, correct deformities, and mobilize the upper extremities using casting and neurophysiological treatment techniques. The typical resting position of the left extremity was 105 degrees of elbow flexion, with the wrist and fingers flexed. The right elbow is positioned in 60 degrees of elbow flexion, with the wrist flexed, and tightness of the lumbricals. Bilateral casts were indicated, but the casting schedule needed to be coordinated to avoid simultaneous casting of the upper extremities.

Significant range-of-motion gains, as well as increased volitional movement, were achieved after the casting program, right more than left upper extremity.

1. Because of the severe increased tone of the left arm, which two casts are the most appropriate to use initially?
   a. Rigid circular elbow cast
   b. Rigid circular wrist cast
   c. Long arm cast
   d. Rigid circular elbow cast with use of a cone or roll orthosis to position hand
2. The right arm was moderately involved. Which cast is the most appropriate to use initially for the right upper extremity?
   a. Rigid circular elbow cast
   b. Rigid circular wrist cast
   c. Metacarpophalangeal wrist cast
   d. Wrist cast with thumb enclosed
3. Which of the following is/are the most appropriate baseline assessment(s) during the initial inpatient rehabilitation stay? Select all that apply.
   a. Range of motion
   b. Modified Ashworth Scale
   c. Stereognosis
   d. Manual muscle test
   e. Functional arm and hand placement
4. Between the series of casts, which of the following should be focused on? Select all that apply.
   a. Remove and replace cast to incorporate gains from one cast to the next.
   b. Remove cast and let the skin breathe overnight, and cast the next morning.
   c. Measure range of motion.
   d. Evaluate the skin for any red areas or breakdown.

APPENDIX 19.2 LABORATORY EXERCISE

Laboratory Exercise 19.1

Choose one of the casts described in the chapter, and ensure that you have the necessary materials to apply and remove the cast. Before starting, determine the correct position to place your partner's hand, wrist, forearm, elbow, etc. After fitting the cast, practice educating your partner on the cast care and precautions using Table 19.4.

---

[a] See Appendix A for the answer key.

APPENDIX 19.3 REVIEW[a]

Upper Extremity Casting Competency Checkout

Therapist _____

Date: _____

1. Why are casts applied?
2. What are two contraindications for application of a cast?
3. What three factors may necessitate special consideration in application and monitoring?
4. What type of cast would you choose for the following problems?
   a. Ninety-degree elbow contracture, moderate muscle tone
   b. Humeral internal rotation, elbow flexion, pronation contracture, mild spasticity
   c. Wrist contracture with thumb-in-palm
   d. Spasticity/tightness/weakness of the lumbricals and posturing in metacarpophalangeal flexion
   e. Hypertropic scarring at anterior crease of elbow, elbow flexion contracture from burns
5. Indicate the removal technique for each of the materials listed. Options are cast saw, unravel, cutting strip, bandage scissors.
   a. Fiberglass _____
   b. Semirigid soft cast _____
   c. Delta-Cast Conformable (functional cast therapy) _____
   d. Plaster _____

6. Match the number with the letter with the use of the casting saw procedure.
   1. Explanation of cast cutter procedure
   2. Holding cast cutter and cutting
   3. Use of cast spreader
   4. Cutting padding
   5. Cutting stockinette
   6. Bivalve technique for elbow bivalve
   a. Place the bandage scissors onto the stockinette to assist with cutting so the bandage scissors do not contact the skin.
   b. Press firmly down and in.
   c. Insert in the cut area of the cast, and spread apart.
   d. Pull up the stockinette so there is no bandage scissor felt on skin.
   e. Draw on the medial and lateral epicondyles.
   f. The cast saw blade oscillates back and forth.

APPENDIX 19.4 CHECKOUT PROCEDURE

Name: _____ Date: _____

Laboratory: Application procedure staff checkout.

Choose one of the following casts to be checked out:
- Rigid circular elbow cast
- Rigid circular wrist cast
- Long arm cast
- Wrist cast with thumb enclosed
- Metacarpophalangeal (MCP) wrist cast—intrinsic plus
- MCP wrist cast—intrinsic minus
- Functional cast therapy (FCT)
  - Precast evaluation documented, physician's order, nursing notified (if inpatient)
  - Preparation of materials

---

[a] See Appendix A for the answer key.

20

Upper Extremity Prosthetics

Debra Latour
Kris M. Vacek

CHAPTER OBJECTIVES

1. Differentiate between various levels of upper extremity amputation as it relates to function.
2. Describe the many causes of an upper extremity amputation.
3. Differentiate the roles of the prosthetic team members.
4. Explain the unique role of the occupational therapist as a team member in upper extremity prosthetic rehabilitation.
5. Identify the characteristics of numerous upper extremity prosthetic devices.
6. Identify advantages and disadvantages of various upper extremity prosthetic devices.
7. Describe the phases of rehabilitation from an occupational therapy (OT) perspective.
8. Provide examples for OT intervention.
9. Explain why individuals with upper limb acquired loss or congenital difference are likely to develop secondary conditions.
10. Describe the physical and psychosocial disparities often experienced by the population.
11. Discuss strategies for marketing upper extremity prosthetics specialty area to the wider community.

KEY TERMS

biofeedback
body-powered prosthesis
componentry
contralateral limb
electrodes
externally powered prosthesis
grip force
harness
hook rubbers
hybrid prosthesis

myoelectric prosthesis
nerve entrapment
osseointegration
overuse syndrome
pattern recognition
phantom pain
phantom sensation
prosthesis
"prosthosis"
psychosocial-emotional impact

radio-frequency identification (RFID)
residual limb
socket
targeted muscle reinnervation (TMR)
terminal device (TD)
3-D printed device
voluntary closing
voluntary opening

Gary is a 52-year-old man who owns and works on his farm. Unfortunately, the drawstring to Gary's sweatshirt hood got caught in an auger and pulled his left, non-dominant hand into the auger. The surgeon completed a transhumeral-level amputation. The team of physicians caring for him sent a referral to occupational therapy to see Gary. What does the occupational therapist do? What should be expected of the occupational therapist's contribution to Gary's rehabilitation?

Orthotics and prosthetics are closely interrelated fields. This chapter serves as a resource for those therapists who serve this historically underserved population. There are approximately 2 million people in the United States who are living with a limb loss.[60,61] Approximately 185,000 amputations

occur in the United States each year.[60] The incidence of upper extremity amputation is lower than the incidence of lower extremity amputation (1:4 ratio).[5] In the population with upper limb loss, the most common loss is a partial amputation of one or more digits, with loss of one upper extremity as the next most common loss (60% at the transradial level). Every year approximately 2000 Americans experience new upper limb amputations at, or proximal to, the wrist.[4]

Approximately 50% of individuals with amputations are fitted with prostheses.[58] Of the 50% fitted with prostheses, only half actually wear the device. Experts cite numerous reasons for this trend.[76] Fit and prosthetic training appear to be the most salient factors that affect prosthetic wear.[13] Prostheses may be heavy and awkward to use. If the fit is

461

not tolerable, or if the potential wearer has not been properly trained to use the device, the prosthesis may end up on the closet shelf. The purpose of an upper limb prosthesis depends on the client's goals. However, most prostheses assist in restoring participation in meaningful functional activities, as well as improving body image and cosmesis.[86] In collaboration with the health care team, the role of the prosthetist is to provide well-fitting prosthetic devices. It is the role of the occupational therapist (OT) to assist individuals in becoming independent users of their devices. In addition, the OT can be instrumental in helping to determine the most appropriate technology to be provided and in assisting the client with developing realistic expectations of the technology.[2,3]

Unfortunately, only a small number of health care providers have extensive knowledge of the rehabilitation of the person with an upper extremity amputation. Typically, therapists may encounter few individuals with upper extremity amputations. Thus it is difficult to remain abreast of the current prosthetic trends and technological developments that affect how therapists promote the maximal level of independence for clients with upper extremity amputations. However, OTs can make a substantial difference in the lives of individuals with amputations if they possess knowledge of the various factors that impact the life of a person with an amputation.

Individuals with upper limb loss or congenital difference (ULL/D) are at risk for experiencing further disparity due to overuse of the sound side. Several studies have documented the presence of pain and musculoskeletal conditions affecting the function of the sound arm in individuals with unilateral ULL/D.[9,46,62] Gambrell[38] conducted a review of the literature noting the consequences and importance of prevention of overuse syndrome with recommendations for a team approach, emphasizing practitioner responsibility to educate patients to the likelihood of overuse and methods that impede development.

Many individuals who experience acquired limb loss report that they were given little to no information by medical professionals.[4,5] Recently Sheehan and Gondo[74] reported on the effect of limb loss in the United States, recognizing that each well-trained member of the specialized amputee rehabilitation team has a specific and important role in the care and recovery of people with limb loss. They cited the need for interventions to address secondary conditions affecting physical and mental health because current standard medical treatments often exclude psychosocial interventions. The authors emphasized that "those with limb loss in America have been forgotten in the health care system"[74](p. 9) because there is no active medical surveillance.

Therapists who treat persons with orthotic needs will naturally be called upon to provide services to persons with upper extremity amputations. Thus it is important for therapists to know how to access the information needed to provide OT to individuals with upper extremity amputations.

This chapter addresses the following content:
- Reasons and causes for amputations
- General knowledge of upper extremity amputations and their impact on function
- Roles of team members and the importance of collaboration
- Various prosthetic options and components
- Goals for OT intervention throughout the prosthetic rehabilitation process
- Psychological and social issues of clients with amputations
- Upper extremity prosthetic intervention for children
- Marketing strategies and recommendations:

REASONS AND CAUSES FOR UPPER EXTREMITY AMPUTATIONS

The causes of upper extremity amputations differ from lower extremity amputations. Lower extremity amputations are largely a result of vascular disease. Most of upper extremity amputations result from trauma (69%), and a majority of these are due to war causalities[30,31] with other causes attributed to disease (27%) or congenital malformation (4%).[30] It is estimated that the number of individuals living with limb loss will more than double by 2050. This is largely due to the rise of vascular disorders.[30,89]

GENERAL KNOWLEDGE OF UPPER EXTREMITY AMPUTATIONS AND THEIR IMPACT ON FUNCTION

Amputation Levels

Fig. 20.1 provides an outline of the various amputation levels, along with their abbreviations. Older terminology included above elbow (AE) and below elbow (BE); however, newer terminology cites the anatomical level of amputation.[40,77] For example, AE is referred to as *transhumeral,* and BE is referred to as *transradial.* The level of amputation directly impacts function.

With levels of amputation there is an inverse relationship between the amputation level and function. The more distal the amputation, the greater the functional ability of the extremity remains. Consequently, less is demanded of the prosthesis with increasingly distal amputations.[40] For example, an individual who has an amputation at the midhumeral level may be functionally able to use shoulder internal and external rotation along with other shoulder motions. However, the individual lacks the functional motions of elbow flexion/extension and forearm supination/ pronation, causing functional limitations. In addition, amputations through the joint, such as at the shoulder, elbow, or wrist, present challenges of fit with componentry to provide the function of the particular joint. For example, if the residual limb is amputated through the elbow (or too close to it), there is not enough space for a prosthetic elbow component; the concern is that the prosthetic device will appear to be asymmetrical to the contralateral limb. Regardless of level,

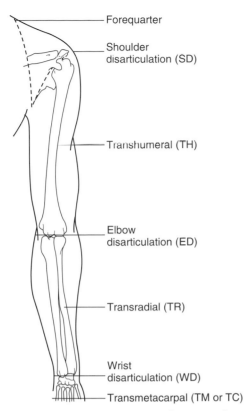

- Forequarter
- Shoulder disarticulation (SD)
- Transhumeral (TH)
- Elbow disarticulation (ED)
- Transradial (TR)
- Wrist disarticulation (WD)
- Transmetacarpal (TM or TC)

Fig. 20.1 Levels of upper extremity amputation.

prostheses help to compensate for the lost motions, but limitations remain. For example, when an individual with a midhumeral amputation wants to receive money from a cashier, more effort is required because of the functional limitations in motion. Compare this with someone whose limb loss is at the transradial level, where often some forearm motion is retained, allowing greater functional capacity of the upper extremity. More specifically, positioning and locking the elbow in flexion is necessary for the individual with the transhumeral loss. Next, the person manually rotates the **terminal device (TD)** to the palm-up position with the sound side. Finally, the person is ready to perform the act of receiving the money. Conversely, an individual with an amputation at the wrist level is functionally able to pronate and supinate, flex and extend the elbow, and retain full shoulder function in the completion of activities of daily living (ADLs). The ability to pronate and supinate serves as a substantial advantage. Supination and pronation enable the person with the amputation to turn the prosthetic hand palm up as if to receive money from a cashier without the substitution movements of shoulder external rotation.

If an individual chooses to wear a prosthesis, the level of amputation appears to impact satisfaction. In a survey conducted in 2006, 93% of 109 respondents with an upper extremity amputation reported owning a prosthesis, whereas 12% of those respondents reported they did not wear it regularly.[4] A majority of those surveyed reported satisfaction with their prosthesis, but one-third reported dissatisfaction with it.[4] Contributing factors to dissatisfaction specifically include socket fit, comfort level, appearance, weight, and ease of use.

Additionally, one-fourth of those surveyed received therapy, and the average number of visits was 25. Twenty percent of those who did not receive therapy reported cost as the leading factor preventing them from receiving the services they needed.[4]

ROLE OF TEAM MEMBERS AND THE IMPORTANCE OF COLLABORATION

The team treating clients with amputations must have knowledge of the diverse upper extremity prosthetic technology to facilitate success. The key team members consist of the client with the amputation, the prosthetist, and the therapist. Other important members include the surgeon, case manager or life care planner, psychologist, physical therapist, and the insurer/reimbursement source. A team approach combines expertise and experience, creating a synergy of professionalism, with team members working together and promoting the maximal level of independence for the individual. The primary goal of therapy is to provide the individual with the proper tools and techniques to regain independence; however, OT is only one dimension of the entire process. The best results in upper extremity rehabilitation include interdisciplinary collaboration.[12]

The Client

The most important member of the team is the person with the amputation. Throughout the assessment and intervention process, several key factors of the client are considered, including specific abilities, characteristics, or beliefs.[3] Factors such as the level of amputation, musculature, skin condition, range of motion, ability to learn, motivation, and values all contribute to the degree of participation in occupations.

The client's goals, desires, and needs establish the foundation for which the team develops the intervention plan. Clients' priorities for rehabilitation vary. It is important to ensure that clients are realistic with their expectations and are well educated in the prosthetic options available to them. Education can come from both the prosthetist and OT. The prosthetist discusses the various prosthetic options available, whereas the OT discusses the functional aspects of each device. This process is important because it helps the key team members formulate the individual intervention plan necessary for successful prosthetic delivery and use.[55] For example, an individual with a transhumeral amputation who works full-time in a factory and desires to return to work will have different needs from an individual with a transradial amputation who is a homemaker. The type of prosthesis selected differs, depending on a precise analysis of the client's desire to participate in meaningful occupations.[3]

The Prosthetist

Orthotics and prosthetics are closely interrelated fields. Forty-one percent of practitioners certified by the American Board for Certification in Orthotics, Prosthetics and Pedorthics hold credentials in both orthotics and prosthetics, and fewer practitioners specialize in upper extremity prosthetic fabrication.[2] Because the incidence of upper extremity amputations is less than lower extremity amputations, it is important for the prosthetist to have specialized training and experience in fabricating and fitting upper extremity prostheses. Prosthetists have knowledge of the technology and prosthetic **componentry** available. Technology for upper extremity prosthetics has significantly evolved since 1976 due to research and development in related technology, such as cell phones, computers, and video games.[17] Prosthetists are experts when it comes to fit and fabrication. Upon prosthetic delivery, prosthetists introduce, educate, and orient the clients about the controls and functions, all of which should be reinforced by the OT. In an ideal setting, prosthetists and therapists collaborate throughout the entire intervention process from assessment of prosthetic needs to return to occupational performance.

The Occupational Therapist

Unfortunately, only a small number of therapists have extensive knowledge of the rehabilitation of the person with an upper extremity amputation. In many practice settings, therapists rarely treat clients with upper extremity amputations. Thus, it is difficult to remain abreast of the current prosthetic and technological developments. Such advances affect how therapists promote the maximal level of independence for these clients. However, OTs can make a substantial difference in individuals with amputations when they possess knowledge of prosthetic intervention.

Occupational therapists' expertise relates to function and occupational performance. Therapists typically work with clients throughout the entire prosthetic rehabilitation process. Each phase of recovery presents its own challenges and demands. Without proper therapy the benefits of prosthetic use may be limited. For example, the therapist may see the client immediately following surgery to address postsurgical issues, including pain, edema, wound healing, and shaping of the residual limb. In addition, OT interventions may beneficially impact successful transfer of hand dominance, awareness and prevention of secondary conditions, and changes in body image. The OT plays an important role as the client explores the various prosthetic devices. Finally, the therapist provides prosthetic rehabilitation upon delivery of the prosthesis and assists the client in achievement of occupational performance.[50]

The therapist reinforces and builds on residual movement, developing functional applications of the prosthesis to address the distinct ADLs (e.g., brushing teeth) and instrumental ADLs (IADLs; e.g., driving) of everyone.[80] The therapist is responsible for ensuring that the client knows how to clean and maintain the prosthesis. In addition, the therapist provides opportunities for the client to practice using the prosthesis in specific daily activities. The therapist focuses on bilateral activities. Often after amputation the individual becomes successful in performing some ADLs unilaterally. Thus therapy must begin early in the rehabilitation process to facilitate use of the prosthesis in bilateral activities.[73]

Initial prosthetic training begins with a reorientation to the prosthesis and basic open-and-close control. Training then includes controlled grasp, such as opening the close control in small increments to grasp small items and then more fully to grasp larger items. Training emphasizes grasping objects of varied texture and density to be handled. Sessions incorporate work on prehension and timing of release. Functional and appropriate tasks are encouraged and require the client to use the prosthesis for gross and fine motor activities. Training also emphasizes drills and tasks to achieve these skills at different heights and in a variety of planes and positions.[47,63] With the combined efforts of the team members, the appropriate prosthetic components are chosen so that the individual can achieve goals through therapy, practice, and education.

PROSTHETIC OPTIONS AND COMPONENTS

A prosthetic device cannot mechanically duplicate the amount of function, reliability, and aesthetic quality that the human upper extremity naturally provides. However, prostheses can improve functional abilities. To provide the appropriate prosthesis, a fundamental understanding of the components is necessary. Health care providers must continually stay abreast of prosthetic developments.

Generally six categories of prosthetic options are available for the person with an upper extremity amputation. The options include (1) no prosthesis; (2) a passive functional aesthetic prosthesis; (3) activity-specific prosthesis; (4) a cable-driven body-powered prosthesis; (5) an externally powered, electrically controlled prosthesis with myoelectric sensors and specialized switches; and (6) a **hybrid prosthesis** that may combine types of control. Table 20.1 outlines the pros and cons of each prosthetic option.

No Prosthesis

Wearing no prosthesis is one approach, and for some individuals it is the best option. For example, an individual may not be able to tolerate the prosthesis for reasons such as residual limb hypersensitivity, soft tissue adhesions, and excessive scarring.[9] Reasons documented in the literature for prosthetic rejection include limited usefulness, weight, and residual limb and socket discomfort.[54,87] Individuals choosing not to wear prostheses may find advantages and disadvantages with this option, which are found in Table 20.1.

Advantages of no prosthesis include increased proprioceptive and sensory input. Disadvantages include limited functional ability, bimanual task difficulty, and the potential for development of **overuse syndrome, nerve entrapment,** or vascular damage in the **contralateral limb.**[68] Some individuals do not wear prostheses because (1) they do not know their options, (2) they had a negative first prosthetic experience, (3) they lack funds, or (4) they are reluctant to undergo surgery for a prosthetic fit and reduction of hypersensitivity.[4]

Passive Functional Aesthetic Prosthesis

A passive prosthesis option is common for individuals who have had amputation distal to the elbow in that they may

TABLE 20.1   Advantages and Disadvantages of Prosthetic Options

Prosthetic Option	Advantages	Disadvantages
No prosthesis	Maintain full proprioception and sensation	Limited functional ability Difficult to perform bimanual tasks
Passive prosthesis	Lightweight Minimal (if any) harnessing No cables; low maintenance Static function: support, stabilize Social function	Prosthesis has no prehension abilities Difficult to perform bimanual tasks
Activity-specific prosthesis	Lightweight Minimal (if any) harnessing No cables; low maintenance Static function: support, stabilize Quick disconnect Crossover functional purposes Robust Reduced maintenance, costs	
Body-powered prosthesis	Heavy-duty construction and function Reduced maintenance cost Proprioception Refer to specifics of VC vs VO terminal devices	Restrictive/uncomfortable harness Poor cosmesis Restrictive functional work area Limited grip force (VO)
Externally powered prosthesis	Unlimited work area Function cosmetic restoration Increased grip force Harness system reduced or absent Increased comfort More modern, high-tech appeal Interchangeable components Development of technology to provide for individual custom fabrication	Battery maintenance Increased weight Susceptible to damage from moisture Increased cost Battery life

VC, Voluntary closing; *VO,* voluntary opening.

maintain elbow flexion and extension and forearm pronation and supination. In this case the obvious purpose may appear to be aesthetic. However, a passive prosthesis provides some degree of function, such as to support and stabilize objects, and digits of a passive prosthesis can be adjusted to assist with activities, such as typing, carrying a purse or a document, or operating the gearshift in an automobile.[67] This type of prosthesis is often used as a first prosthesis for children as young as 4 months of age. A passive prosthesis has many benefits, including its light weight, minimal (if any) harnessing, no cables, and low maintenance. Disadvantages include lack of active grasp and difficulty in performing some bimanual tasks.[52]

Activity-Specific Prosthesis

Many individuals are interested in completing a specific activity. Sometimes the OT fabricates a tool of thermoplastic material or other material that can be attached to a cuff or to the existing TD to serve a specific function. At other times, collaboration with the prosthetist is necessary to obtain a specific TD or a sophisticated adaptation. Activity-specific upper limb prosthetic technology is typically static. The TD attaches to the forearm unit and allows for function to perform specific activities that may include personal care tasks

(e.g., feeding and grooming), instrumental tasks (e.g., cooking, woodworking, and gardening), and diverse recreational activities.[67] Some of the devices have "crossover" functions. For example, a device used for bicycling may also be used to grasp the handles of a shopping cart, a stroller, or even a lawnmower, thus enhancing the functional envelope of the technology. This technology often is robust and lightweight and offers quick release. It typically does not require harnessing or cables and is low maintenance. The activity-specific prosthesis is often suspended with a pin-lock style of liner or a Neoprene sleeve.

Body-Powered Prosthesis

The **body-powered prosthesis** is sturdy and allows for prehension. Body-powered upper limb prostheses are actuated by body motion, which generates tension in a cable. The cable courses from a shoulder harness through a housing to a prosthetic component, such as a hook or elbow. In other words, the active movements of the shoulder and arm cause the tension in the cable to open and close the hand or hand-like component (hook) as shown in Fig. 20.2. Therapists help individuals with the amputation learn the names of the basic components, such as the figure-eight harness, cable, elbow unit, wrist unit, and TD.

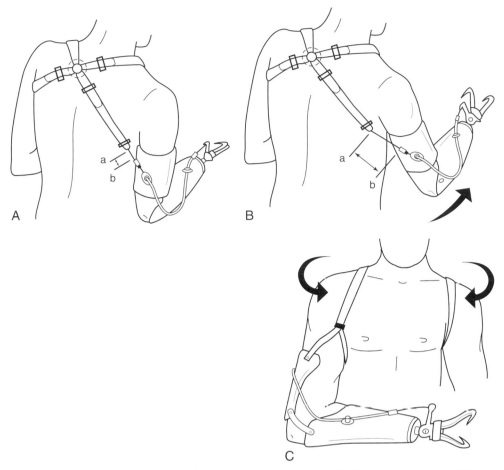

Fig. 20.2 Body motions used to transmit force to terminal device (TD). A, Glenohumeral flexion. B, Biscapular abduction. C, Scapular adduction/retraction.

Benefits of a body-powered prosthesis include its heavy-duty function and construction, decreased maintenance cost, and increased proprioceptive input. Disadvantages may include the restrictive uncomfortable harness, potential for nerve entrapment or compression, decreased aesthetic appearance, restricted functional work area (Fig. 20.3), and limited **grip force** (see Table 20.1). Body-powered TDs generally weigh less than the externally powered prostheses because they lack the heavy motors and circuitry placed within them to operate the myoelectric signals.

The Harness

The purpose of the **harness** is to suspend the prosthesis on the **residual limb.** It transmits force from the body to the prosthesis for independent operation of the prosthetic components.[57] The body-powered prosthesis always requires harnessing. There are two primary types of harness: a figure-eight and a chest strap. The figure-eight harness passes over the shoulder, across the back, and under the contralateral axilla. "The ring lies flat in the back, inferior to C7 and just to the sound side of the center of the spine."[76]

The standard figure-eight shoulder harness for the upper extremity has an axilla loop on the sound side that is commonly uncomfortable and can cause numbness and nerve damage.[24] The chest strap offers an alternative method of

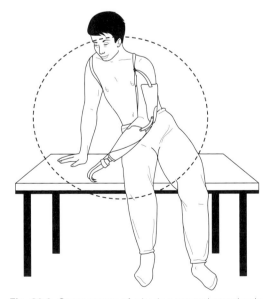

Fig. 20.3 Components of a body-powered prosthesis.

harnessing. It travels across the back, under the contralateral axilla, and across the chest. It is important that the harness, most commonly figure-eight, figure-nine, or chest strap, be tight enough to activate the TD without excessive effort and loose enough to be comfortable, allow freedom of movement of both arms and shoulders, and not entrap the thoracic outlet.

Long-term wear and inappropriate fit may cause discomfort or physical damage. The harness has been found to limit the functional work envelope, which is the space in front of the person who is able to use the prosthesis successfully for functional tasks. Harness systems limit successful prehension when the TD is outside the functional work area. With the body-powered prosthesis, function can be limited above the head, behind the back, and near the ground, primarily because of the restricting harness (see Fig. 20.3). The prosthesis functions because of the ability to move in these planes.

An alternative to traditional harnessing is the Scapular Cutaneous Anchor technology, developed by an OT who also presents with upper limb congenital difference and who is a long-term prosthesis user. The Scapular Cutaneous Anchor is simple technology that adheres to the back in the area between the spine and the scapula on the same side as the limb difference or loss. This location on the back allows movement of the scapula and shoulder to control the TD, thus displacing discomfort or damage in the opposite axilla. It also permits function above the head, at the waist, behind the back, and near the ground.

Discomfort and neurological and musculoskeletal disorders can result from inefficient harness design[21] and long-term wear. After the user has worn a harness for years, the axilla of the sound side experiences increased force and pressure to operate the prosthesis repetitively throughout the day. This can result in neurological and/or vascular damage. A strong case can be made for providing an externally powered prosthesis that either eliminates or reduces the harnessing. This prevents the risk of long-term nerve damage on the sound side. More importantly, use of diverse prosthetic technologies adds to the functional toolkit of the user as no one prosthesis can replicate the diverse functions of the hand.

The prosthetist is responsible for fabrication of the harness, and the therapist occasionally may make minor adjustments to improve function. Sometimes several harness options are attempted to find the type of system that best fits the amputee. It is often a trial-and-error process. Another important factor is the awareness of the increased workload in the remaining arm, which may produce symptoms ranging from minor aches to serious conditions, such as nerve entrapment and overuse syndrome.[46]

The Socket

The **socket** is the part of the prosthesis that intimately fits over the individual's residual limb. It is the connection between the prosthesis and the individual's body. The socket is fabricated from an exact mold of the residual limb, and it is fabricated from various types of laminate or thermoplastic material. Development of high-temperature rigid plastic materials has made it possible to have total contact on the skin and allow decreased weight and increased durability. The use of carbon graphite and the introduction of flexible thermoplastics have resulted in sockets that are more comfortable, lighter, and more durable and have made soft sockets with windows possible. The prosthetist makes modifications over bony prominences and areas susceptible to torque and shear forces.[6] Typically three to four sockets will be fabricated before the final one is delivered.

Intimate socket fit provides a stable foundation of support necessary to transfer forces from the TD. It provides evenly distributed pressure on the residual limb, which prevents skin breakdown or pressure sores. In the past decade a multitude of design innovations have been incorporated, which have resulted in developing better comfort, suspension, stability, and range of motion. The new fitting techniques and socket designs appear to be more efficient for force of transmission and motion capture and more functionally consistent than traditional sockets.[1] Occasionally the prosthetist instructs the individual to wear the socket before all components are attached because it increases wearing tolerance and facilitates reshaping of the residual limb.

As the person with the amputation ages, physical and physiological changes occur. The person may experience weight loss or gain or muscle bulk increase or decrease. These changes have an impact on the size and condition of the residual limb, and the socket may no longer fit as it should. A new socket must be fabricated to fit the exact shape of the residual limb when changes occur. When a new socket is fabricated, it replaces the poorly fitting one in the individual's current prosthesis. An entirely new prosthesis is not needed because the socket is removable and replaceable. This saves on cost. The wearer of a body-powered prosthesis may benefit from using a second sheath or sock made of either a fabric or a gel-like substance to manage poor skin integrity, prevent breakdown, absorb moisture, or provide padding.

The Liners

Liners may be used for comfort and/or for suspension. Liners may be as simple as a sock or fabricated from silicone or other such materials. Depending on several factors, including the level of limb loss/difference, and other componentry, liners with a pin-lock system help to keep the prosthesis on the residual limb. Some individuals opt to not wear a liner or sock and prefer what is called a "skin fit."

The Cable

The harness allows placement of the cable, which is the transmitting force that operates the prosthesis. Body-powered prostheses are operated by body motion that generates tension in the cable. The cable is routed from the harness through a housing to the TD or elbow.[21] The primary movement to operate the prosthesis is glenohumeral flexion. As the individual flexes the humerus, the TD opens. As the individual returns the humerus to neutral, the hook rubbers cause the TD to close. When the individual wishes to open the TD closer to the body, biscapular abduction is used, and adduction or retraction of the scapula allows the TD to close (Fig. 20.4). The following quotation from a client with an upper extremity amputation who uses a voluntary-opening

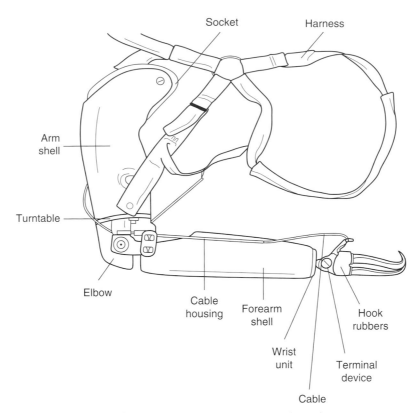

Socket   Harness

Arm shell

Turntable

Elbow   Cable housing   Forearm shell   Hook rubbers

Wrist unit   Terminal device

Cable

Fig. 20.4 Functional work area (body-powered prosthesis).

(VO) TD highlights the importance of the cable system for functional tasks:

The rubber bands on my hooks regulate tension I put on objects. To force the hook open, I first lock the elbow in the desired position. Then I proceed to bring my shoulder forward, putting tension on the cables. After I have grasped the desired object, I bring my shoulder back to the original position.[27]

Cables need periodic replacement when they fray or break. Cable replacement is generally the most common repair needed for the body-powered prosthesis wearer.[27] The OT and the client should know how to replace an old cable with a new one. The process is simple, involving removal of the old cable and reattachment of the new cable to the TD and the harness. It is beneficial for the client to have two or three spare cables at home so that replacement is convenient.

Terminal Device

The TD is the hand component and appears in the form of a hand or a hook. Most body-powered prosthetic hands open and close in a three-point prehension pattern. The prosthetic hooks open and close in a lateral or tip pinch prehension pattern, depending on positioning of the TD. Therapists should be familiar with TD options because they will most likely introduce the person with the amputation to the available options and provide education in their use.

Generally the initial goals of the prosthetist are to fit the person who has had an amputation with a standard prosthesis. The person with the amputation then requires time

to adjust and become an independent user of the prosthetic device. There are two basic TD options, and each is available in two different control systems. Typically an individual has some form of a hand and/or a hook, which can be interchangeable if using the same control system. For example, the client uses the hand-like TD for basic ADLs and uses the hook-like TD for more challenging activities such as quilting or changing a tire. Every TD has its pros and cons. Differences exist between the hand and hook TDs (Table 20.2). The hand-like TD may appear to some to be more aesthetically pleasing. However, digits 3, 4, and 5 are not movable, often occluding vision, impairing function, and providing increased bulk. The hook-like TD allows for successful fine motor prehension, access to visual input, less bulk, and more durability. However, it may be less aesthetically appealing than the hand-like TD.

Voluntary-Opening and Voluntary-Closing Terminal Devices

Important to the type of function is the method of control. The TD may be **voluntary opening** or **voluntary closing.** VO devices are positioned in a closed position, and the user works to open it against the resistance of elastic bands. Closure is implemented by relaxing the control and allowing the elastic bands to pull the opened TD closed. Grip strength with this technology is dependent on the number of elastic bands being used. Each elastic band is equivalent to approximately 1 to 1.5 pounds of force. One must remember that the user has to work against this force to open the TD. For example, five bands might lead to more than 5 pounds of pinch strength,

TABLE 20.2 Advantages and Disadvantages of the Hand and Hook Terminal Devices

Terminal Device	Advantages	Disadvantages
Hand	Cosmetically appealing	Digits 3, 4, and 5 are nonfunctional
		Tendency to impair fine motor manipulation
		Vision obstruction
Hook	Superior fine motor prehension	May be aesthetically unappealing
	Less bulky	
	Durable	
	No vision obstruction	
Voluntary-opening		Must resist force to open
		Limited grip strength
Voluntary-closing	Efficient, ergonomic operation	
	Grip strength control	
	More intuitive control	

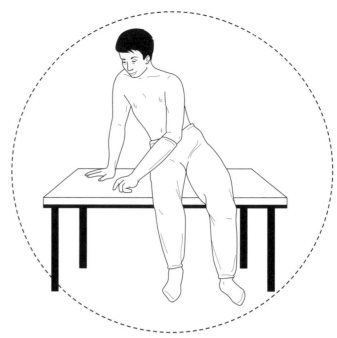

Fig. 20.5 Functional work area (externally powered prosthesis).

but the user must consistently and repetitively resist the force to access use of the device. Voluntary-closing (VC) devices are positioned in the open position, resembling the at-rest position like the natural hand. The user works to close the device and can regulate the amount of grip strength exerted. The user can control the device to use a light grasp (such as when holding a child's hand) or stronger grasp (such as to hold a shopping bag). For sustained closure the user might use a locking system that conserves energy. VC systems appear to offer greater efficiency because they exert less load on the user to access function.

Using a body-powered VO device, the grip can vary from 5 to 20 pounds, depending on the number of hook rubbers used. **Hook rubbers** are like thick, wide rubber bands providing resistance to the grip of the TD. Each rubber band provides 1 pound of grip force, consequently increasing the amount of pressure placed in the axilla on the contralateral side. VC devices can generate grip strength of 60 pounds or greater and are often actuated using bungee-type cords or springs. New technology is emerging that incorporates the features of both VO and VC devices.

The Glove

The glove is the cosmetic covering of the hand-like TD. Gloves are made of either latex or silicone substances and are removable and replaceable. Differences exist between the two types of glove. Latex gloves are sturdy and come in 10 to 15 shades of color. Individuals are matched to the shade that corresponds to their skin tone. Latex gloves easily absorb stains that do not wash off. However, latex gloves are more durable than silicone gloves.

A silicone glove is custom fabricated to match the individual in terms of shape, size, and coloring. It is difficult to differentiate between a silicone glove and a human hand by

sight. Such a glove is truly a work of art. Silicone gloves are more costly and fragile than latex gloves. It is more difficult to permanently stain a silicone glove. However, they tear easily. Persons who have had an amputation generally request the silicone glove because of its life-like appearance. Because silicone gloves are more expensive, funding for a silicone glove is difficult to obtain.

Externally Powered Prosthesis

The **externally powered prosthesis** is another prosthetic option. The externally powered prosthesis is also called a **myoelectric prosthesis** because it operates from the electromyographic (EMG) signal transmitted from the muscles of the residual limb. An externally powered prosthesis has several differences from the body-powered prosthesis, which are outlined in Table 20.1. Beneficial characteristics of a myoelectric prosthesis include an unlimited work area (Fig. 20.5),[25] functional cosmetic restoration, increased grip force, elimination of harnessing, increased comfort, interchangeable componentry, and individualized custom fabrication. Thus myoelectric control is most commonly used when possible.[26,43] Disadvantages of a myoelectric prosthesis include increased weight, increased cost, increased maintenance, and increased risk for damage.

The externally powered prosthesis is composed of various components, as shown in Fig. 20.6. The components include a socket, a forearm shell, electrodes, battery, glove, and TD.

The Harness

Most myoelectric prosthetic devices do not require a harness. Occasionally a harness system is required if it is difficult to fit and maintain contact between the electrodes and the muscle signal or if the socket is loose because of weight loss or other factors. Because the harness system is either eliminated or

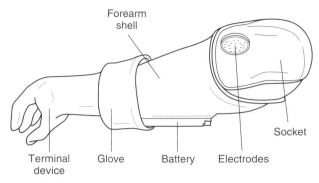

Fig. 20.6 Components of an externally powered prosthesis.

reduced, the functional work area is expanded to include the areas above the head, behind the back, and near the ground compared with the body-powered prosthesis. The Scapular Cutaneous Anchor can also be used to secure electrodes and linear transducers and may be a compelling option because it does not limit the functional envelope.[45,46]

Externally Powered Prosthetic Controls

The externally powered prosthetic socket is unique in that it has **electrodes** that detect the EMG signals of the muscle. The electrodes are mounted directly in the walls of the flexible socket. The EMG signal stimulates the motor in the prosthesis to produce a desired motion. Prosthetic technology for clients with upper extremity acquired loss or congenital differences has dramatically changed over the past decade. The main changes have occurred in components, socket fabrication, fitting techniques, suspension systems, and sources of power and electronic controls.[34,51]

There are a variety of electrodes available. Some are more sensitive than others in detecting the muscle EMG and controlling the movement of the TD. Through the collaborative effort of the team, the best-suited electrodes are determined. Single- or dual-site control systems are available as well as pattern recognition and radio-frequency identification. A single-site system is used if the client cannot differentiate and isolate control of two separate and opposing muscles for electrode sites. This may be beneficial for persons who are cognitively unable to control the dual-site system, such as with young children. For example, the TD remains in the closed position when the individual's muscles are relaxed and open when the muscle contracts. Thus if the individual wanted to grasp an object, he or she would contract the muscle to open the TD, position it around the desired object, and relax. Upon relaxation the TD automatically closes and remains closed until the next muscle contraction.[66]

Commonly a dual-site control system is preferred over a single-site system. The dual-site control system is activated by two separate muscle contractions. For example, the individual with a transradial amputation will most likely contract the wrist extensor muscle group to open the TD and the wrist flexor muscle group to close the TD. The TD can remain in any position if the muscle signals are absent. For example, the same individual can open the TD with contraction of the wrist extensors. Once the muscles are relaxed, the TD will

stay open as if to shake the hand of a friend. As soon as the wrist flexors are contracted, the TD will close. With this system electrodes can be embedded in the liner to offer contact, suspension, and comfort. A sheath or sock cannot be worn because it would interrupt the connection between the muscle and the electrode.

Pattern recognition. Many muscles work in concert to move the arms and hands. The muscles contract in unique ways and generate small amounts of electrical activity called myoelectricity. The patterns of electrical activity are unique for each movement and can be detected by electrodes placed on the surface of the skin. For example, the pattern of myoelectric activity recorded on the forearm during hand opening is different than the pattern recorded while the hand is closing.[15] For those with upper limb loss or difference, remaining muscles can produce these signal patterns. This is called **pattern recognition.** Specialized software interprets the signals to control the arm and hand movement of a prosthesis. Because the command signals can be unique to each user, the technology provides intuitive control of multiple prosthetic movements.[23]

Pattern recognition works best when it has many myoelectric signals to listen to and to interpret. Thus electrode placement is not the same as with conventional single- or dual-site prostheses. For example, there is not an exclusive "hand open" or "hand close" electrode; rather, the system interprets the information from all electrodes. It then accurately decodes the user's intent for movement. The system currently reads eight myoelectric signals using passive electrode dome contacts (sometimes called remote electrodes) and a single wire harness to connect them all.[23]

Like traditional myo-systems, pattern recognition requires (1) the ability to achieve good skin-electrode contact within a prosthesis and (2) the ability of the user and practitioner to learn and understand the mechanism of control. Pattern recognition is currently used by individuals with upper limb loss or congenital difference at the levels of shoulder disarticulation, transhumeral, and transradial.

Radio-frequency identification. Some externally powered TDs are controlled by using wireless communication known as **radio-frequency identification (RFID).** This system involves an RFID reader and a tag. The tag has information stored in its memory, and the reader (using an antenna) interprets this information. RFID technology is used by the public in many ways, such as to control building access, manage stock, and bill for use on toll roads. It is now applied to control the upper limb myoelectric prosthesis. Each tag is programmed with a specific grip pattern. The tag is strategically placed in an area where the user will implement the particular grip. For example, a tag programmed with a trigger grip pattern will be placed on a bottle of window cleaning solution. The RFID system works well with multiarticulating TDs.[44]

Terminal devices. Like body-powered TDs, myoelectric TDs are available in hand- and hook-like presentations and may be VO or VC. The standard myoelectric hand offers a basic open-close function with a three-jaw chuck type of grasp. The fourth and fifth digits do not move. Electric hooks are available in different styles and configurations. Generally these devices are not waterproof, although some manufacturers may offer a protective sleeve. Externally powered TDs have a greater opening range, allowing for the ability to grasp objects of larger size. The externally powered prosthesis provides the ability to use prehension capabilities in all planes. This contributes to the expansion of the functional work area to include space above the head, behind the back, and near the ground. The externally powered TD generally provides grip strength of approximately 20 to 30 pounds.

Multiarticulating terminal device. Advancements in technology offer exciting options in the form of multiarticulating hands. Although these prosthetic hands cannot replicate all the functions of the natural hand, they do offer access to more grip patterns with greater articulation. All the digits in these hands move and are integrated into the diverse patterns. These hands integrate with the pattern recognition and RFID control systems.

The battery. The battery provides the energy for the externally powered prosthesis. Lithium-polymer battery technology advancements have improved the ease of externally powered prostheses. The lithium-polymer batteries are 80% lighter and 70% smaller and offer 30% more storage capacity than nickel-cadmium batteries.[17]

Other joints. The singular prosthesis is made up of many components and is relative to the level of loss or difference experienced by the user. The individual with transradial difference will likely benefit from componentry that offers wrist function and hand function. This chapter is focused on the TDs, but other joint movements are important for the total function of the upper limb. Individuals with higher levels of loss need elbow flexion and extension and shoulder movement. These functions are vital to being able to accomplish ADLs and IADLs. It is important that the OT incorporate these movements and functions of the prosthetic components into the plan of care.

Elbow. Elbow components offer flexion and extension and are available for body-powered and myoelectric control. The body-powered options may require a shoulder shrug or a ballistic forward flexion to activate, or there may be a pull switch or locking mechanism. Although the body movements described may seem unnatural, it may be inconvenient to use the intact hand to actuate the elbow control, particularly during bimanual tasks. Electric options may offer smoother and more efficient movement, but the components add weight to the prosthesis.

Shoulder. Shoulder joints are available for body-powered and myoelectric control, but the movement offered is limited primarily to forward flexion/extension and internal/external rotation. There are different ways to control the body-powered technology, such as a nudge switch or scapular movement. Although the electric options may offer smoother and more efficient movement, the components add weight to the prosthesis. Cumulatively, the externally powered prosthesis could weigh more than 10 pounds.

New Technologies

Emerging technologies impact the performance and the functional outcome for users of prosthetic devices. One such intervention is **osseointegration.**[56] Osseointegration is a surgical procedure that provides "the structural linkage made at the contact point where human bone and the surface of a synthetic, often titanium based implant meet."[56] A type of pin is implanted into the end of the bone and extends through the skin to lock into a prosthesis.

Another intervention is **targeted muscle reinnervation (TMR)**, in which residual nerves from the amputated limb are surgically transferred to reinnervate new muscle targets that have otherwise lost their function. The results of this procedure work well with pattern recognition and improve the control of the upper limb prosthesis.[22]

3-D Printing

Advances in upper limb prosthetic technology offer the consumer added options that may even include access to the technology itself. Additive manufacturing (AM), also known as 3-D printing, has many benefits as well as limitations. AM permits the production of shapes that are complex and that would likely be expensive, if not cost-prohibitive, to reproduce. It has the potential to reduce both the costs and the time associated with manufacturing. There are many forms of AM; one method, fused deposition modeling, has been used to create technology for children with upper limb differences. With this method, plastic is heated and transferred through a hose to create a model one layer at a time. The temperature and humidity of the manufacturing environment must be strictly controlled to manage the structural integrity of the device. If the plastic cools too quickly, the model becomes brittle; however, if it does not cool quickly enough, the model's shape can deform. In either case these factors can negatively affect the quality of the device and its usefulness.[88]

3-D printing technology is referred to as "disruptive" because the impact of reduced costs and decreased time from design to production has disturbed the manufacturing process. This technology has been disruptive to the providers and users of prostheses. Medical devices must meet U.S. Food and Drug Administration (FDA) regulations to help ensure patient safety. Prosthetic componentry are medical devices approved by the FDA and are fit to the user by a prosthetist who has undergone the rigors of academic and clinical preparation as well as national professional certification. **3-D printed devices** are not always fabricated or fit by such professionals. The orthotics and prosthetics (O&P) organizations, with the FDA, are addressing areas related to:

1. "Provision of clinical O&P services by untrained, uncertified, and unlicensed individuals;
2. Manufacturing and distribution of unregulated 3D-printed medical devices; and
3. Lack of institutional review board (IRB) oversight for human subjects testing of 3D-printed investigational medical devices."[11]

Although these devices are not typically provided by OTs, practitioners may be requested to train its usage with particular relevance to addressing ADLs. As with a more traditionally fabricated prosthesis, the OT practitioner should check the fit of the device and inspect the functionality of it. Clients should be advised and counseled about issues such as independent donning and doffing, care of the device, and skin inspection. Depending on the fabrication and features of the device, the OT may use different techniques, such as tenodesis-type action, to control the 3D-printed hand. Should the device offer a body-powered or an externally powered feature, the relevant training strategies would apply. Users of the device should immediately contact the fabricator if there are any problems with fit or function of the device.[11]

THE PROSTHETIC REHABILITATION PROCESS

The educational background of OTs includes motor control, motor learning, and movement as they relate to the upper extremity function required for occupational performance. Education in the psychological and social adjustment to disability is also the OT's area of expertise. The sooner therapy is initiated, the faster the client will be prepared for prosthetic fitting and the chances of engaging in bimanual activities will increase. Many long-lasting deficits are prevented with early intervention from therapy.

PHASES OF REHABILITATION

Prosthetic rehabilitation is categorized into nine phases of evaluation and intervention (Box 20.1). Each phase contains specific items to evaluate along with typical areas to address.[33] The phases are:

1. Preoperative
2. Amputation surgery and dressing
3. Acute postsurgical
4. Preprosthetic
5. Prosthetic prescription and fabrication
6. Prosthetic training
7. Community integration
8. Vocational rehabilitation
9. Follow-up

Preoperative Phase

Ideally the assessment and intervention process begins before the amputation. The health care team forms a plan and educates the client in what to expect after surgery and during rehabilitation. Therapists ensure realistic expectations and outline the typical rehabilitation process. Phantom pain and phantom sensation are explained because they are common occurrences for individuals post amputation. The preoperative phase is a good time to assess hand dominance and determine the need for adaptive equipment. Adaptive equipment is provided on an as needed basis only, because clients will eventually use their prostheses with daily activities, and adaptive equipment may interfere with the transition to prosthetic use.[33]

Amputation Surgery and Dressing Phase

Surgeons determine residual limb length before and during the surgery. Myoplastic closure of the wound is completed, ensuring soft tissue coverage of any distal bone. A rigid dressing or removable rigid dressing can assist in controlling pain.[33]

> **BOX 20.1   Nine Phases of Prosthetic Rehabilitation and Intervention Focus**
>
> 1. Preoperative phase
>   - Team formulates a plan
>   - Educate client on expectations
>   - Provide adaptive equipment
> 2. Amputation surgery and dressing phase
>   - Surgery
>   - Determine length of residual limb
>   - Wound care
>   - Dressing wound
>   - Pain control
> 3. Acute postsurgical phase
>   - Pain control
>   - Range of motion
>   - Wound healing
>   - Contracture prevention
>   - Emotional support
>   - Address phantom sensation/pain
> 4. Preprosthetic phase
>   - Limb shrinkage and shaping
>   - Increase muscle strength
>   - Foster sense of control
>   - Realistic expectations
> 5. Prosthetic prescription and fabrication phase
>   - Prosthetic options considered
>   - Prosthesis is delivered
> 6. Prosthetic training phase
>   - Prosthetic fitting and training
>   - Desensitization of residual limb
>   - Unilateral independence
>   - Educate client in prosthesis controls, etc.
> 7. Community integration phase
> 8. Vocational rehabilitation phase
> 9. Follow-up phase
>   - Purposeful activities
>   - Participation in meaningful activities and occupations
>   - Bilateral activities

Acute Postsurgical Phase

The goals after surgery for the team are pain control, maintenance of range of motion, and wound healing. Postsurgical therapy often incorporates wound care and contracture prevention. Emotional support to the client is essential. Discussions about phantom sensation and phantom pain continue.[33]

Wound Healing and Contracture Prevention

In addition, therapists assist persons in adjusting to the amputation in many ways. Postsurgical goals include early motion, wound healing, scar management, desensitization, pain management, edema reduction, limb shrinkage/shaping, and unilateral independence (change in hand dominance). Many interventions for motion, wound healing, scar management, desensitization, and pain management are the same interventions as used with other diagnoses. Interventions for edema reduction, limb shrinkage/shaping, and change in hand dominance are more specific to this population.

Phantom Pain and Phantom Sensation

Clients with amputations often experience phantom sensation and phantom pain. The role of the health care team is to prepare clients and assure them that these phantom sensations and pain are to be expected and are normal.[29] **Phantom sensation** occurs when the individual feels as if the nonexistent limb is still present. The amputated extremity may feel exactly like the original limb in terms of shape, size, position, and ability to move. Rings or watches that were previously worn may be part of the sensation. Phantom sensation is described as a pins-and-needles or tingling sensation. Phantom sensation diminishes over time.

Phantom pain is different from phantom sensation. The phenomenon of phantom pain is not completely understood. It is common for an individual to experience pain in the phantom limb early on after amputation and have it fade over time. It is reported that 80% of individuals with an amputation experience phantom pain.[4]

Intervention related to phantom sensation and phantom pain is implemented as soon as possible. One study surveyed 65 individuals with upper amputations about phantom pain. Results suggested the best intervention for phantom pain was active participation in functional activity.[81] Other interventions include gentle massage, prosthetic wear, and transcutaneous electric nerve stimulation (TENS). As therapists, we are well equipped to work with clients to optimize the functional use of the extremity with an amputation.[29]

Preprosthetic Phase

The primary goals during the preprosthetic phase are to shape the residual limb, increase muscle strength, and restore the person's sense of control over what is happening.[33]

Limb Shrinkage and Shaping

Limb shrinkage and shaping is addressed for this population. Custom compression garments are available for the client. Edema can be controlled through wrapping the residual limb in a diagonal design, so as not to compromise circulation. Compression garments or wraps should be worn as much as possible to ensure proper shaping of the residual limb. Compression has a direct impact on residual limb shrinkage and shaping. Elevation and retrograde massage are useful alternatives to decrease edema. It is important for the therapist to reinforce the importance of edema management because it has a direct impact on socket fit and comfort. The reduction of edema is a prerequisite for prosthetic fitting.[29]

Time during the preprosthetic phase is crucial for reinforcement of realistic expectations. Individuals with amputations may be under the assumption that they will perform all activities at the same level of independence they had before the amputation. This assumption needs to be discussed. Therapists explain that the prosthetic device will not replace the arm. Rather, it is an assistive tool used to stabilize, support, and hold objects during bimanual activities.

Prosthetic Prescription and Fabrication Phase

The prosthetic prescription and fabrication phase is the time when the team comes to consensus on the type of prosthesis that will best meet the client's needs and condition.[33] The preprosthetic period begins when the individual with the amputation begins exploration of prosthetic devices. The phase concludes upon prosthetic delivery.

Prosthetic Training Phase

During the prosthetic training phase, individuals frequently visit the prosthetist for fittings and modifications of the socket. Clients also see therapists for rehabilitation services. Individuals receiving body-powered prostheses move much more quickly through the fabrication and rehabilitation process because electrodes are not required and muscle sites and signals do not need to be identified. Therapy continues to address any lingering issues from the acute postsurgical phase. Additional goals of therapy during this phase include preparation of the individual to tolerate wearing the prosthesis and using it independently for daily activities. Specifics include electrode training; desensitizing the residual limb to pressure, pain, and weight; maintaining range of motion; eliminating contractures; and unilateral independence.[33]

Electrode Training

If individuals receive an externally powered prosthesis, the best muscle sites are identified and trained to operate the prosthetic features.[38] Finding the sites and training the muscles for electrode placement are primarily the responsibility of the therapist. During this phase, therapists provide extensive training using **biofeedback** to teach individuals to contract the identified muscle or muscles on command. The therapist facilitates the improvement of muscle site control and focuses on isolated muscle contraction, strength, and endurance. Special biofeedback machines are available from prosthetists. It is important for clients to practice muscle contractions in a variety of positions, including lying, standing, and sitting. Practicing muscle contractions in different positions with the extremity in various planes enhances maximal success after delivery of the prosthesis.

Once electrode sites are established, the prosthetist is informed of the exact and most appropriate electrode location for the individual to obtain the most function. Locating and training for electrode sites is often a lengthy, rigorous, and trial-and-error process. Once the socket and electrode sites are sufficient to work the prosthesis, the prosthesis is ready for final fabrication. There may be a period after the preprosthetic phase when the individual is discharged from therapy with a home program until the prosthesis is delivered and therapy can resume.

Desensitizing the Residual Limb to Pressure, Pain, and Weight

Clients may experience disappointment when the prosthesis is delivered and they are unable to use it as they imagined. It is the duty of the health care team to inform individuals of the advantages and disadvantages of the various prosthetic components to provide a realistic picture of rehabilitation. Clients are usually surprised when they realize that the prosthesis is hard, cold, heavy, and not an exact replacement for the hand. With establishment of realistic expectations and acceptance, use of the device greatly improves.[7]

Clients commonly experience residual limb sensitivity. Therapists intervene by teaching and implementing the following desensitization techniques: wrapping, massage, weight bearing, and pain management. Desensitization and pain management are additional components of therapy. Therapists provide modalities for pain and educate clients in managing their pain independently. Each client presents with different complaints, and the treatment is individualized.

In some instances, prosthetists provide clients with sockets to wear as precursors to full-time prosthetic wear. Sockets reshape the residual limb and allow clients to experience how the devices feel. Weights can be added to the distal ends of sockets for increasing tolerance to the weight of the devices as well as readjustment to extended limb length. Prosthesis simulators can be used to help the client adjust to the changes in limb length and to the prosthesis weight and can also be used to initiate controls training toward functional application.

Unilateral Independence

Unilateral independence involves using environmental adaptations and one-handed techniques. It may be necessary to teach clients to switch hand dominance if the dominant hand was amputated. Generally therapists work to promote the maximal level of independence for the individual. Assistive devices and adaptive strategies are often used. For clients with amputations, it may promote better prosthetic success if therapists do not issue adaptive equipment until after prosthetic training, because clients may become efficient with the adaptive equipment and may not be motivated to learn to use the prosthesis. However, many assistive devices used in tandem with prosthetic technology can augment and improve function.

Bilateral Involvement

Clients with bilateral involvement present with unique challenges that are dependent on multiple factors. It is important to understand that the individual's presentation may not be symmetrical and that differing technology—or no technology—may be used. Many individuals with bilateral loss or difference, particularly at a high level (such as shoulder disarticulation) engage in footwork using the toes to accomplish dexterous tasks.

Orientation and Control Training

Upon prosthetic delivery the prosthetist educates clients about the prosthesis and its components. Therapists reorient clients to their prostheses. Prostheses are complex devices, and they cannot be mastered in one therapy session. Clients will not be independent with use of the prosthetic unless there is a complete understanding of all the components.

Client orientation includes education in donning, doffing, operating switches and batteries, and caring for the prosthesis. Therapists ensure that prosthetic fit and function are adequate. Therapy includes evaluation of independence with prosthetic donning and doffing. Clients must be able to properly care for their prosthesis to prevent damage and maximize its potential.

Community Integration, Vocational Rehabilitation, and Follow-Up Phases

The final three phases of community integration, vocational rehabilitation, and follow-up[33] are composed of purposeful activities and participation in meaningful occupation-based activities.[3] These phases are intensive. Clients' visits to other members of the team decrease, and therapists act as liaisons to the teams. These final phases are progressive and evolve as clients' skills develop. During this time, clients learn to operate the controls of their prostheses and practice until they become proficient. Depending on the prosthetic features, clients practice tasks, such as opening and closing the TD, elevating and lowering the elbow, and rotating the wrist on command. Practicing such activities is graded (e.g., controlling the TD to open in three, four, or five separate steps).

Purposeful Activity

With purposeful activity, clients learn how to operate prostheses by engaging in repetitive tasks to facilitate eventual functional use and endurance. Purposeful activity includes using the prostheses to grasp and release objects of various sizes, textures, and weights in different planes and positions. Objects above the head can be difficult to grasp because individuals must relax the wrist extensors and contract the flexors while the hand is elevated. Overhead grasp is difficult to accomplish because of the prosthetic weight. Examples of other activities practiced during this stage include holding and placing a tomato on a counter without crushing it or playing a card game with the cards held by the TD.

Bilateral activities are also a focus in therapy. Often after amputation individuals become successful in performing some ADLs unilaterally. Thus therapy must begin early in the rehabilitation process to facilitate use of the prosthesis in bilateral activities. Training includes controlled grasp, such as opening in small increments to grasp small items and then more fully to grasp larger items. Training emphasizes grasping objects of varied textures and density. Sessions incorporate work on prehension and timing of release. Functional and appropriate tasks are encouraged and require clients to use their prostheses for gross and fine motor activities in various planes.

Occupational-Based Activity

Occupational-based activity involves engaging the client in occupations that match clients' goals. Clients practice skills related to their lifestyle and interests. Training may include grooming and hygiene, meal preparation, dressing, child care, return to work activities, or other meaningful tasks. Tasks may also include preparation for return to employment or recreation.

The primary focus of therapy should include bilateral activities for occupational performance. Box 20.2 lists examples of bilateral tasks.[54] Individuals with amputations usually do not realize the functional benefits of their prostheses until they experience success with bilateral tasks. Bilateral task training may be difficult for some clients who became proficient with one-handed techniques early in rehabilitation.

BOX 20.2 Examples of Bilateral Activities

- Insert a garbage bag into a trash receptacle
- Dry dishes with a towel
- Use cell phone
- Butter bread
- Put toothpaste on a toothbrush
- Lace and tie shoes
- Access currency (coins, bills) from a wallet
- Fold a letter and seal envelope
- Use power tools
- Use scissors to cut along a line and shapes
- Crack eggs and separate the yolks from the whites
- Fold laundry
- Wash dishes in a sink
- Remove lids from jars
- Manage separating zippers or buttons
- Peel oranges
- Sweep and use a dustpan
- Rake and bag leaves
- Peel and cut vegetables/fruits
- Cut meat
- Sewing on buttons
- Thread needles
- Use screw drivers
- Hammer a nail
- Drive a vehicle
- Play sports or card games

As stated earlier, clients are active participants in the rehabilitation process. Therapists design home programs for clients. The programs are continually updated as individuals progress to greater function and independence. Scheduling periodic follow-up visits with the client to review progress and prosthesis function is important. Often therapy will be reinitiated when clients find new skills they need or desire to learn. Therapists are resources for clients, enabling them to achieve maximal function and independence for participation in meaningful activities during a lifetime.

SECONDARY CONDITIONS

Individuals who experience unilateral ULL/D are likely candidates for experiencing secondary conditions related to overuse of the sound upper limb. Several studies documented the presence of pain and musculoskeletal conditions affecting the function of the sound arm in individuals with unilateral ULL/D.[19,46,62] Their findings agree that continual patient follow-up is essential to prevent further disparity and that more studies should be conducted to investigate the effects of prosthesis wear and to determine possible preventive measures. Gambrell[38] conducted a review of the literature noting the consequences and importance of prevention of overuse syndrome with recommendations for a team approach, emphasizing practitioner responsibility for educating patients about the likelihood of overuse and methods that impede development.

PSYCHOLOGICAL AND SOCIAL ISSUES OF CLIENTS WITH AMPUTATIONS

At any of the rehabilitation stages, psychological and social issues may arise, and it is important to make appropriate referrals to specialists as necessary. Persons with amputations voiced that they experience more difficulty dealing with their social worlds than with their physical worlds.[29] Common issues can center around relationships with family, friends, coworkers, and significant others. Specific issues may include posttraumatic stress, body image concerns, loss of sense of wholeness, social isolation, decreased sexual activity, and depression.[71] One of the most common secondary conditions associated with limb loss is depressed mood.[4]

Some research suggests that the valued personal identities and the self-management of patients' ability status should be a priority for the health professionals involved in prosthesis users' medical care and personal development.[59] To users, prostheses may be more than tools, which is suggested by the industry. When embodied, the prostheses represent deeply personal meanings that revolve around mastery of the technology, management of personal information, and self-identity. Earlier research explored factors toward adjustment and social meanings surrounding the use of prostheses and particularly sought perceptions of limb users.[58] Several themes emerged, including actual prosthesis use, social rituals, the perceptions of social isolation, the reactions of others, social implications of whether to conceal or disclose the limb difference, and perceptions or experiences relative to social and intimate relationships. Factors that influence adjustment and successful rehabilitation were early prosthetic fitting, prosthetic satisfaction associated with increased self-esteem, increased social integration and absence of emotional challenges, and the need for individual expression, including social expression, person-first language, societal acceptance, and personalizing the appearance of the prosthesis. Exploration into the psychosocial aspects of persons with amputations serves as the impetus for development of a platform to heighten health care professionals' consciousness of social challenges faced by the population of individuals with ULL/D, to raise the voices of the consumers, and to heighten the hearing of the funding stakeholders.

Family Dynamics

The dynamics of the family may be altered when a family member loses a limb. Significant others or direct family members of the injured person experience a series of losses and adjustments. Family members may fear that the individual is suffering and at risk of dying. Fear and anxiety may become overwhelming at times. Family members may worry about how the individual will adjust to his or her changed body. Issues about intimacy and dependency are common concerns. The therapist should encourage a reconnection between the person who has sustained an amputation and his or her partner.[48,49]

Impact on Rehabilitation

The rehabilitation team should become knowledgeable about the individual's response to the injury. Psychosocial aspects include change in self-image and body image, acceptance of the residual limb, and feeling comfortable in society as a person with an amputation. Some clients may be medically prepared to begin rehabilitation, but they are not psychologically ready. Health providers should not label the client as uncooperative and unmotivated. Rather, they should facilitate and reinforce good communication among the client and health care team. The client should be an active partner in establishing rehabilitation goals.

Counseling People Who Have Amputations

According to Price and Fisher, issues addressed during counseling sessions include depression, distress, sleeplessness, anxiety, changed body image, effects on relationships and intimacy, and feelings of anger and resentment[65]. According to Kohl,[48,49] complaints of emotional distress in the early stages of rehabilitation seemed to be most apparent from 6 to 24 months after surgery. As stated previously, researchers suggest the importance of psychosocial-emotional health[48,49] and that behavioral health issues are often overlooked and unaddressed in this population.[64]

UPPER EXTREMITY PROSTHETIC INTERVENTION FOR CHILDREN

Early gross motor movements in children (such as prone and sitting) emerge between 4 and 6 months.[28] These movements directly involve the use of hands to balance, support, and stabilize the trunk. As a result, fitting children with prostheses is considered necessary to maintain and preserve normal development.[73] Exner[35] stated that "[t]he development of visual perception and eye-hand coordination skills in conjunction with cognitive and social development allow the child to engage in increasingly complex activities."

Early Fitting

According to Hanson and Mandacina,[39] "The single most important advantage of early fitting is the immediate acceptance of the prosthetic arm by the child." The most beneficial age range to receive a prosthesis is from 2 months to 2 years.[36,72,78] Children fitted with prostheses at a young age who wear their prostheses regularly will demonstrate spontaneous use in daily activities.

Children fitted at later ages are less spontaneous and more inclined to use the prosthesis passively.[8,16,39] In addition, because hand skills develop gradually, children should be fitted early so that the prosthesis becomes naturally integrated with bilateral activities. While wearing their prostheses, children must practice activities that require crossing midline, hand position in space, grasping, bilateral tasks, and bringing hands to midline.[8] Table 20.3 suggests types of prostheses, goals, assessments, and interventions for children of different age-groups.

Family Involvement

Acceptance of the prosthesis involves the family. The family should be involved in donning and doffing the prosthesis, playing with the child while the prosthesis is on, and developing wearing schedules. The family should be educated about the importance and advantages of early and consistent prosthetic use. Furthermore, children who have myoelectric prostheses require substantial one-to-one training and attention.[8,32]

TABLE 20.3	Suggestions for Age-Appropriate Prostheses, Goals, Assessment, and Interventions			
Age	**Type of Prosthesis**	**Goals**	**Assessments**	**Intervention**
2 months to 18 months	Passive fitting suspension socket with no harnessing	Weight bearing in sitting and standing Crawling and pulling to stand Rolling front to back Stabilizing toys Bilateral activities	PUFI Typical screening assessments for age range	No different than reaching all appropriate developmental milestones Gross motor skills using the prosthesis Fine motor skills with unaffected upper extremity
12 months to 24 months	Body-powered prosthesis Cookie Crusher myoelectric prosthesis	Using prosthesis as an assist Discovering that the device opens and closes Opening hand upon request Placing toys in the myoelectric hand	University of New Brunswick test U-BET Assisting Hand Assessment Typical screening assessments for age range	Carrying large balls Weight bearing on the prosthesis while playing Stabilizing the body while completing tabletop activities Holding objects Riding toys Musical instruments Self-feeding (beginning)

PUFI, Prosthetic Upper Extremity Functional Index; *U-BET*, Unilateral Below Elbow Test.
Data from Shaperman, J., Landsberger, S. E., & Setoguchi, Y. (1996). Early upper limb prosthesis fitting: When and what do we fit, *Journal of Prosthetics and Orthotics 15*(1):11–17, 2003; Stocker, D., Caldwell, R., & Wedderburn, Z. (1996). Review of infant fittings at the Institute of Biomedical Engineering: 13 years of service, *ACPOC News 2*,1–5.

MARKETING STRATEGIES AND RECOMMENDATIONS

To specialize in upper extremity prosthetic rehabilitation, therapists must be motivated and persistent, just as in any area of practice. There are many avenues for gathering basic information on upper extremity prosthetics, such as journals, books, agencies, other therapists, and the Internet (see the Evolve website for information about client resources, manufacturer resources, and tests and measures). Important information from these resources augments basic prosthetic knowledge. Therapists should establish relationships with prosthetists who specialize in upper extremity prosthetics. Because the number of upper extremity amputations is generally low, it may be difficult for therapists to work full-time in this area unless they are willing to travel regionally or nationally. Some companies employ therapists who cover a designated region and provide prosthetic rehabilitation exclusively. If travel is not an option, therapists can network with prosthetic providers to be the primary referral for prosthetic rehabilitation in a geographical area. Typically therapists who take this route work in an outpatient upper extremity rehabilitation facility.

Spending a week with a prosthetist to learn about the process of reimbursement, fabrication, and orientation to various prosthetic options is valuable. The reimbursement process can take much time, depending on the source of reimbursement and the insurance company's specific benefits regarding prostheses. It is important to remain focused on clients and to serve as advocates for individuals with the amputation. Phone calls and letters from health care professionals may expedite approval of prosthetic devices. Therapy can proceed without approval for the prosthetic devices to accomplish goals from the preprosthetic phase.

In addition, it is important to locate area case managers and physicians who work with this population. Case managers and physicians assist in establishing a referral base. It has been the experience of the author that physicians, prosthetists, and case managers are happy to know that therapists exist who want to work in upper extremity prosthetic rehabilitation. They are also often happy to refer clients. Upper extremity prosthetics is a rewarding field.

👤 SELF-QUIZ 20.1[a]

Answer the following questions.

1. The term *above elbow (AE) amputation* is now called
   a. Transfemoral
   b. Transhumeral
   c. Transradial
   d. Transtibial
2. The term *below elbow (BE) amputation* is now called
   a. Transfemoral
   b. Transhumeral
   c. Transradial
   d. Transtibial
3. The primary cause for an upper extremity amputation is
   a. Congenital malformation
   b. Disease
   c. Trauma
   d. Vascular disorders
4. Which prosthetic option allows individuals to maintain grasp and release within an unlimited work area with full range of motion of the proximal upper extremity?
   a. Body-powered prosthesis
   b. Externally powered prosthesis
   c. No prosthesis
   d. Passive prosthesis
5. Which prosthesis allows individuals to maintain proprioception for grasp and release?
   a. Body-powered prosthesis
   b. Externally powered prosthesis
   c. No prosthesis
   d. Passive prosthesis
6. Which prosthetic option typically allows for increased grip/pinch strength?
   a. Body-powered prosthesis
   b. Externally powered prosthesis
   c. No prosthesis
   d. Passive prosthesis
7. Often therapists establish electrode sites and provide myoelectric training to use externally powered prostheses. In which phase of the rehabilitation process does this typically occur?
   a. Acute postsurgical
   b. Preoperative
   c. Preprosthetic
   d. Prosthetic training
8. A therapist receives an order to evaluate and treat an individual with a transhumeral amputation. The prosthetist indicates the client received the prosthesis 1 week ago. Rank in order the steps of the therapy intervention:
   Step 1: _____
   Step 2: _____
   Step 3: _____
   Purposeful activity
   Occupation-based activity
   Orientation and control training
9. In which phase of postprosthetic training does the client learn to operate the controls of the prosthesis and practice until proficient?
   a. Purposeful activity
   b. Occupation-based activity
   c. Orientation and control training
10. Which secondary condition is most commonly associated with limb loss?
    a. Depressed mood
    b. Isolation
    c. Loss of sense of self
    d. Posttraumatic stress disorder

[a]See Appendix A for the answer key.

REVIEW QUESTIONS

1. What is the relationship between the level of amputation and functional ability? List three reasons for prosthetic dissatisfaction.

2. What are the primary causes for upper extremity amputation?

3. Clarify the specific roles of the client, prosthetist, and OT when treating a person with an amputation?

4. What are the six types of prosthetic options available for people with upper extremity amputations?

5. How would you explain in lay terms the advantages and disadvantages of passive aesthetic functional, activity-specific, body-powered, and externally powered prostheses?

6. What is one therapy goal for each phase of prosthetic rehabilitation? What is one specific intervention for each phase?

7. What are the psychosocial impacts of an amputation that may arise?

8. What are the diverse types of secondary conditions that are likely to arise, and why is it important to advise the client about protective/preventative strategies?

9. How might peer networking be helpful to individuals with either congenital difference or acquired loss of the upper limb(s)?

10. What are some barriers individuals with upper limb acquired loss/congenital difference experience when trying to access specialized intervention?

REFERENCES

1. Alley RD: *Advancement of upper extremity prosthetic interface and frame design, From "MEC '02 The Next Generation. Proceedings of the 2002 MyoElectric Controls/Powered Prosthetics Symposium Fredericton New Brunswick,* Canada, 2002, Copyright University of New Brunswick. Retrieved from http://dukespace.libduke.edu/dspace/bitstream/handle/10161/2684/r_alley_paper01.pdf?sequence=3.

2. American Board for Certification in Orthotics: *Prosthetics & Pedorthics, Inc. Annual report [Brochure].* Available for download at www.abcop.org, 2011.

3. American Occupational Therapy Association (AOTA): Occupational therapy practice framework: domain and process, *Amer J Occup Ther* 68(Suppl):S1–S48, 2014.

4. Amputee Coalition: Home page. Retrieved from http://www.amputee-coalition.org.

5. Amputee Coalition of America: People with amputation speak out. Retrieved from http://www.amputee-coalition.org/people-speak-out/index.html.

6. Andrews KL, Bouvette KA: Anatomy for fitting of prosthetics and orthotics, *Physical Medicine and Rehabilitation* 10(3):489–507, 1996.

7. Atkins DJ: Prosthetic Training. In Smith D, Michael J, Bowker J, editors: *Atlas of amputations and limb deficiencies: surgical, prosthetic, and rehabilitation principles,* Rosemont, IL, 2004, American Academy of Orthopaedic Surgeons, pp 275–284.

8. Atkins DJ: Pediatric prosthetics: a collection of considerations, *Motion* 7(2):7–17, 1997.

9. Atkins DJ: *Comprehensive management of the upper-limb amputee,* Springer London, Ltd., 2011. 2012.

10. Bagley AM, Molitor F, Wagner LV, Tomhave W, James MA: The unilateral below elbow test: a function test for children with unilateral congenital below elbow deficiency, *Developmental Medicine & Child Neurology* 48(7):569–575, 2006.

11. Baschuk, C: *Perspective: the synergistic potential of embracing 3d printing.* The edge. Retrieved from: www.oandp.com/edge.

12. Baumgartner R, Bota P: Upper extremity amputation and prosthetics, *Medicine Orthotic Technology* 1:5–51, 1992.

13. Bennett JB, Alexander CB: Amputation levels and surgical techniques. In Atkins DJ, Meier RH, editors: *Comprehensive management of the upper-limb amputee,* New York, 1989, Springer-Verlag, pp 28–38.

14. Billock JN: Clinical evaluation and assessment principles in orthotics and prosthetics, *J Prosthet Orthot* 8(2):41–44, 2003.

15. Bouwsema H, Van Der Sluis CK, Bongers RM: Changes in performance over time while learning to use a myoelectric prosthesis, *Journal of NeuroEngineering and Rehabilitation* 11(1):16, 2014.

16. Bowers R: Facing congenital differences, *First Step Magazine* 4:23–26, 2003.

17. Bowker JH, Pitham CH: The history of amputation surgery and prosthetics. In Smith D, Michael J, Bowker J, editors: *Atlas of amputations and limb deficiencies: surgical, prosthetic, and rehabilitation principles,* Rosemont, IL, 2004, American Academy of Orthopaedic Surgeons, pp 3–19.

18. Brouwers MAH, Roeling IEM, van Wikjk I, Mooibroek-Tieben EPH, Harmer-Bosgoed MW, Plettenburg DH: *Development of a test prosthesis: An important tool in the decision-making process in providing patients with an upper limb prosthesis, Myo-Electric Controls Symposium (MEC), Fredericton New Brunswick,* Canada, August 2014.

19. Burger H, Vidmar G: A survey of overuse problems in patients with acquired or congenital upper limb deficiency, *Prosthetics and Orthotics International* 40(4):497–502, 2015.

20. Burger H, Brezovar D, Marincek C: Comparison of clinical test and questionnaires for the evaluation of upper limb prosthetic use in children, *Disability & Rehabilitation* 26(14/15):911–916, 2004.

21. Carlson LE, Veatch BD, Frey DD: Efficiency of prosthetic cable and housing, *J Prosthet Orthot* 7(3):96–99, 1995.

22. Cheesborough JE, Smith LH, Kuiken TA, Dumanian GA: Targeted muscle reinnervation and advanced prosthetic arms, *Semin Plast Surg* 29(1):62–72, 2015.

23. COAPT Complete Control. Retrieved from https://www.coaptengineering.com.

24. Collier M, LeBlanc M: Axilla bypass ring for shoulder harnesses for upper-limb prostheses, *J Prosthet Orthot* 8(2):130–131, 1996.

25. Corathers C, Janczewski M: *The orthotic and prosthetic profession: a workforce demand study,* Prepared for the National Commission on Orthotic and Prosthetic Education and the American Orthotic and Prosthetic Association, 2006. Retrieved from www.ncope.org/assets/pdf/final-report-publishing_3-07.pdf.

26. Corbett EA, Perrault EJ, Kuiken TA: Comparison of electromyography and force as interfaces for prosthetic control, *J Rehabil Res Dev* 48(6):629–642, 2011.

27. Crane V: Amputee adjusts, *Probe Magazine* 4:10–14, 1979.

28. Cronin A, Mandich MB: *Human development and performance throughout the lifespan*, New York, 2005, Thomson/Delmar Learning, pp 139–164.

29. Davidson JH, Jones LE, Cornet J, et al.: Management of the multiple limb amputee, *Disabil Rehabil* 24(13):688–699, 2002.

30. Dillingham TR, Pezzin LE, MacKenzie EJ: Limb amputation and limb deficiency: epidemiology and recent trends in the United States, *South Med J* 95(8):875–883, 2002.

31. Dougherty PJ: Wartime amputee care. In Smith D, Michael J, Bowker J, editors: *Atlas of amputations and limb deficiencies: surgical, prosthetic, and rehabilitation principles*, Rosemont, IL, 2004, American Academy of Orthopaedic Surgeons, pp 77–100.

32. Egermann M, Kasten P, Thomsen M: Myoelectric hand prostheses in very young children, *International Orthopaedics* 33(4):1101–1105, 2008.

33. Esquenazi A, DiGiacomo R: Rehabilitation after amputation, *J Am Podiatr Med Assoc* 91(1):13–22, 2001.

34. Esquenazi A, Meier R, Sears H: *The state of upper limb prosthetics*, Presentation at Orlando, FL, 2002, National Prosthetic and Orthotic Conference.

35. Exner CE: Development of hand functions. In Pratt PN, Allen AS, editors: *Occupational therapy for children*, St Louis, 1989, Mosby, pp 235–259. (ed 2.

36. Fisher A: Initial fitting of the congenital below-elbow amputee: are we fitting early enough? *Inter-Clinic Information Bulletin* 15:7–10, 1976.

37. Gallagher P, MacLachlan M: The trinity amputation and prosthesis experience scales and quality of life in people with lower-limb amputation, *Arch Phys Med Rehabil* 85(5):730–736, 2004.

38. Gambrell CR: Overuse syndrome and the unilateral upper limb amputee: consequences and prevention, *Journal of Prosthetics and Orthotics* 20(3):126–132, 2008.

39. Hanson WJ, Mandacina S: Microprocessor technology opens the door to success, *The O&P Edge* 5:36–38, 2003.

40. Hartigan BJ, Sarrafian SK: In Smith D, Michael J, Bowker J, editors: *Atlas of amputations and limb deficiencies: surgical, prosthetic, and rehabilitation principles*, Rosemont, IL, 2004, American Academy of Orthopaedic Surgeons, pp 101–116. 2004.

41. Hebert JS, Lewicke J: Case report of modified box and blocks test with motion capture to measure prosthetic function, *Journal of Rehabilitation Research & Development* 49(8):1163–1174, 2012.

42. Hill W, Kyberd P, Hermansson LH, et al.: Upper limb prosthetic outcomes measures (ULPOM): a working group and their findings, *Journal of Prosthetics and Orthotics* 21(4):69–82, 2009.

43. Huinink HB, Bouwsema H, Plettenburg DH, van der Sluis CK, Bongers RM: Learning to use a body-powered prosthesis: Changes in functionality and kinematics, *The Journal of Neuro-Engineering and Rehabilitation* 13:90–101, 2016.

44. Infinite Biomedical Technology (IBT) (n.d.). Retrieved from http://www.i-biomed.com/.

45. Jebsen RH, Taylor N, Trieschmann RB, et al.: An objective and standardized test of hand function, *Arch Phys Med Rehabil* 50(6):311–319, 1969.

46. Jones LE, Davidson JH: Save that arm: a study of problems in the remaining arm of unilateral upper limb amputees, *Prosthet Orthot Int* 23(1):55–58, 1999.

47. Keenan DD: Myoelectric prosthesis protocol, *American Occupational Therapy Association Physical Disabilities Newsletter* 18(1):1–4, 1995.

48. Kohl SJ: Emotional coping with amputation. In Krueger DW, editor: *Rehabilitation psychology: a comprehensive textbook*, New York, 1984, Aspen, pp 272–281.

49. Kohl SJ: The process of psychological adaptation to traumatic limb loss. In Krueger DW, editor: *Emotional rehabilitation of physical trauma and disability*, ***, Spectrum Publications, 1984, pp 113–119.

50. Latour D: *Use of prosthesis simulators to educate occupational therapists as effective team members*, Chicago, IL, 2016, American Occupational Therapy Association (AOTA) Annual Conference.

51. Latour D: *Impact of bilateral upper limb prosthesis simulators in pre-prosthetic training: a case study*, Boston, MA, 2016, American Orthotics and Prosthetics Association (AOPA) Annual Conference.

52. Law HT: Engineering of upper limb prostheses, *Orthop Clin North Am* 12(4):929–951, 1981.

53. Lindner YHN, Langius-Eklöf A, Hermansson LM: Test-retest reliability and rater agreements of Assessment of Capacity for Myoelectric Control version 2.0, *Journal of Rehabilitation Research & Development, 2014* 51(4):635–644, 2014.

54. McFarland LV, Hubbard Winkler SL, et al.: Unilateral upper-limb loss: satisfaction and prosthetic-device use in veterans and service members from Vietnam and OIF/OEF conflicts, *J Rehabil Res Dev* 47(4):299–316, 2010.

55. Miguelez JM: Critical factors in electrically powered upper-extremity prosthetics, *American Academy of Orthotics and Prosthetics* 14(1):36–38, 2002.

56. Muderis MA: Osseointegration, Orthopaedic Surgeon. Retrieved from http://www.almuderis.com.au/osseointegration.

57. Muilenburg AL, LeBlanc MA: Body-powered upper limb components. In Atkins DJ, Meier RH, editors: *Comprehensive management of the upper-limb amputee*, New York, 1989, Springer-Verlag.

58. Murray CD: The social meanings of prosthesis use, *Journal of Health Psychology* 10:425–441, 2005.

59. Murray CD: Being like everybody else: The personal meanings of being a prosthesis user, *Disability and Rehabilitation* 31:573–581, 2009.

60. National Limb Loss Information Center: Fact sheet—amputation statistics by cause: limb loss in the United States (n.d.). Retrieved from http://www.amputee-coalition.org/fact_sheets/amp_stats_cause.html.

61. National Center for Health Statistics. (n.d.). https://www.cdc.gov/nchs/index.htm.

62. Ostlie K, Franklin R, Skjeldal O, Skrondal A, Magnus P: Musculoskeletal pain and overuse syndromes in adult acquired major upper-limb amputees, *Archives of Physical Medicine and Rehabilitation* 92(12):1967–1973, 2011.

63. Patterson DB, McMillan PM, Rodriguez RP: Acceptance rate of myoelectric prosthesis, *Journal of the Association of Children's Prosthetic-Orthotic Clinics* 25(3):73–76, 1991.

64. Pizzi M: The pizzi holistic wellness assessment, *Occupational Therapy in Health Care* 13(3/4):51–66, 2001.

65. Price EM, Fisher K: How does counseling help people with amputation, *J Prosthet Orthot* 14(2):102–106, 2002.

66. Probsting E, Kannenberg A, Conyers DW, et al.: Ease of activities of daily living with conventional and multigrip myoelectric hands, *Journal of Prosthetics & Orthotics (JPO)* 27(2):46–52, 2015.

67. Radocy B: Upper-extremity prosthetics: considerations and designs for sports and recreation, *Clinical Prosthetics and Orthotics* 11(3):131–153, 1987.

68. Reddy MP: Nerve entrapment syndromes in the upper extremity contralateral to amputation, *Arch Phys Med Rehabil* 65(1):24–26, 1984.

69. Resnik L, Adams L, Borgia M, et al.: Development and evaluation of the activities measure for upper limb amputees, *Archives of Physical Medicine & Rehabilitation* 94(3):488–494, 2013.

70. Ryll UC, Bastiaenen CHG, Eliasson AC: Assisting hand assessment and children's hand-use experience questionnaire –observed versus perceived bimanual performance in children with unilateral cerebral palsy, *Physical & Occupational Therapy in Pediatrics* 37(2):199–209, 2017.

71. Saradjian A, Thompson AR, Datta D: The experience of men using an upper limb prosthesis following amputation: positive coping and minimizing feeling different, *Disabil Rehabil* 30(11):871–883, 2008.

72. Scotland TD, Galway HR: A long-term review in children with congenital and acquired upper limb deficiency, *J Bone Joint Surg Br* 65(3):346–349, 1986.

73. Shaperman J, Landsberger SE, Setoguchi Y: Early upper limb prosthesis fitting: when and what do we fit, *J Prosthet Orthot* 15(1):11–17, 2003.

74. Sheehan TP, Gondo GC: Impact of limb loss in the United States, *Physical Medicine and Rehabilitation Clinics of North America* 25(1):9–28, 2014.

75. Shirley Ryan Ability Lab. (nd). Retrieved from: https://www.sralab.org/

76. Shurr DG, Cook TM: *Prosthetics and orthotics*, Norwalk, CT, 1990, Appleton & Lange.

77. Smith DG, Micahel JW, Bowker JH: *Atlas of amputations and limb deficiencies*, ed 3, Rosemont, IL, 2004, American Academy of Orthopaedic Surgeons.

78. Stark G: Upper-extremity limb fitting, *Motion* 12(4):47–52, 2001.

79. The DASH Outcome Measure (nd). Retrieved from: http://dash.iwh.on.ca/.

80. Toren S: Upper extremity, *First Step Magazine* 3:7–9, 2002.

81. Vacek KM: *Phantom pain and phantom sensation, Research Platform Presentation*, Kansas City, MO, 2001, Amputee Coalition of Americas National Conference.

82. van Dijk-Koot CA, van der Ham I, Buffart LM, et al.: Current experiences with the prosthetic upper extremity functional index in follow-up of children with upper limb reduction deficiency, *Journal of Prosthetics & Orthotics (JPO)* 21(2):110–114, 2009.

83. Whelan LR, Farley J: Functional outcomes with externally powered partial hand prostheses, *Journal of Prosthetics & Orthotics*, 30(2):69–73, 2018.

84. Wijdenes PA, Brouwers MAH, van der Sluis CK: *PPP-Arm: the implementation of a national prescription protocol 2016*, Glasgow, Scotland, 2016, Trent International Prosthetic Symposium (TIPS).

85. Williams 3rd TW: Progress on stabilizing and controlling powered upper-limb prostheses, *J Rehabil Res Dev* 48(6):ix–xix, 2011.

86. Wright FV, Hubbard S, Naumann S, Jutai J: Evaluation of the validity of the prosthetic upper extremity functional index for children, *Archives of Physical Medicine & Rehabilitation* 84(4):518–527, 2003.

87. Wright TW, Hagen AD, Wood MB: Prosthetic usage in major upper extremity amputations, *J Hand Surg Am* 20(4):619–622, 1995.

88. Young E: The 3D-Printed Prosthesis. Amplitude; Sept-Oct; pp26-29. www.amplitude-media.com. Retrieved 25 November 2017, 2016.

89. Ziegler-Graham K, MacKenzie EJ, Ephraim PL, Travison TG, Brookmeyer R: Estimating the predvalence of limb loss in the United States: 2005 to 2050, *Archives of Physical Medicine Rehabilitation* 89:422–429, 2008.

APPENDIX 20.1 CASE STUDIES

Case Study 20.1[a]

Read the following scenario, and answer the questions based on the information in this chapter.

Michael is a 6-month-old baby who sustained a vascular trauma resulting in the amputation of his right wrist and hand at the age of 3 days. Recently Michael began sitting and trying to hold his bottle. He was seen by the prosthetist for consideration of his first prosthesis. Michael was referred to occupational therapy for input and recommendations regarding his developmental milestones.

1. What did the occupational therapist advise?
2. What were the considerations?
   Following delivery of the prosthesis, Michael and his caregivers were referred to occupational therapy for prosthetic training.
3. What might have been included in the occupational therapist's plan of care?

Case Study 20.2[a]

Amy is a 13-year-old girl who presents with a unilateral congenital left upper limb difference at the transhumeral level. She has been wearing a body-powered prosthesis that is cumbersome to wear and to operate. She complains about the traditional harnessing used to suspend and to control the components of the device. The prosthetist is planning to provide Amy with an externally powered device and would like occupational therapy to work with her before delivery for readiness with this technology.

1. What goals will occupational therapy address in the plan of care?

Case Study 20.3[a]

Nick is a 22-year-old man who works as a butcher. His left dominant hand was caught in a meat grinder. The surgeon who was scheduled to perform the amputation of the hand called the Department of Occupational Therapy to have an occupational therapist quickly consult on the best level of amputation for function.

1. What did the occupational therapist advise?
   After the amputation surgery, Nick was referred to an occupational therapist for preprosthetic intervention.

Case Study 20.4[a]

Matt is a 64-year-old man with a right congenital upper limb difference (transradial level). He wears and uses his prosthetic technology daily and for different purposes. For example, Matt uses an activity-specific device that allows him to fish and to shoot archery. He uses an externally powered multi-articulating hand to accomplish tasks at work, where he is a salesman. He uses a body-powered voluntary-closing device for home and property maintenance. Despite all of this, he has been experiencing pain in the left upper limb, neck, and trunk. In addition, he reports that he sometimes feels uncomfortable socially because of the stares and questions asked by strangers in the community. His primary care physician referred him to occupational therapy with the order that states, "Evaluation and Treatment."

1. What might be included in the occupational therapist's plan of care?

---

[a] See Appendix A for the answer key.

21

Professional Development in Upper Extremity Rehabilitation

Tara Ruppert

CHAPTER OBJECTIVES

1. Describe the practice settings where upper extremity rehabilitation occurs.
2. Define hand therapy.
3. Identify the knowledge and skills required to become a certified hand therapist.
4. Describe the process for certification.
5. Identify the benefits of obtaining a specialist credential.
6. Identify the resources available for preparing for the hand therapy credential.
7. Identify pathways of service for experienced therapists to continue professional development.

KEY TERMS

certified hand therapist (CHT)
fellowship program

hand therapy
mentoring

Threaded Case Study A: Owen took a full-time position with a rehabilitation company that served a four-county rural area near his small hometown upon graduation from his occupational therapy program. His job duties consisted of treating clients in a subacute rehabilitation facility, an acute care hospital, an outpatient rehabilitation clinic, and in home health. Owen enjoyed treating clients in these medical settings because he followed many people through the rehabilitation continuum. Within the first year of employment, Owen developed a strong interest in upper extremity orthopedic rehabilitation, especially in fabricating custom orthotics. He enjoyed helping people recover from traumatic or degenerative conditions and return to fulfilling occupations.

Threaded Case Study B: Nicole began a full-time position in an outpatient multidisciplinary rehabilitation clinic attached to a large hospital immediately after graduation. She had the opportunity to work with a variety of clients in that setting: people with neurological, orthopedic, and degenerative conditions. This clinic had a wide variety of referral sources both internal and external to the hospital, and the physical and occupational therapists worked side by side. This environment allowed her to learn from experienced therapists in both disciplines. After practicing for 2 years, Nicole had developed a good relationship with a hand surgeon who had recently joined the orthopedic group. The surgeon approached the

rehabilitation team about providing walk-in services for custom orthotic provision for his patients. Nicole took on this role with some trepidation but soon found an interest and aptitude in custom orthotic fabrication.

ENTRY-LEVEL PRACTICE IN UPPER EXTREMITY REHABILITATION

Entry-level occupational therapists are trained in the rehabilitation process of common upper extremity orthopedic conditions and in the art of custom orthotic fabrication. This skill set is an important part of the identity of occupational therapy and has been part of the occupational therapy scope of practice since the 1970s.[1] However, like many other skills, becoming proficient at fabricating a custom orthosis requires practice. Knowing what to do for someone with an orthopedic impairment also involves experience. Therefore entry-level occupational therapy practitioners who work with clients with upper extremity impairments—whether from orthopedic, neurological, or some other cause—should focus on expanding knowledge and skills throughout their career.

There are multiple medical settings in which an entry-level occupational therapist would be expected to treat people of any age with upper extremity orthopedic conditions. Some of these settings include acute care hospitals, subacute rehabilitation centers, outpatient therapy clinics, home health services, and long-term care facilities. An occupational therapist working in any of these settings is expected to treat a variety

BOX 21.1 Common Upper Extremity Conditions for Entry-Level Practice

Common Upper Extremity Orthopedic Diagnoses
Arthritis
Joint trauma or instability
Burns
Peripheral neuropathy
Connective tissue disorders
Tendinopathy
Cumulative trauma disorders
Tissue contractures
Fractures
Wounds

of conditions that impair upper extremity function (Box 21.1) and needs to provide effective interventions to help clients return to their daily activities. Provision of custom orthotics is one intervention that is commonly indicated for many upper extremity impairments.[2]

The Accreditation Council for Occupational Therapy Education (ACOTE) sets the standards for entry-level education. Standard B.5.11 requires that master's degree and doctorate occupational therapy programs teach "design, fabrication, application, fitting, and training in orthotic devices used to enhance occupational performance and participation."[3] Occupational therapy assistant education programs have a similar standard; "Provide fabrication, application, fitting, and training in orthotic devices used to enhance occupational performance and participation."[3] Occupational therapy programs decide to what degree this standard is met, so the actual content and exposure to orthotic fabrication varies among programs. The majority of entry-level education programs address only the tip of the iceberg in regard to treating upper extremity impairments. The pursuit of continual education beyond initial certification is an essential piece of professional development.

Threaded Case Study A: Within the first year of practice, Owen was surprised by the number of referrals he received to treat people with upper extremity orthopedic conditions. He enjoyed working with this population because clients were often able to return to their previous level of function after occupational therapy interventions. However, Owen quickly realized that he needed more education to treat this population. He attended continuing education courses that addressed upper extremity rehabilitation. At one of these courses he met Cindy, a certified hand therapist who worked in an outpatient rehabilitation clinic 50 miles away from him. At the end of the course they exchanged contact information, and Cindy invited Owen to contact her whenever he had questions about upper extremity rehabilitation. Owen was glad to have found a mentor in this specialty area.

SPECIALTY AREAS IN OCCUPATIONAL THERAPY

With greater experience comes the opportunity to specialize. Occupational therapists have many potential specialty areas, both internal and external to the profession. The American Occupational Therapy Association (AOTA) developed

pathways for board certifications in four different practice areas: pediatrics, mental health, gerontology, and physical rehabilitation. Occupational therapists must have 5 years and 5000 hours of experience in the specific practice area, including at least 500 hours of direct therapy service provision, to apply for the board certifications. AOTA also developed specialty certifications for occupational therapists and occupational therapy assistants in specific intervention areas: driving and community mobility; environmental modification; feeding, eating, and swallowing; low vision; and school systems. The process for obtaining these certifications involves peer review of professional portfolios as evidence of advanced knowledge in the designated practice area. The specialty certifications require various lengths of practice experience.[4]

AOTA offers **fellowship programs** and mentoring programs in specific practice areas. The intent of these programs is to allow graduates to continue didactic education immediately after entry-level certification while working under a clinician mentor. These programs may involve a research and scholarship focus. The areas of fellowship offered under AOTA are geriatrics, low vision, neurorehabilitation, pediatrics, physical rehabilitation, burn recovery, and **hand therapy**. Fellowship programs last from 9 to 12 months. Graduates are eligible to sit for AOTA specialty certification in the related field with 3 years of experience rather than 5 years after successful completion of a fellowship program.[5]

Occupational therapists are eligible for other specialty certification areas outside those offered by AOTA. A nonexhaustive list of potential rehabilitative specialty areas includes[6]:

- Assistive technology (Assistive Technology Professional ([ATP])
- Stroke rehabilitation (Certified Stroke Rehabilitation Specialist [CSRS])
- Ergonomics (Board of Certification in Professional Ergonomics [BCPE], Certified Ergonomic Evaluation Specialist [CEES], or Certified Ergonomic Assessment Specialist [CEAS])
- Lymphedema therapist (Lymphology Association of North America [LANA] Certified Lymphedema Therapist [CLT])
- Neurodevelopmental treatment (NDT)
- Upper extremity orthopedic rehabilitation (**certified hand therapist** [CHT])
- Women's health (Pelvic Rehabilitation Practitioner Certification [PRPC])

These specialty areas are available for occupational therapists or physical therapists. Each clinical specialty identifies the specific requirements for entry, which typically include clinical experience before eligibility and some form of competency assessment, such as a certification examination.

Hand Therapy Certification

Occupational or physical therapists who demonstrate advanced knowledge in upper extremity orthopedic rehabilitation can pursue a **certified hand therapist (CHT)** credential (Box 21.2). The CHT credential is overseen by the Hand Therapy Certification Commission (HTCC), which sets eligibility requirements, administers the initial

BOX 21.2 Definition of Hand Therapy

Hand therapy is the art and science of rehabilitation of the upper limb, which includes the hand, wrist, elbow, and shoulder girdle. It is a merging of occupational and physical therapy theory and practice that combines comprehensive knowledge of the structure of the upper limb with function and activity. Using specialized skills in assessment, planning, and treatment, hand therapists provide therapeutic interventions to prevent dysfunction, restore function, and/or reverse the progression of pathology of the upper limb in order to enhance an individual's ability to execute tasks and to participate fully in life situations.

From Hand Therapy Certification Commission. (2017). *Recertification*. https://www.htcc.org/recertify.

BOX 21.3 Hand Therapy Scope of Practice[a]

Upper Extremity Diagnoses Treated by Hand Therapists

- Adhesions or tightness
- Amputations
- Arthritis and rheumatic diseases
- Congenital anomalies/differences
- Crush injuries/mutilating trauma
- Cumulative trauma disorders
- Cysts and tumors
- Developmental disabilities
- Dislocations and subluxations
- Dupuytren's disease
- Edema
- Factitious disorders
- Fractures
- Infections
- Ligamentous injury and instability
- Lymphedema
- Muscular strains, tears, and avulsions
- Nerve injuries and conditions
- Neuromuscular diseases
- Pain
- Replantation and revascularization
- Spinal cord and central nervous system injuries
- Tendon injuries and conditions
- Thermal and electrical injuries
- Vascular disorders
- Wounds and scars

[a]Printed with permission from the Hand Therapy Certification Commission, Scope of Practice and Domains of Hand Therapy. Hand Therapy Certification Commission. (2017). *Recertification*. https://www.htcc.org/recertify.

certification examination, and tracks the recertification process. The CHT credential originated in 1991 after years of work by the founders of the American Society of Hand Therapists (ASHT) to establish and define the field.[7] Now hand therapy is a recognized specialty in the United States, Canada, Australia, and New Zealand. The HTCC reports that 85% of all CHTs are occupational therapists, 14% are physical therapists, and 1% have both occupational therapy and physical therapy licenses. As of 2017 there were 6284 certified hand therapists in the world.[8] This specialty is somewhat misnamed because these practitioners are experts in treating conditions of the entire upper extremity, not just the hand.

Hand therapists practice in a variety of settings, but the majority work in outpatient therapy clinics in urban or suburban areas.[8] The outpatient therapy setting allows a hand therapist to develop a close working relationship with orthopedic surgeons who specialize in the upper extremity. Some hand therapists work alongside a hand surgeon, providing multidisciplinary treatment in a single clinic setting, whereas others work in clinics near the surgeons' clinics and are able to provide walk-in services. This close interprofessional relationship between surgeon and therapist benefits everyone involved, especially the client, and creates an environment of mutual respect. Hand surgeons often rely on their associated hand therapists to further educate the client in the rehabilitation processes and timelines, and the hand therapists consult with surgeons on complex cases.

The HTCC published a nonexhaustive list of diagnoses that hand therapists can treat within the hand therapy scope of practice (Box 21.3). This information is beneficial to include in the scope of practice because it further clarifies and explains the level of expertise of therapists with the CHT credential. Hand therapists use a wide variety of interventions to treat clients, including but not limited to orthotic fabrication, manual therapy, physical agent modalities, therapeutic exercise, scar management, edema reduction, work hardening, and occupation-based therapy. This level of care requires a solid foundation in many areas, including anatomy, physiology, kinesiology, ergonomics, psychosocial development, learning styles, and research principles.

An occupational or physical therapist who has at least 3 years of clinical experience and 4000 hours of practice with upper extremity rehabilitation is eligible to apply for the certification examination. The examination is administered two times each year throughout the United States. The 4-hour examination is computer based and consists of 200 questions. The HTCC offers a blueprint that outlines the domains addressed by the examination. Applicants must demonstrate knowledge of evaluation, treatment planning, therapeutic interventions, and basic scientific concepts related to the upper extremity.[9] HTCC conducts field research every 5 years to ensure that the examination reflects current practices, skills, conditions, and evidence. Examination pass rates for each testing period over the past 15 years are posted by the HTCC, and the average pass rate for the CHT examination is 56.8%, with a range of 51% to 63%.[10] The pass rate indicates that the examination is thorough, rigorous, and requires a high level of knowledge, all of which are necessary to protect the integrity of the CHT credential.

Benefits of the Hand Therapy Credential

A practitioner with the CHT credential has proven advanced knowledge in the realm of upper extremity rehabilitation. The CHT credential informs referral sources, clients, and payers that the therapist is an expert in the rehabilitation of a wide variety of issues related to the complex upper extremity. The HTCC website offers this quote from a hand surgeon: "In my experience, those with the CHT certification are more experienced, more knowledgeable about anatomy and are willing to 'work outside the box' with complex patients."[8] Hand surgeons rely on hand therapists to provide patient education, fabricate custom orthotics, and use manual therapy interventions. Surgeons especially value the rapport that a hand therapist can build with a patient. As one hand surgeon stated, "A certified hand therapist has demonstrated their commitment, over many years, to develop their fund of knowledge and skill set focused entirely on improving the lives of patients with hand dysfunction. The synergy of a hand therapist and hand surgeon working together is a beautiful and necessary team approach to optimize the outcomes for our patients."[11]

Becoming a clinical specialist can potentially assist with career focus and advancement. The HTCC reports the results of a salary survey every 5 years, which outlines the salaries, benefits, and practice settings of CHTs in the United States. The survey results are beneficial in salary negotiations. The 2017 survey reported that the average salary of a hand therapist had a greater increase than the average salary of a non–hand therapist.[12] The relative rarity of CHTs can provide a competitive edge in the job market. Of course, the CHT credential does not guarantee career or salary advancement.

Threaded Case Study B: Nicole enjoyed treating people with upper extremity impairments and was proud of the improvements she was making with fabricating custom orthoses. She met Dale, a certified hand therapist, at an annual conference for her state's occupational therapy association. They discussed common interests and practices over lunch. As Nicole learned more about the CHT credential, she began to appreciate the impact that specialization could have on her career. She wanted to continue working in the outpatient therapy setting with people who had orthopedic conditions. What she was not sure of was how to begin preparing for specialization.

Becoming a Certified Hand Therapist

The requirements to apply for the hand therapy credential are straightforward. The route to preparing for the certification examination can vary significantly. There is no one preferred track for preparation, so therapists who pursue the CHT must tailor an approach to fit their personal learning styles. Some may choose an independent track, using resources and self-study approaches. Others may decide to seek out more directed guidance for their preparation, such as fellowship programs and mentoring. In either case a critical step for preparation includes pursuit of continuing education courses that address topics related to hand therapy. Because entry-level occupational therapy education must prepare graduates to be generalists, there is not enough didactic time to cover clinical areas in depth. Therefore occupational therapists must take it upon themselves to advance their knowledge after graduation. Courses related to the foundational content of the hand therapy certification examination are critical for success. The ASHT, American Hand Therapy Foundation (AHTF), and the Hand Rehabilitation Foundation (HRF) each hold annual conferences that focus on upper extremity rehabilitation practice and research. These multiday conferences are open to hand therapists and nonspecialists alike and offer information on evidence-based practice and current knowledge. The time spent pursuing continuing education is invaluable for the future hand therapist.

There are a multitude of resources for the clinician who wants to specialize in upper extremity rehabilitation. Textbooks related to upper extremity rehabilitation are important components of a clinician's library and should be referred to frequently in early practice. One essential piece for the developing hand therapist is *Rehabilitation of the Hand and Upper Extremity* by Skirven and colleagues.[2] This two-volume set addresses current research in upper extremity conditions, surgical management, and treatment. Many CHTs consider this resource to be the epitome of essential knowledge. There are many other resources related to development of upper extremity rehabilitation, and both the HTCC and the ASHT websites offer suggestions. The HTCC offers a self-assessment tool that can help applicants identify areas of strengths and areas that need further study before taking the certification examination. The ASHT offers CHT test preparation courses several times each year.

Joining a study group is an effective option for developing further knowledge in a clinical specialty area. Some states have organizations of hand therapists who meet regularly, and these groups can be extremely beneficial for the novice therapist. If this type of specialty group is not immediately available, a therapist can network to find other practitioners interested in pursuing the CHT. The ASHT offers an online community forum, and this type of virtual interaction can be just as effective as meeting face-to-face. Study groups often conduct journal reviews, hold case study discussions, or work through mock examination questions together. Sharing clinical experiences and working through the clinical reasoning process for treatment planning is another powerful approach that study groups employ.

Some practitioners may prefer a more directed approach to mastering upper extremity rehabilitation concepts, rather than preparing independently or with other nonspecialists. One path for guided learning is through a formal fellowship program. Fellowship programs at major U.S. hand surgery centers exist whereby licensed occupational or physical therapists obtain experience in upper extremity rehabilitation under the guidance of expert hand therapists and hand surgeons. These full-time fellowships are typically a minimum of 6 months in length and are highly competitive for entry.

Mentoring is an effective way to develop knowledge and advance practice skills. Mentoring can be an informal or a formal partnership between two or more people, where one practitioner serves as the expert and helps the other practitioner gain a deeper understanding of specific content, treatment practices, and skills. The HTCC supports formal mentorship as part of its mission and has developed a self-assessment tool for mentees and a handbook for mentors to facilitate preparation to become a hand therapist. However, mentoring does not have to be a formal process. Some of the most successful mentoring environments are those that develop informally between coworkers or acquaintances. Upon entering practice, new therapists gain immeasurable benefit from working alongside and learning from more experienced therapists. This type of informal mentoring allows easy communication and idea exchanges when mentors work in close proximity. In some instances, new therapists may work in more isolated environments with limited contact with experienced therapists. In these cases the new clinician must be more self-directed and should find a mentor in the field with whom to interact with on a regular basis. The ASHT facilitates mentoring by connecting willing mentors with available mentees through an online community.

Mentoring offers mutual benefits for the involved parties. Mentors can use their experience and knowledge to help mentees advance in clinical practice but also benefit by learning through teaching. Mentees can benefit from the experiences of their mentors, and exploring new topics together can update the mentor's knowledge. Mentoring does not have to be profession-specific either—a new physical therapist can learn from an experienced occupational therapist and vice versa. This interprofessional exposure is especially beneficial in hand therapy, where the two professions overlap and complement the rehabilitation process. The field of hand therapy developed as a result of mentoring when orthopedic surgeons began to work alongside therapists in the treatment of complex upper extremity cases.[1] Mentoring may be the most important step in preparing to specialize in any area, but especially in hand therapy.

Whichever path a therapist chooses, there is an essential process that should be used routinely to refine clinical reasoning. This process, called experiential learning, was outlined by Kolb in 1984 and is well supported throughout educational research. Kolb outlined four distinct steps to complete when learning new concepts: concrete experience, reflective observation, abstract conceptualization, and active experimentation.[13] The first step is gaining authentic experience related to specific concepts. For the new therapist these experiences are a daily occurrence, but even a seasoned therapist encounters new situations. The second step involves deliberate reflection of the experience and the related outcomes. Specifically, the learner notes any contradictions between prior knowledge and new observations. Making connections from past experiences can then lead to new understanding about how to approach similar situations in the future. This process of active reflection and conceptualization is essential for all practitioners to develop clinical reasoning, especially when pursuing specialization.[14]

Threaded Case Study A: After learning about the CHT credential, Owen set a goal to become a hand therapist as soon as he met the application requirements. For the next 3 years, he tracked the number of hours he spent working with people who had upper extremity impairments. He met the 4000 hour requirement after 4 years of practice due to his mixed case load in the rural setting. During these 4 years, Owen dedicated himself to advancing his knowledge through multiple approaches. He joined the ASHT as a nonspecialist and read the Journal of Hand Therapy *routinely. He obtained continuing education credit by completing the quizzes associated with the articles and sought out as many continuing education courses as possible. Owen focused on attending courses that focused on treatment of conditions that affected the shoulder and the wrist and other courses that elaborated on specific treatment interventions, such as manual therapy skills and custom orthotic fabrication.*

He was fortunate that his employer had a generous policy regarding reimbursement for continuing education courses and clinical resources, but he also budgeted his own money to purchase books for his professional library. He found an online study group consisting of other clinicians who intended to take the CHT examination and became a leader in suggesting activities for the group. Owen kept in contact with Cindy, a CHT, via email and video chat due to the physical distance between them. He found her input and guidance invaluable in his preparations. At her suggestion, Owen attended a CHT examination preparation course 1 year before his goal date for the examination. One of his proudest moments in his career was the day he passed the CHT examination and could add "CHT" to his signature.

Threaded Case Study B: Nicole discussed her aspirations to pursue the CHT with her direct manager at the outpatient clinic where she worked. The manager was supportive of Nicole's desire to specialize in hand therapy. Together they agreed to direct all appropriate upper extremity orthopedic referrals to her whenever possible, including shoulder diagnoses after Nicole completed an in-depth continuing education course on the treatment of common shoulder conditions. Nicole approached the orthopedic surgeons in her facility and informed them of her developing knowledge in treating upper extremity conditions, including shoulder conditions, and encouraged them to refer appropriate patients to her for occupational therapy services. Her confidence grew along with her case load, and she incorporated reflective practice into her routine to ensure that she was delivering proper care. This reflective practice included journaling, building her resource library, dedicating time to reading peer-reviewed journals, and using the HTCC Self-Assessment Tool. Her manager took notice of how often Nicole sought out the more experienced physical and occupational therapists to gain their insight into questions or problems she was encountering. Nicole's greatest step was applying for a fellowship at a renowned surgical center and research hospital in her state. When she was selected for the fellowship, she had to make the hard decision to leave her position with the outpatient clinic, but her manager was supportive of the move. The 6-month fellowship offered Nicole a chance to immerse herself in hand therapy, and although she felt mentally exhausted at the end of each day, her understanding of complex upper extremity rehabilitation grew exponentially. She applied for the CHT examination within 3 months of completing the fellowship and proudly added "CHT" to her credentials.

PROFESSIONAL DEVELOPMENT FOR EXPERIENCED THERAPISTS

Upon successful completion of the hand therapy certification examination, a therapist can begin a new path in his or her career. However, certification is only the first step. The HTCC requires hand therapists to recertify every 5 years by completing 80 hours of continuing education and 2000 hours of work experience within the realm of upper extremity rehabilitation. This recertification piece is essential for ensuring that the hand therapist continues his or her evolution of

BOX 21.4 Pathways of Service for Experienced Therapists

Become a fieldwork educator	Mentor new therapists at place of employment
Join local and national associations	Mentor in an area of clinical specialty
Conduct and publish research	Serve as an adjunct instructor in an OT education program
Present at conferences	Volunteer with state or national associations

OT, Occupational therapy.

knowledge and remains current on best practices.[15] Therefore the dedication to ongoing continuing education and refinement of knowledge is a critical factor for all therapists, specialist or not.

Once a therapist has obtained the designation of specialist in any field, the onus shifts from self-directed learning to self-directed service. The scope of occupational therapy is too great to fully cover in entry-level education, so dedication to the profession predicates sharing knowledge and assisting new generations of clinicians in their progression from student to generalist. Fortunately, there are many ways an established therapist can contribute to the education of future therapists (Box 21.4).

Service to the field is mutually beneficial. When sharing clinical experiences and verbalizing clinical reasoning, the experienced therapist gains a deeper understanding of the concepts while simultaneously assisting the novice therapist. One of the most direct ways to support the discipline is to serve as a fieldwork educator. Licensed therapists with 1 year of experience can become fieldwork educators and directly assist occupational therapy students during Level II Fieldwork experiences.[16] Experienced therapists can also share their knowledge through presenting at local, regional, or national conferences. These types of presentations do not have to address groundbreaking content; what some therapists see as commonplace may be completely new to another therapist, so sharing that information has an impact. Agreeing to formally mentor clinicians in an area of specialty is another path that can significantly influence the mentee as well as contribute to the discipline. One critical way to share knowledge is to instruct in an entry-level occupational therapy education program. Occupational therapy is a high-demand field with nearly 200 programs throughout the country,[17] and these programs are dependent on clinician educators to teach, mentor, and influence students.

Choosing occupational therapy as a career has a multitude of benefits and opportunities and should be viewed as a lifelong journey. Becoming an occupational therapy professional entails a commitment to developing deep understanding of ways to assist people in recovery from ailments or conditions that impact their occupational performance, and this understanding can only be achieved through the pursuit of continual education. Many therapists choose to become specialists in some form: either through long-term experience in a specific practice area, with specific populations, or through formal certifications. Those who choose to become hand therapists are selecting a credential that communicates their level of knowledge to all parties and allows focused practice with people experiencing physical impairments of the upper extremity—from shoulder to fingertip. This field is incredibly rewarding, and professionals who obtain this level of specialization are highly sought and well-respected within the medical community. No matter the credentials, experienced therapists who are dedicated to professional development are a wealth of knowledge and essential leaders for the advancement of occupational therapy.

Threaded Case Study A: Owen went on to start a hand therapy organization within his state, which completed quarterly virtual meetings for journal reviews, case discussions, and advocacy work. He also agreed to present at his state occupational therapy association conference, and although he was nervous about speaking in front of other professionals, he found a receptive audience when presenting on treatment of common upper extremity conditions. This experience bolstered his confidence, and he continued to present at regional and state meetings. Within 6 years of becoming a CHT, he was approached by a local occupational therapy education program about teaching a course on upper extremity rehabilitation, and soon found a new passion for educating future occupational therapists.

Threaded Case Study B: Nicole was fortunate enough to return to her original employer 2 years after obtaining the CHT credential, when the hospital opened an outpatient orthopedic surgery center. Here Nicole worked alongside two other hand therapists and had direct access to two hand surgeons. She worked with people who had complex traumatic conditions involving the upper extremity and provided in-house orthosis fabrication during the hand surgeons' clinic hours. Over the years, Nicole and the other hand therapists participated in clinical research on various upper extremity rehabilitation topics and had the research published in peer-reviewed journals. When she was first approached about completing research, Nicole was concerned about the time demands but soon found that it was manageable with a team approach and with good support from their administration. Over the years Nicole always made time to accept fieldwork students from the regional occupational therapy education program and enjoyed watching these students advance in their understanding of upper extremity rehabilitation.

REVIEW QUESTIONS

1. Do any of the specialization areas mentioned in this chapter interest you?
2. Where do you see your career in 5 years? 10 years?
3. Which path of education interests you—self-directed or guided?
4. Which path of service interests you? Which options do you see yourself doing in 10 years?

REFERENCES

1. Fess E: A history of splinting: to understand the present, view the past, *J Hand Ther* 15(2):97–132, 2002.
2. Skirven T, Osterman AL, Fedorczyk J, Amadio P, eds.: Rehabilitation of the hand and upper extremity, ed 6, Philadelphia, 2011, Elsevier, pp 1565–1580.
3. American Occupational Therapy Association: *2011 Accreditation Council for Occupational Therapy Education standards and interpretive guide.* Retrieved from https://www.aota.org/~/media/Corporate/Files/EducationCareers/Accredit/Standards/2011-Standards-and-Interpretive-Guide.pdf, 2011.
4. American Occupational Therapy Association: *Board and specialty certifications.* Retrieved from https://www.aota.org/Education-Careers/Advance-Career/Board-Specialty-Certifications.aspx, 2011.
5. American Occupational Therapy Association: *AOTA fellowship programs.* Retrieved from https://www.aota.org/Education-Careers/Advance-Career/fellowship.aspx, 2017.
6. Lyon S: *The ABCs of occupational therapy specialty certifications and credentials.* Retrieved from https://www.verywell.com/occupational-therapy-degrees-and-training-2509970?utm_source=pinterest&utm_medium=social&utm_campaign=mobilesharebutton2, 2016.
7. Chai S, Dimick M, Kasch M: A role delineation study of hand therapy. *J Hand Ther* 1(1):7–17, 1987.
8. Hand Therapy Certification Commission: *Consumer information.* Retrieved from https://www.htcc.org/consumer-information, 2017.
9. Hand Therapy Certification Commission: *Certification.* Retrieved from https://www.htcc.org/certify, 2017.
10. Hand Therapy Certification Commission: *Passing rates for the CHT exam.* Retrieved from https://www.htcc.org/certify/exam-results/passing-rates, 2017.
11. Rhodes D: *Personal interview via email,* September 22, 2017.
12. Hand Therapy Certification Commission: *Salary & benefits survey.* Retrieved from https://www.htcc.org/htcc/salarysurvey, 2017.
13. Atkinson G Jr, Murrell P: Kolb's experiential learning theory: a meta-model for career exploration. *J Couns Dev* 66(8):374–377, 1988.
14. Lin S, Murphy S, Robinson J: Facilitating evidence-based practice: process, strategies, and resources, *Am J Occup Ther* 64:164–171, 2010.
15. Hand Therapy Certification Commission: *Recertify.* Retrieved from https://www.htcc.org/recertify, 2017.
16. American Occupational Therapy Association: *COE guidelines for an occupational therapy fieldwork experience – level II.* Retrieved from https://www.aota.org/~/media/Corporate/Files/EducationCareers/Educators/Fieldwork/LevelII/COE%20Guidelines%20for%20an%20Occupational%20Therapy%20Fieldwork%20Experience%20-%20Level%20II–Final.pdf, 2013.
17. American Occupational Therapy Association: *Find a school.* Retrieved from https://www.aota.org/Education-Careers/Find-School.aspx, 2017.

GLOSSARY

A

acromion Forms the summit of the shoulder and connects with the clavicle to form the acromioclavicular joint.

activity-specific devices Terminal devices that are intended for a function or types of functions; often oriented to activities of daily living, work, and recreation.

adherence The extent that a client follows agreed-upon intervention without close supervision.

agonist A muscle that contracts while the other muscle relaxes.

alignment Arranging of anatomical structures so that they are in proper relative position.

AMBRI Multidirectional bilateral shoulder instability, caused by a combination of microtraumas with rehabilitation being the treatment of choice.

Antagonist A muscle that opposes the action of another muscle.

anterior elbow immobilization orthosis Elbow immobilization orthosis positioned on the anterior aspect of the arm.

anterior instability of the shoulder Increased abnormal movement of the humeral head anteriorly, partially displacing the humeral head from the glenoid labrum.

anterior transposition of the ulnar nerve A surgical procedure with two main methods to reposition the ulnar nerve. The procedure includes subcutaneous and submuscular transposition. The subcutaneous method includes moving the ulnar nerve anteriorly medial to the median nerve and below subcutaneous fascia in the forearm.

anticoagulants A substance that hinders the clotting of blood; blood thinners.

antideformity position One positional option includes the wrist in 30 to 40 degrees of extension, the thumb in 40 to 45 degrees of palmar abduction, the thumb interphalangeal (IP) joint in full extension, the metacarpophalangeals (MCPs) at 70 to 90 degrees of flexion, and the proximal interphalangeals (PIPs) and distal interphalangeals (DIPs) in full extension.

aponeurosis A strong sheet of fibrous connective tissue that serves as a tendon to attach muscles to bone or as a fascia to bind muscles together.

appendicular skeleton Bones of the upper and lower extremity, excluding the head, trunk, and vertebrae.

area of force application Area that force is supplied with an orthosis.

arteriovenous anastomosis A blood vessel that connects directly to a venule without capillary intervention.

arteriovenous fistula Surgically created fistula are typically located on the forearm and used for vascular access for hemodialysis.

arthrogryposis Or arthrogryposis multiplex congenita typically involves all four extremities.

A pronounced lack of muscle mass and flexion creases is apparent. Joints have decreased ROM with an inelastic end range. Typical posturing includes internally rotated and adducted shoulders, extended elbows, pronated forearms, flexed and ulnarly deviated wrists, partially flexed fingers, and adducted thumbs.

Assessment of Motor and Process Skills (AMPS) A functional assessment that requires the client to perform an instrumental activity of daily living (IADL) and assesses motor and process skills.

axial skeleton Bones of the head, trunk, and vertebrae.

axonotmesis An interruption of the axon with subsequent degeneration of the distal nerve segment.

B

Bankart An injury to the shoulder resulting in a detachment of the anterior inferior glenoid labrum. This is most often caused by an anteriorly dislocating humeral head.

biofeedback A training technique by which a person learns how to regulate certain muscle functions; one example of usage is to develop control of a prosthesis.

biofeedback machine Equipment used to identify muscle signals and sites.

biomechanical Considering the mechanical aspect of the body such as forces and muscle exertion.

biomechanical principles Principles that include assessment of normal and pathological gait patterns in a clinically observable evaluation.

biopsychosocial approach Involving the interchange of biological, psychological, and social factors.

body-powered prosthesis Prosthesis activated and operated by body movements.

boutonnière deformity A finger that postures with proximal interphalangeal (PIP) flexion and distal interphalangeal (DIP) hyperextension.

brachial plexus palsy Paralysis or paresis of the brachial plexus, a nerve plexus originating from the anterior branches, including the last four cervical and first four thoracic spinal nerves. Plexus innervates the shoulder, chest, and arms.

buddy straps Soft straps used to promote motion and support an injured digit to an adjacent digit.

C

camptodactyly Permanent flexion of one or more of the interphalangeal finger joints usually caused by congenital factors.

Canadian Occupational Performance Measure (COPM) A client-centered outcome measure used to assess self-care, productivity, and leisure.

carpal tunnel syndrome (CTS) A common painful disorder of the wrist and hand induced by compression on the median nerve

between the inelastic carpal ligament and other structures in the carpal tunnel.

central slip This structure crosses the proximal interphalangeal (PIP) joint dorsally and is part of the PIP joint dorsal capsule.

centralization A surgical procedure to realign the wrist to correct a wrist deviation.

cerebral palsy (CP) A condition resulting in a nonprogressive movement and postural disorder because of abnormal neural development or damage to the motor centers of the brain before, during, or after birth.

certified hand therapist An occupational or physical therapist who has demonstrated advanced knowledge in the treatment of upper extremity impairments.

circumferential An orthosis that fits around the circumference of an extremity.

clasped thumb Refers to a classification of thumb anomalies that range from mild deficiencies of the thumb extensor mechanism to severe abnormalities of the thenar muscles, web space, and soft tissues.

clavicular facet Hollow articulation on the sternum that articulates with the clavicle connecting the axial to the appendicular skeleton for the upper extremity.

client-centered intervention Treatment that focuses on meeting client goals as opposed to therapist-designed or protocol-driven goals.

client safety Approach to client care that considers safety.

clinical considerations Presentations or conditions that must be accounted for planning intervention (e.g., lack of sensation, skin breakdown, etc.).

clinical reasoning The in-depth deliberation and decision process that therapists apply in clinical practice involving several approaches toward thinking.

clinodactyly A congenital condition resulting in permanent and abnormal lateral or medial flexion of one or more fingers.

collateral ligaments Ligaments on each side of the joint that provide joint stability and restraint against deviation forces. The radial collateral ligament protects against ulnar deviation forces, and the ulnar collateral ligament protects against radial deviation forces.

complex regional pain syndrome (CRPS) A chronic pain condition thought to be a result of impairment in the central or peripheral nerve systems.

componentry The compilation of components toward assembling a prosthesis.

composite extension Extension of all fingers together.

compression socks Socks used to reduce swelling formation at an amputation site.

concomitant injury Injury that occurs impacting two or more places simultaneously.

congenital hand anomalies Hand deformities found at birth.

congenital trigger finger Condition found at birth in which the finger is pulled into flexion.

constriction band syndrome   A congenital disorder caused by entrapment of fetal parts, usually a limb or digits, in fibrous amniotic bands while in utero.

context   A variety of interrelated conditions within and surrounding the client that influence performance, including cultural, physical, social, personal, spiritual, temporal, and virtual aspects.

contracture   An abnormal, usually permanent, condition of a joint characterized by flexion and fixation and caused by atrophy and shortening of muscle fibers or by loss of the normal elasticity of the skin, such as that from the formation of extensive scar tissue over a joint.

contralateral limb   Limb on the opposite side to the referent.

convection   Transfer of heat between a surface and a moving medium or agent.

coracohumeral ligament   A ligament that forms a ridged support of the anterior shoulder.

creep   Response of soft tissue to prolonged stress. Can be with pain or inflammation or can be managed with controlled stress.

cubital tunnel syndrome   Ulnar nerve compression in the upper extremity located between the medial epicondyle of the humerus and the olecranon resulting in pain and paresthesias in the fourth and fifth digits.

cumulative trauma disorder (CTD)   Musculoskeletal disorder resulting from repetitive motions (usually occupation) that develop over time. Symptoms include pain, inflammation, and function impairment.

D

degrees of freedom   The number of planes in which a joint axis(es) can move.

de Quervain tenosynovitis   The most commonly diagnosed wrist tendonitis that may be recognized by pain over the radial styloid, edema in the first dorsal compartment, and positive results from the Finkelstein test or other assessments for the condition.

distal humerus   Fracture at the end of the humerus bone.

documentation   Professional writing in a formal medical record.

dorsal   Pertaining to the back or posterior.

double crush   Nerves that are compressed at more than one site.

dual site   The use of an externally powered prosthesis from two muscle sites.

Dupuytren contracture   A contracture characterized by the formation of finger flexion contractures with a thickened band of palmar fascia.

dynamic orthosis   A mobilization orthosis that has a stable static base and an elastic mobilizing component.

E

ecchymosis   A subcutaneous hemorrhage marked by purple discoloration of the skin.

elbow arthroplasty   The resurfacing or replacement of the elbow joint.

elbow instability   Injury that results from a dislocation of the ulnohumeral joint and injury to the varus and valgus stabilizers of the elbow and to the radial head.

electrodes   Conductors through which muscle electricity is transmitted to control prosthetic technology.

end feel   Assessed by passively moving a joint to its maximal end range.

Erb palsy   Paralysis of the upper arm and shoulders but not hands caused by a lesion of the upper trunk of the brachial plexus or roots to the fifth and sixth cervical nerves.

Essex-Lopresti fracture   Fracture of the radial head along with dislocation of the distal radioulnar joint and accompanying issues with the interosseous membrane resulting from a fall from a height.

evidence-based practice   The process of reviewing a body of literature to select the most appropriate assessment or treatment for an individual client.

extensor lag   The joint can be passively extended but cannot be fully actively extended by the client.

externally powered prosthesis   Prosthesis that is controlled or powered outside the body; also referred to as myoelectric prosthesis.

F

fellowship program   Post-professional training programs that advance a practitioner's knowledge and skills in a focused area or practice.

figure-eight orthosis   Support straps used with injury to the clavicle and/or acromioclavicular joint. It prevents upward migration of the proximal clavicle and assists in alignment during healing.

finger loops   A method of applying dynamic force to a joint.

finger sprain   Stress or ligamentous injury to a joint. Occurs in varying grades of severity.

flexion contracture   A joint that cannot be passively extended to neutral.

forearm trough   A component of the wrist immobilization orthosis that rests proximal to the wrist on one or more surfaces of the forearm. It provides counterforce leverage to support the weight of the forearm.

functional envelope   Area of work in front and around a person's hands.

functional position   A position that includes the wrist in 20 to 30 degrees of extension, the thumb in 45 degrees of palmar abduction, the metacarpophalangeal (MCP) joints in 35 to 45 degrees of flexion, and all proximal interphalangeal (PIP) and distal interphalangeal (DIP) joints in slight flexion.

fusiform swelling   Fullness at the proximal interphalangeal (PIP) joint and tapering proximally and distally. Often seen following finger PIP joint sprains.

G

glenoid fossa   A shallow depression on the lateral scapula that increases the surface area contact with the head of the humerus.

grasp   The result of holding an object against the rigid portion of the hand that the second and third digits provide. The flattening and cupping motions of the palm allow the hand to pick up and handle objects of various sizes.

grip force   Strength applied by the terminal device to grasp objects.

H

handling characteristics   The properties of thermoplastic material when heated and softened.

hand therapy   Hand therapy is the art and science of rehabilitation of the upper limb, which includes the hand, wrist, elbow, and shoulder girdle. It is a merging of occupational and physical therapy theory and practice that combines comprehensive knowledge of the structure of the upper limb with function and activity. Using specialized skills in assessment, planning, and treatment, hand therapists provide therapeutic interventions to prevent dysfunction, restore function, and/or reverse the progression of pathology of the upper limb to enhance an individual's ability to execute tasks and to participate fully in life situations.

hard end feel   An abrupt hard stop to movement when bone contacts bone during passive range of motion (PROM).

harness   Strapping used to suspend or to help to control the prosthesis.

Health Insurance Portability and Accountability Act (HIPPA)   Health Insurance Portability and Accountable Act regulates privacy standards that protect medical records and other health information.

heat gun   An instrument used to make adjustments to thermoplastic materials.

hook rubbers   Elastic bands used to control a voluntary-opening terminal device.

hybrid prosthesis   Prosthesis with components that are controlled or powered by the body and external to the body.

hypertonicity   Being hypertonic or having excess tone.

hypoextensibility   Lack of ability for muscles to extend or stretch in a typical manner.

hypoplasia   Unfinished or underdevelopment of an organ or part.

hypothenar bar   A component of the wrist immobilization orthosis that palmarly supports the ulnar aspect of the transverse metacarpal arch.

I

immobilization   Orthoses designed to immobilize primary or secondary joints.

integumentary system   A system encompassing the integument (skin) and its derivatives.

intervention process   Process provided by therapist with intervention.

L

lamination   Hard, permanent finish of prosthetic socket.

lateral bands   Contributions from the intrinsic muscles that join dorsal to the proximal interphalangeal (PIP) joint axis. They displace volarly in a boutonnière deformity and dorsally in a swan neck deformity.

lateral epicondyle   The tissue at the lower end of the humerus at the elbow joint.

M

mallet finger   A finger that postures with distal interphalangeal (DIP) flexion.

McKie thumb orthosis   A prefabricated Neoprene orthosis designed to position the thumb in opposition and to which a supinator strap may be added. The primary function is to provide biomechanically sound weight bearing, grasp, and manipulation of objects.

mechanical advantage   The ratio of the output force developed by the muscles to the input force applied to the body structures the muscles move, especially the ratio of these forces associated with the body structures that act as levers.

mechanoreceptor   Sensory nerve ending that responds to mechanical stimuli, such as touch, pressure, sound, and muscular contractions.

medial epicondyle   The part of the humerus that gives attachment to the ulnar collateral ligament of the elbow joint, to the pronator teres, and to a common tendon of origin (the common flexor tendon) of some of the flexor muscles of the forearm.

median nerve   One of the terminal branches of the brachial plexus, which extends along the radial parts of the forearm and the hand and supplies various muscles and the skin of these parts.

memory   The ability of thermoplastic material to return to its preheated (original) shape and size when reheated.

mentor   Experienced practitioner who assists in the professional development of a novice practitioner.

metacarpal bar   A component of the wrist immobilization orthosis that supports the transverse metacarpal arch dorsally or palmarly.

minimalist design   A basic simplified orthotic design.

mobilization orthosis   Orthosis designed to move or mobilize primary or secondary joints.

monteggia fracture   Dislocation of the proximal radioulnar joint along with a forearm fracture.

myoelectric prosthesis   Prosthesis that is controlled or powered outside the body; also known as externally powered prosthesis.

myostatic contracture   Shortening of muscle typically due to immobilization and without pathology.

N

Neoprene   A soft orthotic material consisting of rubber with nylon lining on one side and pile material on the other, thus making the Velcro hook attachment quick. Neoprene retains warmth, has some degree of elasticity, and has contour for a snug fit.

nerve entrapment   A medical condition caused by direct pressure on a nerve, also referred to as a trapped nerve, or may refer to nerve root compression.

neurapraxia   A condition in which a nerve remains in place after a severe injury, with a short-term loss of nerve conduction.

neurophysiological   Branch of physiology that addresses the nervous system.

neurotmesis   A peripheral nerve injury in which laceration or traction completely disrupts the nerve.

normal gait   Smooth, rhythmic patterns of motion requiring little effort involving a gait cycle from initial contact of one foot to the next initial contact of the same foot

O

oblique retinacular ligament (ORL)   Also called the *ligament of Landsmeer,* this structure is determined to be tight if there is limitation of passive distal interphalangeal (DIP) flexion while the proximal interphalangeal (PIP) joint is extended.

occupational deprivation   A state wherein clients are unable to engage in chosen meaningful life occupations due to factors outside their control.

occupational disruption   A temporary and less severe condition than occupational deprivation that is also caused by an unexpected change in the ability to engage in meaningful activities.

occupational profile   The phase of the evaluation process that involves learning about a client from a contextual and performance viewpoint.

Occupational Therapy Code of Ethics and Ethics Standards   The professional code of ethics established by the American Occupational Therapy Association (AOTA). This code sets forth the minimal expectations for occupational therapists.

occupation-based orthotic intervention   A treatment approach that supports the goals of the treatment plan to promote the ability of clients to engage in meaningful and relevant life endeavors.

occupation-centered   An overarching paradigm for conducting occupational therapy assessment and intervention that promotes the ability of the individual with dysfunction to engage in desired life tasks and occupations.

occupation-focused approach   The attention to the occupational desires and needs of an individual, coupled with knowledge of the effects or potential effects of pathological conditions and managed through client-centered interventions.

olecranon process   A proximal projection of the ulna that forms the tip of the elbow and fits into the olecranon fossa of the humerus when the forearm is extended at the proximal extremity of the ulna.

open reduction internal fixation (ORIF)   Two-part surgical procedure for a broken bone, including putting the bone back into place (reduction), followed by using a means of internal fixation (screws, plates, rods, pins) to hold the bone.

orthosis   A device that can support, place in alignment, or help correct the positioning of a body part.

orthotic design principles   Principles that consider the interaction of anatomical and mechanical structures as well as functional considerations of orthotic components and materials.

orthotic terminology   Terminology derived from the anatomical area affected by the orthosis.

orthotic treatment objectives   Objectives that establish short- and long-term goals that enhance functional level with minimal orthotic intervention.

osseo-integration   The structural link at which human bone and the surface of a synthetic, often titanium-based, implant meet.

osteoarthritis (OA)   The most common form of arthritis, in which one or many joints undergo degenerative changes—including loss of articular cartilage and proliferation of bone spurs.

osteoporotic fracture   Low-trauma or fragility fracture, which occurs from a fall from a standing height or less, affecting those with low bone mineral density.

outrigger   A projection from the orthosis base that the therapist uses to position a mobilizing force.

overuse syndrome   Type of injury common to the contralateral side among individuals with upper limb acquired loss or congenital difference, typically caused by repetitive movements or awkward postures and also known as repetitive strain injury (RSI). Symptoms include swelling, pain, and weakness in the affected joints.

P

passive functional aesthetic device   Static prosthesis that appears to look like a hand; functions include stabilizing, supporting, and social tasks.

pathological gait   Abnormal gait that may develop from neuromuscular deficits, joint instabilities, pain, disease, or congenital impairment.

pattern recognition   Control requires a set of myoelectric signals, corresponding to each possible movement of the user's prosthesis, to be recorded and used to calibrate the control system.

pediatric trigger thumb   Presentation typical in early childhood; palpable nodule at the volar aspect of the metacarpophalangeal (MCP) joint flexion crease, known as a Notta nodule.

performance characteristics   The properties of thermoplastic material after the material has cooled and hardened.

phantom pain   Pain that feels like it is coming from a body part that is no longer present; once believed to be a psychological problem, it is now recognized that these real sensations originate in the spinal cord and brain.

phantom sensation   Sensation that an amputated or missing limb is still attached.

physical agent modality (PAM)   Modality that produces a biophysiological response through the use of light, water, temperature, sound, electricity, or mechanical devices.

plaster bandage   Material used for casting.

plasticity   The quality of being plastic or formative.

positioning   Place a joint or extremity in a desired position for optimal healing.

posterior elbow immobilization orthosis   A custom-molded thermoplastic orthosis positioned in 80 to 90 degrees of flexion.

posterior interosseous nerve syndrome   A condition that includes weakness or paralysis of any muscles innervated by the posterior interosseous nerve and does not involve sensory loss.

prefabricated off-the-shelf (OTS)   A commercially-purchased orthotic device that is not custom-fitted.

preformed orthoses   Factory-produced orthoses premolded to a specific design.

prehension   The use of the hands and fingers to grasp or pick up objects.

pressure   Total force divided by the area of application.

principles   The universal nature of obligations and duties and their application to moral decisions.

pronator tunnel syndrome   The compression of the median nerve in the forearm between the two heads of the pronator teres muscle.

prosthesis   An artificial device to replace or augment a missing or impaired part of the body.

prosthosis   A hybrid device accessing the qualities and/or functions of a prosthesis and an orthosis for a retained limb with lost/impaired function.

protocols   Written plans specifying the procedures for giving an examination, conducting research, or providing care for a particular condition.

psychosocial-emotional impact   The effect caused by environmental and/or biological factors on an individual's social and/or psychological aspects.

R

radial   Pertaining to the radius or radial side of the forearm or hand.

radial head   The disk-shaped portion of the radius closest to the elbow.

radial longitudinal deficiency   A longitudinal deficiency of the radius associated with abnormal genetics resulting in missing or malformed radius and a small or missing thumb.

radial nerve   The largest branch of the brachial plexus, supplying the skin of the arm and forearm and their extensor muscles.

radial nerve injuries   Injuries commonly occurring from fractures of the humeral shaft, fractures and dislocation of the elbow, or compressions of the nerve.

radial tunnel syndrome   A condition in which a nerve in the forearm is compressed, causing elbow pain and weakness of the wrist or hand but without causing a loss of sensation.

radialization   A surgical procedure to move the hand closer to the radial border of the forearm.

radio-frequency identification (RFID)   A type of wireless communication that typically involves an RFID reader and a tag. The tag has information stored in its memory, and the reader (using an antenna) can read this information.

reliability   The consistency of an assessment.

residual limb   The remnant limb of a congenital difference or following amputation.

responsiveness   An assessment's sensitivity to measure differences in status.

rheumatoid arthritis (RA)   A chronic systemic disease that can affect the lungs, cardiovascular system, and eyes. Joint involvement resulting from inflammatory disease of the synovium is the primary clinical feature. The disease may range from mild to severe and can result in joint deformity and destruction of varying degrees.

S

scaphoid fracture   A break in the boat-shaped bone of the hand.

sensory system modulation   The brain's ability to regulate and balance excitation and inhibition of sensory input.

serial casting   Casting used to gradually increase range of motion.

serial-static orthosis   A type of mobilization orthosis that positions a joint near its elastic limits to overcome a loss in passive range of motion.

single site   The use of an externally powered prosthesis from one muscle site.

socket   A hard material (resin and plastic) used to make temporary or permanent prostheses.

soft end feel   Soft compression of tissue felt when two body surfaces approximate each other.

soft orthosis   Prefabricated or custom orthosis made from various soft materials.

spasticity   A form of muscular hypertonicity with increased resistance to stretch.

splint   Refers to casts and strapping applied for reductions of fractures and dislocations.

stages of tissue healing   Refers to wound healing stages, such as the proliferative stage, which influence orthotic provision.

static-progressive orthosis   An orthosis that uses nonelastic tension to provide a constant force.

stress   Any emotional, physical, social, economic, or other factor that requires a response or change.

stretch reflex   Reflex that is elicited through passive stretch used with orthotic fabrication for a person who has muscle tone.

subcutaneous   Under the skin.

subluxation   A partial separation or dislocation of the articular surfaces of a joint.

submaximum range of motion   Placement of an orthosis 5-10 degrees below maximum passive range.

submuscular   Under the musculature.

superficial agents   Heating agents or thermotherapy agents that penetrate the skin to a depth of 1 to 2 cm. They include moist hot packs, Fluidotherapy, paraffin wax therapy, and cryotherapy.

superior labrum tear from anterior to posterior (SLAP)   An injury to the glenoid labrum of the shoulder affecting the top of the labrum. The injury can occur in front and back of the attachment of the biceps tendon.

suspension systems   Straps used to suspend or hold a prosthesis.

swan neck deformity   A finger that postures with proximal interphalangeal (PIP) hyperextension and distal interphalangeal (DIP) flexion.

syndactyly   Webbing between finger digits creating fusion of the digits.

T

targeted muscle reinnervation (TMR)   Surgical procedure in which residual nerves from the amputated limb are transferred to reinnervate new muscle targets.

task-oriented approach   Approach toward intervention that encourages hand use with functional tasks.

tendinopathy   Injury to a tendon, including tendonitis, tendinitis, tenosynovitis, and tendinosis.

tendinosis   Noninflammatory degenerative condition of the collagen tissue due to aging, microtrauma, or vascular compromise.

tendonitis   An inflammatory condition of a tendon, usually resulting from strain.

tennis elbow   Also known as lateral epicondylitis, overuse of the forearm extensor muscles causing strain or microtears in the extensor muscles, especially the extensor carpi radialis brevis.

tenosynovitis   Inflammation of a tendon sheath caused by calcium deposits, repeated strain or trauma, high levels of blood cholesterol, rheumatoid arthritis, gout, or gonorrhea.

terminal device (TD)   Hand, hook, or tool used at the end of a prosthesis.

terminal extensor tendon   This delicate structure is formed by the uniting of the lateral bands and provides distal interphalangeal (DIP) extension.

"Terrible triad" injury   A coronoid avulsion fracture resulting in elbow instability and dislocation of the ulnohumeral joint and injury to the varus and valgus stabilizers of the elbow and radial head.

thermoplastic material   Material that softens under heat and is capable of being molded into shape with pressure and then hardens upon cooling without undergoing a chemical change.

3-D printed device   A three-dimensional device that resembles a prosthesis, fabricated from computer-aided manufacturing (CAM).

three-point pressure   A system consisting of three individual linear forces in which the middle force is directed in opposite direction to the other two forces.

torque   The effect a force has on rotational movement of a point. It can be calculated by multiplying the force by the length of the movement arm.

torque transmission   Orthoses that create motion of primary joints situated beyond the boundaries of the orthosis itself or that harness secondary "driver" joint(s) to create motion of primary joints that may be situated longitudinally or transversely to the driver joint(s).

transhumeral amputation   Amputation across the humerus bone.

transradial amputation   Amputation across the radius and ulna bones.

transverse humeral ligament   Forms a bridge between the lesser and greater tubercle of the humerus enclosing the canal of the bicipital groove.

transverse retinacular ligament   This ligament helps prevent lateral band dorsal displacement and thereby contributes to the delicate balance of the extensor mechanism at the proximal interphalangeal (PIP) joint.

treatment protocol   Written plan specifying the procedures for treatment.

trigger finger   A condition when a tendon becomes inflamed and swollen, limiting its ability to slide freely, and the finger locks when attempting to extend the finger after making a fist. Bending the finger or thumb can make a snapping or popping sound.

TUBS   Acronym that stands for Traumatic etiology, Unidirectional instability, Bankart lesion, whereby Surgery is required for the shoulder instability.

U

ulnar   Pertaining to the long medial bone of the forearm or ulnar side of the forearm or hand.

ulnar collateral ligament (UCL) injury   A common injury that can occur at the metacarpophalangeal (MCP) joint of the thumb. This is also known as *skier's thumb* or *gamekeeper's thumb.*

ulnar nerve   One of the terminal branches of the brachial plexus that supplies the muscles and skin on the ulnar side of the forearm and hand.

ulnarization   A surgical procedure to move the hand closer to the ulnar border of the forearm.

V

valgus   Deformed joint with the more distal of the bones deviating from the midline of the body.

validity   The extent to which an assessment measures what it is intended to measure.

values   The internal motivators for an individual's actions.

varus   Deformed joint that is bent inward with the angulation toward the midline of the body.

verbal analog scale (VeAS)   A scale used to determine a person's perception of pain intensity. The person is asked to rate pain on a scale from 0 to 10 (0 refers to no pain, and 10 refers to the worst pain ever experienced.)

viscoelasticity   The skin's degree of viscosity and elasticity, which enables the skin to resist stress.

visual analog scale (ViAS)   A scale used to determine a person's perception of pain intensity. The person is asked to look at a 10-cm horizontal line. The left side of the line represents "no pain," and the right side represents "pain as bad as it could be." The person indicates pain level by marking a slash on the line, which represents the pain experienced.

volar   Also called *palmar,* this term pertains to the palm of the hand or the sole of the foot.

volar plate (VP)   A fibrocartilaginous structure that prevents hyperextension of a joint.

voluntary-closing   Terminal device oriented in the open position; user must actuate to close the device.

voluntary-opening   Terminal device oriented in the closed position; user must actuate to open the device.

W

Wallerian degeneration   When a nerve is completely severed or the axon and myelin sheath are damaged, the segment of axon and the motor and sensory end receptors distal to the lesion suffer ischemia and begin to degenerate 3 to 5 days after the injury.

Wartenberg neuropathy   Compression of the superficial radial nerve that usually includes numbness, tingling, and pain of the dorsoradial aspect of the forearm, wrist, and hand.

wearing schedules   Planned schedules for donning and doffing orthoses.

working memory   The short-term storage of information in the brain.

Z

zones of the hand   The division of the hand into distinct areas for ease of understanding literature, conversing with other health providers, and documenting pertinent information.

A APPENDIX

Answers to Self-Quizzes, Case Studies, and Laboratory Exercises

CHAPTER 1

Self-Quiz 1.1

1. b
2. c
3. a

Case Study 1.1

1. c
2. a
3. 1: b; 2: c; 3: a

CHAPTER 2

Self-Quiz 2.1

1. The therapist should learn about the culture of the client, either through a personal interview with the individual or family or through reading. If the client speaks a language that you do not speak, ensure that a translator is present so that information is accurately transmitted between you and the client. Different cultures may have views about illness and disability that are unique. They may also be of a different faith or have family obligations and responsibilities dissimilar from those you are accustomed to. Wearing an orthosis during certain ceremonies or religious events may not be acceptable to your client. Discuss the orthotic plan, and appropriately explain the importance of compliance. If you learn that cultural difference may be a barrier to compliance, work with the client to arrive at a workable solution.

2. The areas of occupation of play and education as well as developmentally appropriate activities of daily living (ADLs) and instrumental activities of daily living (IADLs) functions should be considered. Personal context factors such as age and gender may impact color selection and the level of independence the child may have with orthotic donning/doffing and care. A younger child may need to have additional straps applied to prevent unwanted orthotic removal or shifting. An older child may be able to independently monitor an orthotic schedule.

Case Study 2.1

1. Natasha's husband, who is her primary caretaker, has accompanied her to treatment sessions. As an important part of her social context, and his role as caregiver, he can assist Natasha with accurate completion of the intake interview. To ensure that Natasha is empowered and her family role as primary home and family caretaker is preserved to the fullest extent possible within this traditional family, the therapist should first address questions to Natasha and verify responses with her husband, only if needed.

2. The orthotic care sheet should be written in large, bold font. Instructions should be written in simple phrases and line drawings used as appropriate to illustrate orthosis and strap placement. Black-and-white or photocopied photos should be avoided because they may not provide high contrast. High-contrast color photos taken of the orthosis on Natasha's hand may assist with accurate placement but should not be used as the only pictorial representation. Orthotic care instructions must be reviewed with Natasha and her husband using the orthotic care sheet before issuing the device. Natasha should be asked to repeat instructions and precautions back to the therapist with the assistance of her husband.

3. As with the orthotic care sheet, large font and line drawings can be used to assist with low vision. Instructions should be phrased simply, and the order of the exercises should be clearly indicated. Line drawings can be effective, as can color photographs of Natasha's hand. Exercise instructions must be reviewed with Natasha and her husband using the handout. Natasha should be asked to demonstrate the exercises and verbalize repetitions and frequency with the assistance of her husband.

4. Following consultation with the treating physician, a removable volar component could be added to the orthosis to statically maintain the alignment of her digits with MCPs secured in neutral. This volar component should be easily removed and applied by Natasha and her husband frequently throughout the day for active exercise regime. The volar component will secure the delicate MCP joints if Natasha were to become unclear about the purpose of the dynamic outrigger and attempt to remove it. The dynamic orthosis with volar component will be replaced with a resting pan orthosis at night. The resting pan orthosis has a lower profile and secures joints for safety during sleep.

Case Study 2.2

1. Graysen indicated that he is not satisfied with his ability to complete independent bill paying, use the computer to communicate with friends and family or social networking websites, and prepare his plate for independent eating. These areas scored poor in performance and satisfaction. Despite these issues being caused by limited

hand function, they should be addressed during the first treatment sessions to enhance the quality of life for Graysen. Although these functions should return eventually as hand function improves, waiting for eventual hand movement, strength, and coordination will create an unnecessary lack of ability to complete meaningful life tasks. Computer use and social communication and bill paying are reported to be the most difficult and least satisfactory areas for Graysen.

2. A client-centered treatment model and a rehabilitative approach will expedite Graysen's return to function. The client-centered model focuses attention on his immediate concerns (bill paying, computer use and social communication, eating/plate preparation). The rehabilitative approach uses adaptations and modifications as treatment methods to enhance function.

3. The Canadian Occupational Performance Measure (COPM) was used to investigate the functional capabilities of the client within all areas of daily functioning. Issues were discovered within the patient's social, personal, and virtual contexts.

4. A suggested orthosis would be one that facilitates his ability to type and hold onto objects, such as flatware and pencils, as well as to provide digital support for typing. The dorsal hand-based orthosis extending from wrist to PIP joints holds all digits in flexion. The long, ring and small fingers would be held in more flexion than the index finger to provide isolated digit for typing and securing tools. This orthosis would be applied to the dominant hand, a second orthosis could be fabricated for the non-dominant hand to facilitate typing and food management during eating.

Case Study 2.3

1. The therapist should conduct an occupational profile (AOTA,2017) with the client to determine the impact that her elbow fracture and current orthotic device are having on her roles, habits and routines. It should also be determined what aspects of her environment and context may be barriers or supports for her current level of occupational participation. The goals of the client should also be clearly identified during this process.

2. The Canadian Occupational Performance Measure

3. A lightweight thermoplastic orthosis should be fabricated to replace the plaster device provided by the physician. Why? Due to the ongoing healing status of her elbow, it is important to continue with intermittent immobilization during occupations and other activities that are meaningful to the client. In addition, due to the heavy and ill-fitting nature of the plaster orthosis, a custom thermoplastic splint can reduce the potential for further harm to the wrist and shoulder.

4. The intervention itself would not change, a custom elbow orthosis must be fabricated. However, the ability of the client to engage in her desired leisure occupation of swimming and attending church activities should be considered. In other words, the device should be created to enable her to safely swim in her pool with her friends, and independently engage in ADLs required to attend church activities. Not engaging in these meaningful activities may lead to isolation, lack of physical activity and detrimental changes to her daily routine.

Citation for occupational profile:

American Occupational Therapy Association. (2017). AOTA occupational profile template. *American Journal of Occupational Therapy*, 71(Suppl. 2), 7112420030. https://doi.org/10.5014/ajot.2017.716S12

Matching

1. E
2. C
3. J
4. I
5. G
6. A
7. F
8. D
9. B
10. H

CHAPTER 4

Self-Quiz 4.1

Part I

1. d
2. a
3. b
4. a
5. c

Part II

1. Distal palmar crease
2. Proximal palmar crease
3. Thenar crease
4. Distal wrist crease
5. Proximal wrist crease

Part III

1. Longitudinal arch
2. Distal transverse arch
3. Proximal transverse arch

Self-Quiz 4.2

1. F
2. F
3. T
4. T
5. F
6. T
7. F
8. T
9. T
10. F

CHAPTER 5

Self-Quiz 5.1

1. F
2. T
3. T
4. F
5. F
6. T
7. F
8. T
9. F
10. F
11. T
12. F
13. T
14. F

CHAPTER 6

Self-Quiz 6.1

1. F
2. T
3. T
4. T
5. F
6. T
7. F
8. F
9. F
10. T
11. T
12. F
13. F
14. T

Case Study 6.1

1. Steven has a radial nerve injury, which he sustained from falling asleep with his arm positioned over the top of a chair.
2. Never hesitate to call the physician's office. If the physician is not available, leave your question with the nurse.
3. The therapist should suggest an orthosis for radial nerve and research orthoses for that condition. He or she should review both textbooks and evidence-based practice articles, time permitting.
4. Steven should be educated about orthotic precautions, such as monitoring the orthosis for pressure sores, and about an orthotic-wearing schedule, including removal for hygiene and exercise, so the orthotic provision is safe and effective.
5. As discussed, adherence can be complicated because so many factors need to be considered for why a person is nonadherent. Is Steven's nonadherence related to a self-image problem with the orthosis or for some other reason that he has not stated? Refer to Box 6.2 for ideas of factors contributing to nonadherence. The therapist

should provide open-ended questions to get Steven's perception about his nonadherence and what it would take for him to become adherent with orthotic wear. More specific education, including sharing of research evidence about the importance of orthotic wear with a radial nerve injury for regaining function, would be helpful. This education would also help Steven understand the slow process of nerve regeneration. Due to Steven's history of alcohol abuse leading to the development of the condition, he may need psychosocial support beyond the therapy clinic. Psychosocial support can be tactfully suggested by the therapist, and Steven can request a referral from his primary physician for intervention.

Case Study 6.2

1. Many areas were missing from the charting. Charting initially did not specify the extremity. It did not include client history of having de Quervain tenosynovitis or prior level of function. It did not mention prior treatment of receiving a prefabricated orthosis and did not specify where the reddened area was on the thumb. It provided an opinionated comment about client adherence. It would have been better to have provided factual information, such as a direct quote from Marie. The inclusion of normal measurements for range of motion, grip, and pinch strengths would make it easier for the reader to have a better understanding of deficits. It did not address the impact of the condition on doing work and home occupations. It did not address Marie's current level of pain. It should include the type of orthosis, position, and location. It should include a statement on fit, comfort, and function of the fabricated thumb immobilization orthosis. Goals are vague and not related to function. It would have been helpful to involve Marie with the goal setting, perhaps through administering the Canadian Occupational Performance Measure (COPM).
2. In every situation, questions using the interactive clinical reasoning approach will be different. The following are a few of many suggested questions:
   - What questions do you have about wearing this fabricated orthosis? (This question may open up discussion, considering that Marie did not continue to wear the prefabricated orthosis due to developing some chafing on the volar surface of the thumb interphalangeal [IP] joint.)
   - How will you go about following an orthotic-wearing schedule based on the home and work demands in your life? (This question may be helpful, considering Marie's history of nonadherence with the first orthosis.)
   - What type of support do you need to help you with your orthosis and hand injury? (This question may help you better understand how Marie is coping with her condition.)
3. For this discussion, respect Marie's confidentiality by moving to a private area if in a large therapy room. You might assume that one reason Marie was nonadherent with the prefabricated orthosis was because it caused a reddened area on the thumb IP joint due to fitting

improperly. However, you should tactfully question Marie for her reasons for nonadherent, which might be different from your assumption. Refer to Box 6.2 for ideas of factors that contribute to nonadherence and to Box 6.3 for ideas for open-ended questions to ask Marie. In any case, you should fabricate a well-fitted comfortable orthosis and monitor the fit carefully for potential pressure sores. Clear education about the reason for orthotic wear along with any evidence from research may help Marie's adherence. It will be important to check with Marie regularly about follow-through with the orthotic-wearing program. Consider making a phone call or emailing Marie to check on her level of compliance and to answer any questions.

4. Marie likely has workers' compensation insurance.

CHAPTER 7

Self-Quiz 7.1

1. T
2. T
3. F
4. T
5. T
6. F
7. F
8. T
9. F
10. F
11. F

Case Study 7.1

1. (1) The thermoplastic strip was not the best choice because it was not providing enough wrist support. (2) The thermoplastic strip may have placed the wrist in the wrong wrist position.
2. The wrist should be positioned as close to neutral as possible.
3. There are a variety of options for an orthotic-wearing schedule. The American Academy of Orthopaedic Surgeons (AAOS) suggests nighttime wear at the minimum and daytime wear during activities that aggravate the condition.
4. The therapist should observe areas such as the ulnar styloid, the first web space, and the volar and dorsal aspects of the hand over the metacarpal bones for skin irritation. Angela should notify the therapist immediately if irritation occurs. In addition, Angela should be educated to not perform full finger flexion in the orthosis due to that motion causing increased pressure on the carpal tunnel.
5. In this case, trust was violated because Angela dutifully followed a wearing regimen for an orthosis that did not correctly fit and was exacerbating her condition. As McClure[45] suggests, providing research evidence specific to her situation might help her better understand the rationale for a custom-fabricated orthosis in a neutral position. Conservative management with using an orthosis may help because the condition was caught early.[53]

6. A custom orthosis may provide more stability to the wrist and overall a better fit. A pre-fabricated orthoses may not position the wrist in neutral.

Case Study 7.2

1. The therapist should use an orthosis to put Diane's wrist in neutral to provide a low-load stretch.
2. The therapist should continue to use a serial orthosis to get Diane's wrist into a functional wrist extension position.
3. This decision for discontinuation is made in collaboration with Diane's physician based on her progress. Discontinuation of using an orthosis could occur when Diane obtains more functional wrist extension because wearing the orthosis too long will result in muscle weakness and/or joint stiffness. Once the orthosis is removed, the therapist will continue to work on obtaining increased active wrist extension and normal wrist motions for function.

Laboratory Exercise 7.2
Orthosis A

1. The wrist is positioned in extreme ulnar deviation. The wrist strap is placed incorrectly.
2. This extreme position stresses the wrist joint and possibly contributes to the development of other problems, such as wrist pain, pressure areas, and de Quervain tenosynovitis.

Orthosis B

1. The wrist is positioned in flexion instead of a functional hand position of extension. Positioning in wrist extension helps with digital flexion. If the wrist is flexed, the client loses functional grasp. The wrist strap is placed incorrectly.

Orthosis C

1. Metacarpophalangeal (MCP) flexion is inhibited because the orthotic metacarpal bar is too high. The wrist appears to be radially deviated. The wrist strap is placed incorrectly.
2. Potential development of skin irritation or pressure areas exists with digital flexion, and the person does not have a full functional grasp.

Laboratory Exercise 7.4

1. Hypothenar bar
2. Metacarpal bar (palmar bar)
3. Forearm trough

CHAPTER 8

Self-Quiz 8.1

1. T
2. F
3. F
4. T
5. F
6. T
7. T
8. F
9. F

Case Study 8.1

1. The hand is placed in a hand-based thumb immobilization orthosis (MP radial and ulnar deviation restriction orthosis) with the CMC joint in 40 degrees of palmar abduction and the MCP joint in neutral to slight flexion and ulnar deviation. It is important to place the thumb CMC joint in a position of comfort and that position may not be exactly in the suggested degrees
2. To provide rest and protection during healing.
3. Precautions may include: 1) Not restricting IP joint movement by extending the thumb post too high. 2) Monitor for skin irritation and for pressure sores especially at the radial base of the first metacarpal and the first web space. 3) Make sure that the thumb post is supportive and not too restrictive.
4. As Jack is a 10-year-old male he may not adhere to wearing the orthosis, which is essential for proper healing of the ulnar collateral ligament. Perhaps to make the orthosis more acceptable for Jack to wear the therapist might fabricate it out of colored thermoplastic material that Jack selects, decorate the orthosis, or make it look like a cartoon character. The therapist needs to work with Jack's mother to encourage adherence.
5. Jack will need to wear the orthosis continuously for 4 to 5 weeks except for removal for hygiene.
6. An option as suggested by Ford et al.[25] is to fabricate a hybrid orthosis with a circumferential thermoplastic mold around the thumb covered by a neoprene wrap. This orthosis will provide stability to the MCP joint and allow for functional movements during skiing. Other options exist based on therapist clinical reasoning.

Case Study 8.2

1. Based on Margaret's symptoms, the therapists should fabricate a hand-based orthosis. Because only the carpometacarpal (CMC) joint is involved, the orthosis designed by Colditz[17] which immobilizes only the CMC joint—would be appropriate.
2. To provide stability and to control subluxation and pain.
3. Based on Colditz's recommendations,[17] Margaret should wear the orthosis continuously for 2 to 3 weeks (with removal for hygiene). After that time, she should wear the orthosis during times when the thumb is irritated by activities.
4. Because of the wrist and thumb involvement, the therapist would consider fabricating a forearm-based thumb orthosis.
5. Because the thumb metacarpophalangeal (MCP) joint is involved, consider fabricating a hand-based orthosis that includes the MCP joint.
6. The therapist should position the thumb MCP joint in 30 degrees flexion and in palmar abduction as tolerated.

Laboratory Exercise 8.1

1. Thumb post
2. Metacarpal (palmar) bar
3. Forearm trough

Laboratory Exercise 8.3

1. The two problems are the following: (1) The metacarpal bar is too high to allow full finger metacarpophalangeal (MCP) flexion and (2) the thumb interphalangeal (IP) joint flexion is limited because the material around the thumb extends too far distally.
2. An irritation might develop at the thumb IP joint (where the thumb opening is too high) and at the base of the index finger (where the metacarpal bar is too high). The orthosis limits full finger flexion.

CHAPTER 9

Case Study 9.1

1. b
2. c
3. b
4. c
5. b

Case Study 9.2

1. Diabetes mellitus is associated with Dupuytren disease.
2. Either a resting hand orthosis or a dorsal forearm-based static extension orthosis is appropriate to use after a Dupuytren contracture release.
3. The therapeutic position includes wrist in neutral or slight extension and metacarpophalangeals (MCPs), proximal interphalangeals (PIPs), and distal interphalangeals (DIPs) in full extension. The thumb does not need to be included in the orthosis.
4. Ken should wear his orthosis well after the wounds have completely healed. After healing, he should wear the orthosis several weeks or months thereafter during the nighttime to provide stress and tension to counteract the scar contraction. (He may discontinue his resting hand orthosis in favor of individual finger orthoses.) The orthosis can be removed for hygiene, exercise, and activities of daily living (ADLs).
5. To accommodate for bandage thickness, the design of the orthosis should be wider. As bandage bulk is reduced, the orthosis should be modified to maintain as close to an ideal position as possible. Therefore thermoplastic material that has memory will assist with the modification process. In addition, because this is a fairly long orthosis, a material with rigidity is helpful to adequately support the weight of the forearm, wrist, and hand.
6. Assuming no major complications in Ken's rehabilitation, he may require outpatient therapy. At a minimum, Ken should be seen for a home exercise program and monitored until the wound heals. The therapy may entail a minimum of one visit per week.
7. Ken may require assistance for any wound care and dressing changes initially. In addition, if he has difficulty with any one-handed techniques, he may require some assistance with ADLs or instrumental activities of daily living (IADLs) (particularly writing). Temporary accommodations may be required at work or when driving if the automobile has a manual transmission.

Laboratory Exercise 9.2

1. Thumb interphalangeal (IP) joint is flexed rather than extended; incorrect strap placement at distal forearm trough.
2. Radial deviation at the wrist; incorrect strap placement at distal forearm trough.
3. Poor wrist support; incorrect placement of straps at distal forearm trough.

CHAPTER 10

Self-Quiz 10.1

1. T
2. F
3. F
4. T
5. F
6. F
7. F
8. T
9. T
10. F
11. T

Case Study 10.1

For Laura

1. Posterior elbow immobilization orthosis: Elbow in 120 degrees of flexion, forearm in neutral, and wrist in 15 degrees of extension.
2. Supine on a plinth, with the shoulder in 90 degrees of forward flexion, elbow in 120 degrees of flexion, forearm in neutral rotation, and wrist in neutral extension of 15 degrees.
3. Protect the olecranon, medial and lateral epicondyles, and radial and ulnar heads by padding the bony prominences and molding the orthosis over the padding.
4. The orthosis is worn at all times and removed for protected range-of-motion (ROM) exercises only in a protected environment.

Case Study 10.2

For Marissa

1. Orthosis: A commercial brace that can be blocked at 90 degrees of flexion and allow for active flexion from 90-degree position as tolerated.
2. Wearing schedule: To wear the brace always, and to perform the exercises within the brace. The brace will be adjusted in therapy every week to increase the flexion angle by 10 to 15 degrees.

For Frank

1. A posterior elbow splint with elbow in approximately 70 to 90 degrees of flexion would be appropriate to allow for the transpose ulnar nerve and the surgically manipulated soft tissues to heal. Because this procedure included an ulnar nerve submuscular transposition, slight pronation in the forearm is recommended. The orthosis should support Frank's wrist but keep the fingers and thumb free to move.
2. At 10 days after surgery it is expected that Frank's inflammation will have subsided. For this reason the wearing schedule will depend on Frank's activity-rest cycle. In the first 2 weeks of orthotic use, Frank should keep the orthosis on during daytime activity and off at rest and during exercise. Nighttime orthotic wear may be indicated depending on Frank's preferred posture (e.g., excessive flexion). Orthotic use should be prescribed with intermittent ROM exercise to prevent stiffness. Typically, clients such as Frank will need 6 weeks to heal. The orthosis should be gradually weaned off and used as a tool for behavior modification (i.e., to prevent vigorous activities too soon).

For Bob

1. Bob may need two forms of orthoses for contracture management—one for flexion, one for extension. However, the priority at this time is to increase Bob's elbow extension using a static progressive turnbuckle orthosis with the goal of increasing Bob's outward reach. The turnbuckle orthosis may be discharged once Bob achieves elbow extension of −30 degrees because at this position the orthosis loses its leverage. However, with the remaining −30-degree limitation, Bob could benefit from an anterior elbow orthosis to continue stretching the elbow into extension.
2. Static progressive splinting depends on low-load passive stretch principle and therefore the therapist should consider prescribing a wearing period of gentle but prolonged stretch of 4-6 hours daily total. The periods may be broken up and interspersed with activities. Since Bob just had his external fixator removed and has significant contractures/stiffness of the elbow, it is imperative that the therapist prescribes a high-repetition, low-intensity exercise and activity program that maximizes and challenges the available ROM. Night time-splinting is no longer indicated.

CHAPTER 11

Self-Quiz 11.1

1. T
2. T
3. F
4. T
5. F
6. T
7. T
8. F
9. F
10. T

Case Study 11.1

1. Traditional adduction and internal rotation (IR) sling
2. Less than 4 weeks
3. Scapula dyskinesis and frozen shoulder syndrome

4. Lauren should be educated about proper wearing positioning, including scapula alignment. Her shoulders should be at an equal height, and there should not be excessive compression of the humeral head. Lauren should remove the orthosis when not in the community and perform a light range of motion (ROM) and isometric-based home exercise program (HEP).

CHAPTER 12

Self-Quiz 12.1

1. T
2. F
3. F
4. F
5. T

Self-Quiz 12.2

1. Swan neck deformity and/or rheumatoid arthritis, distal interphalangeal (DIP) joint osteoarthritis (OA), or trigger finger
2. Volar plate injury
3. Trigger finger
4. Proximal interphalangeal (PIP) collateral ligament injury

Case Study 12.1

1. The orthosis should cross the distal interphalangeal (DIP) joint.
2. Marge needs to wear the orthoses during sleep.
3. Marge needs to continue using the devices as long as she is still having pain.

Case Study 12.2

1. The distal interphalangeal (DIP) joint of the right long finger.
2. All of the time except for skin care, during which time the joint needs to be supported in extension.
3. Dip gutter orthosis, dorsal-volar DIP orthosis, or stack orthosis.
4. Ryan is likely to need to wear his orthosis for 6 to 8 weeks.

Case Study 12.3

1. Debbie should have a dorsal proximal interphalangeal (PIP) orthosis because the injury involved the volar plate.
2. The orthosis should cross the PIP joint in 20 to 30 degrees of flexion to protect the injured volar plate.
3. The index and long fingers should be buddy taped to support the injured long finger and maintain alignment. With injury to the radial collateral ligament, the middle phalanx would tend to ulnarly deviate, and the buddy strap helps correct this tendency.
4. Teach Debbie how to use self-adherent compressive wrap to treat the edema. Consider building up the girth of her tennis racquet handle to minimize stress on her injured joint.

Case Study 12.4

1. Yes, Alexa would benefit from proximal interphalangeal (PIP) hyperextension block orthoses to improve her active PIP flexion.
2. You could fabricate trial thermoplastic orthoses for a few fingers and assess if they help.
3. Important client factors are Alexa's job dealing with the public and what she finds to be most cosmetically appealing. Orthoses will be needed for multiple fingers and will be used long term, and thus streamlined fit and durability are desired qualities. Orthosis adjustability may also be beneficial because PIP size may fluctuate from swelling related to her arthritis.
4. Alexa should wear her orthoses during the daytime only, because these are functional orthoses.

Laboratory Exercise 12.1

1. It blocks the proximal interphalangeal (PIP) joint.
2. It blocks the distal interphalangeal (DIP) joint.
3. It does not prevent the PIP from hyperextending, allowing the finger to still posture in a swan neck deformity.

CHAPTER 13

Self-Quiz 13.1

1. T
2. T
3. F
4. F
5. T
6. T

Case Study 13.1

1. a. Y
   b. Y
   c. Y
   d. Y
   e. Y
2. b
3. d
4. a
5. c

CHAPTER 14

Self-Quiz 14.1

1. T
2. T
3. F
4. T
5. F
6. T
7. T
8. F
9. F
10. T
11. T
12. F

Self-Quiz 14.2

1. B
2. F
3. A
4. G
5. D
6. E
7. C
8. H

Case Study 14.1

1. Activities that require grasp and pinch will be affected.
2. An elbow orthosis is appropriate. Due to interosseous weakness, the hand should be monitored for a possible hand-based orthosis for the ulnar nerve.
3. The elbow is flexed 30 to 45 degrees, and the wrist, if included, is in neutral to 20 degrees of extension.
4. There are a couple of options that the therapist may consider. The first option is lining the orthosis to make it more comfortable. Another option would be to consider the comfort benefits of a prefabricated elbow orthosis. Care must be taken, however, that the prefabricated orthosis correctly positions his elbow in the appropriate amount of flexion.
5. Because symptoms are continuous, the therapist should suggest that Mark wear the orthosis all the time.
6. Mark must become aware of activities that irritate his condition, such as sleeping with his elbow bent.

Case Study 14.2

1. b
2. b
3. b
4. b
5. a

Laboratory Exercise 14.1

S: "My pain has decreased."

O: Pt. reports that pain has decreased with resisted pronation from a score of 5 out of 10 to 2 out of 10. Manual muscle testing for the pronator quadratus, pronator teres, flexor carpi radialis, palmaris longus and flexor digitorum superficialis, flexor pollicis longus, and flexor digitorum profundus to index and long fingers were all 4 (good). The long arm orthosis was discontinued on [date] with physician order.

A: Pt. was receptive to continue doing ADLs and home exercise program. Pt. plans to modify work and home activities to decrease repetitive pronation and supination. Pt. has been instructed in a light strengthening program.

P: Occupational therapist will continue to monitor home exercise program.

CHAPTER 15

Case Study 15.1

1. d. A volar forearm-based hand immobilization orthosis that stretches and positions the wrist and the fingers in composite extension at or slightly greater than 5 degrees is most appropriate. Over time the angle of wrist extension with the fingers in composite extension may be adjusted. Because Rose also has edema, the orthosis facilitates edema reduction by keeping the hand upright and in a nondependent position. A dorsal-based forearm platform with a volar hand component that positions the wrist and fingers in tolerable composite extension may position the hand in a desirable manner, but with Rose's edema, donning the orthosis will be difficult. A volar finger spreader with volar forearm component is a viable alternative because it provides the added benefit of keeping the web spaces aerated. However, since Rose reports pain with passive extension greater than 5 degrees, the position of maximum passive extension may increase the pain and compromise orthotic adherence. With Rose's condition still in the acute stages of recovery, a rigid cast is not appropriate at this time. Finally, a volar cone orthosis is not appropriate because it may accentuate the edema and skin breakdown. In addition, placing the fingers in flexion over a cone and the wrist at submaximal stretch promotes contractures.

2. Before altering or discontinuing the orthosis, the therapist monitors how caregivers and the nursing staff apply the orthosis. A common pitfall is when the straps are applied tightly, creating choke points, especially at the wrist. The therapist reinforces the importance of proper carryover for the orthotic program to be successful. The therapist considers interventions to manage edema and evaluate other potential reasons for the swelling.

3. e. When a client has early signs of active control of hand movement, the therapist considers using orthoses to facilitate better hand control so that the client can engage in intensive, repetitive task practice. With the edema resolved the appropriate orthosis is a Neoprene thumb abduction and extension orthosis that extends to the forearm radially. The forearm component supports the wrist with emerging stability. Once the client is more capable of stabilizing the wrist during grip, the therapist may switch to a short opponens orthosis. Both Neoprene-based and short opponens orthoses restrict the thumb from assuming flexion-adduction. These orthoses prevent contracture formation and facilitate a greater repertoire of prehensile patterns. A finger spreader, a hard cone, and an inflatable orthosis are inappropriate substitutes because they only restrict hand use in a functional, task-oriented manner. If Rose's spastic tone continues to pose problems with hand function, the therapist may provide a hand immobilization orthosis to provide wrist and hand flexor stretch during intervals of rest.

4. While Rose is using a Neoprene-based orthosis or a short opponens orthosis, family and caregivers encourage Rose to use her affected hand during activities, such as eating or drinking (e.g., holding a cup, picking up dense finger foods) and leisure (e.g., playing cards). The therapist considers active strategies and modalities to further develop strength and stability of grasp and maintain range of motion.

Case Study 15.2

1. d. The most immediate goal is to ensure that the hand and wrist are not kept in a composite flexion position. Because of the Modified Ashworth Scale grade, a comfortable composite stretch of the finger and wrist flexors is warranted. The volar design ensures ease of wear especially during the acute rehabilitation phase.

2. a. This orthotic design allows Brian to practice reaching to grasp by assisting the fingers and wrist in appropriate extension. Repetitive resistance at maximum stretch of the flexors will promote muscle inhibition over time.

CHAPTER 16

Self-Quiz 16.1

1. T
2. F
3. F
4. T
5. F
6. T
7. F
8. T
9. F
10. T
11. T
12. T
13. T

Self-Quiz 16.2

1. A material that has high drapability and moldability is not a good choice for making antigravity orthoses. A material that has resistance to drape and memory is suitable. A slightly tacky orthotic material that lightly adheres to underlying stockinette may be helpful. Preshaping techniques assist in molding.

2. A positioning orthosis places the involved joints in submaximum extension. This position permits adequate skin hygiene.

3. An orthosis should not limit the use of uninvolved joints. An arthritis orthosis immobilizes only the affected joints and positions the thumb in a resting position. When there is bilateral hand involvement, the client may need to alternate wearing right and left orthotics.

4. Pad the outside of the orthosis.

5. The straps should be soft, wide foam straps that are cut a little long to adjust for edema. The orthotic design should be made wide enough to accommodate the edema.

Self-Quiz 16.3

Matching

1. b
2. d
3. c
4. a
5. e

Case Study 16.1

1. c
2. a and c
3. b, c, and d
4. d

Case Study 16.2

1. a and d
2. d
3. a
4. d
5. c

Laboratory Exercise 16.1

1. The orthosis blocks the wrist and thumb interphalangeal (IP) joint.

2. The figure-eight is not properly positioned to effectively prevent hyperextension of the thumb IP joint. The figure-eight orthosis should be rotated and placed on the finger to prevent IP hyperextension.

CHAPTER 17

Case Study 17.1

1. Option A would probably not be adequate to address concerns of losing range of motion (ROM) of the wrist and fingers. Once range is lost, it can be difficult (if not impossible) to regain. Therefore prevention is paramount. Relying on passive range of motion (PROM) may be disruptive to other activities and occupations during the day. The constant effects of moderately to severely increased tone will be difficult to overcome with activities alone. The thumb orthoses alone would not be adequate to address concerns with the wrist and finger flexors.

2. Option B would probably best meet Mathew's needs at this time. Prolonged stretch to the wrist and finger flexors could occur at night. Active functional movement during play, z-care, communication, and school activities could be emphasized during his waking hours. Because the left upper extremity is tighter and less functional, it would also be prudent to wear the left resting orthosis on this hand periodically during the day. A thermoplastic thumb orthosis for the right hand would control some of the increased tone in the hand but leave the wrist and fingers free for active and functional movement. ROM measurements would be required to determine optimal wearing schedules. You will contact Matthew's parents to discuss your recommendations for using the orthoses and the purpose of the orthoses and to get their input. Assuming they are in agreement, you arrange a meeting with his parents before the orthoses are taken home. At this time you will review the purpose of the orthoses, demonstrate how to apply the orthoses, and provide an opportunity for the parents to practice donning and doffing the orthoses. You will also give the parents written instructions, precautions, and your phone number. Photographs of the orthoses on Matthew's hands will be included if needed.

3. Option C would be excessive use of resting hand orthoses at the present time. Matthew should continue to experience active movement and sensory feedback as much as possible during the day, especially with the right hand.

4. Option D would unnecessarily restrict active use of the hands during the day while leaving the wrist and finger flexors shortened during the night and on weekends. This family is involved in Matthew's programming, and you will address the issue of correct application at home by meeting with the parents as described in Option B. If you have questions regarding follow-through at home, you should obtain more information about the family's strengths and limitations, the parents' understanding of intervention, and family routines. You should then individualize your style of collaboration and provide instruction for that family.

Case Study 17.2

1. Option A, a resting hand orthosis, would not be appropriate because Luke has full passive range of motion (PROM) in the left wrist and hand. Elongation of wrist and finger flexors is desirable but could be accomplished through weight-bearing activities.

2. Option B, a standard wrist cock-up (immobilization) orthosis, would not adequately address the problem of thumb adduction into the palm. It is likely that positioning the thumb in opposition will have an inhibitory effect on the wrist and hand. If the wrist flexion continues to be a problem after the thumb is addressed, other orthotic or treatment options could be considered.

3. Option C, issue a Neoprene thumb abduction orthosis for daytime wear to facilitate a functional thumb position during grasp and prehension activities. Consider a thermoplastic "C" bar insert attached to the Neoprene orthosis if needing a firmer material to adequately position thumb in more challenging cases. A thermoplastic thumb spica may be considered for night wear in those patients who would benefit from more continuous intervention.

4. Option D, fabricating a resting-hand orthosis for both hands would immobilize all digits unnecessarily and would result in Luke being unable to use his hands for exploration, play, and to assist in self-feeding activities. Luke has full range of motion in all digits, except for the right thumb and orthotic intervention should aim to be as least restrictive as possible, while facilitating continued use of his hand for play.

Laboratory Exercise 17.1

Two fabrication problems are present in this orthosis. First, the C bar does not fit into the web space of the thumb and provides inadequate positioning of the thumb between radial and palmar abduction. Second, the sides of the forearm trough are too high, resulting in bridging of the straps.

Laboratory Exercise 17.2

The straps are not keeping the wrist positioned in the orthosis. The distal forearm strap should be placed just proximal to the ulnar styloid, and a second strap should be added just distal to the ulnar styloid, preventing the flexor action of the wrist from lifting the wrist away from the orthosis' surface. The orthosis does not fit snugly into the thumb web space.

CHAPTER 18

Case Study 18.1

1. The occupational therapist could assist with donning and doffing of the device, developing wear schedules based on the client's needs, and develop skills to integrate the device into activities of daily living (ADLs).

2. An optimally provided orthosis could address the client's concerns with mobility and ADLs that require lower extremity (LE) functionality.

3. Total contact, three-point pressure systems, and kinaesthetic reminder could each play a role in this particular client. Three-point pressure systems could address the client's paralytic equinus in swing phase, total contact would distribute the pressure throughout a larger area of the limb, and the sensation of wearing an orthosis could enhance proprioception.

4. This client would most benefit from a thermoplastic ankle-foot orthosis (AFO). The AFO would enable a heel strike at initial contact, modulate forward progression of the tibia during stance phase, and eliminate equinus positioning throughout swing phase.

Case Study 18.2

1. Neuropathy can negatively affect the sensory, motor, and autonomic functions. Sensory deficits could result in diminished protective sensation, making the client unaware of injury. Motor neuropathy can result in atrophy of the intrinsic muscles of the foot, resulting in an imbalance of the muscles that facilitate locomotion and other weight-earing activities. Autonomic neuropathy can result in diminished function of the glands within the feet, compromising skin integrity, which may compromise the soft tissue envelope, increasing the risk of infection.

2. Extra-depth footwear has the ability to be adjusted to achieve an optimal fit to the client's foot, creating additional volume for deformities such as clawed toes.

3. Accommodative foot orthoses create an interface for the diabetic foot that conforms to the client's present alignment, ensuring pressure is distributed over the largest possible surface area. A corrective orthosis applies specific forces to achieve an alignment different from the client's in situ presentation, which could potentially result in skin breakdown where forces are excessive.

Case Study 18.3

1. The common peroneal nerve bifurcates into the deep and superficial peroneal nerves, which innervate the anterior and lateral compartments of the leg.

2. Swing phase functionality would be affected in a similar manner, but the solid ankle trimline would not allow for the client's tibia to progress forward to 10 degrees of relative dorsiflexion at terminal stance, forcing the client to either take a shorter contralateral step or hyperextend the knee on the ipsilateral side to maintain step length symmetry.

Case Study 18.4

1. The anatomical knee joint is a polycentric joint. The application of a single-axis joint would not accurately follow the knee's axis of rotation as it moves through normal range of motion, which could result in the orthosis migrating and placing less than optimal forces through the client's knee.
2. The three-point pressure system is exemplified in the coronal plane to create an unloading of the client's osteoarthritic lateral compartment.

Case Study 18.5

1. Both sensation and proprioception are unaffected by paralytic postpolio syndrome as polio affects the anterior horn of the spinal cord, resulting in only motor deficits.
2. The client should be provided a knee joint that locks as the posterior offset joint on the provided orthosis relies on maintaining the weight line anterior to the knee joint, which cannot consistently be done with a client who does not achieve terminal extension.

Case Study 18.6

1. This position seats the prosthesis into the socket, encouraging joint stability. Relative adduction or excessive hip flexion could encourage the prosthesis to shift out of the socket.
2. Sitting and transferring would be more difficult and require modifications to perform these tasks.

Case Study 18.7

1. A client with a thoracic-level lesion would not have adequate volitional strength at the hips or knees to facilitate ambulation with just ankle-foot orthoses.
2. Ambulation with the hip-knee-ankle-foot orthosis (HKAFO) would require a swing-through gait versus the much more natural reciprocating pattern that is enabled by the reciprocating gait orthosis (RGO).

CHAPTER 19

Case Study 19.1

1. Baseline evaluation includes range of motion, manual muscle test, functional use, Modified Ashworth Scale, and sensation.
2. The rigid circular wrist cast can assist with improving range of motion into wrist extension, where the wrist flexors are more dominant and lead to myostatic contracture. A roll or small cone can be placed if the fingers require positioning. The metacarpophalangeal (MCP) wrist cast can improve range of motion into wrist extension and increase the MCP range into extension due to spasticity of the lumbricals.

However, care must be taken that the intrinsic musculature is not overstretched and causing microtear.

3. After the client receives a botulinum toxin type A (BtA) injection, the therapist should wait 2 to 7 days for the BtA to take effect. The wrist and fingers may feel extremely loose, and caution should be taken on the initial position of the wrist for casting. Remember, nerves and blood vessels have been in a shortened position. Placing the wrist in an overstretched position may cause pain. Ella's stretch reflex was felt at 85 degrees of wrist flexion, at the beginning of range. Position the cast at the point of stretch reflex or submaximal range to prevent overstretching, microtearing, and pain.
4. An increase of at least 5 to 10 degrees in passive range of motion is expected when each cast is removed. The casting program is discontinued when range of motion has not increased or there is no improvement in volitional movement.
5. An orthosis can be fabricated to maintain the range of motion.
6. The primary goal for Ella is that the caregiver will be able to place her arms through a sleeve of a shirt or coat with ease and for her to wear a splint to maintain her range of motion.

Case Study 19.2

1. a and/or d
2. c
3. a, b, e
4. a, c, d

Competency Checkout Review 19.3

1. Casts are applied to improve range of motion, to improve movement that may interfere with task performance, to assist with contracture and spasticity management for impairment of muscle or absence of opposing force, hygiene care for washing and bathing, and for wearing a definitive splint.
2. Contraindications for casting include severe skin redness, open wounds, edema, heterotopic ossification, and severe rigidity.
3. Special monitoring of the cast may be required for a client with burns, and the need to change the cast within 2 to 3 days to allow monitoring of skin needs to be considered. Pediatric clients and clients at risk for edema require additional diligence to ensure that they do not get the cast wet, place items in the cast, or have restricted circulation.
4. Types of casts
   a. Rigid circular elbow cast
   b. Long arm cast
   c. Wrist cast with thumb enclosed
   d. Metacarpophalangeal (MCP) wrist cast
   e. Rigid circular elbow cast (monitor for swelling distally)
5. Cast removal
   a. Cast saw
   b. Unravel
   c. Cutting strip, bandage scissors
   d. Cast saw

6. Casting saw procedure
    1. f
    2. b
    3. c
    4. a
    5. d
    6. e

CHAPTER 20

Self-Quiz 20.1

1. b
2. c
3. c
4. b
5. a
6. b
7. c
8. Step 1: C
   Step 2: A
   Step 3: B
9. a
10. a

Case Study 20.1

1. Following an evaluation that included developmental assessment, and given that Michael is progressing along a developmental continuum, the OT would likely have recommended a passive prosthesis to assist with weight-bearing during sit, quadruped and transitional movements, and for bimanual activities such as clapping and fingering hands, holding a cup or bottle, and self-feeding finger foods.
2. Findings from the evaluation, parent goals, available technology
3. Relevant play and self-care activities; parent education; play group, peer support

Case Study 20.2

1. The OT will want to prepare Amy for the differences in the features of this technology, how it will be controlled and what tasks for which it might be most beneficial. It will be important for the OT to communicate with the prosthetist to understand the difference in weight and to use a pre-prosthetic progressive weight tolerance program to facilitate. In addition, the OT will access information from the OT evaluation to determine the activities most meaningful to Amy and incorporate them into the plan of care.

Case Study 20.3

1. Given best available information available from current evidence, the OT recommends that the surgeon avoid an amputation through a joint (such as the wrist), but consider an amputation proximal to it. Individuals with trans-radial level of loss appear to manage well with prosthetic technology, and have more options. Should the amputation occur as a wrist disarticulation, the options become limited.

Case Study 20.4

1. The OT will likely complete the OT evaluation and consider all areas of reported pain as well as the a query into how Matt completes most tasks and what compensatory methods he uses. The OT will want to focus on education to prevent further disparity such as joint protection, other adaptive strategies, conditioning exercises, assistive devices, and peer support to prevent isolation. The OT may want to role play social circumstances that are awkward or uncomfortable to help Matt develop his own responses that are comfortable and that he can be confident using.

Web Resources and Vendors

SOCIETIES, ORGANIZATIONS, EDUCATION

American Academy of Orthopaedic Surgeons
   http://www.aaos.org/

American Association for Hand Surgery
   http://www.handsurgery.org/

American Hand Therapy Foundation
   http://www.ahtf.org/

The American Occupational Therapy Association, Inc.
   http://www.aota.org/

The American Occupational Therapy Foundation
   http://www.aotf.org/

American Orthotic & Prosthetic Association
   http://www.aopanet.org/

American Physical Therapy Association
   http://www.apta.org/

American Society of Hand Therapists
   http://www.asht.org/

American Society for Surgery of the Hand
   http://www.assh.org/

Canadian Association of Occupational Therapists
   http://www.caot.ca/

E-hand.com The Electronic Textbook of Hand Surgery
   http://www.eatonhand.com/

Exploring Hand Therapy
   http://www.exploringhandtherapy.com/

Hand Therapy Certification Commission
   http://www.htcc.org/

International Federation of Societies for Hand Therapy
   http://www.ifsht.org/

Journal of Hand Therapy
   http://journals.elsevierhealth.com/periodicals/hanthe

World Federation of Occupational Therapists
   http://www.wfot.org/

ORTHOTIC MATERIALS AND ACCESSORIES SUPPLIERS

The following list is of course not exhaustive. Neither is the quality and/or service of products implied, and company contact information is subject to change.

AliMed
1-800-225-2610 http://www.alimed.com/online-catalog.aspx

Allegro Medical
1-800-861-3211 https://www.allegromedical.com

Benik Corporation
1-800-442-8910 http://benik.com/

Biodynamic Technologies
1-800-879-2276 https://www.biodynamictech.com

Chesapeake Medical Products
1-888-560-2674 http://www.chesapeakemedical.com

Core Products International, Inc.
1-877-249-1251 http://www.coreproducts.com/

DeRoyal
1-800-251-9864 http://www.deroyal.com/

3-Point Products
1-410-604-6393 http://www.3pointproducts.com/

Dynasplint
1-800-638-6771 http://www.dynasplint.ca/en/

Joint Active Systems
1-800-879-0117 https://jointactivesystems.com/

Joint Jack Company
1-860-657-1200 http://jointjackcompany.com/

North Coast Medical, Inc.
1-800-821-9319 http://www.ncmedical.com/

Performance Health
1-800-323-5547 http://www.performancehealth.com

Restorative Care of America, Inc. (RCAI)
1-800-627-1595 http://www.rcai.com/

Smith & Nephew, Inc.
1-800-558-8633 http://smith-nephew.com/us/professional/

Tetra Medical Supply Corporation
1-800-621-4041 http://www.tetramed.com/

SOFT CAST VENDORS

3M Scotchcast Soft Cast (Fiberglass)
3M Health Care
3M Center Building 275-4E-0
Saint Paul, MN 55144-1000
1-888-364-3577

Delta-Cast Soft (Polyester Cast Tape)
Delta-Cast Conformable—Functional Cast Therapy (Polyester Cast Tape)
BSN Medical, Inc.
5825 Carnegie Blvd.
Charlotte, NC 28209-4633
1-800-552-1157

INDEX

Note: Page numbers followed by "f" indicate figures, "t" indicate tables, and "b" indicate boxes.